Principles of Clinical Decision-Making

By

H.F. Jeejeebhoy MBBS (Lond.), PhD (McGill), FRCS, FRCPC (Path.).

Phases 3 and 4 Consultants

Ottawa, Canada

TRAFFORD PUBLISHING™

Note for Librarians: A cataloguing record for this book is available from Library and Archives Canada at www.collectionscanada.ca/amicus/index-e.html
ISBN 1-4120-8654-X

Printed on paper with minimum 30% recycled fibre. Trafford's print shop runs on "green energy" from solar, wind and other environmentally-friendly power sources.

TRAFFORD PUBLISHING™

Offices in Canada, USA, Ireland and UK

This book was published *on-demand* in cooperation with Trafford Publishing. On-demand publishing is a unique process and service of making a book available for retail sale to the public taking advantage of on-demand manufacturing and Internet marketing. On-demand publishing includes promotions, retail sales, manufacturing, order fulfilment, accounting and collecting royalties on behalf of the author.

Book sales for North America and international:
Trafford Publishing, 6E–2333 Government St.,
Victoria, BC V8T 4P4 CANADA
phone 250 383 6864 (toll-free 1 888 232 4444)
fax 250 383 6804; email to orders@trafford.com
Book sales in Europe:
Trafford Publishing (UK) Limited, 9 Park End Street, 2nd Floor
Oxford, UK OX1 1HH UNITED KINGDOM
phone 44 (0)1865 722 113 (local rate 0845 230 9601)
facsimile 44 (0)1865 722 868; info.uk@trafford.com
Order online at:
trafford.com/06-0410

10 9 8 7 6 5 4 3

An Ackowledgment

I am indebted to my wife, Adeline for her invaluable help in the writing of this book.

It could not have been written without her assistance in editing, indicating errors of language and identifying comissions and omissions of punctuation. She is not a qualified medical practitioner and this was valuable. Each time she found the language of the text difficult to understand she told me so. An alteration in the text was always an improvement.

There were others who helped in my general education on the topics in this book. I acknowledge them in the Introduction.

Introduction

Correct therapy must not only treat the presenting disease or dysfunction but also ensure preservation or restoration of the coordinated integration of all systems. This coordinated integration is a requisite for every animate. It is essential for smooth, precise and purposeful voluntary movements. It is also needed for the correct reception and recognition of new information, for its integration with new and remembered multimodal information and selection of information for storage in long-term memory. Abstract and logical thinking, reasoning, responses and decision-making need and use information stored in long-term memory. The coordinated integration of systems is a quality common to all animates. The objective of this book is the development and description of a frame which shows how biological systems interact and coordinate and how such a frame can be used by physicians to improve clinical decision-making.

Last night I observed coordinated integration of systems at close quarters. A ladybug covered with a closed pink shell with black dots was wandering on my desk. Six legs were moving in precise, purposeful and coordinated sequences which directed the insect in whatever direction it wished to move. I pushed it off the table with the edge of a sheet of paper. What followed was a surprise. Suddenly, when pushed to the edge of the table the pink carapace opened as a bivalve would, two gossamer thin wings emerged from its posterior and then swung vertically. They vibrated at blurring speed and the insect flew away with speed and precision to another destination. Everything was perfectly coordinated and smooth. If a single component of these actions had not worked disaster and possibly death would have followed.

The inception of this book was two conversations I had with the late Norbert Wiener during his visits to India in the late 1950s. At the time he was the founder of a new science termed "Cybernetics". On the first occasion he asked me how medical decisions were made. I replied that I did not know and that I had not thought about the subject. Also that I was a surgeon and the essential clinical decisions had been made before I saw the patient. On the second occasion I told him that I had thought about his question but was daunted by its complexities. Thinking and discussions continued when I was in the USA in the early 1960s. Unfortunately, later discussions were not possible as I left Boston in 1963 and he died in the next year while visiting Stockholm.

Wiener's biographer, Steve Heins (Steve Heins. The Cybernetics Group. Cambridge, Mass. MIT Press, 1991) has very correctly observed that Wiener had "an obsession with finding predictability through chaos and signal through noise". This came through very clearly during our discussions about decision-making in clinical medicine. He insisted that all analyses must start with the identification of basic principles. Gradually build an edifice on these principles till the final objective is reached; in this instance a frame which shows how biological systems interact and coordinate and how such a frame can be used by physicians to make good clinical decisions.

However, the task of formulating a frame that depicts the totality of physiological and pathophysiological integration is not simple and this has been recognized by many authors. Thus, Porter in his book, "Cybernetics Simplified" (The English Universities Press Ltd., London, 1969.) wrote:

> "It must be emphasized and re-emphasized that the most complex control process known to man is man himself. Man is controlled by a vast coordinated network of neurons, nerves and muscles, which carry out his thought processes and activate his behavior with almost negligible power requirements, and in a manner which is far beyond our comprehension at present. As a decision-making system man is supreme."

Later in the same book he added:

> "Of all control the fantastic network of interconnected neurons in the brain, the communicating nerve fibers, the countless chemical reactions, and the vast array of human muscles all together constitute by many orders of magnitude the most complex system with which man is confronted. How this system manages to be self-stabilizing in the presence of a multiplicity of disturbances of all kinds, including severe brain damage, is far beyond the present status of control theory to explain."

The facts of our daily existence are immutable proof that this coordinated integration exists.

For the last three decades I have attempted to analyze the process of clinical decision-making on the bases suggested by Dr. Wiener. This book is the result of these three decades of cogitation and yet it is not perfect. Why has it taken so long? There are many reasons. The first task was to identify the basic requirements. The totality of available information on all physiology, biochemistry, clinical medicine, pathology and cognitive psychology is immense. It was necessary to abstract the essentials hidden in much verbiage. This took time for without extensive reading and prolonged cogitation the abstraction of essentials is not possible.

Secondly, every time a hypothesis was developed it had to be revised because of obvious flaws. Third was the time limitations imposed by a medical practice. Lastly, and most important, it was often difficult to get accurate information. Inadequate peer reviews of publications were one cause. The other was the normal conflicts of research which are research followed by presentations, disagreements, additional research on the topic and a final consensus. Some time later (at times, many years later) information which has the imprimatur of general usage and acceptance is recorded in standard textbooks. By that time the information could have become obsolete or incorrect. Then the whole cycle must restart.

Many of the statements made in this book are, of necessity, subjective compromises of conflicting views. The views on ethics are subjective but dogmatically expressed because they often color the statements made. It is necessary for physicians to understand that their clinical decisions are often colored by their personal views on correct ethics. These are considerations which enter into almost every clinical decision. Personal views on ethics vary from one individual to another and the frequent consequences are disputations on correct therapy.

The first half of my career as a physician was spent in specialty medicine; surgery, research on tissue transplantation and tumor biology, and finally pathology. This conditioned the way I reasoned and practiced. Admittedly, throughout this period general primary care medicine was also practiced but only on an ad hoc basis. The big picture only began to become evident when I practiced every form of medicine (general medicine, general surgery, obstetrics, gynecology, psychiatry, etc.) in a small hospital staffed by two nuns in a desolate rural area. One left because of the despair born of helplessness. Diagnosis was possible but there were no drugs or monies for therapy. Surgery was limited by a lack of anesthetics, assistance and equipment. All was done under spinal or local anesthesia with a relative or one of the nuns providing solace and encouragement at the other end. Oxygen was not available and blood pressures during surgery were maintained by tiltings of an antiquated operating table. The one redeeming feature was that for the first time I learnt how to deliver babies with difficult presentations. The superb teachers were the local ladies who specialized in delivering babies. Their training was excellent for they used techniques handed down from one generation to the next over centuries. When they told me that a Caesarean delivery was needed because of a difficult presentation they were always right. Caesarean deliveries were a luxury they did not have previously. All pregnant women with impossible fetal presentations used to die. Postoperative infections killed many Caesarean deliveries but many survived.

An additional awakening was a locum done for a sick general practitioner friend. It was only then that I realized that the first and most important clinical decisions were made by primary health physicians. The practice of specialty medicine stopped and for the last 28 years I have worked as a primary care general practitioner and, at the same time, attempted to analyze the processes used by physicians to make clinical decisions. Practice as a primary care physician was a deliberate choice For me it was (retirement was six months ago - hence, the past tense) the most satisfying way of being a doctor and of studying the methodology of clinical decision-making. My thanks are first directed to the hundreds of patients, some with extremely complicated physical and psychiatric problems, who consulted me. They unwittingly educated me on the basics of clinical decision-making and I unknowingly received this education by progressive osmosis into my thought processes.

This introduction would be incomplete without some additional thanks. The first is to the late Dr. John Merrill. He was the head of the Cardio-Renal Unit at the Peter Bent Brigham Hospital in 1962 and 1963 while I was in Boston as a research fellow in his department at the Harvard Medical School and an Instructor in Medicine at the Peter Bent Brigham Hospital (now Brigham and Women's, I think). My fellowship was as a surgeon wanting to do research on transplantation biology and learn about the postoperative medical care of these patients. Instead, Dr. Merrill taught me all the basics of the physiology and clinical features of cardiac disease and nephrology that I needed to know. Any subsequent additions to my knowledge are only new therapies and the more precise investigations now possible. I thank him.

I am also indebted to the many professional associates I met during the eight years I spent in the Department of Surgery at McGill from 1965-1973 as a full time researcher on transplantation biology and tumor immunology. Most were not surgeons. The Professor of Physiology allowed me to teach physiology as an Instructor on a moon-lighting unpaid basis. Each term I was assigned a new topic and at the end of the eight years found myself quite knowledgeable about physiology.

Especially valuable at the time was the opportunity to attend some of the conferences and seminars at the Montreal Neurological Institute. Much neurology was learnt and, for the first time, I was introduced to the subject of cognitive psychology. A belief common to most physicians is that psychology and its sub-disciplines are topics not relevant to the practice of medicine. This is an erroneous view. Clinical decision-making is very reliant on assessments of the verbal, gestural and prosodic responses of patients and a knowledge of basic cognitive psychology often eases the difficulties when making these assessments.

The list of acknowledgments would not be complete without mention of the period spent at the Fox Chase Institute for Cancer Research in Philadelphia. In 1973 I was awarded a one year Eleanor Roosevelt Fellowship by the IUCC. It was spent in the laboratory of Dr. R.Prehn and was a fruitful year. I thank him. An additional three years were spent at the Institute at their kind invitation to stay on as a Visiting Scientist. There were many interactions with the Oncological Hospital across the yard. The four years spent at the Institute were especially valuable for learning the rigorous thought processes of researchers in these areas. They were not the same as the intuitive processes used by most physicians to make decisions.

Theoretically, a book on clinical decision-making requires the detailing of the clinical features, methods for diagnosis, for assessments and for choosing and monitoring the responses to therapy of all diseases. This is a daunting and impossible task in a monograph of this size; description of the essential diagnostic features of every clinical disease would require numerous large volumes of text. A simple abbreviated alternative is used in this book. First, one has only included clinical conditions which might be seen by a general practitioner at some time during a working life of medical practice. Inevitably, they include the conditions most commonly seen by specialists for many patients initially assessed and diagnosed by general practitioners are subsequently referred to specialists for confirmation of the diagnosis and/or for therapies which are beyond the capabilities and/or facilities available to the general practitioner. An occasional rare condition is included but only where necessary to make a point. Second, one only describes the symptoms and signs which must be present when a diagnosis or clinical assessment is correct. Those which are not essential for validity of the diagnostic assessment are not detailed unless they are integral to the text. As long as the physiologically desired and permissible norms are known the qualitatives of any dysfunction, the choice of optimal therapy and the response to it can be determined by their deviations from these norms or, when therapy is given, the extent of return, or failure to return, of the clinical features to the desired and permissible limits of normal physiology.

Assessments which are based on comparison with desired and permissible physiological norms need summaries of reasonable size which encompasses the facts of normal physiology, biochemistry, cognitive psychology and pathology that are relevant to the practice of clinical medicine. In every chapter which treats clinical problems a summary of this type precedes or is included and incorporated in the text on clinical dysfunctions. The word "relevant" is not used to derogate the writers of texts on physiology or biochemistry or pathology. Each is mandated to provide comprehensive texts about their subject. Thus, a text on physiology meets the needs of physiologists but only a small portion is needed for the day-to-day practice of clinical medicine. It is these small but relevant facts of physiology, biochemistry and protective pathology that provide the bases for comparisons between clinical features and the permissible and desirable limits of systems functions. Perhaps the word "essential" is better used in this context rather than the word "relevant". These comparisons can provide the bases for assessments of the qualitatives of the symptoms and signs of disease or syndrome of dysfunction, and for choosing and monitoring optimal therapy. Admittedly, the nature of the problems mean that many of the judgments made are subjective and disputable but that is integral to a discipline which has clinical features which present as subjective qualitatives and not as specific quantitatives.

Incidentally, the clinical case histories presented were all patients seen and treated by me. Many were treated over long periods in collaboration with specialists. I retired about six months ago but have not changed the descriptions of the case histories to the past tense as most of this book was written when I was in an active medical practice. I specifically indicate those who were patients of colleagues and friends.

At the end of each chapter that details clinical information there is a section which summarizes the therapeutic options available for that system. These sections are usually small in size and short on details. This is deliberate. Therapy and methodologies currently in vogue often have a short shelf life. The text of these sections on therapeutic options tend to concentrate on detailing the conceptual bases for therapy rather than on their specifics. The clinical features which are needed for diagnoses are less mutable and are expressed in greater detail.

Contents

1

Clinical Decision-Making: Some Basics

1. Definitions, Ethics, Evidence-Based Medicine, and Computers

Table of Contents

Decisions defined.

To decide is to choose. Even if a decision is obvious inaction is always an option. It is an option that patients frequently choose.

People make decisions all the time. They range from those that are simple to others that are complex. For example: what time to wake up in the morning; how to interrelate with family members; how to provide for the needs and the futures of any children; what time to leave for work; how to respond to the demands of employers and optimize performance at work; alternatively, if unemployed, how to get money for daily needs and how to deal with prospective employers. The list is much longer. Some relate to matters affecting the relationships within the family. Others are concerns for items related to employment, the work place and coworkers. The decision or decisions made might not be ideal but are the ones the individual thinks best in the circumstances existing at the time.

The clinical decision.

The clinical decision is a bit different from the decisions of daily living as the margins for error are smaller. It has two sequential components. The first is diagnosis and the second is the decision on optimal therapy.

The practice of medicine is not an intellectual exercise with the solution of a diagnostic problem as the desired result. People only consult physicians when they need relief or cure of sickness. Hence the final and most important component of the clinical decision is the one that identifies the best therapy.

Diagnosis is an essential preliminary but determination of specific etiologies is not always possible. Often therapy based on assumptions of etiology will control or cure. I have many elderly patients with congestive heart failure controlled by therapy, some for more than 10 years, and without precise determination of etiology. In these patients the assumption is that the failure results from a combination of coronary artery narrowing and the decreased cardiac contractility that accompanies aging. As a rule, unpleasant invasive procedures are only needed for such patients when control is not possible with available therapies.

Wrong decisions and right ones.

Usually, decisions are neither completely right nor completely wrong. Individuals make decisions that they consider best in the circumstances existing at the time. The ideal decision may be different. The patient's subjective views and values are the main reasons for these differences. The following are some examples of these constraints: age; cultural values; financial circumstances; family ties; education; religious beliefs; concomitant disease (e.g., chronic, acute or preterminal); obedience to the requirements of moral law and legislated constraints. Additional considerations are variations in desires for security, for hedonistic satisfaction, for different sexual mores and of abilities and inabilities to love and to hate. Many other considerations temper decisions, some tangible, others not.

Regarding proposed therapy, important considerations for the patient are the ability to afford and to obtain. The patient also considers other factors before deciding. Is the proposed therapy likely to be beneficial? Is it necessary? Will I comply? Only the patient can answer these questions.

Maxim:

There is a single basic constant required for making good clinical decisions:

Every clinical decision must strive to restore or maintain the functional integration of all biological systems as a single coordinated unit. This integration is essential for smooth, precise and purposeful voluntary movements. It is also needed for the correct reception and recognition of new information, for its integration with new and remembered multimodal information and eventual selective storage in long-term memory. Abstract and logical thinking, and reasoning and decision-making need information stored in long-term memory.

The coordinated integration of systems is a quality common to all animates.

How does one know when the objectives are attained? The objectives are attained when the features of organ or systems dysfunctions have returned to the permissible limits of normal physiology and biochemistry. In order to determine whether the response to therapy is acceptable the physician only needs to know the relevant facts of normal biochemistry and physiology. The response to therapy is acceptable when clinical features of the dysfunction or dysfunctions have returned, or are returning to these desirable and permissible ranges of function.

The clinical features of common dysfunctions should be basic constants in the selection of material taught during medical training. This is knowledge that should remain with every practicing physician throughout their working lives. In this book the sections on "Diagnosis" concentrate on detailing the facts of normal biology as the basis for clinical assessments and therapy. Most of the clinical conditions detailed try to demonstrate this. In addition, most are those likely to be encountered by a general practitioner in day-to-day medical practice. An occasional uncommon condition is included when needed to illustrate a principle. The permutations and combinations of the abnormals are too many to detail. Assessments and therapy are only possible by comparisons with the biological norms that are permissible and desirable.

Ethics for clinical medicine

Dictionaries define the word "ethical" in different ways. Perhaps one of the best is in Webster's New Riverside Dictionary, (Mifflin, 1984): "Conforming to accepted principles of right and wrong". The definition is good because of its implication that ethical values will differ from time to time, from nation to nation, and even from one part of a nation to another. Unfortunately, at times, many of these differences are the result of disagreeable racial and religious differences.

The patient's role in clinical decision-making.

The routine daily decisions made by all individuals differ from those made in a clinical setting. A sick person does not have the knowledge or training needed to identify the priorities related to the illness, or to decide on the best therapy. It is the function of the physician, to provide that information. The same applies to individuals practicing other specialized occupations. The physician must study and analyze the problem, assess probabilities, recognize priorities, identify choices, and present them to the patient.

In an ideal world the sick person, in collaboration with the professional adviser, would then decide on what course of action to take. Often this ideal is not realized, or cannot be realized. The patient often tells the physician to "do what is best". Alternatively, consent is given verbally, or implied by silence. At times this silence implies dissent that the patient is reluctant to express. When there is silence it is a good idea to get a verbally expressed consent or dissent. Often the patient is too embarrassed to express dissent to the doctor. At times communication between physician and patient is not ideal. Sometimes because of lack of time. At other times because of the physician's failure to recognize that this is an important part of clinical practice.

Patients rights.

Once a physician has identified and informed the patient of the available therapeutic options, it is the prerogative of the patient to choose the desired option. A prerogative that the patient may delegate to the physician ("do what you think is best"), to another person, or to both. A prerogative that an appropriate delegated surrogate may assume if the patient is mentally incompetent or unable to comprehend or communicate. Alternatively, a prerogative that a mentally competent patient might decide to exercise without delegation or assistance, even if the choice differs from the one the physician has recommended. This often happens. Physicians must learn to accept such dissents because the wishes and the choices of the patient must always prevail.

At times the physician might strongly disagree with a decision made by the patient. The usual reason is a belief that the life of the patient, or that of a dependent minor is at grave risk if therapy is refused. The physician must once again apprise the patient of the pros and cons of the contemplated decision. If the patient's opinion remains unchanged this decision must be accepted. Recourse to the judiciary is only indicated if the physician feels that the patient cannot make reasonable decisions because of mental incompetence, confusion, delirium or coma, and is without delegated surrogate. Alternatively, if it is felt that the decision of a guardian jeopardizes the life of a minor, especially if there is a feeling that self interests or seemingly unreasonable religious dogmas are intruding.

In some circumstances there might not even be enough time for a judicial decision. A patient with a severe infection and high fever is often delirious and unable to understand or to respond with intelligence and comprehension. Alternatively, a patient with a medical problem requiring urgent and radical therapy could be mentally incompetent, or in a coma, and without delegated responsibility. At times there are no delegated surrogates or family members willing to assume responsibility. In such situations the physician has a dilemma if there is not enough time for an appeal to the judiciary. Resolutions are usually based on personal views and conscience. Some physicians would feel an obligation to do whatever is needed to try to save life, regardless of the consequences - these are often situations with major clinical hazards and uncertain chances of a successful outcome. Others might feel that the code of their profession does not necessarily require the acceptance of such responsibilities as unpleasant consequences might flow from their actions. I write from personal experiences. Even if the patient dies, unpleasant consequences are uncommon. As long as relatives feel satisfied that the best was done, given the circumstances existing at the time, criticisms are unusual. Gratitude is more common. It might also be necessary to satisfy peers that the actions were appropriate and had the sanctions of general acceptance and usage. At times this is more difficult than dealing with relatives of a deceased.

In the doctor-patient relationship some absolutes do exist. It is tempting to state that the Hippocratic oath embodies these absolutes. This is no more true. The passage of time and changing mores and therapies must accommodate revisions of some of the original verities. However, the most important of these remains and is summarized by the phrase: **"Primum non nocere".**

> "I will prescribe regimens for the good of my patients according to my ability and my judgment and never do harm to anyone."

In other words, if you cannot help the patient do not do anything that can cause harm, and that includes physical as well as mental harm. This postulate is well put, though needing a small modification for present times. Currently, many therapies must be given despite known toxic effects - a common example is anti-cancer chemotherapy.

Incidentally, books by Withington[1] published in 1894 and another by Garrison[2] published in 1914, claim that the Hippocratic oath did not start with Hippocrates but with the Asclepiads, a cult that worshipped Apollo and also ran a complex of temple-spas for the affluent. Visitors received recitations of the deeds of Aesculapius (one of Apollo's sons) and enthusiastic statements about the therapies of the Asclepiads. These included purges, emetics and bleedings. The records note that all were cured (one suspects that most were self-curing, non-existent or imagined ailments).

However, another injunction of the Asclepiads is as appropriate today as it was when first made.

> "In every house where I come, I will enter only for the good of my patients, keeping myself from all intentional ill-doing and all seduction, and especially from the pleasures of love with women or with men, be they free or slaves"

Hm!

Informed consent.

How much should a physician tell a patient and what is "informed consent"? The answer to the first part of this question is that, in theory, the physician should always tell the patient about all probable benefits and all possible risks of any proposed investigation or therapy. In practice this is impossible. Almost every treatment can result in any possible complication and it would be impossible to detail all to a patient. Even if it were possible, the relating of all possible complications could paint such a bleak picture that a refusal of all invasive investigations and all therapy would almost certainly result.

The Nuremberg code helps to define "informed consent". The code was formulated in 1947 by a judiciary that tried 23 physicians and scientists. All were accused of torture and murder in Nazi death camps. A book by Annas and associates[3] and comments in the Dictionary of medical ethics[4] are comprehensive guides for protection of humans and their rights in clinical medicine and research. The guiding principles for obtaining informed consent are not complex and are well expressed in the first item of the Nuremberg code:

> "The voluntary consent of the human subject is absolutely essential. This means that the person involved should have legal capacity to give consent; should be so situated as to be able to exercise free power of

choice, without the intervention of any element of force, deceit, duress, constraint or coercion; and should have sufficient knowledge and comprehension of the elements of the subject matter involved as to enable him to make an understanding and enlightened decision. The latter element requires that before the acceptance of an affirmative decision by the experimental subject there should be made known to him the nature, duration, and purpose of the experiment; the method and means by which it is to be conducted; all inconveniences and hazards reasonably to be expected; and the effects upon his health or person that may possibly come from his participation in the experiment.

The duty and responsibility for ascertaining the quality of the consent rests upon each individual who initiates, directs or engages in the experiment. It is a personal responsibility which may not be delegated to another with impunity."

Does this first tenet of the Nuremberg code have any relevance in clinical medicine? It certainly does. The unpredictabilities and uncertainties of clinical practice are detailed in Chapter 16. It suffices to say that uncertainties and unpredictables are always present in clinical medicine and research. All but the most trivial form of therapy is an experiment with an uncertain outcome and also, at times, unpredictable adverse effects and complications.

The first Declaration of Helsinki by the World Medical Association[5] reaffirmed the principles of the Nuremberg Code. There were some differences in wording. Annas[6] has criticized these differences because of a feeling that they permit inappropriate justifications. Perhaps they do.

Incidentally, the Nuremberg Code did not specify that a patient should have all available information, only that there should be sufficient information to make a reasonable decision. The patient who has been advised to have therapy that has the sanction of general acceptance and usage does not need as much information as do participants in clinical trials. In any clinical trial patients must receive all available information about the objectives of the trial and of possible consequences, favorable and especially, the unfavorable. In experimental trials all complications are possible. Almost certainly some will occur. The subjects of these experiments must be aware of all favorable and unfavorable possibilities before consenting to participate.

Unqualified commitment to the principle of informed consent can sometimes result in absurd and undesirable consequences. No physician can predict how long a patient with a preterminal medical condition will live. It is absurd to tell patients or relatives that there is only three or six months left. Some will confirm the prediction while others may pursue a lingering course over a long period.

There are some patients who do not want to know what is wrong with them or that a recurrence of malignancy is present. Respect their stated and often unstated views. Spouses, offspring and close friends will communicate these unstated views to the physician. Reticence is acceptable as long as those close to the patient are told all the details. I have often told a sick person that she looks much better today and that I would see her the next day despite the belief, usually correct, that she would be dead by the next day. Of course, when sickness is preterminal relatives must be told that no therapy is available and the only medical consideration is relief of pain and suffering. It also helps to tell them that the dilaudid or morphine for relief of pain may create disorientation and even coma and death. I have not known anyone who has contended that this was euthanasia. All accept the inevitability of death and all hope that the passing will be quick and painless, or pain free if it is a prolonged illness. The practice of medicine certainly requires adherence to basic principles, but adherence tempered by judgment, sensitivity and common sense.

In days gone by there were probably few concerns about "informed consent". Human experimentation, masquerading as therapy, was probably widespread. One suspects that the results were often disastrous. Legions of individuals must have died from the repeated therapeutic bleedings practiced through the centuries. The stated objectives were removal of evil spirits, and other imagined afflictions. Fortunately, experiments on humans without their informed consent is now almost unknown in civilized societies. Physicians of the latter part of this century have developed greater respect for the autonomy of patients, and the laws and mores of most societies enforce respect for it.

Unethical, marginally unethical and ethical clinical studies

Unethical studies.

Some valuable anecdotal findings would be considered unethical by present day standards. I cite two examples.

— **The first** was the reduction in the incidence of puerperal fever deaths because of the work of Semmelweiss. In the description of his studies I include details of the final disaster when his investigations resulted in eleven unnecessary deaths and his subsequent confinement in an asylum.

— **The second** is Jenner's discovery of the protective effects of vaccination against smallpox. The benefits to humanity were great but only after experimentation on a minor and with the real possibility of transmitting active, and potentially lethal smallpox to a child. Why did he not test his hypothesis on himself? Hopefully, it was because he had previously contracted smallpox and, as a consequence, was immune to the disease.

Questionably unethical studies

Next I detail two which are not unquestionably unethical but verge on the borderline of inappropiate experimentation. They are the actions of Domagk, the discoverer of prontosil and the work of Lykoudis in treating peptic ulcers.

Domagk gave prontosil to his direly ill daughter who obviously could not give informed consent but was near death. A redeeming factor was the recovery of the child. At the time no clinical studies had shown that prontosil was an effective antibacterial. Lykoudis' subjects were consenting adults and his medications cured many with peptic ulcers but without any proof that peptic ulcers were caused by bacteria.

Unquestionably ethical studies.

Lastly I present one study that does not present ethical problems, even by current standards. Itt is William Withering's observational study of the effects of digoxin. Some have suggested that even observational studies are unethical without informed consent of all those studied. In 1963 Bradford Hill (Hill, A.B. Medical ethics and controlled trials. Brit. Med. J. 1963; i:1043.) in a lecture decried the labeling of observational studies as experimental even if no experimentation was involved - this seems to be a valid objection.

Currently, strict controls ensure that most clinical studies are ethical. The evaluations of results are often difficult and controversial

1. Unethical studies

Semmelweiss and the eradication of puerperal fever.

Semmelweiss discovered the cause of puerperal fever and introduced antisepsis to clinical medicine. Puerperal fever is fever following childbirth and due to uterine and pelvic infections. The following summarizes his life and achievements. His studies were based on simple observations, small groups of patients and a methodology that was initially harmless. The conclusions reached saved thousands of lives in his lifetime and in future generations but the story ended unhappily. He based his final study on incorrect reasoning and it resulted in the deaths of eleven otherwise healthy women.

Ignaz Semmelweiss was a Hungarian educated at the Universities of Pest and Vienna. He received his doctor's degree in 1844 from Vienna and lived there from 1818-1865. In 1844 Semmelweiss was appointed assistant at the obstetric clinic in Vienna and this is where his work began. Well-to-do women delivered babies at home. Hospitalization was for the poor, for those with illegitimate children or for those with obstetric complications. The mortality for the hospitalized was 25-30%, mostly from puerperal fever. At that time the presumed causes for puerperal fever included "miasma", overcrowding, poor ventilation, and the onset of lactation.

Semmelweiss noted that the mortality in the first division of the clinic was two to three times that in the second division. The two divisions were identical except in one respect; students got instruction in the first and midwives in the second. The students came to the maternity wards immediately after dissecting dead bodies. He hypothesized that the students carried something from the dissecting rooms to the maternity wards and that this was the cause of puerperal fever. Meanwhile a friend died from a wound infection that had occurred during examination of a woman with puerperal fever. The autopsy findings were similar to those found in women who had died of puerperal fever. This strengthened his belief that students were carrying the disease from autopsied cadavers to pregnant women. They were instructed to wash their hands in chlorinated lime before vaginal examinations of pregnant women. The mortality rates from puerperal sepsis rapidly dropped and from March to August 1848 no women in his division died from puerperal fever.

During Semmelweiss' lifetime he, his views and his findings were reviled by peers (including the well-known pathologist, Rudolf Virchow). Only later generations recognized his seminal influence on antisepsis and infection control. One of them, the renowned Joseph Lister wrote:

> "I think with the greatest admiration of him and his achievement and it fills me with joy that at last he is given the respect due to him".

The story ends on a sour note. The following are word for word quotations from Sinclair's biography of Semmelweiss[7] (I have asked the publishers for permission to use quotations from this book but they say they have no records of its existence; publication was almost a century ago but surprisingly, remains in the library of our local medical school in Ottawa):

> "Every visitor to the labor ward (Kreissezimmer) who might have to make an examination must, on entering, wash his hands in a solution of chlorinated lime, and this chlorine disinfection once for all was considered sufficient for that visit. After making the first examination the student was required, before proceeding to another patient to employ merely soap and water for the cleansing of his hands. The practice was based on the assumption that cadaveric particles adhering to the hands were the only cause of infection, and the cadaveric poisoning could be destroyed once for all. But a further extension of the doctrine of infection had soon to be made, and the practice of disinfection modified accordingly. ...."
>
> "In October 1847 a woman was admitted to the Labor Ward and placed in Bed No. 1. This patient was discovered to be suffering from foul-smelling medullary carcinoma of the cervix uteri and Bed No. 1 was that with which the daily visit of the staff and students always began. After examining this parturient patient (presumably all first washed their hands with the chlorinated lime before examining this first pregnant patient who also had an advanced, ulcerated and infected cervical malignancy - my comment) we all washed our hands merely with soap and water: the consequences of these proceedings was that of twelve women confined at the same time eleven died from puerperal fever."

The explanation was that washing with soap and water had not destroyed the "putrid matter". As the examinations proceeded the putrid infecting material (presumably, bacteria) was conveyed to the genitals of the other women who were in labor, and so the puerperal fever spread.

Sinclair continues as follows:

> "From this experience the inference had to be drawn that not only cadaveric particles adhering to the hand, but that putrid matter derived from living organisms produces puerperal fever. Consequently it is necessary that the examining hands, not only after manipulating the cadaver, but even after examination of individuals from whom putrid matter might foul the hands, must also be disinfected by the chlorine process before another patient is examined. At last the conclusion was drawn that not only cadaveric particles adhering to the hand, but that putrid matter derived from living organisms produces puerperal fever. Thereafter hands were washed with chlorinated lime before any patient was examined."

He further records:

> "we never again spread the childbed fever by conveying putrid matter by means of the examining fingers from one individual to another."

Puerperal fever was almost eradicated but at the expense of eleven women who died without knowledge of what was being done. In 1865 Semmelweiss died in a mental hospital.

Nowadays chlorinated lime is not used. Instead physicians use (or should use) disposable plastic gloves for pelvic examinations and wash their hands before and after with soap and water. The disposable gloves are discarded.

Comment.

This was an example of the disastrous consequences that can result from uncontrolled clinical experiments done by a person who believes in the correctness of his personal views. It is probable that neither peer review nor informed consent preceded any of the studies done by Semmelweiss. In his favor one must admit that, at the time, peer pressure probably dissuaded any physician willing to collaborate or interact with him.

The contribution of Semmelweiss to clinical medicine was immense but will always be shadowed by the eleven unnecessary deaths in the final studies. Most communities now insist on informed consent for invasive investigations and all experimental procedures. At the time when Semmelweiss practiced medicine it is possible that this would have sounded ridiculous. The then current attitudes about the rights of women, especially indigent women, and women with illegitimate pregnancies, probably did not exceed minimal tolerance. Another description of Semmelweiss and his times is by Hempel[8]. I have not been able to find this book anywhere. Can one conclude that Semmelweiss was a medical pioneer whose observations have saved thousands of lives? Does this redeem the human experimentation that resulted in unnecessary deaths of eleven women? It is a conundrum that I leave the reader to ponder for these are often difficult questions to answer. The times were different and so were the customs and attitudes.

Edward Jenner and vaccination against smallpox.

Edward Jenner[9,10] was born in 1749 and died in 1823. It was a time when smallpox was widespread in England. The mortality rates were high and the disfigurements of survivors were unpleasant. It was known that inoculation with material taken from the lesions of an infected person would confer immunity. This practice was widely used throughout Asia at the time. Unfortunately the inoculum could and did sometimes produce clinical smallpox that killed the recipient. Additionally, if the inoculated person developed smallpox the disease could spread to the uninfected.

A related disease, cowpox, could be contracted from cattle and was relatively benign. Those infected with cowpox were subsequently immune to smallpox. These facts were used by Jenner as the basis for his experiments. In May 1776 he took material from cowpox lesions on the hands of a dairy maid, Sarah Nelmes, and inoculated an eight year old boy, James Phipps, with this material. On July 1 he inoculated the boy with smallpox matter. Fortunately the boy did not develop the disease. The control of smallpox by vaccination began and the incidence of the disease rapidly declined.

The disease has killed hundreds of thousands, if not millions through the centuries. Vaccination and the particular epidemiology of smallpox have now permitted global health workers to almost eradicate the disease. Unlike Semmelweiss, Jenner received approval and recognition in abundance during his lifetime.

Comment.

One doubts if in present times any form of consent, informed or otherwise, could ever be obtained to do experiments of this sort on eight year old boys. It is probable that in days gone by many other such experiments were performed but with less fortunate results. One suspects that many subjects of such experiments died. Presumably money was paid to parents or guardians of these unfortunate children, or to adults if they themselves were to be the subjects of experimentation. The reader must ponder the ethics of this problem. An unnecessary death is never justifiable nor is the possibility of one. Yet the whole world has gained much from Jenner's discovery. Perhaps the real hero, and the one who should receive all our plaudits is the eight year old boy, James Phipps. The experimenter can always experiment on himself and many of the illustrious names in medicine have done so. Some have suffered for it. Perhaps Jenner could not do so because he had previously contracted smallpox and become immune to further infection by the virus.

2. Marginally unethical studies.

Gerhard Domagk - the discoverer of prontosil.

Domagk was a physician and a professor of pathology at the University of Munster. In 1927 he was given a two year leave of absence to do research in a new Pathology laboratory built by IGFarbenindustrie. During this period he found that a red dye (later called prontosil) protected mice and rabbits from streptococci and staphylococci.

Soon after this discovery his daughter became seriously ill with a streptococcal infection. Death was imminent and the father, in desperation, gave his daughter some prontosil. Complete and rapid recovery ensued. He did not report on this episode till 1935 when clinical studies had confirmed the anti-bacterial properties of prontosil. A new weapon against disease had arrived - the chemical antibacterial. Over the next fifty years many variations of prontosil were synthesized and used for different diseases. Domagk was honored by a grateful public and in 1939 received the Nobel Prize for Medicine or Physiology.

Domagk gave prontosil to his daughter before its clinical effectiveness was proven. She, of course, could not give informed consent even if the father has asked for one. Was the discoverer justified in giving it to his daughter before clinical trials had demonstrated its effectiveness in clinical sickness? Most parents would answer in the affirmative. Some would not. The reader must judge.

Hindsight tells us that the discovery of the first antibacterial agent was an event of epochal importance in clinical medicine. Subsequent research has produced many antibacterials and saved thousands of lives. But nationalist feelings continue the debate on who was the first to discover an antibacterial.

Actually the first antibacterial discovered was penicillin. The Oxford dictionary defines an antibiotic as a "substance capable of destroying or injuring bacteria or similar organisms" so that there is really no difference between an antibiotic and an antibacterial.

Alexander Fleming discovered this antibiotic in the 1920s but it was not till World War II that it was used to treat human infections., especially battlefield infections. Development for large scale use resulted from the works of Florey and Chain. Fleming did not seem to have any interest in being actively involved in the industrial production of penicillin in large quantities. Fleming, Florey and Chain received the Nobel Prize for Medicine in 1945. Production, clinical trials and dissemination of information to physicians are as equally important as discovery. The latter is often the product of academic institutions, the former needs the resources of the pharmaceutical industry. It is difficult to assign priorities as between Fleming and Domagk. Fleming was the first to discover and Domagk the first to apply antibacterials to clinical sickness. Let us leave it at that. Both were great benefactors of humanity.

I have personal experience of prontosil as in that same year (1939) my life was saved by the drug. A mastoid infection had become an abscess that had eroded the temporal bone. I remember that the pain was excruciating. So bad that morphine injections had to be given to this nine year old boy. My father hunted all over town for prontosil. All was hoarded in anticipation of an imminent war with Germany. Eventually some was found. Within a day the pain had gone and in five days I was up and about.

Was Domagk justified in giving his daughter a drug not previously shown to be effective in humans? Most parents would answer that he certainly was. Some would not. Was he justified in waiting till 1935 before reporting on prontosil's effectiveness on his own daughter - probably not. I leave the reader to judge.

.John Lykoudis and the discovery of the cause of peptic ulcers.

Until the early 1980s vagotomy and pyloroplasty for disabling peptic ulceration was a common major surgical procedure. Today it is uncommon because of the discovery that most peptic ulcers are caused by Heliobacter Pylori, an infection that is easily eradicated by antibiotic therapy with subsequent resolution of the ulceration. Warren and Marshall[12] are usually credited with the discovery that peptic ulceration results from bacterial infection. In fact it was John Lykoudis[13] who first postulated that the cause of peptic ulceration was bacterial infection of the stomach.

The subjects of his therapies were consenting and informed patients. He successfully treated thousands of mostly Greek patients with combinations of anti-bacterial agents that he called Elgaco (the Greek word for ulcer is elkos). However, his findings were repeatedly rejected by other physicians, his Government, by many pharmaceutical companies, and at least one prestigious journal: the JAMA. Rigas and associates[14] record part of the response of this journal: "[it] does not seem appropriate for our journal". The use of acid inhibitors for peptic ulceration was the dogma of the medical hierarchy at that time and the use of antibiotics instead had no chance of receiving their imprimatur.

The activities of Domagk and Lykoudis are only marginally unethical as they did break some rules on clinical experimentation The patients that Lykoudis treated were willing consenters. In most jurisdictions there are many givers and takers of unproven therapies and medications. As a rule no laws are broken as long as the recipients are consenting adults. The givers may be qualified physicians., naturopaths, homeopaths, vitamin peddlers or, it seems, anyone on the street who can persuade consenting adults to take the latest cures for cancer and other diseases.

An obviously ethical clinical study.

William Withering (1741-99) and digitalis.

William Withering[11] was a man who had the good fortune to have his experiments done for him by others. He noted the remarkable ability of a family of Shropshire farmers to treat dropsy (currently described as edema of the legs and usually caused by congestive heart failure) by drinking a herbal infusion. He traced this to the presence in the infusion of a product of the foxglove plant. He called the active agent digitalis and established the proper ways to administer digitalis and also, the connection between dropsy - previously considered a primary disease - and cardiac failure. These were not experiments but observational studies. Though not sanctioned by peer review, they were conducted on agreeing and otherwise fatally ill people. A valuable therapeutic agent had been discovered, one that continues to be widely used. No criticism of these observational studies are justified.

Abuse of patients

The following are examples of the different ways physicians abuse patients:

Experiments on humans.

Experimentation on humans without informed consent is a horrible and revolting practice. A clinical trial is also an experiment on humans but one always preceded by peer review and genuine informed consent.

Many examples of experimentation on humans without any consent have been described by Pappworth[15]. Most were done by state supported organizations as acts designed to combine cruelty, pain and degradation prior to a previously made decision to kill. Unfortunately many human experiments were done without any desire to harm or degrade. Pappworth has described a study in which cardiac catheterization was done on patients anesthetized for dental extractions. A cardiologist felt that asking the patients to allow a small sample of blood to be taken during the extractions sufficed as informed consent for cardiac catheterizations!

Human experimentation without informed consent is usually an act authorized by the State and carried out by physicians. Therefore, it is appropriate to examine State, physician, and patient interactions.

State, physician, and patient interactions.

It is not only in this century that physicians have acted on behalf of established authority to the detriment of patients. However, the enormity of disgraceful conduct by physicians in the twentieth century has been astounding. They experimented on humans during the second World war, experiments that usually ended in the deaths of their subjects. It was physicians who maintained the penal so-called psychiatric institutions of Soviet Russia (I do not know if these institutions still exist). It was, and continues to be, physicians who provide a facade of respectability and consent to institutionalized coercion, torture and death. These were, and continue to be common in this world. In democracies with Constitutions that defend human rights legal officers appointed by the state often defend and justify these actions by convoluted legal rationalizations.

I have personally spoken with physicians who, in my opinion, abused their positions in the interests of the State. One conversation with a Soviet psychiatrist was easy to understand. There were no regrets. The State that had been established was the best of all possible States (this was before the recent disintegration of the Soviet Union). Hence, anyone who disapproved of the State and wished to complain about its way of functioning was having paranoid delusions. If supportive psychotherapy could not cure this mental aberration hospitalization and treatment as an in-patient of a psychiatric Institution was needed till a change of attitude was demonstrable.

There were no regrets nor attempts at justifying conduct that the physician thought was appropriate and justifiable. I suppose there was a certain Kafkaesque logic to her responses.

The other conversation was more difficult and personally, most disturbing. The physician had been involved in Nazi death camp experimentation. When we spoke alcohol had reduced his inhibitions to negligible levels. The experience was neither pleasant nor edifying. I heard incredible things, about events and about people and about the unbelievable ways humans can behave. At times the tone was one of justification, at others of remorse, and at others, of: "What would have happened to my family and me if I had not complied?" This was a difficult question to answer, and for me it is still a difficult question. We all like to think we would act honorably under pressure but without being tested one can never be sure. Self-preservation is a basic and often overpowering instinct. On the other hand physicians are privileged people. We have received the wisdom and learning of the centuries, we have received honor and respect from our fellows, and our patients trust us with their lives for they have no others to trust. At times the consequence of not cooperating with the State is death or even worse (torture before death), not only for oneself but also one's family. Death is the inevitable finale to life. Often the question of how and when is a choice between honor and survival. Each person will balance the two and make a choice when under pressure. No one can predict with certainty what the decision will be. If one has never been tested one never knows. The Tokyo Declaration of the World Medical Associations is detailed later in this chapter. It provides specific injunctions to doctors about resisting participation in torture. The injunctions are equally applicable to all humans.

The Tuskegee Syphilis Study.

Dictatorships and undemocratic countries are not responsible for all the inappropriate human experimentation that takes place. The Tuskegee Syphilis Study is an example of disgraceful human experimentation in a country where human rights and democratic mores are constitutionally enjoined, and usually respected: the United States of America. A book by Jones[16] contains a detailed description of this experiment on humans.

In 1932 the United States Public Health Service initiated a study to document the natural history of syphilis. They recruited black sharecroppers in Macon County, Alabama; 399 with syphilis and 201 other individuals without the disease. All were given free meals, free medical services and burial insurance! No treatment was given to any of those with syphilis - a rigid requirement of the study. When the study began the standard treatment for syphilis was injections of arsenicals and topical applications of mercury or bismuth ointments. This was not given to those with syphilis in the "study". When penicillin became available for effective treatment of syphilis this also was withheld.

Jones estimates in his book that between 28 and 100 men died of causes directly related to untreated syphilis. Undoubtedly, men with syphilis passed on their disease to sexual partners and offsprings[17] - the exact number we do not know.

This is an example of human experimentation strictly prohibited by constitutional mandates but ignored, presumably because the subjects were poor, hungry and black. Moreover, it was a stupid and unnecessary investigation because, at the time when the experiment was initiated, the natural history of syphilis was the subject of many textbooks dedicated to this single topic and incorporating centuries of knowledge about the disease. Even when I was in medical school in the early 1950s the library had many thick volumes describing every aspect of syphilis, books written at various times in the preceding 50 years.

Appropriate state-physician interactions.

What should be the correct relationship of physician and State as regards patients. The following is a summary answer to this question. It needs no elaboration.

In 1985 the South African Medical and Dental Council barred Benjamin Tucker from practicing medicine for "disgraceful conduct" because of circumstances relating to the death of Stephen Biko from head injuries. Mr. Biko had been a fighter for human rights and at the time of his death was a prisoner. In 1991 the license of Dr. Tucker was restored following a letter of apology he sent to the council. I first saw this letter in a summary of material published in the New York Times. The following excerpts from Dr. Tucker's letter summarize the correct and desirable relationship between the State, the individual physician and the physician's patient. They also detail the probable consequences when these guidelines are breached. Dr. Tucker wrote:

> "In failing to make full and proper inquiries from the patient himself, from members of the South African Police, and from colleagues about matters relevant to Mr. Biko's condition, and in failing and neglecting to examine Mr. Biko thoroughly and adequately, I was the author of my own misfortune." .... "On reflection on the cause of this failure, I came to realize that, over the period of 30 years I had at that time been employed by the State as a district surgeon, I had gradually lost the fearless independence that is required of a medical practitioner when the interests of his patient are threatened. I had become too closely identified with the interests of the organs of the state, especially the police force, with which I dealt practically on a daily basis. In the circumstances of Mr. Biko's case, I too readily accepted the decisions of the Security Police, without safeguarding the interests of my patient. .... As a result of my conduct, not only the interests of my patient suffered, but also those of the medical profession and my country."

Torture.

Torture or "vigorous interrogation" as its practitioners call it is common. It would not be useful to name the guilty countries - it seems to be ubiquitous, and often dismissed by those who are guilty as being for the public good. The World Medical Association in its Tokyo declaration[18] on torture states:

"For the purposes of this Declaration torture is defined as the deliberate, systematic, or wanton infliction of physical or mental suffering by one or more persons acting alone or on the orders of any authority, to force another person to yield information, to make a confession, or for any other reason."

The following were its specific injunctions to physicians.

Article 1: The doctor shall not countenance, condone or participate in the practice of torture or other forms of cruel, inhuman, or degrading procedures, whatever the offense the victim of such procedures is suspected, accused, or guilty, and whatever the victim's beliefs or motives, and in all situations, including armed conflict and civil strife.

Article 2: The doctor shall not provide any premises, instruments, or knowledge to facilitate the practice of torture or other forms of cruel, inhuman, or degrading procedures or to diminish the ability of the victim to resist such treatment.

Article 3: The doctor shall not be present during any procedure during which torture or other forms of cruel, inhuman or degrading treatment is used or threatened.

Article 4: A doctor must have complete clinical independence in deciding upon the care of a person for whom he or she is medically responsible. The doctor's fundamental role is to alleviate the distress of his or her fellow men, and no motive whether personal, collective or political shall prevail against this higher purpose.

Article 5: Where a prisoner refuses nourishment and is considered by the doctor as capable of forming an unimpaired and rational judgment concerning the consequences of such a voluntary refusal of nourishment, he or she shall not be fed artificially. The decision as to the capacity of the prisoner to form such a judgment should be confirmed by at least one other independent doctor. The consequences of the refusal of nourishment shall be explained by the doctor to the prisoner.

Article 6: The WMA will support, and should encourage the international community, the national medical associations, and fellow doctors to support the doctor and his or her family in the face of threats or reprisals resulting from a refusal to condone the use of torture or other forms of cruel, inhuman or degrading treatment.

No addition to these injunctions is needed except to state that all are equally applicable to all citizens in civilized societies.

Sexual and other forms of abuse.

"Sexual abuse" is difficult to define in specific terms. It is often defined as anything of a sexual nature that degrades, even if previous consent has been obtained (minors and the mentally incompetent can never consent). Incidentally, sexual abuse includes heterosexual as well as homosexual abuse. Bizarre and inappropriate actions, the gestural and prosodic language of the physician and other intangibles usually identify sexual abuse by a physician when it is occurring.

Sexual interactions between a physician and an individual who is still a patient is probably not desirable, even if they are consensual. Consensual sexual activity between doctor and patient can be potentially degrading for the latter. This is because the physician is often consciously or unconsciously perceived and acts as a dominant and domineering individual, acting with the authority and power conferred by status. But what is the appropriate interval between severance of the doctor-patient relationship and resumption or start of sexual interactions?

Sexual abuse by physicians is never acceptable but, given the nature of humans, there will always be an occasional physician who tries when circumstances provide opportunities. The only prevention is vigilance and training during the period of training in medical schools. The trainee must be brain-washed to understand that once a doctor-patient relationship begins, the patient is flesh providing information and nothing else. It must be emphasized that the physical examination is analogous to the examination of a machine by a mechanic to find out why it does not work. Physicians may look, touch and examine but may not do anything else.

The abuse of a patient's body or sensibilities is never justifiable or acceptable. Absolute 100% zero tolerance is essential. The teachers have a responsibility to weed out those who cannot develop the necessary conditioned reflexes. Colleagues and peers have a responsibility to restrain and report. Licensing bodies have a responsibility to see that such individuals never have access to similar temptations again. I am told that retraining is possible. This may be true but licensing bodies must always bear in mind that the public trusts doctors and expects licensing bodies to protect them from deviants. Unfortunately, when licensing bodies discipline such physicians the latter turn to the judiciary who often decide that the sexual interaction was consensual and therefore, the discipline was unwarranted and needs reversal.

Euthanasia and assisted death.

The following is a quotation from John Donne's work, the Biathanatos:

> "Death, therefore, is an act of God's justice, and when He is pleased to inflict it, He may choose His officer, and constitute myself as well as any other."

I find this free-wheeling attitude to euthanasia, or, at least assisted euthanasia unacceptable. Others will differ but who decides when "God's justice" is to be inflicted, and who decides on the inflictor?

There is a voluminous literature on the subject of euthanasia and assisted euthanasia. The relief of the pain and suffering of incurable terminally ill patients is not euthanasia even though the relief of pain by narcotics may hasten dying. In a few countries euthanasia is legally permissible, with appropriate safeguards. In many countries suicide is permissible but not in others. It is within the caveats of these restrictions that one writes the following generalities.

If there is pain and suffering from incurable and preterminal disease the physician's obligations are clear. Relief of pain and suffering are the primary considerations. Any drugs administered are for these purposes alone. It is understood that death may be hastened or precipitated by the medications given but this should not (in my opinion) ever be the objective. Pain and suffering can almost always be controlled, even though, at times, it requires sedation to the point where the patient is rendered semi-comatose. Ideally, if a terminally ill patient is mentally competent and sufficiently conscious to communicate intelligently it is a good idea to inform and get consent (at the least, verbal or implied consent) for medication with the more potent narcotics (for example morphine and dilaudid), but with delicacy. I emphasize the word "delicacy" for injudicious talk at this stage can quell the only remaining support - hope.

Even when pain is severe there are patients who refuse narcotics for relief. I have treated two patients who refused any medication for pain relief because they felt it was "God's will" that they die with what I thought was intolerable and extreme pain. Both were members of religious orders and in both instances their wishes were respected. Every individual has the right to refuse recommended therapy and every health professional must always honor this right.

Euthanasia is not justified if the only problems are mental handicaps, severe and inadequately treated psychiatric disease, encephalopathies or dementias from organic brain diseases such as Alzheimer's disease, multiple brain infarcts or prion infections.

When neurological and electroencephalographic opinion confirm brain death the decision to end life-supporting technology is not difficult. At other times the EEG does not show brain death but the comatose patient needs artificial ventilation to remain alive. In these circumstances exercise caution before ending artificial life support. There are two important caveats:

First, be sure that the disease is indeed incurable and terminal. A second, and even a third opinion from respected colleagues are invaluable, and essential if one feels a psychiatric component is present. The involvement and understanding of consenting nursing staff are also essential. Never coerce if conscience says no. The consent of close relatives for termination of life support is always desirable even when not mandated by the Institution or jurisdiction. At least it gives comfort to the bereaved to have participated in the decision.

Second, wrong diagnoses do occur and prognostications of imminent demise from preterminal disease may be incorrect. Always remember that physicians are not fortunetellers and they can make errors just as any other human can.

There are borderline problems. As an example I once had a patient dying with recurrent and metastatic lung cancer who had a stroke. He was unconscious and required a mechanical respirator to keep alive. The electroencephalograh did not confirm brain death. After a few days the attending hospital physicians asked the relatives to permit termination of the life-support respirator even though there was no evidence of brain death. The relatives asked me to opine. I told them it was better to die in this way. The alternative was possible recovery of consciousness and spontaneous respiration only to die later from the increasing suffering of recurrent and metastatic lung cancer. They eventually agreed and the patient died peacefully soon after the mechanical respirator was turned off.

Another more recent example was the patient of a colleague. He had progressive amyotrophic lateral sclerosis, a gastrostomy for feeding, a tracheostomy and assisted respiration for breathing, a catheter to collect urine, diapers to collect feces, and a wheelchair. He made repeated requests for assisted euthanasia that my colleague, quite correctly, was not able to satisfy. Eventually a demand that no liquids or solids be introduced into his gastrostomy was orally expressed with difficulty as he could not talk normally or write at all. A document was drawn up by his lawyer that he signed with an X, helped along with an assisting hand. It was witnessed by three people, including me. His request was met and he died five days later. It is impossible to make rules that cover all eventualities. In borderline situations pressure from relatives is a frequent distraction, especially when one feels that there could be an element of self interest.

Trust.

The use of the word "trust" sounds patronizing. However, most patients accept the therapy advised because they trust the physician. Trust is an intangible based on many factors. Perhaps the most important is verbal, gestural and prosodic language that gives an impression of competence and of indefinable reliability and security. When patients trust physicians they believe that whatever is recommended is correct. They also feel that they have got all the information needed to make good choices and decisions. The converse is the case when the physician does not inspire trust. To write that trust is an important factor in the patient-doctor relationship sounds paternalistic. Perhaps so, but the fact remains that it is a cogent consideration in clinical practice.

How does one inspire trust? The question is difficult to answer. The following are some tentative answers. Physicians inspire trust when they show that they have listened to what patients wish to say and that any statements made by the physician were made after careful deliberation. Also, when they respect the individual patient, listen to any concerns about recommended therapy and show that they have sincerely listened to these concerns. Patients do not like to feel that anything is being concealed. They immediately sense any evasions. Most patients appreciate unvarnished straightforward talk from the physician. Some do not. They prefer evasions rather than the facts. Comply if you feel that the facts would be mentally disturbing. However, a close relative should always have the unvarnished facts; a spouse or an offspring who is a responsible adult. The physician would be wise to record that this has been done and the name of the individual who was informed. They may or may not feel that the patient should be told the truth and they are the best judges in these situations. Close family members are usually best able to evaluate the reactions of the patient to information that could be potentially devastating.

As time passes physicians learn how trust is generated. There is no standard method. Individuals vary widely in their mannerisms and ways of communicating and so do physicians when dealing with patients.

In the interests of expediency physicians do sometimes have to take chances. For example, it would be impossible to function in my medical practice if every patient who needed a blood examination had to be told that after a venipuncture there was a remote possibility of cellulitis of the arm, loss of an arm or even life. Nor could I function if I had to tell every patient who was being sigmoidoscoped that there was a remote chance of bowel perforation, peritonitis and even death (I know that some physicians who are particularly concerned about malpractice suits do tell their patients about these remote possibilities and obtain signed consents before performing such procedures). Such statements are unnecessarily frightening and confusing. Patients are not trained to assess medical risk-benefit probabilities. It is the function of the physician to summarize the more common and real risks and benefits and advise patients of the abstracted pros and cons of proposed procedures and treatments. It is the abstraction that is difficult. It can never be as comprehensive as possible. However, it must and will suffice if it honestly attempts to provide the patient with all information needed to make an informed decision.

Confidentiality.

Patients will not give physicians unqualified trust if they feel that what they impart might be revealed to someone else without their consent. This has been realized by physicians over the centuries and the principles are clearly stated in the Hippocratic oath. The following is a translation from the original:

> "What I may see or hear in the course of the treatment or even outside of the treatment in regard to the life of men, which on no account one must spread abroad, I will keep to myself, holding such things shameful to be spoken about."

In other words, no information about the interaction between a patient and a physician may be revealed to any third party without the patient's consent. Of course the situation is different when the patient is mentally incompetent, confused or comatose. In such situations information must be imparted to a legally delegated surrogate, or if no individual with a power of attorney is available, to one or more close and responsible relatives who agree to assume responsibility.

Evidence-based medicine

Evidence-based medicine uses statistical analyses of clinical trials to determine whether some newly introduced therapy is as effective as its manufacturer claims. It is also used to compare the effectiveness of two or more different clinical practices or therapies. It is often based on meta-analyses. The pros and cons of meta-analyses are contentious topics and some are detailed below.

What is a meta-analysis?

An early paper by Peto[19] summarized the rationale for meta-analyses. It correctly postulated that many clinical trials do not give clear-cut results because the numbers of patients are too small and/or the variables too many. In clinical meta-analyses participants in control and study groups should have comparable variables.

A meta-analysis combines results from many centers to answer one or more specific questions. In any meta-analysis there are many variables: age; gender; nutritional status; socio-economic conditions; and the many different permutations and combinations in the ways that a disease can present. It is presumed that the different groups in the meta-analysis will have comparable variables and thus circumvent effects due to the variables. This may or may not be a correct assumption. It depends on the population base and the location chosen for the study. For example, are the results of meta-analyses that compare groups in the racially heterogeneous populations of North America comparable to similar analyses that compare groups in the essentially homogeneous racial populations of Europe.

Those who decry meta-analyses maintain that they are unjustified statistical manipulations that combine results from studies that are not strictly comparable in order to obtain results that support unjustifiable conclusions[20]. This view has some merits. The opposite view is that meta-analysis provides a method for combining results from several studies in order to obtain statistically significant therapeutic guides. This view also has merit but only if the design of the study complies with the criteria detailed below.

Requirements for clinical trials.

Informed consent. Needless to say all participants in a clinical trial must receive all information about the objectives of the trial and the possible adverse reactions and risks. They must get as much detailed information as possible before their informed consents are recorded.

The baseline characteristics of the participants. The participants in a clinical trial or meta-analysis usually have many variables. For example a meta-analysis of any aspect of breast cancer must include information on many topics: age; tumor histology; premenopausal or postmenopausal status; extent, if any, of lymph node involvement; invasion of vascular and/or nerve tissue; metastatic involvement of other structures; treatment (lumpectomy, mastectomy and/or radiotherapy alone or in combination with surgery and/or chemotherapy); family history; previous use of oral contraceptives; and the number of children and whether one or more were breast fed. The meta-analysis must also remember that long periods often intervene between the first treatment and the first recurrence. For example, I recently had a patient where the interval was 14 years. Four months after the appearance of a single hepatic metastasis (detected by an ultrasound at the time of the routine annual medical examination) she died with disseminated metastases. The variables are the baseline characteristics of the participants. All should be recorded to ensure that control and study groups have comparable variables.

Statistics. The statistics chosen for analysis must be appropriate and have general acceptance. The opinions of independent assessors who are not participants in the trial are valuable adjuncts for those who must judge but are not versed in the complexities of statistical analyses.

Assessments of the numerical data. The probability values of statistics (p values) inform whether control and study groups are different and the chances that this deduction is correct. A p value less than 0.005 means that the chances of an erroneous deduction is 5 in 1000 and one of 0.0005 that the chances are 5 in 10,000. Something is happening but is it clinically important? The p values of an analysis do not provide information about the magnitudes of the differences. They are often small when individuals in each group are many. Statistical significance does not always equate with numerical significance. The numerical differences between control and study groups can be too small for clinical significance and use even when p values are less than 0.0005.

The criteria for terminating the trial. Most trials are ended when the statistical differences between control groups and study groups reach a predetermined level. In large meta-analyses most studies are terminated when the p value between the two groups is less than 0.005 or in other studies less than 0.0005. If all that is required is a statistical determination that control and study groups differ, termination of the study at this point is justifiable. If the object is to determine the clinical value of the results this is not enough. For example the ASCOT-LLA[23] study on statins was terminated after three years because the p value was 0.0005. Yet the numerical difference was a reduction of 1.33 coronary events per 100 patients given the statin for three years.

Perhaps the termination of such studies should not be based on p values alone but on p values as well as previously agreed numerical differences. The latter should have priority as the object of the exercise is not assessments of statistics but of clinical usefulness. Clinical value has priority over statistics.

The subject of clinical trials are discussed once again in the last chapter of this book. It details some of the benefits and some of the adverse consequences of interactions between physicians and pharmaceutical companies in the conduct of clinical trials.

Determination of clinical importance is easy at times but at other times difficult. I shall present an example of each. The first is short because it shows how easy it can be to decide on the value of a proposed therapy. The second is much longer because it shows how difficult assessments of some meta-analyses can be.

Meta-analyses that demonstrate obvious and immediate value

The following is a good example of a meta-analysis that is easy to interpret.

Waksman and the discovery of streptomycin.

The story of the discovery of streptomycin and its use was summarized by Raju in 1999[21]. The discoverer was **Selman Waksman**, a soil microbiologist. After many years searching for antibacterial agents in soil, two of his graduate students, Albert Schatz and Elizabeth Bugie, isolated Actinomyces Griseus from the throat of an infected chicken. Waksman found that the organism could inactivate Mycobacterium Tuberculosis in vitro. He supplied 10g of the bacteria, now called streptomycin, to William Feldman and H. C. Hinshaw at the Mayo Clinic. Both confirmed its ability to ameliorate, and often cure, human tuberculosis. The results were astounding. I was in medical school at the time. Patients with miliary tuberculosis responded best because they had not developed cavities as yet. Before streptomycin a diagnosis of miliary tuberculosis was a death sentence. In my last year in medical school the clinical use of streptomycin for treating tuberculosis began. For the first time we saw the lesions of miliary tuberculosis disappearing and patients with miliary tuberculosis rapidly regaining health and putting on weight. It was not necessary to wait for any publication in a journal to know that the **"eyeball test"** (my definition of a test with a result of unquestionable value) was positive. A miracle was taking place and none of us had doubts that required resolution by statistical analyses. Subsequent clinical trials and analyses were superfluous. All patients with tuberculosis got streptomycin. Many with cavitations, especially tension cavities required supplementary surgical excisions.

Later, potentiating supplements such as isoniazid were added. Current therapy does not use streptomycin as first line therapy but when it first appeared some fifty years ago it saved thousands of lives; including that of my wife who remains fit and well 49 years after treatment with a streptomycin and isoniazid combination. Currently streptomycin is only used as second line therapy for recurrences and treatment failures.

Drugs can cure but cannot prevent recurrences. In poor countries recurrences are frequent and usually associated with poverty, hunger and poor living conditions. Often, another factor is opportunistic infection or reactivation of dormant M.Tuberculosis because of a depressed immune response. Infections with HIV/AIDS is a common cause. Other causes include chronic disease of any sort, long-term corticosteroid therapy and chemotherapy for malignant disease. Between 1.7 and two million individuals die each year from untreated tuberculosis, from disease that does not respond to therapy, or from repeated recurrences of disease.

Meta-analyses that are difficult to assess

At times it is difficult to assess the merits of therapies studied by meta-analyses. Statistical differences are often very significant while the numerical differences are not. Some of the reasons for these disparities were detailed above. A study of the meta-analyses of statins has been chosen to show the frequency of these disparities in some meta-analyses. It is also chosen to show physicians how important it is to determine numerical differences between control and experimental groups before making therapeutic decisions based on the meta-analysis.

The statins.

Statins are drugs that competitively inhibit 3-hydroxy-3-methyl glutaryl-coenzyme A (HMG-CoA) reductase, an enzyme that catalyzes the conversion of HMG-CoA to mevalonate. This is the rate limiting step in the biosynthesis of cholesterol. A voluminous literature supports the original Framingham observation that coronary artery atheromatous disease is often associated with high blood cholesterol and LDL levels. Atheromas contain lipids and this is why a cause and effect relationship is assumed by many. Unfortunately it is impossible to conclusively prove such a relationship. For obvious ethical reasons, the rigorous postulates used by Koch to confirm causations of disease cannot be used in clinical practice.

Most clinical trials show that statins can reduce blood lipid levels. Two questions remain.

First, does the administration of statins sufficiently decrease the numbers of deaths due to coronary artery disease or, at least, the numbers of "coronary events" to justify their long-term administration to those at risk? The phrase "coronary events" is commonly used in these analyses. It denotes the sum of fatal and non-fatal myocardial infarctions in the study.

Second, can statins decrease the progression of coronary artery atheromas? The drugs are not inexpensive and occasional serious adverse effects can and do occur so that the above question needs early resolution.

My interest in this topic dates from seeing a disclaimer by the manufacturer of a well known statin. **The disclaimer was in the small print of a full page color advertisement in the Lancet (June 5, 2004).**

It stated:

> **"The effect of LIPITOR on cardiovascular mortality and morbidity has not been determined."**

A summary of some clinical meta-analyses on statins.

Most clinical meta-analyses confirm that the statins can reduce the lipid levels in blood. With one exception, the ALLHAT-LLT study, most claim a statistically significant reduction in "coronary events" when patients take statins. What about the numerical differences between control and treatment groups in these studies? These should be estimated before deciding that all individuals with risk factors for coronary artery disease, or a previous history of myocardial infarction should receive statins.

The following is a summary of some of the more important meta-analyses that have studied the effects of statins. There was no single dysfunction that was the object of study. The subjects of these studies had one or more of many dysfunctions and risk factors for coronary artery disease: hypertension; diabetes; cigarette smoking; a history of coronary artery disease; and obesity and inactivity. Most had combinations of any one or more of the above but some participants had no previous history of cardiac disease. The results of these meta-analyses were all comparable regardless of the reason for doing the meta-analysis.

The ALLHAT-LLT study[22].

In the ALLHAT-LLT study there were 513 clinical centers treating 10,335 patients. One group was given a statin and the other "usual care" only, i.e., no placebo. Blood cholesterol levels were decreased by statins. However, the study did not show any difference in all-cause morbidity or mortality from coronary heart disease between the two groups. Pravastatin did not confer any additional benefit to usual good care.

The ALLHAT-LLT study was criticized for various reasons in order to explain the differences between the results of that study and those in the ASCOT-LLA investigation detailed below. In fact the differences were almost nonexistent.

Anglo-Scandinavian Cardiac outcomes Trial (ASCOT-LLA)[23].

In the ASCOT-LLA study 10,305 patients were randomly assigned to atorvastatin (Lipitor) or a placebo. There were 5168 individuals in the statin group and 5137 in the placebo group. The primary end point of the trial was the sum of all coronary events: non-fatal myocardial infarctions and fatal CHD. After three years the total coronary events in the group given the statin was 178 versus 247 in the placebo-treated group. The statistical difference between the two groups was estimated as $p=0.0005$.

The numerical difference between the two groups was 69 (247 - 178 = 69). This works out to 1.34 (69 ÷ 5168) x 100 = 1.34) fewer coronary events per 100 patients given the statin for three years or 0.45 (1.34 ÷ 3 = 0.45) per 100 patients taking the statin for a year. The placebo was not described except in general terms. Surprisingly, the investigators felt it was unethical to continue the trial after expiry of the initial three year period because the calculated p value was so low!

An on-line Lancet commentary about this trial was made by Lindholm and Samuelson[24]. They wrote:

> "In absolute terms ...... the incidence of cardiovascular disease in ASCOT-LLA was only 3-4 per 1000 patient years for the primary event and 2 per 1000 patient years for stroke. Hence active lipid-lowering treatment can be estimated to result in only a small increase in the probability of remaining free from a myocardial infarction over 5 years from 95% to 97% in patients with good control of blood pressure.".

They called this a relative risk reduction of 36% which indeed it was. Some physicians might feel that this small decrease in coronary events do not justify giving an expensive and potentially harmful drug to patients. Others might not.

These results are the basis for the latest advertisements for Lipitor in the Lancet (e.g., the issue of February 19, 2005). They write:

> **"ASCOT LLA assessed the effect of atorvastatin ..... the primary end-point was coronary events, a**

composite of nonfatal MI and fatal CHD. Relative risk reduction for the primary end point was 36% (based on incidences of 1.9% for atorvastatin vs 3.0% for placebo) ......".

Absolutely right. A reduction of 3% to 1.9% is a 36% reduction - (3- 1.9)x100=36.66%) reduction in coronary events

The West of Scotland study[25].

The study was published in the New England Journal of Medicine as "Prevention of coronary heart disease with pravastatin in men with hypercholesterolemia". There were 6595 participants divided between two groups, one given pravastatin and the other a placebo (not described).

There were 248 coronary events in the control group and 174 in the group given statins. Thus, 74 fewer coronary events in the group of 3297 participants given the statin for 4.9 years. A reduction of 2.2 fewer coronary events for every 100 individuals who took pravastatin daily for 4.9 years ((74 ÷ 3295) x 100 = 2.2). This is the equivalent of 0.45 less coronary events per 100 patients taking the statin for a year (2.2 ÷ 4.9 = 0.45).

The PROSPER investigation[26].

This study investigated the effects of pravastatin on prevention of CHD in 50% of the participants who had no previous history of heart disease, and retardation of heart disease in the remainder who had had a previous history of heart disease. There were 5804 patients in the study. Placebo was given to 2913 individuals and pravastatin to 2891 (nature and mode of administration of placebo not specified in the report except in general terms). Follow-up was 3.2 years.

There were 356 coronary events in the group given a placebo and 292 in the group given pravastatin. Hence, pravastatin given for three years to elderly individuals reduced coronary events per 100 treated patients by 2.2 in that period ((64 ÷ 2891) X 100 = 2.2); 2.2 ÷ 3 = 0.7 fewer coronary events per 100 patients taking the statin per year. The statistical p value for the primary end-point (fatal and non-fatal coronary artery disease) was 0.006.

The MRC/BHF study[27].

In this study 10269 individuals got simvastatin while 10267 were given a placebo (nature and mode of administration of the placebo not specified in the report except in general terms).

Results.

All cause deaths.

All cause deaths in the group given statins : 1328

All cause deaths in the group given placebo 1507

Difference = 1507 - 1320 = 179.

Therefore, (179 ÷ 10269) x 100 = 1.7 fewer patient deaths per 100 individuals who took statins for five years; or 1.7 ÷ 5 = 0.34 fewer all cause deaths per 100 individuals taking statins per year.

First event non-fatal myocardial infarctions plus first event deaths from coronary artery disease.

First event coronary events in the group given statins for 5 years = 898.

First event coronary events in the group given placebo for 5 years = 1212

Difference = 1212 - 898 = 314.

Therefore (314 ÷ 10269) X 100 = 3 fewer coronary events per 100 individuals who took statins for five years; or 3 ÷ 5 = 0.6 fewer coronary events per 100 patients taking statins for a year. The p value was calculated as 0.0005.

These analyses show.

Calculation of numerical differences are needed for good therapeutic assessments when the numbers in each group are large, even if the p values are small.

Clinical significance can be marginal and of little consequence, even when p values are very low.

Evidence-based medicine and assessments of benefit versus cost plus risk ratios need evaluations of numerical differences between study and control groups, even when p values are very low.

Question 1.

Does statin administration reduce deaths from coronary atheroma?

The answer is a qualified yes. Statistically, the differences between control and treated groups are usually significant but the numerical differences in the incidence of "coronary events" are usually trivial and probably not of clinical importance.

The following are some possible reasons:

- **The numbers of individuals in each group.** It is a well known statistical fact that when large groups of individuals are the subjects of a study, the larger the numbers in each group the smaller the numerical difference needed to produce highly significant p value differences (e.g., $p=0.005$). Something is happening but only numerical calculations of the differences between groups will determine the clinical importance of the difference.
- **Was the correct question asked?** The statins were released for sale as drugs that could lower blood lipids. This they do effectively. The medical community assumed that lowering of blood lipids would decrease "coronary events". No studies on this question were done prior to the release and widespread use of statins by individuals with coronary heart disease.
- **What did the placebo do?** Many meta-analyses do not detail the composition of the placebo or how it was given. They are often described as "matched" or "comparable" placebos. Hence one possibility, perhaps a remote one, is that the increased mortality in placebo-treated groups was due to the placebo, perhaps by negating the benefit of some current medication or by some direct toxic effect. Inconvenient but real possibilities. The ALLHAT study is persuasive. In that study patients did not get any placebo. No difference in coronary events were seen in either the group given a statin and "usual care" and the other given "usual care" alone. In every statistical analysis it is always necessary to consider a null hypothesis or a conclusion opposite to the one expected, assumed and desired.
- **A decrease in coronary events is unlikely because of existing effective and optimal therapy.** Another possibility is that all individuals with coronary heart disease in the studies cited above were receiving optimal care prior to taking statins, albeit as different but equally effective clinical cocktails. If this were the case one cannot expect a numerically significant decrease in coronary events because of the addition of statins to the therapies. The patients are already receiving treatment that provides maximum benefit. An alternative explanation for the failure to show a reduction of coronary events in patients without symptoms is that these individuals did not need any therapy. Atheroma is common and usually begins at an early age. It is often symptomless. Many individuals are fat and have high blood lipid levels. In my search of the literature I have not found any publication that specifically details how many individuals with high blood lipid levels die of coronary artery disease.
- **Perhaps the statins were not given and could not be given in doses sufficiently large to produce a beneficial clinical effect.** The doses given sufficed to produce statistically significant differences, indicating that there was some effect. But, perhaps, they were not large enough to result in numerically significant differences. Manufacturers of statins correctly advise that pregnant women should not take them as the developing fetus needs abundant cholesterol. True. About 85% of body cholesterol comes from endogenous production. The gastrointestinal mucosa normally sheds cells at the rate of 100 million cells per day. New cells form by mitosis in the crypts. The entire gastrointestinal epithelium is replaced every 3-6 days. The skin has a comparable rate of cell death and replacement. The production of new cells requires a lot of cholesterol as this lipid is an essential component of cell walls. Taking statins does not seem to have resulted in specific gastrointestinal or epidermal dysfunctions. Why? Is it because statins are not given in doses sufficient to significantly reduce endogenous cholesterol synthesis. Additionally, cholesterol is an essential initial component in the biochemical sequences that synthesize the sex hormones, the corticosteroids and the mineralocorticoids. Statins, given in current dosage, do not result in demonstrable hormonal deficits. Presumably because

endogenous cholesterol production is not sufficiently depressed by statins in the doses given.

If the musings in the preceding paragraphs are correct the future outlook for the statins is bleak. It looks as if they cannot be given, and should not be given in doses sufficiently large to significantly reduce morbidity and mortality from coronary artery disease. Hazards and adverse effects do exist, even with current dosage. Rhabdomyolysis and renal failure are real risks. Already, one statin has been withdrawn from the market because of such complications However, the dangerous adverse effects currently identified are infrequent as long as the drugs are taken with the appropriate caveats provided by manufacturers.

Question 2.

Does taking statins reduce progression of coronary atheromas? This is a question that is difficult to answer for two reasons. The first is that it is probably excessively optimistic to expect any demonstrable retardation of atheromatous coronary artery disease in the short time the statin is given in the clinical trials.

The second is that many patients in these meta-analyses have had angiograms and when necessary, angioplasties, prior to the start of the trial. Others will have them during the course of the trial if episodes of coronary artery insufficiency develop. Persistent patencies of the stretched vessels may be due to statins but this cannot be proved if there are coexisting previous or recent angioplasties.

If one wishes to prove that statins reduce the incidence and progression of atheromas they must be given from an early age and for long periods. This is because there is much evidence that plaque formation begins at an early age. They have been demonstrated in individuals in their twenties. If these individuals later develop cardiac dysfunctions due to coronary artery atheromas they usually do so in their forties or later - probably some twenty years after the first appearance of atheromas and their subsequent slow growth. It is unrealistic to give medications with potential hazards to young people for such long periods just in order to prove a point.

Possible Phase 4 complications.

Phase 4 complications are unanticipated adverse effects occurring after a drug is in clinical use. They are said to be unpredictable but often are not. Is the final invoice for the Phase 4 complications of long-term statin administration in? The following is relevant to the above question. In the 1970s clofibrate was widely used to lower blood lipids. One trial[28] claimed that clofibrate reduced the risk of cardiovascular disease by 20%. Some years later the WHO[29], presumably to update their list of essential drugs, reviewed the effects of clofibrate. To everyone's amazement the study showed that patients taking clofibrate had an excess overall mortality of 47%. How much of this was the result of starving cells of the cholesterol that is essential for maintaining the integrity of cell wall membranes?

Are we going to see similar effects in individuals taking statins for long periods? All cells need cholesterol for maintenance of the structural integrities of their cell walls and 85% of body cholesterol derives from endogenous synthesis. Long-term statin administration could reduce this synthesis. Admittedly, the effects could be small with the small doses of statins currently given to patients. The effects of a long-term cumulative depression of endogenous cholesterol synthesis remain unknown. Neurons, and the cells of cardiac and skeletal muscle cannot mitose. The possible effects of small long-term depressions of endogenous cholesterol synthesis are disturbing. We already lose some 5000 neurons each day. They cannot be replaced by mitosis. Will exogenous food cholesterol suffice to provide enough cholesterol to maintain the integrities of the cell walls of the remaining cells? Perhaps not if endogenous synthesis is inhibited by statins and the diet is deficient in fats, as it frequently is in the elderly and the poor. Only future generations will be able to answer this question.

Concluding comments on statin usage.

An editorial in a recent issue of the Lancet[30] decried the decision of the UK Health Service to give the statin, simvastatin (Zocor: Merck Frosst) over-the-counter (OTC) status. Perhaps that Health Authority has come to conclusions comparable to those expressed here. I am told that in the UK the State Health Service pays for all prescribed drugs. Giving a drug OTC status absolves the State from requiring prescriptions for the drug and hence, of having to pay for it. The reclassification of simvastatin was recommended by the UK Committee on Safety of Medicines. The British Heart Foundation and the Royal Pharmaceutical Society of Great Britain support the reclassification[31]. Good. The State should not have to pay for medications of marginal clinical benefit when optimal treatment is already being provided. Once patients are informed of the putative benefits and real hazards they can buy or not, as they choose. The State is saved money. Unfortunately, the costs of hospitalizations and treatments of individuals with coronary artery dysfunctions will remain essentially unchanged. This regardless of whether or not individuals take or do not take statins in the doses currently recommended.

The principal difficulty for physicians is persuading patients that they do not need the statin. Vigorous, aggressive and ubiquitous advertising by manufacturers have convinced the public that death from coronary artery disease and raised blood lipids is inevitable if they do not take a statin. No matter. The drugs are not too hazardous. The individual physician can and should advise on pros and cons of statins before prescribing. If the patient still wants to take statins a refusal to prescribe is unreasonable as the desired medication has the sanction of general usage and acceptance and adverse effects are uncommon in the short-term.

This text on the difficulties of assessing the results of some meta-analyses was deliberately detailed and perhaps provocative. The object was to help those physicians who wish to assess the pros and cons of proposed therapies before prescribing the recommended therapies to their patients. Those who do not have the time or inclination to do such analyses have the real and appropriate option of waiting for assessment by peers and then complying with practices that have the imprimaturs of general acceptance and usage. Complying with general acceptance and usage is not always appropriate. The recent HERS study on hormone replacement therapy for menopausal symptoms is an example.

Computers versus the human brain for clinical decision-making

The subject of computers and their role in clinical decision-making is dealt with early in this book because of current interest in the topic.

What is a computer?

On December 23, 1947, after three years of research and the expenditure of more than a million dollars, three researchers at Bell Laboratories announced the development of a transistor. The three were John Bardeen, Walter Brattain and William Shockley and all three were jointly awarded the 1956 Nobel Prize in physics for their achievement. The transistor is a minute semiconductor used as a fast relay switch and/or, as an amplifier. It is comparable to the vacuum tube used in the original computers but is much superior in speed, performance, and reliability, and immeasurably smaller in size. The transistor, in combinations with other transistors and with conduits of electricity, is the basis of the modern computer and of the current electronic industrial revolution. Computers are machines that can receive, store, retrieve and manipulate information on the basis of commands given by software programs devised and written by humans.

Computers do not, cannot, and are not expected to think. They can only take orders from humans. The medium of direction is software written in any one of the languages that computers understand. Most programs in current use are based on logical linearity. Newer programs try to imitate the seemingly illogical way in which the network of 10-100 billion human neurons and their associated connections work. Magical properties are accredited to these so-called "neural networks". However, their development is in its infancy. Their postulated magical qualities could be only the result of bigger memories, better software, more transistors, superior technology, and greater speed.

The potential uses of computers in clinical medicine.

A computer receives and stores information much as the human brain does. Human brains receive information in a variety of forms (examples are pain, and tactile, visual, auditory, gustatory, and olfactory information). The information received is converted into electrical signals, integrated with other new or pre-existing electrical signals, and information that merits retention is stored in long-term memory. Later, when required, the electrical signals are accessed and converted to any one or more of different forms of cerebral activity such as imagery, motor action, sensory perception, mentation and decision-making.

The computer functions in an approximately similar way. Typically, information is typed in at a keyboard and converted into electrical signals that are transmitted along a cable into the computer. There it is converted into binary language. This language is a pattern of magnetic "bubbles". The "bubbles" are magnetic chunks that have polarizations opposite to that of the magnetic films in which they are embedded. The presence of a "bubble" denotes binary 1, its absence, binary 0.

The advantages and disadvantages of the use of computers in clinical medicine.

The computer is superior to the human brain for reception and storage of information. The capacity of human memory is limited and finite. Not so with the computer. Its capacity to receive and store information is only limited by the number of storage devices available. Available floppy discs can each store about 1.5 million characters, the equivalent of about 225 pages of text. CD-ROMs can each store more than 600 million characters (a million characters is roughly equal to 150 pages of a standard textbook).

The computer's ability to record and retrieve with fidelity is far superior to that of the human brain and computers work much faster. The human brain accesses memory at hundreds of milliseconds per item while a computer can access the same information in fractions of milliseconds. The available space for storage in a computer is only limited by the megabytes of disc space that can be added and incorporated. Theoretically, it is infinite. The anatomy of the brain determines its capacity. It is finite but not small because of the large numbers of neurons and synapses it contains.

The computer's role in medicine?

To answer the question it is necessary to detail some of the advantages and some of the disadvantages of using computers in clinical medicine.

The advantages of computer use in clinical decision-making.

Storage. Computer technology allows accurate storage of large amounts of information.

Recall. The computer can recall whatever is needed with equal accuracy.

Manipulation of information. Manipulation of stored information is easy but only possible on the basis of instructions it receives from software created by humans.

Clinical applications.

Available software can analyze ECG data, evaluate laboratory results, and function as teaching aids. Those used as teaching aids are particularly useful when pictorial features are important, e.g., in histopathology. The original IntelliPath system was a laser videodisc with some thousands of pictures of histologic microphotography[32] that were valuable teaching and reference aids for budding and practicing pathologists. Programs that tried to deal with clinical problems were less successful[33,34,35]. The references are to some original programs. Current computer programs for use in clinical medicine are more sophisticated and versatile. However, few that are currently available can approach the ability of a qualified physician to assess clinical problems. Computers can provide flow charts, decision trees and other aids to clinical decision-making. They can also provide a differential diagnosis of a clinical problem when given the symptoms, signs and results of ancillary investigations. At present there are few situations where a competent physician cannot perform equally well and usually better.

What are the reasons for the current inability of computer programs to replace competent physicians?

First results from the inherent unpredictables and uncertainties of clinical medicine. These are detailed in Chapter 16. Programs could probably be devised to respond to the many permutations and combinations that are possible just as programs for playing chess can think thousands of moves ahead. Programs currently available are not as sophisticated and probably never will be. Chess is a single game with set rules. Clinical medicine consists of hundreds of diseases with rules that are flexible and not set in stone.

Second and equally important is the inability of current programs to recognize the gestural and prosodic variations of the interactions between physician and patient. Gestural and prosodic language are extensively discussed in Chapter 3, pages 73-74. For now it suffices to write that they are important elements in making clinical assessments and decisions.

The disadvantages of using computers to make clinical decisions.

There are important disadvantages to the use of computers for making clinical decisions. The **first** mentioned below is probably resolvable by technology. One wonders if **the other** can be resolved.

Inconvenience. The use of computer technology requires availability of a computer, a monitor screen and a keyboard. This may not be convenient in clinical situations, though miniaturizations of these needs by wireless technology will progressively decrease this inconvenience.

Adherence to custom and usage. However, there is one other problem that is possibly greater and is the result of custom and usage. Present generations are accustomed from childhood to use books, to flip to an index to find what is needed, to rapidly scan pages for needed information, and to move rapidly between pages that may be separated by hundreds of other pages. Wireless information technology miniaturizations have the potentials to provide similar rapid access to information. It is possible that another generation will be brought up to use them. I doubt that this generation will ever show such a preference unless the methods of schooling change in radical ways.

The superiority of the human brain for reasoning and deciding.

The nerve impulse

The topics of nerve impulse initiation and transmission should be more correctly described in the chapter on the central nervous system. They are detailed here for two reasons:

First, because an intelligent comparison of the capabilities of the human brain versus the computer is not possible without a description of cerebral neural capabilities. The text includes the requisites for normal neural activity and hypothesizes that an almost infinite numbers of neural transmission patterns are possible.

Second, because the nerve impulse is a fundamental component of biology. Without the nerve impulse the control of systems becomes impossible. Chaos and eventual death is inevitable unless "life" is maintained by artificial technology.

The nerve impulse.

The nerve impulse is the basic unit for coding of biological information and commands. Without the nerve impulse the assessments and judgments of clinical medicine would be impossible. Currently available software does not provide the means for computers to execute these judgments and assessments.

The nerve impulse is an all-or-none discharge and therefore comparable to 1 in the binary code; the absence of a nerve impulse is the equivalent of a 0. Once the mode of generation and transmission of the nerve impulse is described it will be possible to understand why almost infinite patterns of nerve discharges are possible. The consequences of this diversity are transmission of equally numerous and diverse items of information, interaction and command. These compensate for the finite capacity of the brain and its slowness, relative to the computer, in accessing information.

The synapse.

The synapse is the functional unit of CNS activity. The nerve impulse is transmitted along an axon. As it nears its target the axon branches into many terminals. The axon terminals of a single axon can activate many nerve cells because of terminal axon branching. As a corollary there is frequent convergence on a single neuron of nerve impulses from many sources - (the principle of convergence and divergence[38]). The synapse is a small space located between the termination of an axon terminal and its target. When transmitting a nerve impulse the axon terminal discharges a chemical neurotransmitter into this space. After it performs its delegated function the neurotransmitter is rapidly metabolized or returned to the axon terminal. This is a requisite for precise action. In situ persistence of the neurotransmitter would interfere with the effects of subsequent nerve impulses and result in chaos.

The numbers of synapses in the nervous system are estimated to be between 10^{11} to 10^{15}. Estimates of the numbers of neurons in the cerebrum vary from a low of 10 billion (10^{10}) to a high of two hundred billion neurons (2×10^{11}). The actual figure is probably somewhere in between these two extremes. Information comes to the neuron by many synaptic communications between its body and its dendrites, with the dendrites, somas and axon terminals of other neurons.

An amazing number of axon terminals and dendrites end at synapses on the surfaces of many neurons. Eccles estimated that each pyramidal cell receives some 10,000 synapses[39]. Ito has calculated that many of the cerebellar Purkinje cells each communicate with other neurons at more than 100,000 synapses[40]. On the basis of these estimates there must be some 10^{11} to 10^{15} synapses in the CNS. The many terminals at the end of each axon terminal and the many synaptic communications between neurons ensure wide distribution of the information presented by axon terminals. One estimate is that at any one time a single neuron can provide information to some 10,000 others by relays of information along different synaptic communications.

Neurotransmitters.

There are two types of neurotransmitters; those that excite and those that inhibit.

Intracerebral and spinal cord neurotransmitters include dopamine, serotonin, norepinephrine, acetylcholine, and the amino acids, L-glutamate and L-aspartate. The inhibitors include gamma-aminobutyric acid (GABA) and the amino acid glycine.

Outside the brain the principal neurotransmitters are acetylcholine and norepinephrine. **Acetylcholine** is the neurotransmitter acting at neuromuscular junctions, at the preganglionic synapses of sympathetic and parasympathetic nervous systems, and at the post-ganglionic terminals of the parasympathetic system.

Norepinephrine is the neurotransmitter for post-ganglionic sympathetic terminals. Exceptions are sweat glands and muscle blood vessels where the sympathetic neurotransmitter at axon terminals is acetylcholine.

The receptors.

The principal receptors for providing the CNS with information about the external environment are the eyes, the ears, olfactory smell receptors, the taste buds, the vestibular apparatus, the receptors that respond to changes in position, and the cutaneous receptors that record pain, touch and changes in surface pressure and temperature.

The principal receptors for providing the CNS with information about the internal environment are receptors that record pain in the abdominal viscera, and in muscles, joints and ligaments. Other receptors receiving information about the internal environment are baroreceptors, chemoreceptors and osmoreceptors that record changes in pH, pO_2, pCO_2, and the osmotic pressures of body fluids. In addition, information about the internal environment can be transmitted to the CNS by afferent somatic (e.g., to and from the respiratory muscles) and autonomic nerves without initial recording by receptors. The brain also has receptors that respond to local changes in pH. Little information about the internal environment is consciously felt or recognized. The one exception is visceral and musculoskeletal pain. Usually, afferent information from and efferent commands to structures in the internal environment are mediated by the afferent and efferent limbs of automatic long arm positive and negative feedback reflexes centered on brain stem foci.

The generation and transmission of nerve impulses.

A seminal publication in 1952 by Hodgkin and Huxley[36] showed how nerve impulses were generated and transmitted. They both received Nobel Prizes to honor their findings. Hodgkin's later monograph[37] details subsequent studies.

Intracellular negativity with respect to its exterior is the basis for generation and transmission of nerve impulses. When the outer and inner surfaces of a membrane are separated by different concentrations of electrically charged particles an electrical potential difference develops between the two surfaces. This is characteristic of membranes that surround cells because the intracellular concentrations of their positively charged Na^+ and K^+ ions are different from the concentrations of these ions in the extracellular fluids. These concentration differences result from the activity of a membrane pump system known as the sodium-potassium pump. The pump uses an enzyme, $Na^+\backslash K^+$-activated adenosine triphosphatase to extract high energy phosphate bond energy (~P) from cell membrane ATP. It uses this energy to extrude $3Na^+$ from the cell for every $2K^+$ that are retained. The result is a cell interior that is negatively charged with respect to its exterior. The difference is approximately -50mV to -70mV and this decrease in intracellular negativity provides the basis for initiation and propagation of nerve impulses.

The sodium-potassium pump uses a large part of the biologically usable energy produced by aerobic oxidation within cells. One estimate is that as much as 30% of this energy is used by the sodium pumps of cell membranes; in muscle and nerve estimates have been as high as 60-70%. When sufficient energy usable for biological reactions is unavailable the pump cannot be maintained, nerve impulses cannot be generated and unless energy deficits are rectified, death is imminent.

The cell membrane of the neuron also has sodium and potassium ion channels, both normally closed by charged "gating particles". It is believed that in response to changes in potential differences ("gating voltages") across neural membranes, the configurations of the gating particles change to allow passive ion fluxes along concentration gradients. Neurotransmitters that stimulate (those that produce excitatory post-synaptic potentials or EPSPs for short) open the sodium channels. Na^+ flows in and the internal surface of the cell membrane becomes less negative. Neurotransmitters that inhibit (the inhibitory post-synaptic potentials or IPSPs for short) open the potassium channels and potassium moves out of the neuron, thus increasing intracellular negativity. There is usually some leak of Na^+ ions through these channels into the cell. **An important function of the sodium pump is extrusion of excess intracellular $Na^+$and to thus maintain intracellular negativity.**

The change produced by an EPSP or IPSP at a single postsynaptic locus is usually surprisingly small - about 1mV or less[41]. A change of approximately +25mV at the axon hillock is needed before the neuron can generate an action potential. When this point is reached an axon potential is initiated and generates a nerve impulse which has a positive charge with respect to the axon origin. Current which is the nerve impulse, begins to flow along the axon from positive to negative points as each point successively becomes positive with respect to the next; dissimilar electric charges attract each other while similar charges repel.

The action potential can initiate another action potential in a post-synaptic neuron or initiate contraction, via a neurotransmitter, when it terminates on an endorgan in striated, smooth or cardiac muscle. Alternatively, it can induce changes in glandular secretion, also via a neurotransmitter, when it terminates on a receptor in a gland. When peripheral receptors of information are stimulated, basically similar processes transmit information along afferent nerves to the central nervous system. The above has two consequences:

First, the intervals between discharges vary as the algebraic sum of EPSPs and IPSPs acting on the neuron via thousands of synapses. At times this algebraic sum will exceed the +25mv change needed at the axon hillock for generation of a nerve impulse. At other times it might not and this will result in irregularities of transmission.

Second, variations in rates and regularities of transmission can result from the different and often rapid speeds at which nerve discharges can travel. They range from 120m/sec in the Aα motor activity and proprioception fibers to 1m/sec in the slow C fibers of the postganglionic sympathetic fibers and some fibers in the dorsal roots. Small nerves can transmit 100 nerve impulses/sec. Neurons in the central nervous system can fire at 500-1000 times per second. Neurons of interneuron systems can exceed even these fast rates. For example, the discharge rates of neurons in the Renshaw interneuron system can exceed 1500 per second.

The possibility of infinite variations in the patterns of neural discharges.

If one views the neural transfer of information as a binary number system with 1 denoting the transmission of a nerve impulse (the nerve impulse is an all-or-none phenomenon) and 0 by none, an almost infinite numbers of neural discharge patterns of information are possible, depending on the algebraic sum of the EPSPs and IPSPs of the neural impulses reaching the neuron. The patterns of neuronal discharges could be almost infinite because of the many synapses of each neuron. At times the algebraic sum of EPSPs and IPSPs might exceed the +25mv change needed to transmit a nerve impulse at other times it might not. The result would be irregularities of transmission. Additional variables could result from the rates of nerve transfer. As previously detailed, small nerves have the ability to transmit 100 nerve impulses/sec. Neurons in the central nervous system can fire at 500-1000 times per second. In the Renshaw cell interneuron system discharge rates can exceed 1500 per second. This system modulates activity at the motor neuron.

Thus, it is theoretically possible for hundreds of thousands and perhaps millions of items to be stored in long term memory, each with a distinctive binary number. This could provide a neurological basis for an understanding of the mechanisms underlying perception, recognition, remembering and decision-making. Limitations of space and the objectives of this book preclude any further discussion and hypothesizing about these difficult subjects.

Computers versus the human brain.

Computers are the vehicles of choice for storage and recall of information. The brain can reason, remember, recall, command and make judgments and assessments that the computer cannot until software is available to make such judgments and assessments. The nerve impulse moves much more slowly than the electric discharge of a computer but it compensates by the infinitely different patterns of information and commands that it can transmit, at least in theory. In addition, unlike the computer it can decide what needs retention in long-term memory.

Visual recognition is an example of one aspect of brain superiority. When an object is seen the retina transmits almost a million different parallel signals[42]. They pass along the optic nerve and arrive at the lateral geniculate body, then the cortical optic cortex and finally at the tempero-parietal heteromodal association area. Here, complex processes integrate the information with stored multimodal information (sensory, motor, autonomic and limbic) and recognize it for what it is.

It takes about 500msec for a person to respond in a visual recognition test and this represents no more than about 100 synaptic stops between input and output[43]. We know little about how the brain accomplishes these seemingly impossible tasks, only that it does achieve the desired objective or objectives with facility and accuracy. The difficulties of developing software to accomplish similar tasks is well known. Even development of software to recognize human faces remains a challenge!

The human brain has no superior for performing tasks specific to humans.

Admittedly, unlike a computer, the capacity of the brain is limited by its anatomy. The large capacity of the computer results from a theoretically infinite amount of space (by additions of hardware) to do what humans request: storage, recall and manipulations based on orders given by software. In these respects the computer is superior to the brain but it is inferior for assessments, recognitions and commands.

I am aware that there are current software chess programs that can defeat grandmasters. The programs calculate all options and possibilities, often many million times into the future. This is a major undertaking but it involves a single activity, chess, that has set and rigid unchanging rules.

Medicine is much more complicated. The computer is an invaluable tool for storing, receiving and manipulating information on the basis of commands given by software. By contrast, the human brain has, and must have considerable internal plasticity to assess, to change and to interact with sick humans.

Will any computer software ever be able to simulate these attributes of the human brain? Is it really necessary to try creating such programs? Perhaps not. The computer performs superbly at what it is required to do. A well trained and competent physician usually performs equally well at whatever is required for the efficient practice of clinical medicine. It is not necessary to require a computer to imitate cerebral function. Certainly, the brain will never be able to imitate the capabilities of a computer. Leave the two worlds to complement each other. The practice of clinical medicine is not a science but an art with inherent uncertainties and unpredictables, and rules and results that continually change. All who ply this trade have their own unique ways of performing. Current computer programs do not have the plasticity to imitate these capabilities.

The computer does have one additional important attribute. This has appeared since the development of the **Internet**. The Internet can store incredible amounts of information. When the physician needs information on any topic or author, access is easily obtained through one or more pages of the Internet. There is one caveat. The information is not always sufficiently comprehensive or accurate. Often reference to other sites are needed to confirm the correctness, and increase the amount of information received after the first search.

Alternative medicine.

Alternatives and supplements to conventional medicine are numerous. They include chiropratic medicine, homeopathy, naturopathic and herbal medicine, acupuncture and a variety of other disciplines. They seem to satisfy the needs of many patients. I am not able to comment on the pros and cons of these therapies because little literature is available on scientifically verified results. Also, my personal experience of these therapies is non-existent. Before scoffing it is always necessary to remember that many medications used in the practice of medicine were originally derived from plants. Perhaps the best example is a drug widely used in cardiology - digoxin. It is a drug originally derived from a plant, the foxglove, and first used by William Withering[11] for cardiac disease in the late 18th. century and now commonly used for cardiac dysfunctions. Many other drugs were originally derived from the environment. Perhaps the one most commonly used is acetylsalicylic acid (commonly known as aspirin). It originated from the barks of willow trees.

Conclusion.

This conclude an introductory chapter to the processes and problems of clinical decision-making. It introduces some basics. More of these basics of clinical decision-making follow in the next four chapters, Chapters 2, 3, 4 and 5.

References for Chapter 1.

1. Withington, E.T. Medical History, London. Blakiston, 1894.
2. Garrison, F.H. An introduction to the history of medicine. Philadelphia. W.B. Saunders, 1914.
3. The Nazi doctors and the Nuremberg code: human rights in human experimentation. Annas, G.J., and Grondin, M.A. (eds.). New York. Oxford University Press, 1992.
4. Dictionary of medical ethics. Duncan, A.S., Dunstan, G.R., et al. (Eds.) The Nuremberg Code, 1947. London. Longman and Todd, 1981.
5. World Medical Association Declaration of Helsinki. JAMA 1997; 277:925.
6. Annas, G.J. The changing landscape of human experimentation: Nuremberg, Helsinki, and beyond. Health Matrix 1992; 2:119.
7. Sinclair, W.J. In: Semmelweiss - his life and his doctrine. Manchester. University Press, 1909.
8. Hempel, C.G. Philosophy of natural science. Englewoods Cliff, N.J. Prentice-Hall, 1966.
9. Edward Jenner. An inquiry into the Causes and Effects of the Variola Vaccinae. London. 1978.
10. Underwood, E.A. Edward Jenner: The Man and His Work. Brit. Med. J. 1949; 1:881.
11. An account of the foxglove and some of its medical uses: with practical remarks on dropsy and other diseases. London. G.G.J. and J.Robinson, 1785.
12. Marshall, B.J., & Warren, J.R. Unidentified curved bacilli in the stomach of patients with gastritis and peptic ulceration. Lancet 1984; i:1311.
13. Lykoudis, J. The truth about gastric and duodenal ulcer. Athens, Greece. 1966.
14. Rigas, B., Feretis, F. et al. John Lykoudis: an unappreciated discoverer of the cause and treatment of peptic ulcer disease. Lancet 1999; 354:1634.
15. Pappworth, M.H. Human guinea pigs: experimentation on man. London. Routledge and Kegan, 1967.
16. Jones, J.H. Bad Blood: The Tuskegee Syphilis Experiment. New York. Free Press, 1993.
17. Hammonds, E.M. "Your silence will not protect you: Nurse Eunice Rivers and the Tuskegee Syphilis Study". In: Ed. E,C, White: The Black Women's Health Book: Speaking for Ourselves. Seattle. Seal Press, 1993.
18. World Medical Association. Declaration of Tokyo on guidelines for medical doctors concerning torture and other cruel, inhuman or degrading treatment or punishment in relation to detention and imprisonment. Tokyo, 29th. World Medical Assembly, 1975. I could only access the details on the Internet World Medical Association page.
19. Peto, R. Why do we need systematic overviews of randomized trials? Stat. Med. 1967; 6:223.
20. Pocock, S.J. & Thompson, S.G. The role of meta-analyses in clinical and epidemiological research. In: Marmot, M. & Elliott, P. (Eds.): Coronary heart disease epidemiology: from etiology to public health. Oxford. Oxford University Press, 1991.
21. Raju, T.N.K. The Nobel Chronicles. Lancet 1999; 353:1536.
22. The ALLHAT Officers and Coordinators for the ALLHAT Collaborative Research Group. Major outcomes in moderately hyper-cholesterolemic, hypertensive patients randomized to pravastatin vs usual care. JAMA 2002; 288:2998.
23. Sever, P.S., Dahlöf, B. et al. Prevention of coronary and stroke events with atorvastatin in hypertensive patients who have average or lower-than average cholesterol concentrations in the Anglo-Scandinavian Cardiac Outcomes Trial— Lipid Lowering Arm

(ASCOT-LLA): a multicentre randomized controlled trial. Lancet 2003; 361:1149.

24. What are the odds at Ascot today? Lindholm, L.H. & Samuelsson, O. http://image.the lancet.com/extras/03cmt57web.pdf.

25. Prevention of coronary heart disease with pravastatin in men with hypercholesterolemia. Shepherd, J. Cobbe, S.M., et al. NEJM 1995; 333:1301.

26. Shepherd, J., Blauw, G.J., et al. Prospective study of pravastatin in the elderly at risk of vascular disease (PROSPER): a randomized control trial. Lancet 2002; 360:1623.

27. Heart Protection Study Collaborative Group - MRC/BHF. Heart protection study of cholesterol lowering with simvastatin in 20,536 high risk individuals: a randomized placebo-controlled trial. Lancet 2002; 7:360.

28. Committee of principal investigators. A cooperative trial in the primary prevention of ischemic heart disease using clofibrate. Brit. Heart J. 1978; 40:1069.

29. Oliver, M.F., Heady, J.A. et al. for the committee of principal investigators: WHO cooperative trial on primary prevention of ischemic heart disease with clofibrate to lower serum cholesterol: final mortality follow-up. Lancet 1984; 2:600.

30. OTC statins. A bad decision for public health. Lancet 2004; 363:1659.

31. Meek, C. UK MDs oppose selling statins without prescription. CMAJ 2004; 171(1):25.

32. Nathwani, B.M., Heckerman, D.E. et al. Integrated expert systems and videodisc in surgical pathology. Hum. Path. 1990; 21:11.

33. Weed, L. The computer as a new basis for analytic clinical practice: coupling individual problems with medical knowledge. Mount Sinai J. Med. 1985; 52:94.

34. Miller, R., McNeil, M. et al. The INTERNIST/QMR project - status report. West. J. Med. 1986; 145:816.

35. Bankowitz, R., McNeil, M. et al. A computer-assisted medical diagnostic consultation service. Ann. Inter. Med. 1989; 110:824.

36. Hodgkin, A & Huxley, A. A quantitative description of membrane current and its application to conductions and excitation in nerve. J. Physiol. (London) 1952; 117:500.

37. Hodgkin, A.L. Conduction of the Nervous Impulse. Springfield, Ill. Thomas, 1964.

38. Sherrington, C.S. The Integrative Action of the Nervous System. New Haven. Yale University Press, 1906.

39. Eccles, J.C. Evolution of the brain: Creation of the self. London & New York. Routledge, 1989, p.150.

40. Ito, M. The Cerebellum and Neural Control. New York. Raven press, 1984.

41. Pansky, B., Allen, D.J. et al. Review of Neuroscience. New York. Macmillan Publishing Co., 1988.

42. Churchland, P.S. Neurophilosophy: Toward a Unified Understanding of the Mind\Brain. Boston, Mass. The MIT Press, 1986.

43. Churchland, P.S. Neurophilosophy. Cambridge, Mass. & London, England. MIT Press, 1986.

2

Clinical Decision-Making: Some Basics
2. Reasoning and Remembering

Table of Contents

Memory - its importance for reasoning and remembering.

Reasoning and remembering relies on information stored in memory. Many of the references in this chapter are to publications in the 1970-1990 period and some, such as those by Lashley, go back to the 1920s. This choice is deliberate. The object is to give appropriate credit to the original author or authors. Each year dozens of new papers are published on memory and the mechanisms of decision-making. Few unequivocally define new areas of the brain which are responsible for memory storage and use. Investigations of these topics are difficult. Ethical considerations exclude studies by experimental ablations of human cerebral tissue. Information on human brain function is only obtainable from correlations between clinical findings and pathological lesions or surgical ablations. Alternatively from assumptions and hypotheses based on experimental psychology. The assumptions and hypotheses of experimental psychology have the flaws inherent to all such exercises.

Pathology and surgical excisions often define specific areas of brain function. They never exclude the possibility that it is not the pathology or ablation that defines the area but instead, the interruption of tracts passing by on their ways to other areas of the brain.

There are some exceptions. One is the postoperative studies on H.M., a patient who had a surgical bilateral hippocampectomy many years ago. His neurological and psychological deficits have been extensively studied over many years, in particular by Milner who has reviewed many of the findings in a recent revue article[37]. Over the years she has extensively studied and written on the psychological consequences of H.M.'s hippocampectomy. The other is the clinical deficits of memory and behavior that follow prefrontal lobotomies. They are detailed later in this chapter. Disputes continue on how memory is stored, the location of the memory engrams, and the signals that select specific memory composites for use. Many of the references cited in this chapter are old because they refer to papers by originators of ideas. All but a few are accessible in most medical school libraries, albeit, at times, only by microfiche search.

Roland and Friberg used injections of radioactive xenon to locate the areas where memory is stored (J. Neurophysiol. 1985; 53:1219). They concluded that small memory banks are squeezed in wherever there is space in the brain. Presumably, many neural communications between memory banks provide the interactions needed for intelligent and selective retrieval and use of stored material. This model correlates well with the clinical features of progressive dementias such as the multi-infarct dysfunctions, Alzheimer's disease and other degenerative cerebral disorders. Repeated studies with radioactive materials are not possible as they have inherent dangers, some bordering on the unethical.

At present there is little one can add to the invocations of St. Augustine, as recorded in his "Confessions". The following is a quotation from J.G. Pilkington's[1] excellent translation:

> "Great is this power of memory, exceeding great, O my God - an inner chamber large and boundless! Who has plumbed the depths thereof? Yet it is a power of mine, and appertains to my nature; nor do I myself grasp all that I am."

Recent discoveries on long-term synaptic potentiation and inhibition could provide the basis for learning and remembering. These topics are detailed in a later chapter that summarizes the role of the central nervous system in biology. Knowledge about the precise physiological mechanisms for remembering and reasoning may not be known but all know what the brain can do. Use this knowledge as does one who comfortably uses and knows what a computer can do but not how it functions.

Reasoning defined.

Reasoning resolves problems. It can also establish principles and concepts. The first step in reasoning is collection of all relevant information. The next is analysis of the collected information and then the formulation of a conclusion. The conclusion could be an uncertainty, a conviction or a decision. Avoid absurd but logical conclusions, by liberally peppering reasoned decisions with common sense and objective thinking. Faulty conclusions often result from emotional, unobjective, and illogical inputs. These are common but usually unimportant in the ordinary events of daily living. In clinical medicine they can have undesirable and occasionally fatal consequences.

Correct decisions often need modifications because of circumstances. The most frequent considerations are availability, the ability to afford and the acceptance of suggested therapy. Many other considerations often intrude. Examples are moral and cultural values, perceptions of right and wrong, family ties, religious and cultural beliefs, and many other factors, some tangible, others not. Equally important are changes in the aggressiveness of the disease and/or unacceptable or other adverse responses to drugs.

Information needed for reasoning and deciding is information stored in long-term memory in either one of two basic forms. Psychologists term them **episodic and semantic memory**, a classification originally proposed by Tulving[2]. Subsequently, psychologists have proposed other classifications but the simple Tulving classification suffices for the needs of the average clinician. Tulving has provided two excellent reviews of his current views and the current status of memory classifications[3,4].

Recently a third type of memory is postulated, **i.e., implicit memory,** the memory of skills performed automatically; intelligent and grammatically correct speech, bicycle riding, walking, and swimming are examples. Implicit memory is probably only a synonym for preprogrammed movements.

In Tulving's classification **semantic memory** is the memory of factual information. For example, words and their definitions, numbers and calculations, the facts of history, geography, anatomy, physiology, pharmacology and the other disciplines of clinical medicine, and hundreds of other comparable items. Semantic memory contains verified facts. The difference between **semantic** and **episodic** memory is that information in the former is precise and previously verified for correctness. The information in episodic memory is probably correct but unverified. The word **"memory"** is used in this text to describe all aspects of memory. Division into episodic and semantic components is only made where essential to convey a specific meaning. Thus, a reference to factual information stored in semantic memory denotes reference to precise and correct information of confirmed validity. A reference to information in episodic memory does not denote this type of precision or validity but merely a fuzzy probability of correctness.

Episodic memory is the memory of experiences. Each is a multimodal sensory, motor, autonomic and intellectual collection of information about one or more comparable clinical presentations. As detailed above, each includes causes and their consequences, related mnemonics for remembering, protocols for investigations, available therapies, possible adverse drug reactions and a variety of other factors and the times and situations when they occurred. Composites are often linked and used in association with other composites that might contain information not contained in the original. Composites represent information acquired by experience. For this reason the phrase **"experience composite"** and **"memory composite"** are used interchangeably in this book.

A single composite could contain material spanning years, as for example the events that occur from the time of presentation to the time of death of an individual with a chronic and eventually fatal disease. Examples are patients with multiple sclerosis, cystic fibrosis or malignant disease with many regressions, recurrences and treatments over a period of many years.

Recall of composites in episodic memory is often one dimensional, pictorial, and mediated by visual imagery. This view is consistent with the extensive literature on imagery and with observations that suggest that thinking in images is a reality that is not different from thinking in language[5]. The use of episodic memory is not confined to the practice of clinical medicine. More common is its use for deciding on problems of daily life. and family interactions.

Heuristic reasoning.

What is heuristic reasoning?

Heuristic reasoning is problem solving by comparison of a current problem with memories of previous comparable problems and their resolutions. Heuristic reasoning circumvents and avoids information related to other topics. The alternative is sequential linear or parallel searches through vast amounts of information. Both are lengthy and time-consuming.

The units of heuristic reasoning are memory composites. Long term memory contains hundreds if not thousands of these composites. The numbers increase as experience increases. Each composite contains many items; previous decisions, inappropriate and appropriate therapies, their sequelae, expectations of adverse effects and other complications, and prognosis. The composite can also contain mnemonics and protocols for investigating and treating, and information about events extending back over long periods. Examples are the clinical courses of individuals with chronic lung disease or those with malignant disease who have recurrent remissions and recurrences.

Heuristic reasoning is an empirical process. Humans use it to decide on problems with complexities that are beyond the capacity of the human brain to resolve in a reasonable time, or to resolve with certainty. We use heuristic logic for resolution of almost all problems of day-to-day living and also for the special needs of work. Little of the subsequent literature adds to a summary by Dehn and Schank in a book published in the 1980s[6]. The following is a quotation from their text:

> " ...... most people use heuristics for solving most everyday problems. The vast majority of decisions we make each hour are made heuristically, and even when a problem allowing algorithmic solution arises, it is usually surrounded by a great many more problems requiring heuristic solutions."

and later,

> "Realizing that virtually all intelligent problem solving (formal and informal) is done heuristically is

essential to any realistic approach to intelligence."

In clinical medicine the interaction between patient and physician is the most important factor in arriving at a heuristic decision. If the information collected is not accurate nor comprehensive the conclusion is biased to inaccuracy.

Heuristic reasoning does not guarantee a correct answer. It provides reasonable and probable suggestions but it is not infallible. The clinical assessment is faster than one reached by conventional structured and linear logic. When used for the problems of daily living a correct and accurate answer is often unimportant. One may enter a store to purchase an apple. If desired one can use algorithms to compare prices in different stores. The decision on whether to buy the apple is made by informal and unreliable heuristic decisions. The decision may or may not be the best but this does not matter as the choice of which apple to buy is of little importance. An apple is an apple. Some like one variety, others another.

In clinical medicine an incorrect heuristic decision can harm. A decision reached by rapid heuristic reasoning always requires confirmation from precise and verified factual information stored in semantic memory. This information is rapidly accessed by cues which are probably generated by one or more components in the selected memory composite or composites. These cues circumvent and avoid the large amounts information related to other topics. If semantic memory has not stored the needed information books, journals, CD-ROMs, colleagues and specialists should be consulted. Regardless of how it is done, the heuristic assessment always needs confirmation by previously verified facts.

An example of the value of heuristics is the recognition of visual information within a multimodal sensory frame. When an object is seen the retina transmits almost a million different parallel signals[7] along the optic nerve. They reach the lateral geniculate body and then the cortical optic cortex. Finally they arrive at Wernicke's area for integration with other multimodal information and are eventually recognized within a frame of pre-existing knowledge about visual and other modalities; sensory, motor, autonomic and limbic. It takes about 500msec for a person to respond in a visual recognition test and this represents no more than about 100 synaptic stops between input and output. In a linear processing program 100 steps is not enough, especially as coordinated vestibular and motor activities are also required; the vestibulo-ocular reflexes that track objects as the head moves. It is possible that visual information is so rapidly recognized because of parallel processings and heuristic comparisons with items previously seen and stored in memory. This could provide almost instantaneous information on quality, color, and a variety of the other attributes seen. Another possibility is that it results from long-term postsynaptic potentiations and depressions of neural paths (see Chapter 6 which details the normal physiology and the dysfunctions of the central nervous system).

Available information changes or increases from time to time. This information is stored in semantic memory and used, as needed, for confirmation or rejection of a heuristic decision. The memory composite incorporates this new information as well as its consequences when used in clinical medicine. The memory composite also changes as the physician acquires more experience. The resolution of a single problem could require the use of information stored in many memory composites.

Polya's postulates on heuristic reasoning.

Interest in heuristic reasoning began with the work of George Polya in the 1940s. He published his work on heuristic reasoning in 1945. The title of the book was "How to solve it"[8]. He defined heuristics as:

> "reasoning not regarded as final and strict but as provisional and plausible only, whose purpose is to discover the solution of the present problem."

A summary of Polya's postulates on heuristic reasoning.

They are slightly modified by me for use in clinical decision-making:

- Have you seen the problem before? (In other words: "Have you previously seen a patient with similar signs, symptoms and history?" - my addendum).
- Do you know a related problem?

- Try to think of a familiar problem having the same or similar unknown.
- Can you restate the problem (e.g., as in the equation below)?
- Could you think of a comparable problem?
- Can you solve a part of the problem and drop the rest without detriment?
- Check every step as you carry out the plan.
- Review everything as you proceed (the iterative loop to be later described is ideal for this purpose). If the result or method used can resolve other comparable problems, store it in memory.
- Heuristic reasoning is not infallible. Always verify the heuristic decision by accessing relevant factual information stored in semantic memory.

Example.

Baron[9] has posed the following difficult equation for solution and its solution helps to understand how information in semantic memory and heuristics can complement each other for problem-solving. It helps that the formula for solving quadratic equations had been previously determined by medieval Arab mathematicians. The question posed was **what values of x satisfy the equation: $x^4 - 13x^2 + 36 = 0$?**

Information in semantic memory is used first and then heuristic analysis.

By letting $y = x^2$ the equation is converted to a simple quadratic equation: $ay^2 - by + c = 0$, where $a=1$, $b=13$ and $c=36$. Solution of the equation requires determination of y for the quadratic equation $1y^2 - 13y + 36 = 0$; the original equation is solved by determining y which is equal to x^2 and then of x which is the square root of x^2. This shows how a seemingly difficult problem can be converted to a well-known and readily soluble one,

$$y\ (y = x^2) = \frac{-b \pm ((b^2 - 4ac)\ ^\wedge 0.5)}{2a}$$

i.e., a simple quadratic equation. The new generalization regarding solutions of equations of the type $ax^4 \pm bx^2 \pm c = 0$ can now be stored in memory as one to be readily recalled and used when a comparable problem is encountered in the future.

Previously stored generalizations are used for the exact calculation of x. They depend on the discriminant (D) which is $b^2 - 4ac$. If D is greater than 0 there are two solutions to the equation. If D = 0 there is only one solution and if D is less than 0 there is no solution. In this instance the equation $x^4 - 13x^2 + 36 = 0$ has a D value greater than 0 and the equation is satisfied by two values: either x=2 or x=3.

At this point a heuristic decision is needed; does one choose 2 or 3 as the appropriate value for x?

Some caveats about heuristic reasoning.

A voluminous literature on heuristic reasoning has accumulated over the last twenty years. Not much except unproved hypotheses add to two early publications[10,11] and, given the context of this monograph, these suffice to provide enough information for current needs. There are at least two important caveats about heuristic reasoning and decision-making:

First. To identify any information that is incompatible with the clinical assessment.

All analyses and assessments made by heuristic reasoning need confirmation by recourse to factual knowledge stored in semantic memory. It is never permissible to dismiss any one or more items which must be present if the heuristically-generated assessment is correct. If one or more are absent go back to the beginning, reassess all available information and modify or, if necessary, completely alter the assessment. Many of the mistakes in clinical medicine result from dismissal of factors that are inconveniently incompatible with an otherwise perfectly satisfying heuristically-derived conclusion. An objective, unemotional and logical approach is essential.

Second. To identify items which are absent but not essential for using the heuristically-derived assessment.

Such absences uncommonly negate the validity of a heuristically-derived clinical assessment. Watch for their appearance as the disease progresses and treat appropriately when necessary. For example, one does not have to demonstrate every textbook feature of multiple sclerosis or scleroderma for the diagnosis to be correct. Nor does a patient with pain and rebound tenderness in the right iliac fossa, a leucocytosis and fever have to demonstrate all the other classical prodroma and clinical features of acute appendicitis to make the diagnosis.

Case history.

A young man of 32 came to see me with a one week history of abdominal pain located in the right iliac fossa. A palpable tender mass was present in the painful area, with overlying rebound tenderness. There was no fever or increase in neutrophils. Nor were there any symptoms suggestive of intestinal obstruction. The patient was referred to a surgeon who felt the patient had an appendix abscess despite the absence of fever and a normal neutrophil count. There was no change in the clinical picture despite a course of broad spectrum antibiotics and metronidazole. A suggestion was made that this was acute Crohn's disease without obstruction and did not need surgery but therapy from a gastroenterologist. The surgeon disagreed. He felt that surgical drainage was needed. Laparotomy showed an edematous red mass of coiled terminal ileum, cecum and ascending colon. The surgeon did a right hemicolectomy. The pathological diagnosis was Crohn's disease. Unfortunately years of complications, recurrences and invalidism have followed and continue. All due to recurrences of the disease.

The above case history demonstrates that a required and probablyt essential feature of a dysfunction must never be disregarded. In this instance it was the absence of a fever and a leucocytosis.

On the other hand careful questioning and assessment is necessary to distinguish conditions such as transient ischemic attacks from hysterical phenomena, panic attacks, and other trivia that are not due to pathology. Epilepsy must be distinguished from pseudo-epilepsy (hysterical fits), peptic ulcer from stress-induced dyspepsia, night cramps from vascular disease of the legs, and so on.

Tools that complement heuristic reasoning.

The following are some useful tools that help in making heuristic decision:

Inductive and deductive reasoning.

Logicians distinguish two types of reasoning. The one is **deductive reasoning** which is defined as reasoning from premises that suffice to reach a correct, reasonable and logical conclusion. The other is **inductive reasoning** where available information does not suffice to reach a solution that one can confidently conclude to be correct. One or more conclusions may be reached. Any of them could be correct or incorrect. It is a type of reasoning without certainty of correctness.

Logicians have commented on the fuzziness of the difference between deductive and inductive reasoning[12]. But the distinction is important in clinical medicine because few clinical variables are precisely quantifiable and the outcomes of therapy are often unpredictable.

Hence, inductive reasoning is the type of reasoning usually employed for clinical decision-making. Examples of clinical variables where differences are qualitative and not precisely quantifiable include the variations of normal biology, the differences in responses to pathology, unknown functional reserves in affected tissues, in compensating systems and in systems affected by other diseases. An additional important factor is unpredictable temporal change in any one or more of the above. The ideal tool for inductive reasoning is an iterative loop specifically designed for assessments of differences that are qualitative and not mensurable with precision (Chart 2-2).

A few clinical problems do have variables that are quantifiable. Most derive from laboratory investigations. The results are often diagnostic in the appropriate clinical setting. For such items ideal investigative tools for subsequent assessments are algorithms, deductive reasoning, and iterative loops designed for situations where the numbers of iterations can be predetermined (Chart 2-1).

Algorithms.

The word "algorithm" derives from the name of the 9th. century mathematician Abu Ja'far Mohammed ben Musa (also known as alkhwarazmi, i.e., the native of Khwarazm). The algorithm is a way of solving mathematical problems using a finite number of steps. The result should always be correct and predictable on the basis of information provided and for this reason the algorithms have a limited use in clinical medicine where most of the variables are qualitatively different, and prone to change from time to time with often unpredictable outcomes. The quantitative precisions required for algorithmic resolutions are usually absent.

Most studies that claim to have solved specific clinical problems by algorithmic reasoning have actually used flow sheets and statistics rather than algorithms. Algorithms cannot be used to solve problems when the variables are not precisely quantifiable.

Knuth's monograph on algorithms[13] defines them as "a finite set of rules which gives a sequence of operations for solving a specific type of problem". He proposed five rules: The following is a paraphrase of the original:

First, the algorithm must always terminate after a finite number of steps.

Second, each step of an algorithm must be precisely defined, with the required actions rigorously and unambiguously specified for each step.

Third and fourth were that every algorithm must have an input and an output.

The fifth and last requirement was that all required actions in an algorithm should result in a conclusion reached in a finite length of time.

Flow charts.

The flow chart graphically depicts the sequence of events and the decisions that should occur during resolution of specific clinical problems. They depict a desirable procession of events, options and choices required for resolution of the typical clinical problem where variables are qualitative and not quantifiable with precision. Their usefulness is limited by the many possible and unpredictable permutations of virulence, progression of the disease, age related decreases in functional reserve, variations in host resistance, variations in the responses of mechanisms that normally compensate for functional deficits, unacceptable or adverse reactions to therapeutic drugs, and many other factors.

Flow charts and the design of clinical trials.

The flow chart is often used for designing clinical trials. Its usefulness in providing direction can be exceeded by the restrictions it imposes on the judgments of participating physicians. Certainly a clinical trial must be terminated if there are undesirable complications and even deaths.

At other times clinical trials are ended because of statistically significant but numerically trivial differences between groups, especially when large numbers are compared. An example is the PROSPER investigation on the effectiveness of statins in reducing morbidity and mortality from coronary artery disease. The topic was detailed in Chapter 1.

Statistics and Bayesian analysis.

Statistics use calculations to determine the probability (the p value) that future events will eventuate in similar ways. Bayesian analysis predicts on the basis of previous events.

For the record, Thomas Bayes (1702-1761) was a theologian and mathematician who was the first to establish a mathematical basis for inference from statistical probabilities. His observations were posthumously published in 1763 in a monograph titled "Essay Towards Solving a Problem in the Doctrine of Chances". His postulates have become the basis for a statistical technique, called Bayesian estimation. It calculates the probability that a given proposition is correct on the basis of statistics regarding previous comparable situations.

Statistics and Bayesian analysis indicate probabilities about the behaviors of groups, not of individuals. Treat the individual patient in the way one should but do not expect that the response will necessarily correspond to the one predicted by statistics or Bayesian analysis.

Clinical decision analysis.

A somewhat more sophisticated use of flow charts and statistical analysis has been devised by Pauker and Kassirer[14] as an alternative to the simple flow sheet. They use the flow chart and statistical analysis in conjunction to build "decision trees". The decision tree is a graphic depiction of the statistical probabilities that could result from different strategies investigations and therapies.

Iterative loops.

The iterative loop is a repeating loop format for investigating, repeatedly reassessing and deciding on problems.

Every iterative loop must have three components:

A point of entry. In clinical medicine the decision loop is entered as soon as physician and patient interact.

At least one variable. Variables are items which can change quantitatively and/or qualitatively from time to time and from one iteration to the next.

A point for exit from the loop. The point at which one exits from an iterative loop depends on the type of loop used: a quantitative or qualitative iterative loop.

Quantitative and qualitative iterative loops.

The quantitative iterative loop.

The quantitative iterative loop is one where the problem predetermines the numbers of needed iterations. This is the type of loop usually employed for numerical calculations (Chart 2-1).

The format varies according to the problem and many variations of the basic format can be devised to perform extremely complex calculations, especially if nested loops are also used (see later). The numerical problem predetermines the numbers of iterations needed. Once this value has been reached one exits from the loop and outputs the decision.

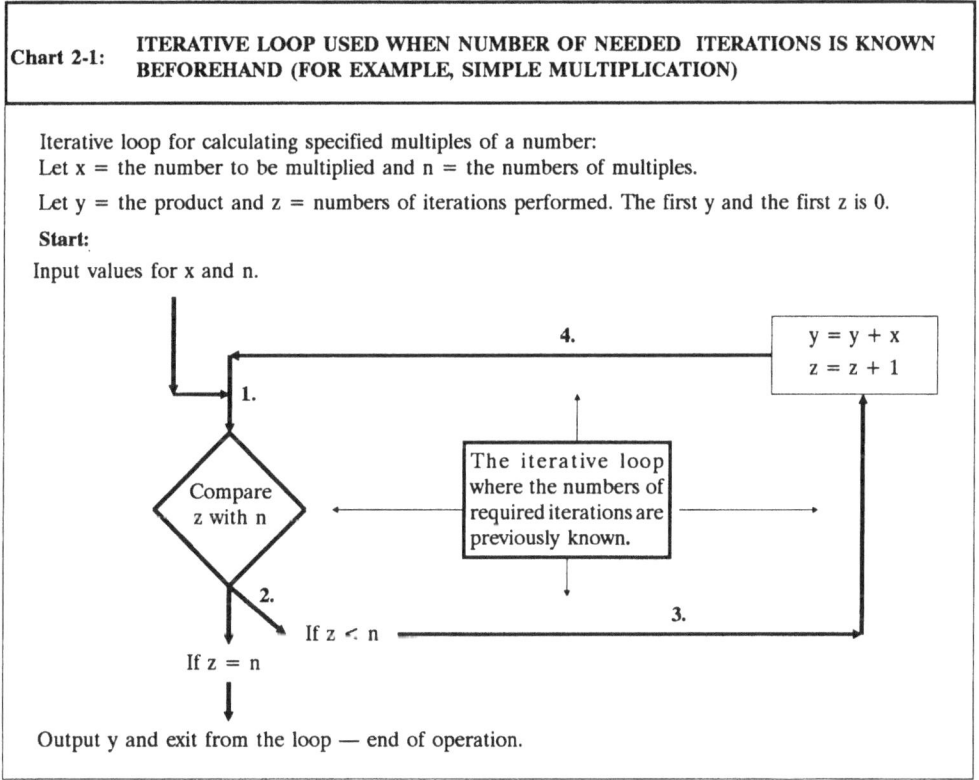

Chart 2-1: ITERATIVE LOOP USED WHEN NUMBER OF NEEDED ITERATIONS IS KNOWN BEFOREHAND (FOR EXAMPLE, SIMPLE MULTIPLICATION)

Iterative loop for calculating specified multiples of a number:
Let x = the number to be multiplied and n = the numbers of multiples.

Let y = the product and z = numbers of iterations performed. The first y and the first z is 0.

Start:

Input values for x and n.

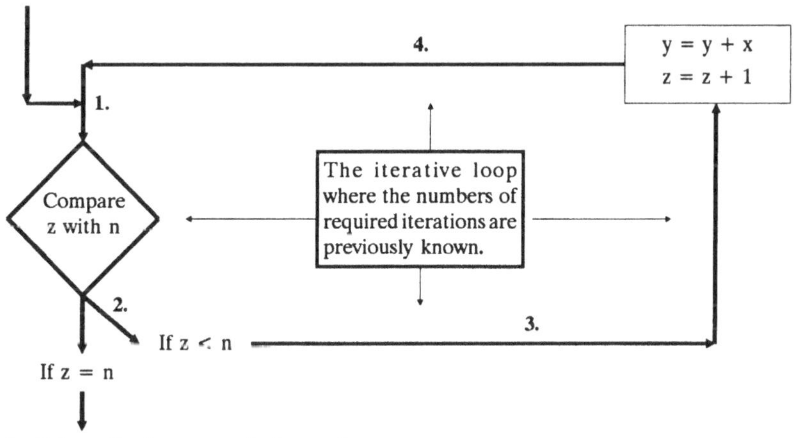
4.
y = y + x
z = z + 1
1.
Compare z with n
The iterative loop where the numbers of required iterations are previously known.
2.
3.
If z < n
If z = n

Output y and exit from the loop — end of operation.

Incidentally, the working of the digital time-piece is based on a loop of this type. A quartz crystal is stimulated by a battery and vibrates at exactly 2^{15} (i.e., 32,768) times per second. A chip in a microprocessor counts the vibrations and instructs the digital display to advance one second each time it has counted 32,768 vibrations. I have not verified these facts but, if correct, it is an amazing phenomenon. I present it unchanged from its description in: “Computer Basics”. The book is the first volume in the Time-Life books series on computers, p. 17.

The qualitative iterative loop.

The qualitative iterative loop is used when differences between variables are qualitative and not quantifiable with precision. Because the variables are not quantifiable the numbers of needed iterations cannot be predetermined. Chart 2-2 hypothesizes on the ways in which qualitative iterative loops are usable in clinical medicine

Chart 2-2: THE ITERATIVE LOOP FOR VARIABLES WHICH CANNOT BE QUANTIFIED WITH PRECISION: THE VARIABLES ARE QUALITATIVE AND THE NUMBERS OF REQUIRED ITERATIONS CANNOT BE DETERMINED BEFOREHAND

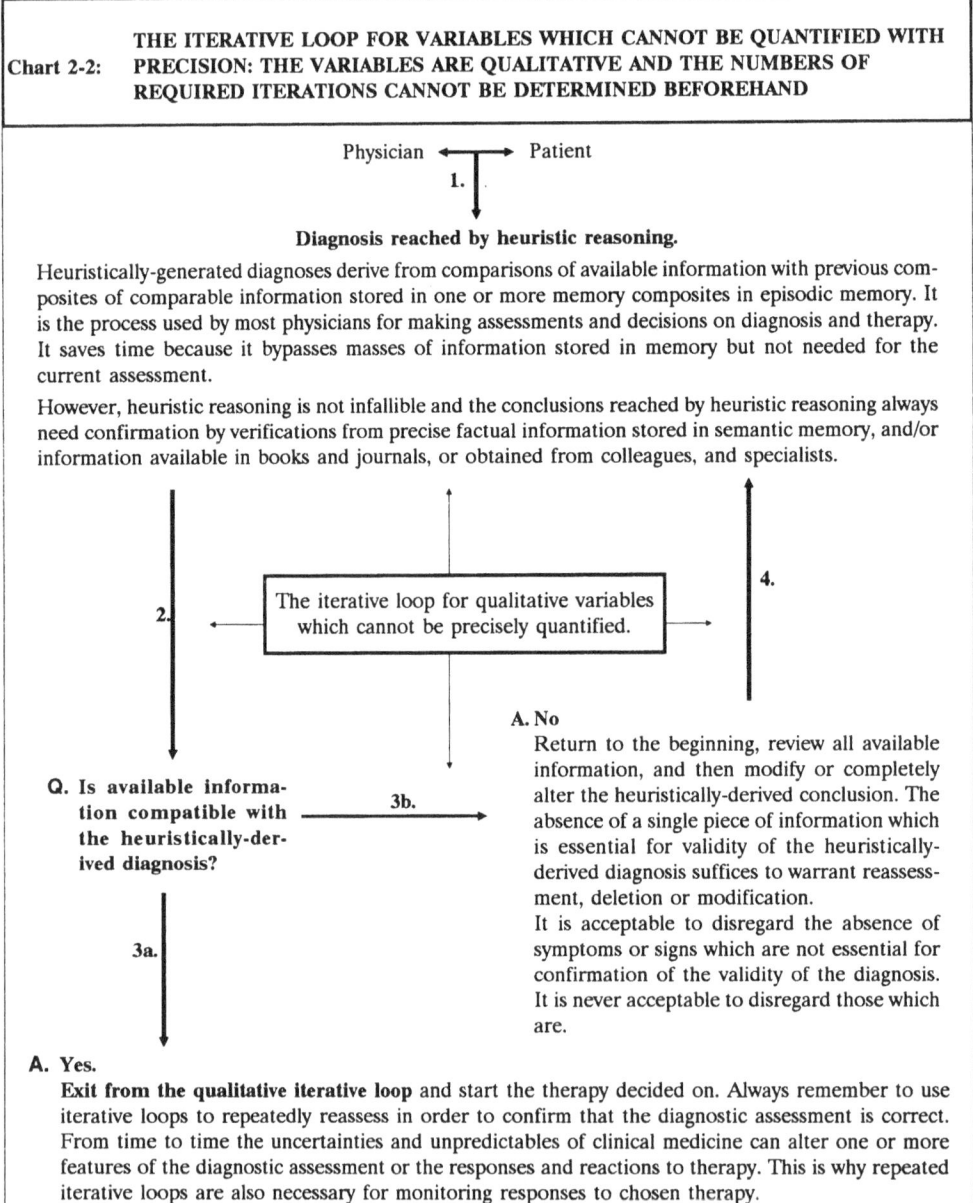

Physician ↔ Patient

1.

Diagnosis reached by heuristic reasoning.

Heuristically-generated diagnoses derive from comparisons of available information with previous composites of comparable information stored in one or more memory composites in episodic memory. It is the process used by most physicians for making assessments and decisions on diagnosis and therapy. It saves time because it bypasses masses of information stored in memory but not needed for the current assessment.

However, heuristic reasoning is not infallible and the conclusions reached by heuristic reasoning always need confirmation by verifications from precise factual information stored in semantic memory, and/or information available in books and journals, or obtained from colleagues, and specialists.

2.

The iterative loop for qualitative variables which cannot be precisely quantified.

4.

Q. Is available information compatible with the heuristically-derived diagnosis?

3b.

A. No

Return to the beginning, review all available information, and then modify or completely alter the heuristically-derived conclusion. The absence of a single piece of information which is essential for validity of the heuristically-derived diagnosis suffices to warrant reassessment, deletion or modification.

It is acceptable to disregard the absence of symptoms or signs which are not essential for confirmation of the validity of the diagnosis. It is never acceptable to disregard those which are.

3a.

A. Yes.

Exit from the qualitative iterative loop and start the therapy decided on. Always remember to use iterative loops to repeatedly reassess in order to confirm that the diagnostic assessment is correct. From time to time the uncertainties and unpredictables of clinical medicine can alter one or more features of the diagnostic assessment or the responses and reactions to therapy. This is why repeated iterative loops are also necessary for monitoring responses to chosen therapy.

for making decisions and for monitoring the consequences of those decisions. The chart is self-explanatory and requires no additional comment except for one; a comment on the use of “nested iterative loops”.

The nested iterative loop.

A nested iterative loop is one that resides within the main loop and is independent of it. It permits the independent evaluation of a variable. An advantage is that many iterations of the nested loop can be performed for each iteration of the main loop with considerable saving of time.

Long-term memory and memory composites

Long-term memory is the repository for all stored information. In contrast to short-term memory the capacity of long-term memory is enormous but not infinite. All that is perceived cannot be stored in long-term memory. Some type of selection is needed and this is performed by the hippocampus, the attention filter and short-term memory. More about these filters later in this chapter.

With respect to long-term memory, two topics need detailing. The **first** is the way in which information travels the neural pathways till it reaches the areas where material is selected for storage in long-term memory. The **second** is how it is stored and best used.

The first describes the anatomical neural pathways from reception to selection of information for storage in long-term memory. It will not knowledge which will improve the processes which select information for storage in long-term memory. This depends on the type of medicine practiced and the unique ways in which individuals make decisions. For example the priorities of a cardiologist will differ from those of a neurologist and those of a general practitioner will differ from both.

Logically, detailing of the first should precede the second. In this text the opposite is chosen. The reason is that the second is more important to the practicing physician than the first. It provides information about how information in long-term memory is stored and best used for clinical decision-making. Once this is known the discriminations that the physician needs for choosing information for storage in long-term memory will improve.

Storage of information in long-term memory.

The brain contains many neurons (estimates vary from 10^{10} - $2x10^{11}$ and each neuron communicates with other neurons by many synapses. According to Eccles[15] 10,000 synapses communicate with each pyramidal cell of the cerebral cortex and Ito[16] has claimed that each Purkinje cell and its climbing fibers have 100,000 synapses with other neurons. The numbers of synapses in the brain is estimated as between 10^{11}-10^{15}. The quantity of information that must be stored in long-term memory is enormous.

The brain can be trained to increase its capacity for storage and retention. An example of what is possible is detailed by Solzhenitsyn[17] in one of his novels - The Gulag Archipelago Three. The following is a quotation from the book (translation by H. Willetts):

> "I discovered later that prose, too, can be quite satisfactorily tamped down into the deep hidden layers of what we carry in our heads. No longer burdened with superficial and frivolous knowledge, a prisoner's memory is astonishingly capacious, and can expand indefinitely. We have too little faith in memory."

Later he wrote:

> "In prisons the composition and editing of verses had to be done in my head ...... Once a month I recited all that I had written. If the wrong line came out I went over it all again and again until I caught the slippery figures." .... "Until the end of my sentence (by which time I had accumulated 12,000 lines), ..."

Where and how is long-term memory stored?

Studies of where the brain stores memories were started by Lashley in the 1920s[18]. On the basis of cortical ablation experiments on mice and rats he proposed the rule of "Equipotentially" which postulated that all areas of the cortex were equally important for learning and remembering. The radio-xenon cerebral blood flow studies of Roland and Friberg (Roland, E.P. & Friberg, L. Localization of cortical areas by thinking. J. Neurophysiol. 1985; 53:1219) suggested that this hypothesis was equally valid in humans and that memories were squeezed into vacant areas scattered throughout the cortex with a preponderance in the prefrontal cortex.

Subsequently, many comparable experiments have confirmed the findings of Roland and Friberg. One assumes that there are many rapid to and fro neural communications between the memory banks.

Lashley's failure to find memory engrams could have resulted from severance of nerve connections between different memory banks during his ablations of mammalian brain tissue. Support for Lashley's original postulate and radio-xenon studies of Roland and Friberg is that they correlate well with post-mortem pathological studies of patients with multi-infarct dementia, Alzheimer's disease and the degenerations of prion infections. These diseases result in deficits of long-term memory while the patients are still alive. The pathological lesions are scattered throughout the brain and the extent of disease as seen on CT scans correlate well with the degree of forgetting but not with any specific forgotten items.

Numerous papers on memory are published each year. Conjectural hypotheses are many but few add much to the original concepts of Lashley, Hebb (The organization of behavior. New York: Wiley, 1949), and Roland and Friberg. Ethical considerations limit the extent of possible studies in humans. Most new ideas derive from assumptions and hypotheses based on experimental psychology or correlations between clinical findings and pathology or therapeutic surgical ablations.

The storage and use of information in memory.

Chart 2-3 on the next page is a basic hypothetical overview of a general plan of memory storage. The literature on the topic of memory storage is large. The references cited here[19,20,21,22,23] are to some of the original publications. Additional references are not cited as most only confirm the original postulates. There is a dearth of precise new information about the minutiae of memory storage.

The general belief is that the brain stores information in hierarchies of inter-related and interacting clusters and nodes. The word "cluster" refers to a collection of items of related information[24,25]. Each cluster is connected with one or more nodes (called control elements in some publications). The nodes are comparable to the memory composites previously described. They are the bases for heuristic reasoning and decision-making.

Associated nodes are interconnected and arranged in a hierarchy of descending importance. Organization and storage of information in clusters and within nodes are also arranged in hierarchies of decreasing importance. This reduces the time needed for assessments of information, and for problem solving and decision-making.

Each physician will develop an individual hierarchical plan that depends on personal assessments of different clinical problems and the type of medicine practiced. Thus, generalists such as general practitioners and pathologists (the generalist pathologist is slowly disappearing) would have hierarchies different from those practicing specialty medicine. Specialists would have hierarchies of importance directed to rapid resolution of problems specific to the specialty practiced. Thus, a cardiologist would have a hierarchical organization of memory in which symptoms suggesting cardiac dysfunction would place high while symptoms related to a disease such as Parkinson's disease or multiple sclerosis would rate low. The converse would be true about a neurologist. Information for identification and treatment of situations with actual or potential dangers should rate high in every hierarchical tree, regardless of the discipline practiced.

Rehearsal.

The term "rehearsal" as used by psychologists does not mean repetition. It is a process that groups clusters and nodes into a better frame for memory organization and use, usually in response to an internal command. The internal command is often incorporated into the memory composite and provides the basis for its reorganization and the reorganizations of related composites.

Rehearsal increases the efficiency and effectiveness of recall by changing the contents of clusters and nodes as well as the ways in which they interact. It can add new information in appropriate places and delete old information that is superfluous or incorrect. It is the mechanism for responding to the continual changes in knowledge, therapies and perspectives that are normal in clinical medicine. Chart 2-4 on page 42 summarizes the basics of rehearsal.

Rehearsal can also effect rearrangement of existing hierarchical arrangements of nodes. Situations and circumstances change from time to time and rearrangements of hierarchical inter-relationships must follow suit. Much of what is effected by rehearsal is done automatically. However, the process becomes more effective and

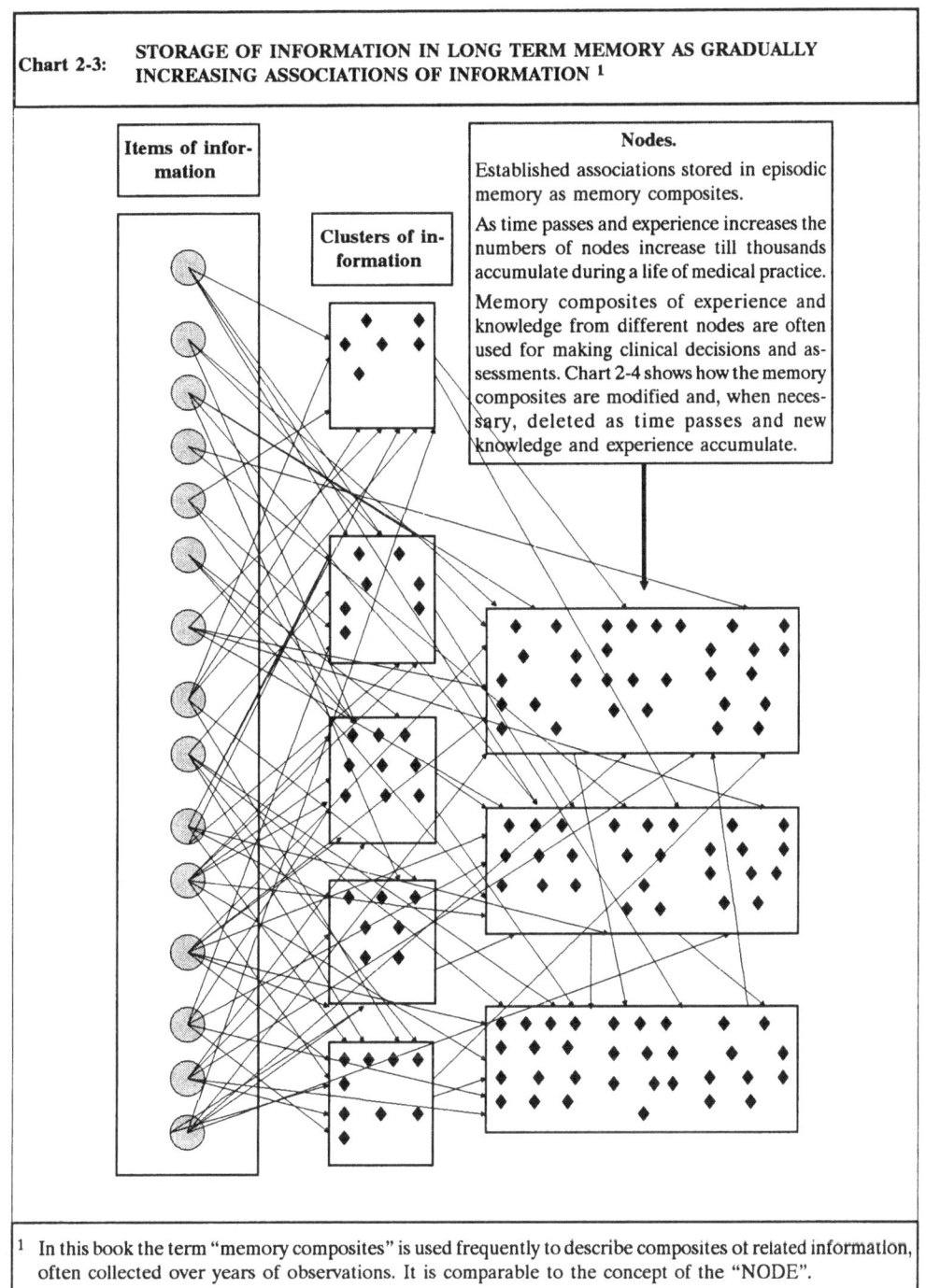

Chart 2-3: STORAGE OF INFORMATION IN LONG TERM MEMORY AS GRADUALLY INCREASING ASSOCIATIONS OF INFORMATION [1]

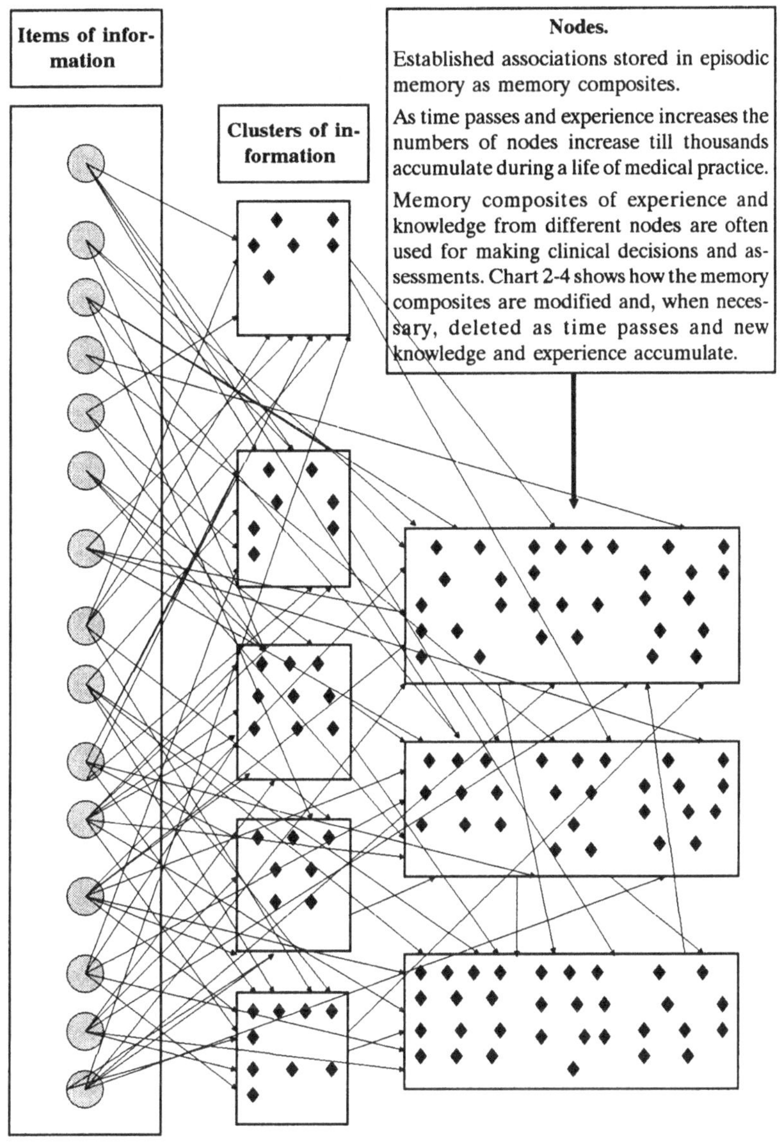
Items of information
Clusters of information
Nodes.
Established associations stored in episodic memory as memory composites.
As time passes and experience increases the numbers of nodes increase till thousands accumulate during a life of medical practice.
Memory composites of experience and knowledge from different nodes are often used for making clinical decisions and assessments. Chart 2-4 shows how the memory composites are modified and, when necessary, deleted as time passes and new knowledge and experience accumulate.

[1] In this book the term "memory composites" is used frequently to describe composites of related information, often collected over years of observations. It is comparable to the concept of the "NODE".

efficient if the physician understands what can be done and what changing needs and circumstances require. The process of rehearsal and modifications of memory composites continues throughout the working life of every practicing physician.

Operational memory.

The term **"operational" or "working" memory** was probably first employed by **(Contd. on page 43)**

Chart 2-4: FORMATIONS AND ALTERATIONS OF MEMORY COMPOSITES BY REHEARSAL

The memory composite

A memory composite is a remembered collection of facts, observations, protocols, mnemonics, treatments, adverse reactions and other items based on the clinical features and course of a previous clinical problem. Diagnosis usually begins with a heuristic assessment which compares the current clinical picture with one or more memory composites with comparable attributes. Access to an appropriate composite or composites is probably by concordance between external verbalized or intellectual commands and internal stored commands. Heuristic reasoning is a fast form of reasoning as it bypasses and circumvents material which is not relevant to the presenting clinical problem. An assessment based on heuristic reasoning should always be verified by subsequent confirmatory referral to precise and correct factual information stored in semantic memory or accessible in books, journals, CD-ROMs and/or from colleagues and specialists.

The memory composites in episodic memory are continuously modified by new information altering or deleting existing composites, and/or generating new memory composites, mnemonics, and protocols for investigations and therapy. Some of the factors responsible for these changes are itemized below.

Alterations, improvements and/or deletion of stored memory composites:

— A previous clinical problem could not be resolved by comparisons with memory composites stored in episodic memory. On that occasion it was only possible to resolve the problem by sequential searches of factual information stored in semantic memory or in books, journals, CD-ROMs and/or from colleagues. The experience gained is stored as a new memory composite and/or incorporated into pre-existing composites. Improved heuristic reasoning should result.

— New protocols for investigations and therapy, new mnemonics, and new generalizations for analysis and decision-making. Some are generated by the physician. Others derive from books and journals, and from discussions with colleagues, specialists and teachers. In general it is usually desirable that new information has general usage and acceptance before incorporation into one or more memory composites.

— Alternatively, the physician might feel that the new information, though widely accepted, does not meet personal criteria for validity and/or safety. An example is the refusal of many physicians, including myself, to provide hormone replacement therapy (HRT) to post-menopausal women despite forceful exhortations[1]. The reasons were our knowledge that HRT increased the incidence of breast cancer[2] in recipients, and a feeling that the putative benefit on cardiac dysfunction remained unproven - a belief now confirmed by clinical meta-analyses[3,4]. Do not incorporate into a memory composite any material which you feel is potentially or actually hazardous, even if it has the imprimatur of general acceptance and usage.

— Memory composites often require modifications when new research, new therapies and previous theories of causations and descriptions of clinical courses change. Deletions or alterations of some composites will become necessary. Changes in available knowledge are continuous and the composites of information stored in long-term memory must reflect this fact.

One or more new and/or altered memory composites stored in episodic memory for resolution of future comparable clinical problems by heuristic reasoning.

The acquisition of new memory composites and the modification or deletion of existing ones should begin on the first day of clinical training and continue through the working life of a physician. As the years pass this will result in more correct and effective clinical assessments and treatments because of the increasing accuracies, complexities and sophistications of stored memory composites.

1 American College of Physicians. Guidelines for counseling postmenopausal women about preventive hormone therapy. Ann. Intern. Med. 1992; 117:1038.

2 Barrett-Connor, E., Stunkel, C.A. Hormone replacement therapy (HRT): risks and benefits. Int. J. Epidemiol. 2001; 30:423.

3 Hulley, S., Grady, D., et al. Randomized trial of estrogen plus progestin for secondary prevention of coronary heart disease in postmenopausal women. JAMA 1988; 280:605.

4 Mosca, L., Collins, P., et al. Hormone replacement therapy and cardiovascular disease. A statement for health care professionals from the American Heart Association. Circulation 2001; 1104:449.

(Contd. form page 41) Posner and Rossman[26]. It refers to a collection of items activated from long-term memory and kept in an activated state during solution of a problem. Posner[27] has commented as follows:

> "All human information-processing requires keeping track of incoming stimuli and bringing such input into contact with already stored information."

This is the function of operational or working memory. It is probably mediated by previously generated internal commands. These internal commands are probably intrinsic to the memory composite or composites being assessed. Operational memory derives from information relevant to solution of the problem. The selected information is moved to the front of long-term memory and kept there as long as a decision on the clinical problem remains unresolved.

Consolidation.

This process permanently incorporates recently acquired information in long-term memory. Young memory patterns are easily disrupted. An example is the retrograde amnesia that often follows trauma to the head. Immediately after the injury the loss may extend back months or years. As the patient recovers memories begin to return. First to return are those that are furthest back in time. Later, more recently acquired information returns. When recovery ceases no additional information is recovered. Amnesia for the period preceding the trauma may be seconds, minutes, hours, days, months or years of information stored in long-term memory. This information is lost for ever when recovery ends. Presumably the shock to the brain occurred before any of this information had a chance to be consolidated in long-term memory.

Complex memories probably never consolidate and need continual repetition for remembering. An example is the concert musician who needs to continuously practice the same musical repertoire, often for many hours a day. The need for remembering and/or reading written music and simultaneously and rapidly executing complex related motor movements and intellectual interpretations of the music seems to exceed the capacity of the human brain to remember without constant repetition.

According to Eccles[15] the studies on H.M. (a patient with bilateral hippocampectomy) showed a retrograde amnesia for the three years prior to surgery in addition to the anterograde amnesia resulting from the operation. He felt that this indicated that one to three years of consolidation are needed before a memory remains unforgotten and retrievable. Similar retrograde amnesia may also result from the electric shocks of electroconvulsive therapy.

Eccles opined as follows:

> "the hippocampal input to the neocortex must be replayed much as in the initial experience in what we may name "recall episodes" for one to three years. Failure of this replay results in the ordinary process of forgetting. After three years the memory codes in the cerebral cortex are much more securely established and apparently require no further reinforcing by hippocampal inputs; hence they are not lost in the disruption of bilateral hippocampectomy or electroconvulsive therapy."

Consolidation needs repetition or repeated use for the first 1-3 years after information enters long-term memory. Priorities, therapies, information, knowledge and concepts are continually changing. Hence, rehearsal and consolidation are tasks that must continue throughout a physician's professional life.

Modifications of stored memories by experience.

Experience is the sum total of all the episodic memory composites acquired during life. At the end of life they probably number over a hundred thousand. There are frequent modifications of parts or all of these experience composites by additions, deletions and rearrangements, from time to time. Most result from repeated rehearsals because of new clinical experiences, and experiences related to the needs of daily living, changing circumstances, domestic needs, and other priorities. The objectives of the rehearsals are rearrangements for optimal use.

Experience is important in heuristic reasoning. The inexperienced tend to use reasoning based on factual knowledge; knowledge stored in semantic memory or derived from books, journals, lectures, colleagues and specialists. They use this information in combination with sequential searches of memory using previously developed protocols for reasoning[28]. Experience is not used for they do not have memory composites related to the presenting clinical problem. The process is usually much slower than those used by physicians with experience. In order to solve problems the latter tend to bypass sequential reasoning by using heuristic reasoning based on episodic composites stored in memory.

The experienced use formal sequential reasoning when resolution is not possible with heuristic reasoning. They also use, or certainly should use, precise factual information obtained from any one or more sources to confirm or refute every conclusion reached by heuristic reasoning. The absence of a single piece of information that is essential for confirmation of a heuristically-derived diagnosis suffices to require reassessment, modification, or deletion of the assessment. The absence of symptoms or signs that are not essential for confirmation of the diagnosis is acceptable. To disregard the absence of those that are essential is not acceptable. Ad hoc heuristic reasoning is never infallible. It must always be confirmed by recourse to information of confirmed validity stored in semantic memory or accessed from books, journals, CD-ROMS or associates. In some unknown way when the heuristically-generated assessment needs confirmation by material in semantic memory it can bypass the facts in semantic memory that are not relevant to its assessment. Perhaps signals are built into the memory composite or composites used and these effect the bypass of irrelevant semantic information.

Experience and the ten-year rule.

Experts are experts because they have a lot of knowledge related to their subjects. They perform well and fast because the knowledge is mainly in the form of chunks of experience. Newell and Simon[29] have postulated that an expert of international standing such as a grand master in chess or a Nobel laureate in chemistry has some 50,000 to 100,000 chunks of experience information stored in memory before reaching such a status. Each of these chunks, as well as their many associations and interactions, can be recalled from episodic memory, examined and used as and when necessary. Psychologists estimate that it will take about ten years or so to acquire 50,000 chunks of information and this estimate approximates biographic data of high-performing experts. This postulate is now designated "the ten year rule". For physicians this "ten year rule" begins when medical school training begins.

It does take time to acquire enough experience to perform with competence. Someone once said to me: "Good medical practice is the result of experience but acquisition of experience results from bad medical practice." A statement which has some truth in it.

The ten-year rule postulates that an apprentice needs some ten years of experience to perform with the competence of an expert. Obviously, this is not all that is needed. To be a competent expert it is necessary to mix experience with common-sense, with individuality, with insight and with the unique intangibles that are specific to the individual and cannot be described in precise terms.

Critics of the ten-year rule have cited the works of Mozart, an individual who composed symphonies before he was 10. Currently there are chess grandmasters who are teenagers. Gifted individuals, so-called geniuses, are few and their abilities do not negate the general postulate of the ten-year rule. Variations between humans have always existed and will continue to exist. In general, to be good at doing anything most people usually need the experience of an arduous ten years during which memory composites are acquired and modified for personal use. Additional needs are qualities unique to the individual, some inherited, others acquired and all wonderfully mixed to produce a human who thinks and acts as all humans should.

Note that ten years of experience will not make an individual a super specialist at anything. A trite pejorative response to those who claim correctness on the basis of experience is to ask whether it is ten (or whatever numbers of years of experience are claimed) years of experience or one year's experience repeated unchanged ten times.

The super-doctor, the super-musician, or the super-anything is the product of experience combined with the indefinable unique quality that is called genius. Ten years of medical practice may result in a competent physician but not necessarily a super-doc. Ten years of piano playing and composing may produce a competent musician but not a Mozart. Ten years of painting could result in a competent artist but not one who paints like a Picasso. Ten years of attempting to write poetry may produce acceptable verse but not those of a William Shakespeare.

Genius is an indefinable quality. A few have it and they are destined to have major influences on humanity.

Its existence certainly does not negate the validity of the ten year rule.

Sensory information: reception to long-term memory

Chart 2-5 summarizes the processes that intervene between cerebral reception and the selection of material for storage in long-term memory. Chart 2-6 illustrates the inputs to the tempero-parietal heteromodal association area for multimodal integrations.

The text of this section may seem unnecessarily detailed for a book of this type. The detailing is deliberate. Material stored in memory is the basis for clinical decision-making. Detailed knowledge of the processes involved in remembering will improve selection and storage of needed information in long-term memory. It will also improve interactions with and the assessments and diagnoses of patients disabled by neurological pathologies.

The brain does not have an infinite capacity and the volume of available medical knowledge is large and continually growing. One estimate in 1976 contended that the core body of general internal medicine alone had a million facts (I have lost the reference). Since then there has been an information explosion. Thousands of new papers are published each year so that the figure quoted above needs multiplication by many factors to provide any reasonable estimate of internal medicine information available at present. To this one must add available information in the other branches of clinical medicine: surgery, obstetrics and gynecology, genetics, pathology, anatomy, physiology and biochemistry. Material to be stored in memory must be selected by every individual physician according to needs as it is impossible to store everything. Necessarily, and inevitably, this selection will be subjective for it depends on the type of medicine practiced.

There is a basic core knowledge of physiology, pathology and clinical medicine that is essential to the resolution of almost every diagnostic or therapeutic problem. It is knowledge that is learnt, or should be learnt, during training in medical school. It needs integration into the thought processes of every physician because it is essential for resolution of most clinical problems. Additions to this core depends on the type of clinical medicine practiced. The needs of a general practitioner will differ from those of a specialist and the specialty practiced will determine the needs of the latter.

There is also a need to identify material that has importance but is not needed for daily use. This type of information does not need detailed storage. One only needs to remember that such information exists and the journals, books, CD-ROMs, Internet web sites and other locations where it is accessible. Once again, the needs of specialists will vary according to the specialty practiced. The needs of a general practitioner are as large as those of any specialist but different in detail.

The plasticity of the brain.

The brain has considerable plasticity. Neurons cannot proliferate and regenerate, yet it is common to find that the functional deficits of a major stroke often decrease with time, occasionally with only a small residual deficit of fine movements. The assignment of dysfunctions to specific areas of the brain requires awareness of this fact. Even though neurons cannot proliferate, some degree of recovery is always possible. At times there are almost complete recoveries of function. The reasons for these recoveries have been debated for more than a hundred years. One possible explanation is sprouting of new axon terminals from damaged but viable neurons. They probably terminate on target cells that are still viable but not normally targeted. Subsequently these newly targeted cells provide the neural basis for re-learning whatever function was lost.

Cerebral reception areas.

Chart 2-5 summarizes the sequences from the cerebral reception of information to the selection and storage of desired material in long-term memory.

The primary reception areas.

Processing of information begins in the primary reception areas. The principal ones are:

- **The motor cortex.** The input is from the cerebellum, the basal ganglia, the vestibular complex, cranial nerve and spinal cord neurons, and all sensory areas (primary, unimodal and heteromodal). It has many neurons,

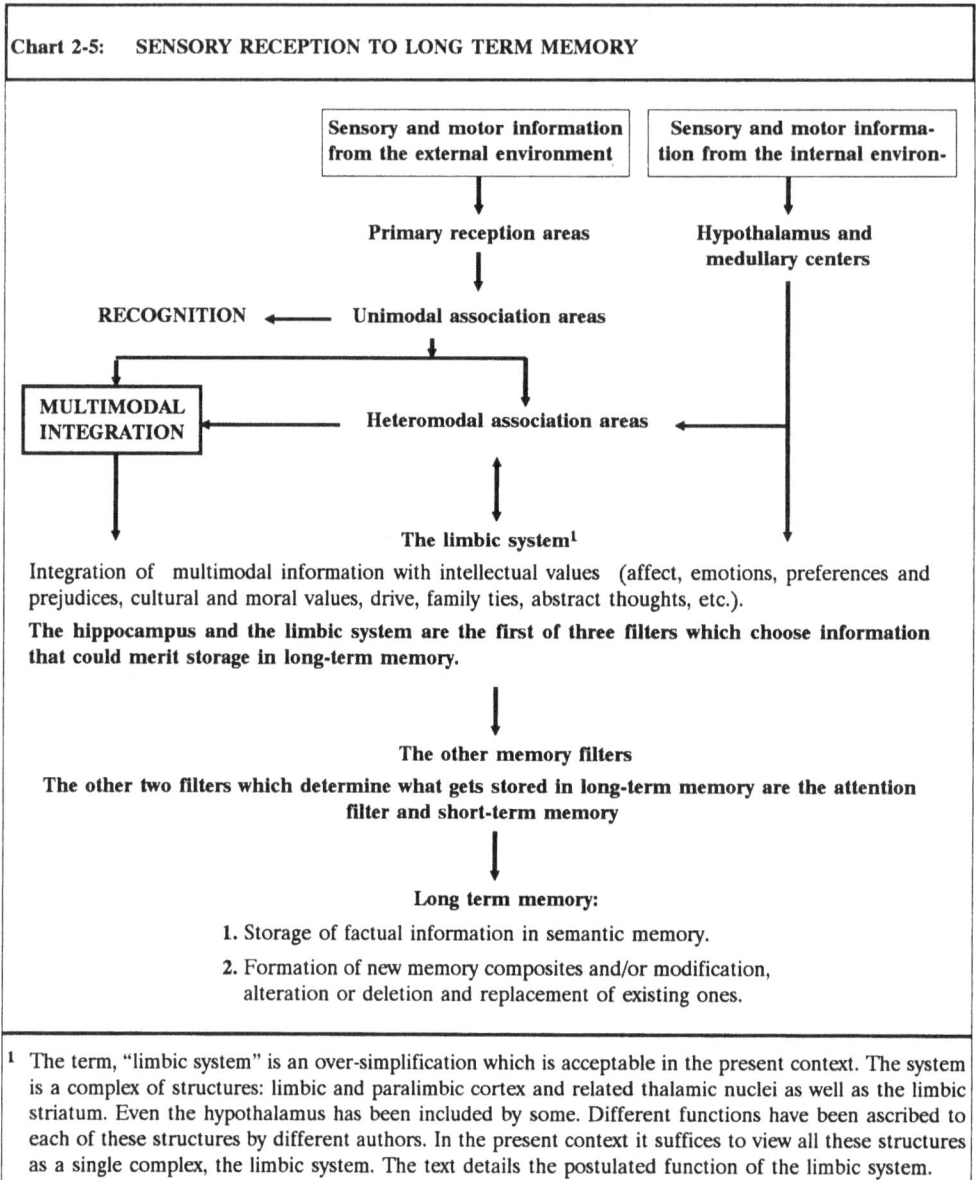

Chart 2-5: SENSORY RECEPTION TO LONG TERM MEMORY

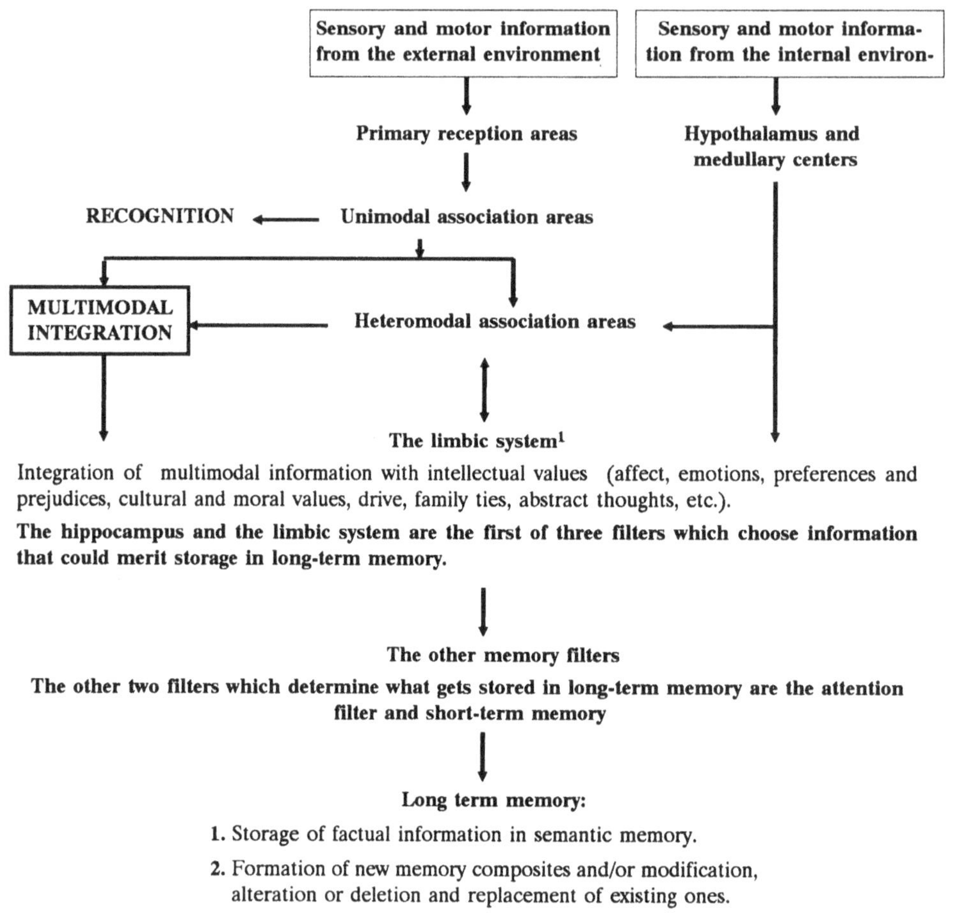
Sensory and motor information from the external environment
Sensory and motor information from the internal environ-
Primary reception areas
Hypothalamus and medullary centers
RECOGNITION
Unimodal association areas
MULTIMODAL INTEGRATION
Heteromodal association areas
The limbic system[1]
Integration of multimodal information with intellectual values (affect, emotions, preferences and prejudices, cultural and moral values, drive, family ties, abstract thoughts, etc.).
The hippocampus and the limbic system are the first of three filters which choose information that could merit storage in long-term memory.
The other memory filters
The other two filters which determine what gets stored in long-term memory are the attention filter and short-term memory
Long term memory:
1. Storage of factual information in semantic memory.
2. Formation of new memory composites and/or modification, alteration or deletion and replacement of existing ones.

[1] The term, "limbic system" is an over-simplification which is acceptable in the present context. The system is a complex of structures: limbic and paralimbic cortex and related thalamic nuclei as well as the limbic striatum. Even the hypothalamus has been included by some. Different functions have been ascribed to each of these structures by different authors. In the present context it suffices to view all these structures as a single complex, the limbic system. The text details the postulated function of the limbic system.

each with many synaptic connections. Eccles[15] has estimated that each pyramidal cell has some 10,000 synaptic connections with other neurons. **The following are the other main primary reception areas:**

- **Subcortical areas for reception of pain sensations;** mainly thalamic and limbic.
- **The cortical post-Rolandic area for sensory information** and for mediating reflex responses to pain sensed in thalamic and limbic areas.
- **The primary visual cortex** in the occipital pole and the banks of the calcarine fissure.
- **The primary auditory cortex** in the superior temporal gyrus.
- **The primary reception areas for vestibular information.** They are the multiple connections between the spinal cord and the cerebellum and the reticular formation.
- **The primary sensory reception areas for olfactory sensations.** The prepiriform cortex in the vicinity of the

uncus.

- **The primary reception areas for gustatory sensations.** The lower end of the postcentral gyrus, the insula and the superior temporal gyrus.
- **The primary reception areas for sensory information from the internal environment.** They are scattered throughout the body: **medullary centers** for respiratory, vasomotor and cardiac function; the **hypothalamus** for autonomic information; and the **peripheral receptors for autonomous hormone** systems; especially the insulin-glucagon system, the renin-angiotensin-aldosterone complex, the parathyroid hormone-serum ionized calcium system, the renal erythropoietin-red cell maturation interaction and the atrial natriuretic peptide hormone-angiotensin interaction.

  As a rule information about the internal environment is not perceived consciously and most responses to this type of information are mediated by automatic long arm negative or positive feedback reflexes centered on the medulla and hypothalamus. The exceptions are pain from abdominal viscera, the bones, joints, ligaments and muscles, and from the body surfaces. They are probably consciously sensed in the region of the thalamus. Any necessary reflex responses are probably mediated by higher centers.

The unimodal association areas.

The initial processing of information is in the unimodal sensory areas where the new input is integrated with pre-existing information about the specific sensory modality.

Location of the unimodal association areas.

There are three unimodal association areas:

- The superior parietal lobule for **somatosensory information.**
- The superior temporal gyrus for **auditory information.**
- The mid and inferior temporal and peristriate areas for **visual information.**

Inputs to the unimodal association areas.

The input is from adjacent primary reception areas. The functions of the unimodal reception areas can only be inferred from neurological dysfunctions that result from pathology or trauma. They are:

A decrease in the complex perceptions that result from integrations of information in the unimodal areas with pre-existing memories pertaining to the information received. Examples are defects in two-point discrimination, in position sense and stereognosis, in localization of touch, in judgment of distance and space, in stereo and color vision, and in discrimination between different sound frequencies and sequences.

Modality-specific disconnection syndromes may result because of the absence or decrease of modality-specific inputs to the heteromodal and limbic areas. Examples are impairment of visual-auditory and motor-sensory patterns, depending on the modality deficit.

The heteromodal association areas.

In the heteromodal association areas multimodal new and previously remembered information is integrated into single recognizable units. Each acquires multiple attributes because of these integrations. There are at least two, and perhaps three principal heteromodal association areas:

Location of the heteromodal association areas.

A tempero-parietal area (Chart 2-6). It occupies the banks of the superior temporal sulcus, the posterior part of the auditory association cortex and part of the inferior parietal lobule. The tempero-parietal association cortex also includes the angular gyrus, the supramarginal gyrus and part of the superior parietal lobule. An **important component** is Wernicke's area where spoken and written language are integrated with pre-existing information.

The prefrontal cortex. It lies anterior to the motor association cortex on the lateral surface of the brain. The prefrontal cortex also has an orbitofrontal component.

The ventral temporal lobe[30]. It is difficult to tell from the literature if this is a heteromodal area that exists in primates but not humans, whether it exists in both, or whether it is merely synonymous with the limbic cortex. One suspects the last and, for this reason, there are no additional comments about this area.

Chart 2-6: THE TEMPERO-PARIETAL HETEROMODAL AREA ON THE BRAIN'S LATERAL SURFACE

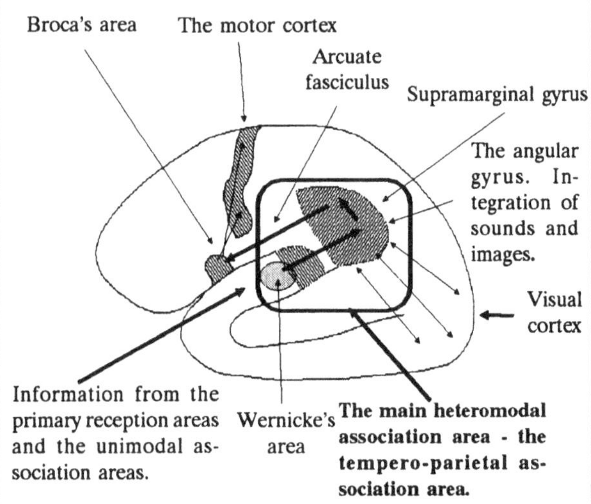
Broca's area
The motor cortex
Arcuate fasciculus
Supramarginal gyrus
The angular gyrus. Integration of sounds and images.
Visual cortex
Information from the primary reception areas and the unimodal association areas.
Wernicke's area
The main heteromodal association area - the tempero-parietal association area.

Lesions of:

1 **Wernicke's area or of the tracts leading to it** result in loss of comprehension of language, both of the spoken and the written word. The ability to speak and to express oneself is retained if Broca's area is unaffected but responses to questions and comments are inappropriate and oral language is nonsensical.

2 **Damage to Broca's area or of the tracts leading to it** results in speech which is inarticulate. There is retention of auditory comprehension if Wernicke's area is unaffected. A lesion of Broca's area is usually accompanied by a left hemiplegia due to an associated vascular lesion affecting the right hemisphere (the left hemisphere is dominant for speech in 90% of right-handed and 50% of left-handed people).

Inputs to the heteromodal association areas.

The input to the heteromodal association areas is from other heteromodal association areas, and the unimodal association areas. In addition there are to-and-fro communications with the limbic cortex for integration of multimodal information with mood, affect, likes, dislikes, drive, and other emotions. In the heteromodal association areas new information, previously processed in the unimodal association cortex, is integrated with pre-existing or new information pertaining to other modalities. Transcription of this integrated information into language probably also occurs in the heteromodal association cortices of the right and left hemispheres.

The heteromodal association cortices of the right and left hemispheres communicate via the corpus callosum because the two hemispheres must communicate for the correction interpretation of language. Broca's speech area is usually in the left hemisphere. It verbalizes processed multimodal sensory information from the heteromodal association areas. The right hemisphere is usually responsible for the paralinguistic components of language (gesture and prosody). These need integration with verbal and written language and with processed multimodal sensory information. Hence, the need for communication between the two hemispheres, a communication provided by the corpus callosum.

The functions of the heteromodal areas.

Once again the functions can only be surmised from dysfunctions due to pathology or trauma. Damage to the heteromodal association areas disrupt multimodal sensory integration and can result in a variety of bizarre and complex syndromes. Of these Wernicke's aphasia is the one most often described. The following are three examples of heteromodal dysfunctions:

Wernicke's aphasia. An important consequence of damage to the heteromodal association areas are deficits in the multimodal integrations of visual, auditory and other sensory information which are needed for the comprehension and speaking of language. Typical of such a deficit is Wernicke's aphasia which is characterized by a comprehension deficit involving all aspects of language. Most single item deficits (e.g., word deafness, alexia, etc.) result from interruptions of one or more modality-specific inputs. Speech is possible if Broca's area is undamaged but it is nonsensical as are the responses to questions and comments.

Visuomotor and visuospatial disturbances. Deficits of this type are seen when the posterior parts of the heteromodal association area are affected, especially if the lesion is bilateral. In its most severe form the deficit may result in a global inability to orientate in space.

Damage to the prefrontal heteromodal association areas. There is rarely any effect on motor performance or sensory perception and recognition. The main consequences are disturbances in behavior and intellectual performance. The symptoms are bizarre combinations of any one or more of the following: unkempt and slovenly appearance and behavior; inappropriate apathy or happiness; poor judgment; decreased insight; inability to think logically; decrease in attention span; inability to organize simple chores; inappropriate and incorrect responses to questions; and other disorderly behaviors and intellectual disturbances.

The limbic system.

There are three filters that select for storage in long-term memory. Chart 2-7 tracks multimodal integrated information as it goes from the tempero-parietal heteromodal area on the lateral surface of the brain to the limbic cortex on its medial surface via the cingulate gyrus. The limbic system adds intellectual components to multimodal information: emotion; likes; dislikes; drive; affect (a medical term that somewhat imprecisely denotes feelings - it really denotes more); cultural and moral values; personal beliefs; autonomic tone; and other sentiments, some tangible, others not. The limbic systems and the hippocampus are the first group of the memory filters.

Inputs to the limbic system.

The principal inputs are from the heteromodal association areas.

Location of the limbic system.

The limbic cortex is a ring of gray matter that surrounds the interventricular foramen. It includes the following; the orbitofrontal cortex, areas of the medial temporal lobe including the hippocampus, the amygdala, the parahippocampal gyrus, the cingulate cortex, the fornix, the stria terminalis, the limbic nuclei of the thalamus, the mammilary bodies and the hypothalamus. These structures are interconnected in a complex manner - the Papez circuit[31] (Chart 2-7).

The role of the limbic system in remembering remains a bit controversial. There are those who maintain that severe amnesias only occur after bilateral involvement of limbic structures. Others maintain that the function of the limbic system is not to store but only to select the events and phenomena destined to reach the attention filters[32]. The correlation of clinical findings with pathological observations suggest that when limbic structures are damaged (especially the hippocampal and mammilary structures) any loss of memory mainly results in deficits involving anterograde memory. This suggests that the initial processing of material for storage in long-term memory takes place in the limbic cortex.

The following clinical syndromes are the result of pathology affecting the limbic structures.

They support the above contentions:

- **Herpes simplex encephalitis.** When mild, the disease may be confined to the amygdala, the hippocampus and parahippocampal gyrus; it has a predilection for limbic structures. The result may be a pure amnestic syndrome. The amnesia is typically anterograde with little loss of retrograde memory. Unfortunately, at times the disease is more severe and can result in what has been called "limbic dementia"[33]. The syndrome comes with disorders of insight, emotion and judgment, and disturbances of sexual behavior and appetite similar to those seen in the Kluver-Bucy syndrome.
- **The often quoted case of H.M.** H.M. was an epileptic subjected to bilateral excision of hippocampal areas. The result was severe anterograde amnesia that has remained unchanged for many years[34]. The cause of the amnesia has been ascribed to bilateral excision of amygdala, hippocampus and parahippocampal gyrus. I use the present tense as I believe H.M. is still alive.
- **Thiamine deficiency.** Thiamine deficiency is often, but not always, the result of excessive alcohol drinking. It is the usual cause of the Korsakoff syndrome. The syndrome is generally ascribed to bilateral lesions of the mammilary bodies, or in some instances, to lesions of the limbic nuclei of the thalamus. The memory deficit is typically one that involves new memories (anterograde amnesia). Indeed, Korsakoff's original patient could play a reasonable chess game but could not remember how any given position on the chess board had appeared. He had, of course, learnt the game previously and stored that information in long-term

Chart 2-7: MEDIAL SURFACE OF CEREBRAL HEMISPHERE: PROCESSED MULTIMODAL INFORMATION FROM THE TEMPERO-PARIETAL AREA ON THE LATERAL SURFACE PASSING TO THE LIMBIC CORTEX ON THE MEDIAL SURFACE [1,2]

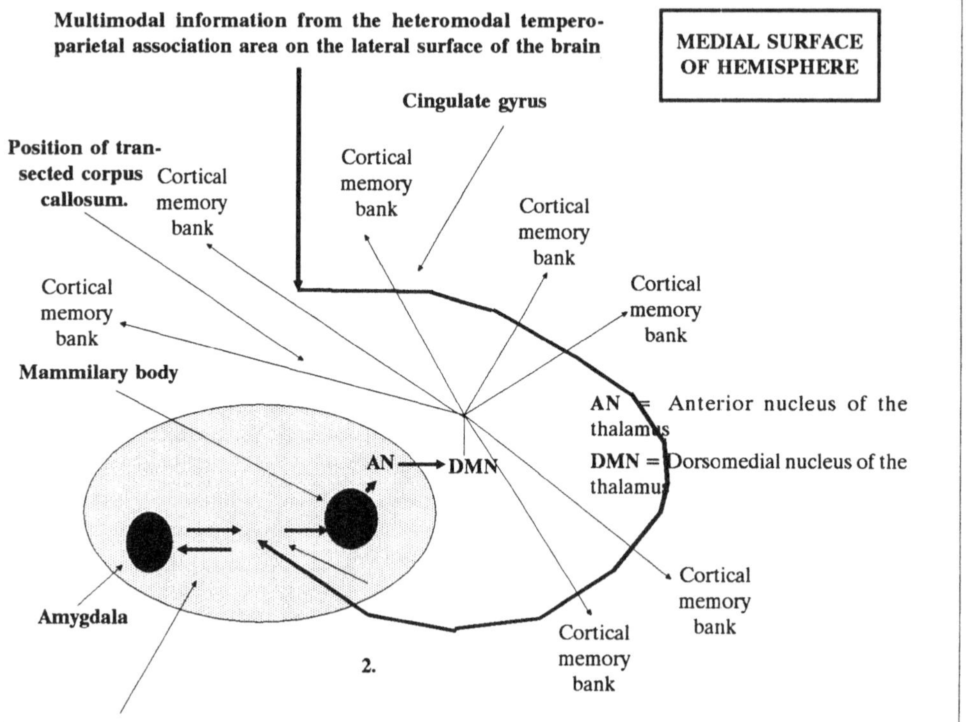
Multimodal information from the heteromodal tempero-parietal association area on the lateral surface of the brain
MEDIAL SURFACE OF HEMISPHERE
Cingulate gyrus
Position of transected corpus callosum.
Cortical memory bank
Cortical memory bank
Cortical memory bank
Cortical memory bank
Cortical memory bank
Mammilary body
AN = Anterior nucleus of the thalamus
DMN = Dorsomedial nucleus of the thalamus
AN → DMN
Cortical memory bank
Cortical memory bank
Amygdala
2.

THE LIMBIC CORTEX

Personalization of memories by integration with emotion, likes, dislikes, drive, affect, cultural and moral values, personal beliefs, autonomic tone, etc. The sequence is:

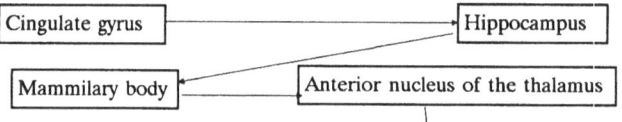

Cingulate gyrus → Hippocampus → Mammilary body → Anterior nucleus of the thalamus

Exit to dorso-medial nucleus of the thalamus (DMN) and then to the cortical memory banks.
Selection for storage in long-term memory depends on filtering by three filters: **the hippocampus and the limbic system, the attention filter and short-term memory.**

↓

Cortical memory banks of long-term memory

[1] The suggested scheme for selection and storage of information in long-term memory is a slight modification of one proposed by Eccles (Eccles, J.C. Evolution of the Brain: Creation of the Self. London and New York: Routledge. p.154. 1989.).

[2] Cerebral blood flow studies using radio-xenon (Roland, P.E., Friberg, L. Localization of cortical areas by thinking. J. Neurophysiol. 1985; 53:1219.) suggest that memories are stored in areas scattered throughout the cortex, with a preponderance in the prefrontal cortex. Controversies on this subject continue.

memory.

Miscellaneous causes of limbic dysfunctions.

Other examples of amnesia due to lesions of limbic structures include tumors of the hypothalamus and of the floor and walls of the third ventricle.

The memory filters.

The capacity of the brain is not infinite and the amount of information it receives continuously is immense. Only a small portion of this information is consciously recognized and of this, only a minute fraction is eventually stored in long-term memory. After the limbic system has chosen, two additional hurdles filter and select information that merits storage in long-term memory. They are the attention filter and short-term memory.

Accurate scientific information on the memory filters is meager. Most discussions of the memory filters are conjectured hypotheses based on the observations of experimental psychology. We know what happens but not how it is done. This is the frame of caveats for appropriate evaluations of what follows.

There are three principal memory filters which identify material which merits storage in long-term memory:

- **The limbic system and the hippocampus.** Destruction or disease of this complex results in an anterograde deficit of memory. The finding derives from studies of a patient called HM who had a hippocampectomy for seizures which were uncontrollable. The studies on HM are well reviewed in a paper by Milner[37]. There is a suggestion that some anterograde memory extends to short-term memory before rapid rejection
- **The attention filter.**
- **Short-term memory**

A hypothetical scheme of the processes that occur between recognition and the final selection of material for storage in memory is depicted in Chart 2-8.

The attention filter.

The attention filter is the second gate through which material must pass. Information that does not merit storage is excluded. All that passes through is next examined by short-term memory.

The attention filter is a theoretical concept with few known anatomical or physiological correlates. The concept is not new. Many neurologists as far back as the late 1800s have viewed attention as an important requirement for intellectual activity[35,36]. An excellent review of current material is by M-M. Mesulam[38].

Sokolov has proposed one of the more plausible hypotheses on the location and mode of action of attention filter components. He postulated[39] that the degree of attention tone is the result of interactions between cortical and reticular brain components. Painful stimuli activate the reticular components without cortical intervention. Stimuli of other types are first recognized in the cortex and after multimodal integration, impulses travel to the reticular system which determines the necessary level of attention tone. Impulses pass back to the cortex and thalamus to generate an orienting reflex: movements of head and eyes to positions that best perceive the new information, set the appropriate level of attention and facilitate responses to the new information.

This reticular activating system is probably an important modulator of levels of sleep and wakefulness and this provides some support for Sokolov's hypothesis. Since Sokolov's postulate other hypotheses have been proposed to explain the attention filter. Their detailing is not germane in the present context.

Dysfunctions of the attention filter.

A confusional state is characteristic of damage to the attention filter. Thinking is confused because of frequent interruptions by unfiltered irrelevant thoughts, ideas and sensations. Individuals become incoherent, easily distracted and incapable of purposeful and coordinated movements. Many areas of the brain in addition to the reticular activating system set attentional tone. Efferents from the heteromodal areas and those generated by movements and thoughts also affect attention tone, probably by connections with the reticular system.

Many different pathologies can affect any one or more of these structures and cause confusional states. Examples are the many metabolic and toxic conditions that act as encephalopathies. The possible causes of such en-

Chart 2-8: THE MEMORY FILTERS

There are three memory filters: the limbic system, the attention filter and short-term memory

Information from the external environment

Perception and reception are not optional. All stimuli are perceived, generate neural impulses (adaptation of receptors is the exception to this rule) and are recognized. The attention filters are one of the gates which select what, if any, of this information merits storage in long-term memory.

Information from the internal environment

Receptors for stimuli originating in the external environment (visual, auditory, cutaneous pain and other sensations, kinesthetic and positional information, and changes in temperature, pressure, and sensations of vibration). →

Primary reception and association areas → hetero-modal association areas → **limbic cortex**

← Receptors for stimuli originating in the body (pain, visceral sensations, osmotic and blood pressure changes, and proprioceptive impulses). Except for pain, most are not perceived consciously but are the afferent limbs of long arm negative and positive feedback reflexes mediated by centers in the medulla and hypothalamus.

↓

The first memory filter: the hippocampus and limbic cortex

The transfer of material which could merit storage in long-term memory is transmitted to the other two memory filters by neurons in the hippocampus and limbic area which together comprise the first memory filter. Studies on H.M. have shown that limbic dysfunction results in anterograde amnesia (i.e., inability to receive and record new information).

↓

The second memory filter: the attention filter and signal

The "attention signal" recognizes information which has been processed and passed along by the limbic cortex. The information which could merit subsequent storage in long-term memory, is passed on to the last memory filter: short-term memory. The rest is deleted and forgotten.

Attention filtering in this filter probably results from neural interactions between the cortex and the reticular system, a hypothesis originally postulated by Sokolov [1].

↓

The third and last memory filter: short-term memory

The capacity of short-term memory is small. The number of packages of information that can be remembered at any one time is between 5-9. Short-term memory determines what material is stored in long-term memory. Whatever is not to be stored is deleted. For example a phone number which requires a response on an occasional basis would be stored in short-term memory, responded to and then deleted. A phone number which is used frequently is stored in long-term memory. Examples are ones home and business numbers and those of close friends and relatives with whom there are frequent communications.

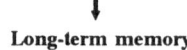

↓

Long-term memory

[1] Sokolov, E.N.: Neuronal models and the orienting reflex. In Brazier, M. (Ed.): The central nervous system and behavior. Madison, N.J. Madison Printing, 1960.

cephalopathies are many: fevers; infections, especially urinary and pulmonary infections in the elderly; hepatic and renal failure; hyperglycemia and hypoglycemia; disturbances of acid-base balance; over-ingestion or withdrawal of alcohol, barbiturates, opium derivatives, cocaine and other so-called recreational drugs; unexpected adverse reactions to therapeutic drugs used correctly and for appropriate reasons; and many brain diseases. Examples are meningitis and encephalitis, cerebrovascular accidents and other vascular lesions, emboli (atheromatous, fat or air), degenerative diseases (e.g., Alzheimer's disease), trauma, subdural hematomas, post-epileptic states, and space-occupying lesions (benign, malignant or inflammatory, e.g., abscesses and tuberculomas), with or without accompanying raised intracranial pressure.

Short-term memory.

Information that has passed through the attention filter is next examined in short-term memory. The capacity of short-term memory is small. It has been estimated that the number of packages of information that can be remembered in short-term memory is between 5 and 9. Indeed most information that enters short-term memory is forgotten and after about 15-20 seconds there is little or no recall of information not transferred to long-term memory. The size of the information package or chunk depends on how the individual processes information. The process of chunking becomes better as individuals learn better ways of remembering and devise more efficient ways of handling information. Determination of what merits remembering and the methods used for remembering seem to be unique to each individual.

Material that passes the attention filter and short-term memory for storage in long-term memory is probably selected automatically by internal commands, previously generated by the individual. They are probably similar to the verbalizations or thought processes of the same individual. Observations and experience are the most likely sources for development of such commands and they could be incorporated in existing memory composites which would know what additions were needed for the composite. Once remembered the individual can improve selection by appropriate modifications of previous commands, or generation of new ones that meet specific needs.

Other aids for selection include protocols, mnemonics, words and phrases. Improvements of remembering are especially important for physicians who, by the nature of their profession, must remember, analyze and make composites of many facts and experiences for future use.

The attention filter and short-term memory are as Scylla and Charybdis, guarding the portal of entry into the vast cavern of long-term memory, turning away what does not merit entrance and, with reluctance, allowing entrance to that which does. The allusion is particularly apt as it is probable that there is a to and fro filtration and deletion of unnecessary information between the attention filter and short-term memory, till the final selection of material that merits entry into long-term memory.

Memory filters and computers compared.

The existence of memory filters highlights the differences between the brain and the computer. The computer operator exercises control by keyboard entry. It is not necessary to enter everything but it is easier to do so than to discriminate. Everything can be entered, stored and accessed because of the speed, the storage capabilities and accessibility of material stored in a computer.

The human brain functions many thousand times slower than a computer. In addition, the information recognized at any one time is immense; consider the numbers of items recognized in a mundane activity such as a short walk along a busy street. Chaos would result if there were no control on material entering long-term memory. This control is exercised by the hippocampus and limbic system, the attention filter and short-term memory. Without them no orderly and sensible brain function would be possible.

In addition, because of different designs, the human brain and the computer store and retrieve information in different ways. In general, the former initially use unplanned and heuristic non-linear rules for reasoning. Computer function is generally based on preplanned linear and parallel-processed algorithmic type reasoning and rapid retrieval.

This ends a short chapter that summarizes the processes of reasoning and remembering.

Chapter 2 References.

1. The Confessions of St. Augustine. Translation by Pilkington, J,G. New York. The Heritage Press, 1963.

2. Tulving, E. Episodic and semantic memory. In: Tulving, E. & Donaldson, W. (Eds.): Organization of Memory. New York. Academic Press, 1972.

3. Tulving, E. Episodic memory: from mind to brain. Annu. Rev. Psychol. 2002; 53:1.

4. Tulving, E. Episodic memory and common sense; how far apart? Philos. Trans. R Soc. London Biol. Sci. 2001; 29:356.

5. Kosslyn, S.M. Image and Mind. Boston, Mass. Harvard University Press, 1980

6. Dehn, N & Schank, R. Artificial and human intelligence. In, Sternberg R.J. (Ed.): Handbook of Human Intelligence. Cambridge. Cambridge University Press, 1982.

7. Churchland, P.S. Neurophilosophy: Toward a Unified Understanding of the Mind\Brain. Boston, Mass. The MIT Press, 1986.

8. Polya, G. How to solve it: A new aspect of mathematical method. Princeton, N.J. Princeton University Press, 1945.

9. Baron, J. Thinking and deciding. Cambridge. Cambridge University Press, 1988.

10. Sherman, S.J. & Corty, E. Cognitive heuristics. In Wyer, R.S. & Skrull, T.K. (Eds.): Handbook of social cognition. (Vol. 1). Hillsdale, N.J. Lawrence Erlbaum Associates, 1984.

11. Kahneman, D., Slovic, P. & Tversky, A. (Eds.): Judgment under uncertainty: Heuristics and biases. New York. Cambridge University Press, 1982.

12. Skryms, B. Choice and chance (2nd. edition). Encino, California. Dickenson, 1975.

13. Knuth, D. Fundamental algorithms. Reading, Mass. Addison-Wesley, 1973.

14. Pauker, S.G. & Kassirer, J.P. Clinical decision analysis. N. Engl. J Med. 1987; 316:250.

15. Eccles, J.C. Evolution of the Brain: Creation of the Self. New York. Routledge, 1989.

16. Ito, M. The Cerebellum and Neural Control. New York. Raven press, 1984,

17. Solzenhytsin, A.I. The Gulag Archipelago Three. (Translated by H. Willetts). New York. Harper and Row, 1978.

18. Lashley, K.S. 1929. Brain mechanisms and intelligence. Chicago. Univ. of Chicago Press. (Reprinted in 1963 with introduction by D.O. Hebb.)

19. Anderson J Bower G. Human associative memory. Washington, D.C. V.H.Winston, 1973.

20. Estes, W. Structural aspects of associative models for memory. In: Cofer, C. (Ed.), The structure of human memory. San Francisco. W.H.Freeman, 1976.

21. Anderson, J. Language, memory and thought. Hillsdale, N.J. Erlbaum, 1976.

22. Collins, A. & Loftus, E. A spreading-activation theory of semantic processing. Psychological review 1975; 82:407.

23. Norman, D. & Rumelhart, D. Explorations in cognition. San Francisco. W.H.Freeman, 1975.

24. Schiffrin, R. Memory Search. In: Norman, D.A. (Ed.), Models for memory. New York. Academic Press, 1970.

25. Simon, H. Information processing theory of human problem solving. In: Estes, W.K. (Ed.), Handbook of learning and cognitive processes. (Vol. 5). Hillsdale, N.J. Erlbaum, 1978.

26. Posner, M. & Rossman, E. Effect of size and location of informational transforms on short-term retention. Journ. Experimental Psychology 1965; 70:496.

27. Posner, M. Short-term memory systems in human information-processing. Acta Psychologica 1967; 27:267.

28. Chi, M., Feltovich, P. et al. Categorization and representation of physics problems by experts and novices. Cognitive Science 1981; 5:121.

29. Newell, A., Simon, H. Human problem solving. Englewood Cliffs, N.J. Prentice-Hall, 1972.

30. Seltzer, B., Pandya, D.N. Some cortical projections to the hippocampal area in the rhesus monkey. Exp. Neurol. 1976; 50:146.

31. Papez, W. A proposed mechanism of emotion. Arch. Neurol. Psychiatry. 1937; 38:725.

32. Signoret, J.L. Memory and amnesias. In: Behavioral Neurology. Ed.: Mesulam, M-M. Philadelphia. F.A.Davis Co, 1985 (a good review of subject).

33. Gascon G.G., Gilles, F. Limbic dementia. J. Neurol. Neurosurg. Psychiatry 1973; 36:421.

34. Milner, B., Corkin, S., Teuber, H.L. Further analysis of the hippocampal amnesic syndrome: 14 years follow-up study of H.M. Neuropsychologia. 1968; 6:215

35. Ferrier, D. Functions of the brain. New York. Putnam, 1880.

36. James, W. The Principles of Psychology. New York. Holt, 1890.

37. r(Milner, B. The medial temporal-lobe amnesic syndrome. Psychiatr. Clin. North Am. 2005; 28:599).

38. Mesulam, M-M. Attention, Confusional States and Neglect. In Mesulam, M-M. (Ed.): Principles of Behavioral Neurology. Philadelphia. F.A. Davis, 1985.

39. Sokolov, E.N. Neuronal models and the orienting reflex. In Brazier, M. (Ed.): The Central Nervous System and Behavior. Madison N.J. Madison Printing, 1960.

3

Clinical Decision-Making: Some Basic Principles

3. The Clinical Assessment

Table of Contents

Disease defined.

The Pocket Oxford Dictionary defines **disease** as an "unhealthy condition of body or mind; illness, sickness, etc.". It is a good definition because it does not imply that disease always results in physiological dysfunction. Disease can exist without demonstrable physiological dysfunctions. This is because mechanisms that compensate for dysfunction can negate the effects of disease (Chart 3-1).

Dysfunction defined.

A dysfunction is an increase or decrease of function which transgresses physiologically permissible and desirable limits. It may affect a single organ or a biological system complex and results from disease, or aging, and often, from a combination of both. When compensation is inadequate dysfunctions present as symptoms and signs.

Syndrome defined.

A syndrome is the concurrent or sequential appearance of symptoms and signs suggestive of a specific clinical disorder. Some symptoms, signs, or both are requisites for diagnosis of a specific dysfunction. Others might not be though they could be concurrent or appear later.

In fact, additional symptoms and signs can, and often do appear later. They may confirm the initial assessment. Alternatively, they could create doubts about its correctness. Additional symptoms and signs could also indicate

Chart 3-1: ALTERNATIVE CLINICAL PRESENTATIONS OF CLINICAL DYSFUNCTIONS

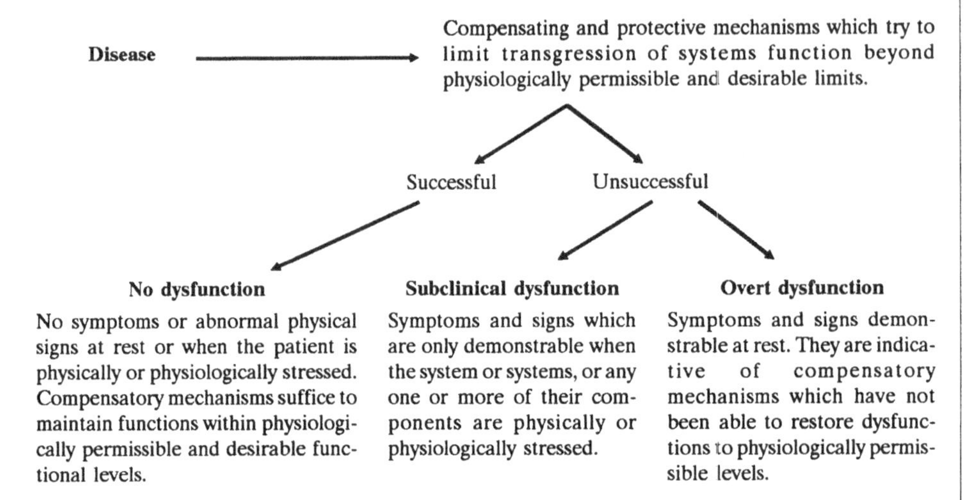
Disease
Compensating and protective mechanisms which try to limit transgression of systems function beyond physiologically permissible and desirable limits.
Successful
Unsuccessful
No dysfunction
No symptoms or abnormal physical signs at rest or when the patient is physically or physiologically stressed. Compensatory mechanisms suffice to maintain functions within physiologically permissible and desirable functional levels.
Subclinical dysfunction
Symptoms and signs which are only demonstrable when the system or systems, or any one or more of their components are physically or physiologically stressed.
Overt dysfunction
Symptoms and signs demonstrable at rest. They are indicative of compensatory mechanisms which have not been able to restore dysfunctions to physiologically permissible levels.

the existence of previously unsuspected problems involving other structures. Incidentally, aging is not a disease but the reductions in physiological function associated with aging often exacerbate the effects of pathology.

Diagnosis.

Diagnosis identifies the nature of a clinical problem. Many have emphasized the importance of accurate diagnosis for making correct clinical decisions. A comment Ryle[1] once made is often cited:

> "the three main tasks of the clinician are diagnosis, prognosis and treatment. Of these diagnosis is by far the most important, for upon it the success of the other two depends."

Ryle's statement is correct only if "diagnosis" means a comprehensive assessment of the clinical status. The word "diagnosis" derives from the Greek verbal combination of "*δια−*" which means "thoroughly" and "*γιγνϖακειν*" which means "to perceive, to learn, or to know" (Oxford English Dictionary).

Diagnosis is not simply the identification of a complex clinical problem by name. It also requires assessment of all related, and seemingly unrelated systems to identify any which might need functional amplification or dampening. The objective is restoration of the coordinated and integrated functions of all systems. This integration and coordination ensures that humans can perform with characteristic smooth, precise and purposeful volitional movements, that they can reason, decide and mentate normally and perceive, recognize, remember, recall and respond to sensory information correctly. At times restoration of systems integration and coordination is not possible. The objective then becomes prevention or retardation of additional deterioration of systems integration and coordination.

Animates are mortal beings. At some point in the life of every individual uncontrollable progression of dysfunction is inevitable. When the condition is preterminal the only functions of the physician are relief of pain and suffering; not additional unnecessary, often unpleasant and useless additional investigations and therapies.

A post-mortem diagnosis at an autopsy or clinicopathological conference helps jog memory on future occasions. A clinical problem that is current requires a thorough and comprehensive premortem assessment. It is essential that all factors relating to the presenting illness are known.

Chart 3-2: CLINICAL ASSESSMENT (STEP 1): THE HISTORY

STEP 1 THE HISTORY		PHYSICIAN
Verbal, gestural and prosodic interactions between patient and physician.	↔	Simultaneous back and forth search in memory for recollections of previously encountered situations which are similar or comparable.
Preliminary heuristic generation of one or more hypotheses on the nature of the clinical problem. Operational memory is generated and kept activated[1].	← / →	Proceed to **STEP 2 (the physical examinations)**.

[1] Operational memory is memorized information, selectively chosen for resolution of the current problem, and kept in an activated state till the problem is resolved (Posner, M & Rossman, E.: J. Exptl. Psychology 1965; 70:496). It lets one bypass masses of irrelevant information while assessing the problem.

Chart 3-3: CLINICAL ASSESSMENT (STEP 2): THE CLINICAL EXAMINATION

STEP 2 THE CLINICAL EXAMINATION		PHYSICIAN
This should be as much an interactive process between patient and physician as was the taking of the history.	↔	Simultaneous back and forth search in memory for factual information and for recollections of previously encountered situations which are similar or comparable.
Deletion or modification of one or more of the heuristic hypotheses generated in Step 1 and/or addition of new ones.	←	
From now on the validity of each hypothesis generated by heuristic reasoning should be verified by factual information in semantic memory or in books, journals, CD-ROMs or by information obtained from colleagues and specialists. Any hypothesis which is not compatible with factual information must be modified or deleted and replaced.	→	Proceed to **STEP 3 (ancillary investigations.)**.

Chart 3-4: CLINICAL ASSESSMENT (STEP 3): ANCILLARY INVESTIGATIONS

STEP 3 ANCILLARY INVESTIGATIONS		PHYSICIAN
They include examinations of blood and urine, and when appropriate, the stools. Other investigations include X-rays, cytology of cervical scrapings, body fluids and aspirates, biopsies, ultrasounds, CT scans, MRIs, electroencephalograms and electromyograms. Practically no patient-physician interaction is involved at this stage, The interaction begins when the information obtained is given to the patient and discussed.	↔	Each and every hypothesis generated by heuristic reasoning, whether in Step 2, or on the basis of the findings in Step 2 plus the results of ancillary investigations, must be compatible with factual information in semantic memory or in books, journals, CD-ROMs, and Internet web sites or obtained from colleagues and specialists. If the hypothesis or hypotheses are not compatible with factual information modifications and, at times deletions are essential. Eventually when the hypothesis or hypotheses on the clinical problem are compatible with the clinical findings and the accepted facts of clinical medicine, physiology and physiological pathology **proceed to Step 4 (the clinical reassessment loop - Chart 3-5)**.

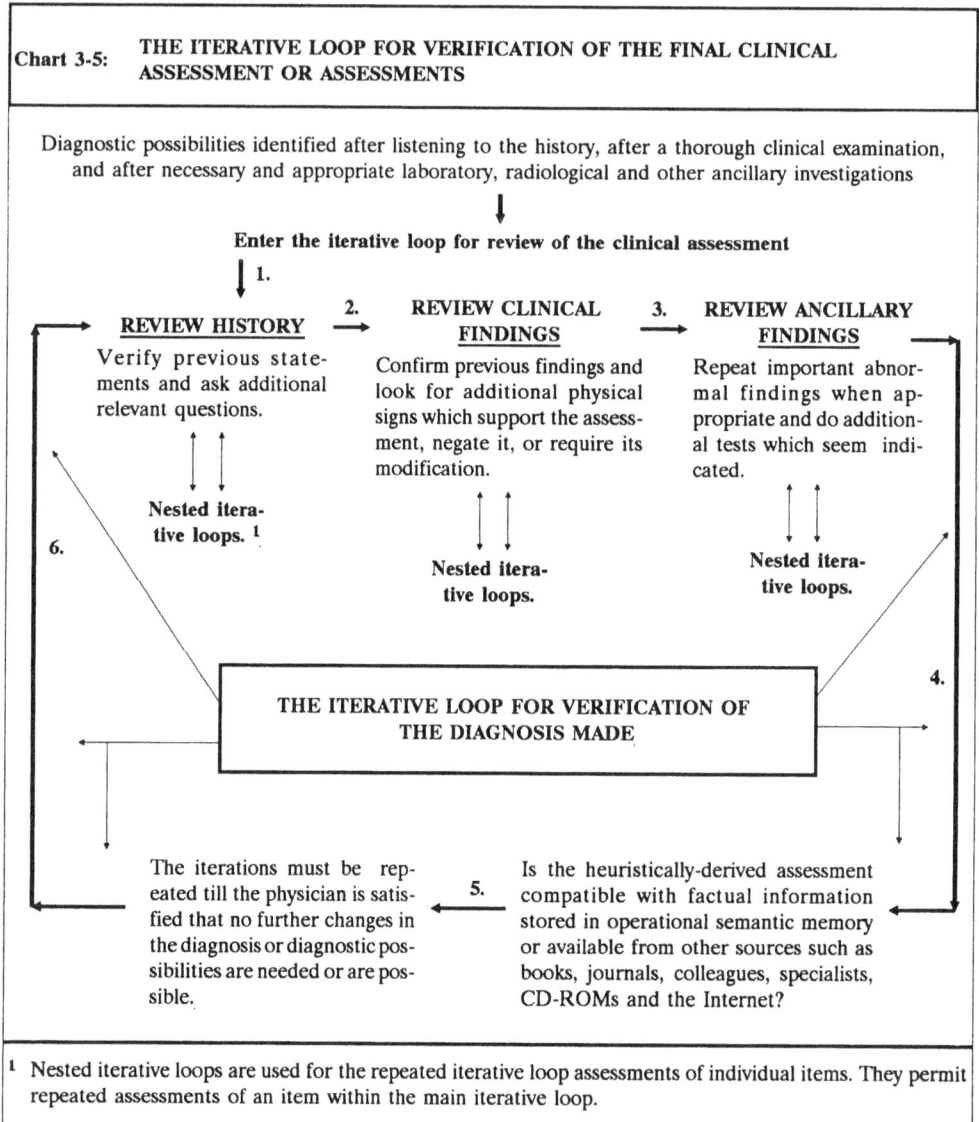

Chart 3-5: **THE ITERATIVE LOOP FOR VERIFICATION OF THE FINAL CLINICAL ASSESSMENT OR ASSESSMENTS**

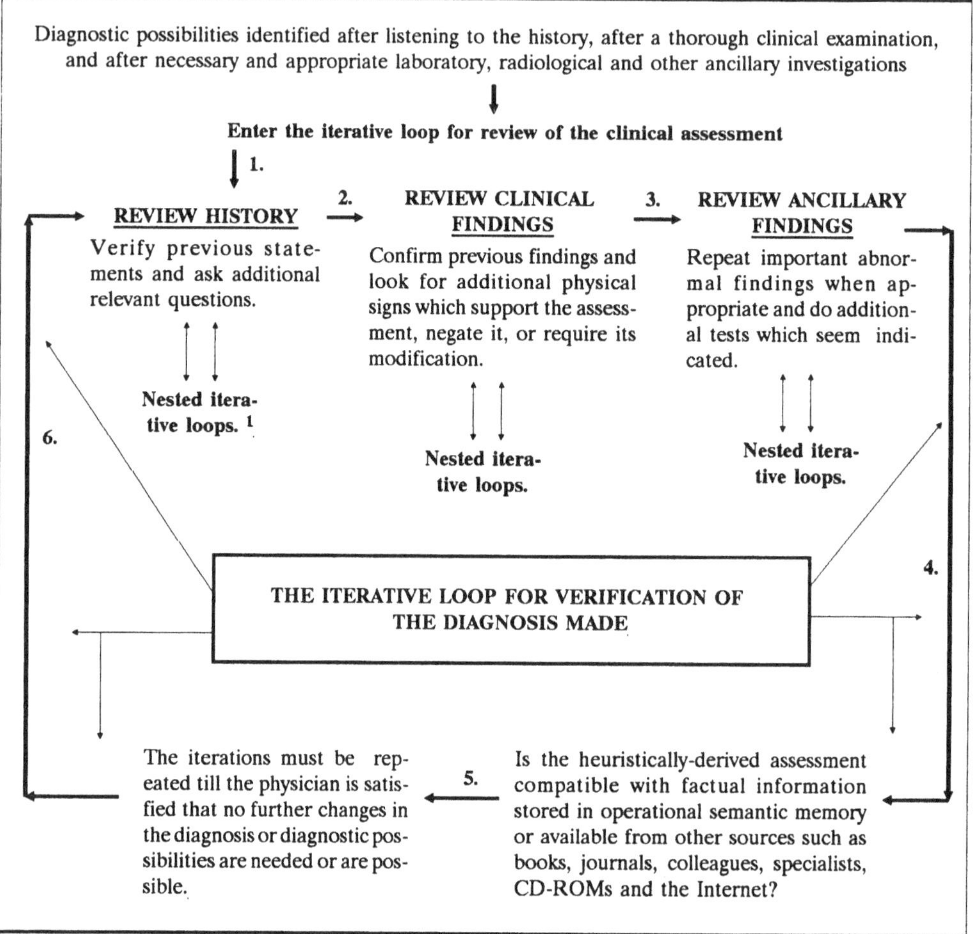
Diagnostic possibilities identified after listening to the history, after a thorough clinical examination, and after necessary and appropriate laboratory, radiological and other ancillary investigations
Enter the iterative loop for review of the clinical assessment
1.
REVIEW HISTORY
Verify previous statements and ask additional relevant questions.
Nested iterative loops. [1]
2.
REVIEW CLINICAL FINDINGS
Confirm previous findings and look for additional physical signs which support the assessment, negate it, or require its modification.
Nested iterative loops.
3.
REVIEW ANCILLARY FINDINGS
Repeat important abnormal findings when appropriate and do additional tests which seem indicated.
Nested iterative loops.
4.
THE ITERATIVE LOOP FOR VERIFICATION OF THE DIAGNOSIS MADE
Is the heuristically-derived assessment compatible with factual information stored in operational semantic memory or available from other sources such as books, journals, colleagues, specialists, CD-ROMs and the Internet?
5.
The iterations must be repeated till the physician is satisfied that no further changes in the diagnosis or diagnostic possibilities are needed or are possible.
6.

[1] Nested iterative loops are used for the repeated iterative loop assessments of individual items. They permit repeated assessments of an item within the main iterative loop.

The assessments of dysfunctions.

The first step is a thorough clinical assessment. Charts 3-2 - 3-6 summarize the requirements. Textual amplification is not needed. Clinical dysfunctions and dysfunctional syndromes can affect any one or more of many system complexes: neurological; cardiac; pulmonary; renal; endocrine; metabolic; and the systems which protect against environmental hazards and environmental pathogens.

Infections remain the most common of all dysfunctions affecting humans. They range from minimal self-limiting viral infections to infections which are difficult to treat and often fatal. Examples of those which can be fatal include infections with virulent pathogens and infections by an overwhelming number of pathogens of normal virulence. Pathogens include bacteria, viruses, rickettsiae and parasites and other pathogenic organisms. When there is decreased immunological competence, for example in people with HIV/AIDS infections, normal body commensals can become pathogenic and cause opportunistic infections.

A diagnostic assessment needs all relevant information. Myocardial infarction is a common affliction and a frequent cause of long-term disability and death. It is chosen to show how much more information is needed for a comprehensive clinical assessment once the physician has made the initial diagnosis.

The patient presents with clinical, biochemical and ECG changes of a myocardial infarct. The basic diagnosis has been made. The following are examples of additional information needed:

- How many hours have passed since the pain of the myocardial infarct started or did the patient go to the hospital immediately after it began.
- Its severity. How bad is the pain? Did it need an opiate such as morphine for control?
- What is the temporal status of any existing cardiac dysfunction? Is it acute, chronic, acute superimposed on chronic, or progressive disease, (Chart 3-6)?

Chart 3-6: THE TEMPORAL PHASES OF DISEASE: POSSIBLE ONSETS AND OUTCOMES

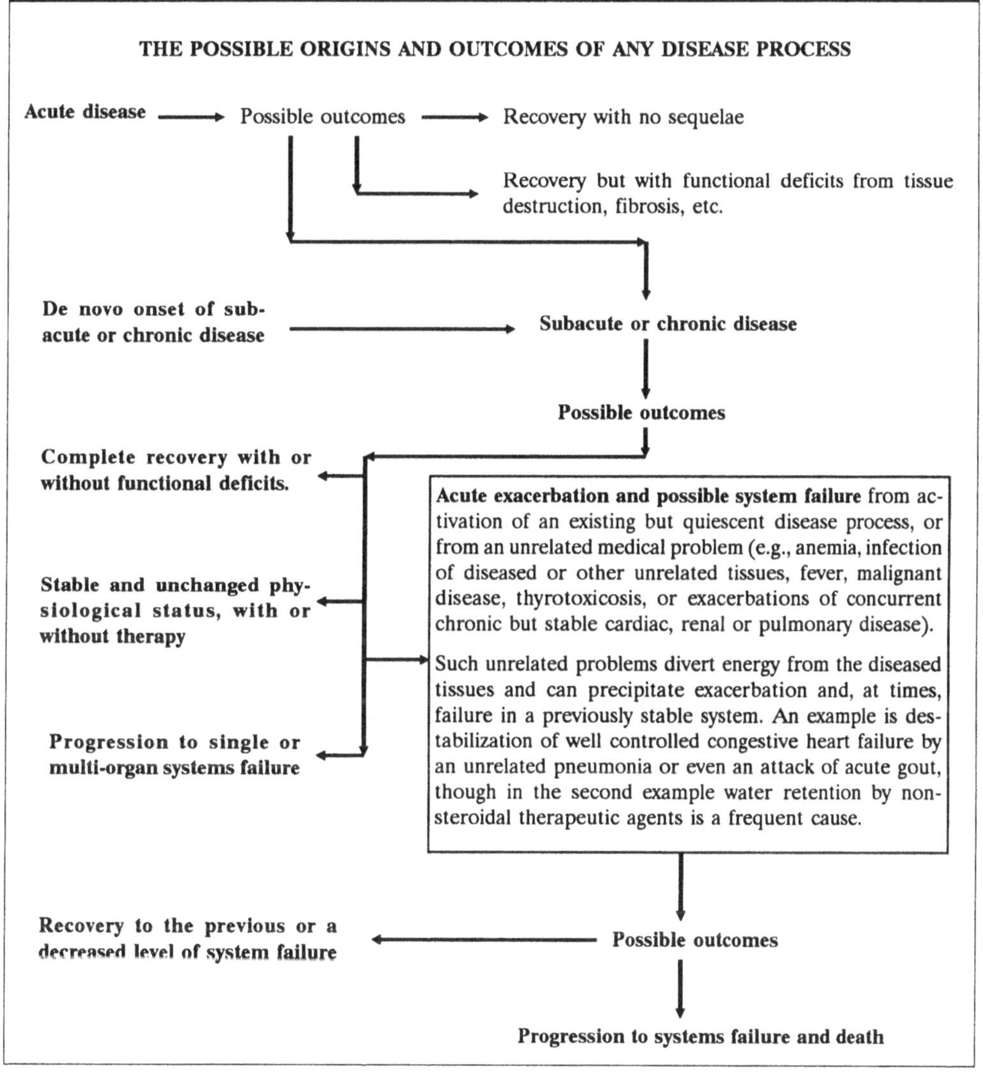
THE POSSIBLE ORIGINS AND OUTCOMES OF ANY DISEASE PROCESS
Acute disease
Possible outcomes
Recovery with no sequelae
Recovery but with functional deficits from tissue destruction, fibrosis, etc.
De novo onset of subacute or chronic disease
Subacute or chronic disease
Possible outcomes
Complete recovery with or without functional deficits.
Stable and unchanged physiological status, with or without therapy
Progression to single or multi-organ systems failure
Acute exacerbation and possible system failure from activation of an existing but quiescent disease process, or from an unrelated medical problem (e.g., anemia, infection of diseased or other unrelated tissues, fever, malignant disease, thyrotoxicosis, or exacerbations of concurrent chronic but stable cardiac, renal or pulmonary disease).
Such unrelated problems divert energy from the diseased tissues and can precipitate exacerbation and, at times, failure in a previously stable system. An example is destabilization of well controlled congestive heart failure by an unrelated pneumonia or even an attack of acute gout, though in the second example water retention by non-steroidal therapeutic agents is a frequent cause.
Recovery to the previous or a decreased level of system failure
Possible outcomes
Progression to systems failure and death

- What is your clinical estimate of the functional reserve of the heart and of effectiveness of existing mechanisms which compensate for cardiac dysfunctions? Is there any evidence of acute cardiogenic failure resulting in marked hypotension? Is there any evidence of milder heart failure manifested by a raised jugular venous pressure?
- Is there any previous history of one or more myocardial infarcts? If the patient has had a previous myocardial

infarct what was the treatment given and what was the response to the therapy? Have there been persistent symptoms of angina or shortness of breath since then?

— Is there any previous history of angina on exertion or at rest?

— Does the patient have any arrhythmia or is there a previous history of an arrhytmia which was resolved by therapy?

— Are there any additional cardiac dysfunctions such as valvular disease, or uncontrolled or poorly controlled hypertension?

— What medications, if any, are the patient receiving for cardiac and/or non-cardiac problems?

— Do you think that atheromatous coronary artery disease has caused the infarct? If you do is there any evidence that similar pathology is also causing dysfunctions in areas supplied by other blood vessels (e.g., the carotid-vertebrobasilar complex, the peripheral limb vasculatures, the blood vessels of the kidneys or the mesenteric blood vessels)? More specifically, is there any previous history of transient ischemic attacks, stroke, or of peripheral vascular disease?

— Is there any evidence of an infection affecting any other organ or system? Is there fever? Is the patient anemic? Is there a coexisting or previous history of any acute or chronic disease affecting other organs or organ systems. For example:

- Pulmonary disease such as acute inflammations, pulmonary emboli, pneumothorax, bronchiectasis, and/or chronic obstructive lung disease or asthma.
- Neurological disease.
- Renal problems, hepatic and/or endocrine disease.
- Malignant disease (primary, metastatic, or both).
- Immunological deficits (e.g., due to AIDS), or abnormal immunological reactions (e.g., autoimmune blood cell or joint disease, and immune complex dysfunctions).

— Is there any history of adverse reactions to specific drugs?

— Is the proposed therapy acceptable to the patient? Is it affordable? Is it available?

— Have all the risks and benefits of proposed therapy been detailed to the patient? Has the patient given informed consent to any proposed thrombolytic therapy (verbally or in writing)?

— Finally, are there any other factors which could have relevance to proposed therapy?

— Does the Institution have any previous medical records about the patient? If they do a review of the records is essential.

The basics of clinical decision-making.

Chart 3-7 summarizes the sequential steps needed for clinical decision-making. It emphasizes the need for liberal use of iterative loops for correct assessments.

Often etiology cannot be identified. No matter. Satisfactory therapy can be provided on the basis of a "most likely" etiology. Many patients with congestive heart failure are adequately controlled without specific identification and demonstration of the cause. Usually it is assumed that cause is myocardial insufficiency due to coronary artery disease.

Chart 3-7: ITERATIVE LOOPS AS USED IN CLINICAL ASSESSMENTS

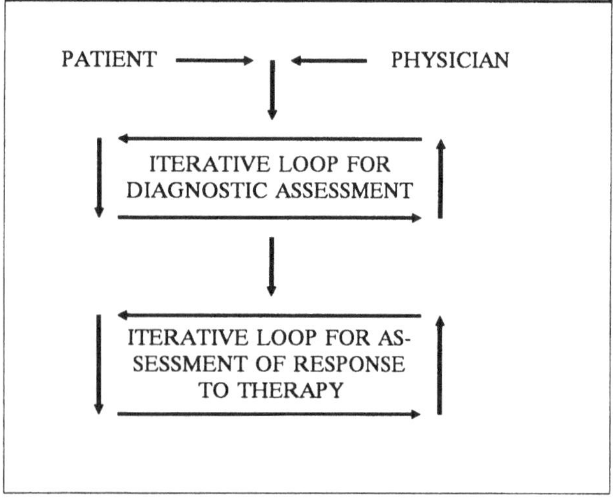
PATIENT
PHYSICIAN
ITERATIVE LOOP FOR DIAGNOSTIC ASSESSMENT
ITERATIVE LOOP FOR ASSESSMENT OF RESPONSE TO THERAPY

The second and more important step is the decision on therapy. This can be a complex problem. The last three chapters of this book discuss this topic in detail.

Diagnostic difficulties.

The clinical assessment will usually provide a fairly good idea of the nature of the disease or dysfunctional syndrome. However, on occasion the clinical picture is difficult to assess, especially in the early stages of a disease. When additional symptoms and signs appear the uncertainties are often resolved. There might remain a few unresolved and puzzling problems for any one or more reasons. The following lists some examples of such difficulties.

The patient's only symptom is shortness of breath.

This is a symptom which can indicate cardiac disease or respiratory disease. A previous history will indicate if it is part of the recovery process from an acute illness, from debilitating anti-cancer therapy, from inadequate nutrition or from a variety of other disorders. The exclusion of cardiac or respiratory disease is of prime importance.

Case history.

Patient age 45 was seen because of shortness of breath. There were no other symptoms and no previous history of any medical problem. Clinical examination was normal as was the chest X-ray and ECG. A treadmill exercise test suggested coronary artery disease and a radionuclear myogram showed significant deficits of myocardial vascularization. An angiogram showed two significant stenoses which were treated with stent angioplasties. There was no positive response to this therapy. Post-angioplasty therapy included a beta blocker and it was only when his dyspnea became worse that one realized that he probably also had a pulmonary disease exacerbated by the beta blocker. A previous chest X-ray, spirometry and CT scan of the chest were normal and I remained puzzled as to the cause of his dyspnea. Beta blockers were stopped but dyspnea continued. The problem remained puzzling and the clinical picture gradually worsened.

The patient was questioned again about his lifestyle, work and history. When initially asked about his work he had said that he worked in a factory which coated metal sheets for others. Physicians know little about industrial processes and initially, this line of questioning was not pursued. Later it was. He told me that he did galvanizing. A friend told me that this was the coating of iron with zinc in order to prevent rusting. The patient was always exposed to zinc fumes even though he used a mask. He then spontaneously told us that dyspnea always disappeared within a week of starting his annual vacation. The pulmonary dysfunction was due to zinc sensitivity. He found another job and is not dyspneic anymore. The cardiac dysfunction was a red herring but one which needed therapy. He has resumed taking a beta blocker each day as a prophylactic against any subsequent coronary incident.

The message of this case is manifold. First, when shortness of breath is the only symptom it can be difficult to determine if the cause is cardiac or respiratory. Second, never prejudge. Third, view every form of therapy as a clinical experiment. If it is not successful go back to the beginning and review other possibilities. Last, but perhaps most important of all, when taking a history inquire about everything, however irrelevant it might seem to you. In this instance I was at fault for not inquiring for more details about his work. I thought coating metal sheets for others was some mysterious procedure unrelated to his dyspnea.

Unusual headaches.

Beware of atypical headaches.

Case history.

Patient of 52 came to the office complaining of headache of two days duration. He assumed it was just a non-specific headache of no importance. On the morning of his visit the pain had become severe and was now mainly on the left side of his head. He had been a patient of mine for the previous 18 years and I knew that he had a high threshold for pain. Thus, I took serious note of his symptoms. There was no history of trauma but the patient was on medication for hypertension. Clinical examination was negative. There were no neurological deficits, pupillary reactions were normal and the blood pressure was 120/80. The headache was atypical and when I saw him it was intense. A CT scan was done. It showed a large subdural hematoma on the left side. Surgical evacuation was done just as he was beginning to lose the ability to speak. There was complete recovery. The cause of the hematoma was never identified; I am told that even straining at stool can cause such lesions.

The message is that most headaches are benign idiopathic reactions but beware of headaches having atypical features. This is especially important if there has been any trauma, if the patient is elderly, if there is history of malignant disease in some other part of the body (hemorrhage from metastatic brain lesions is not infrequent), and if there are concurrent hematological diseases and/or anticoagulation medications. Neurological deficits are often absent in the early stages of a subdural hemorrhage.

Multiple etiologies.

Multiple etiologies can, and often do coexist. They may affect multiple organs and systems. Consequently, a difficult medical problem can result from a complex of multisystem disease; one or more different pathologies affecting one or more organ systems, and often caused by one or more different etiologies. The result is a multisystem dysfunction with each dysfunctional complex contributing some or all of its clinical features to the pool of signs and symptoms. Difficulties in clinical assessments are common in such situations.

Systems failure may be primary, or secondary to failure of another system or systems.

A dysfunction could represent the functional failure of one or more mechanisms which have adequately compensated for the functional deficits of the primary disease. Symptoms and signs from the primary disease could be absent or minimal while clinical features resulting from failure of mechanisms for compensation predominate.

Common and uncommon manifestations of disease.

Usually dysfunctions present in any one of the following ways:

— As an acute hypofunction syndrome.

— As a subacute or chronic hypofunction syndrome.

— As an acute hyperfunction syndrome.

— Or as a subacute or chronic hyperfunction syndrome.

They may not present in any of these four ways and the following are some examples of atypical presentations:

Organ dysfunction without symptoms or physical signs.

Diagnosis is by incidental findings on routine examination. Alternatively, the patient may, on occasion, present with only the most trivial manifestations of dysfunction. The following is an example:

Myocardial infarction.

An estimate is that 15-20% of myocardial infarctions are painless and often symptomless. At annual medical examinations I have occasionally noted that the ECG, when compared with one done a year or so previously, indicated that a silent infarct had occurred during the year. Another example is a myocardial infarction where the only symptom is an episode of profuse sweating.

Case history.

A priest, age 52, consulted me because of increased shortness of breath during his morning walk. He told me this began after Easter Sunday. During the service there was profuse sweating when he raised the chalice. No pain or other symptoms. An ECG showed a fairly recent infarct. Progression eventually required by-pass surgery. He died twelve years later from another acute infarct.

Organ dysfunction identified by unexpected and incidental radiological and/or laboratory findings.

Occasionally organ dysfunction is only recognized from incidental laboratory and/or radiological findings. The following are some common examples:

— The unexpected finding of lung pathology from a routine chest X-ray: examples are tuberculosis, tumors, granulomas, atelectases and pleural effusions.

- The unexpected finding of an impalpable breast tumor on a mammogram.
- A diagnosis of hypothyroidism or hyperthyroidism without characteristic clinical features but with routine blood tests which showed abnormal levels of circulating TSH, free T4 and/or total T3. Even if the TSH is high always check the T4 and T3 blood levels before giving throxine for presumed myxedema.
- An incidental finding of a low hemoglobin during a routine physical examination may be the first indication that the patient is losing blood or is anemic for any one or more other reasons.
- Abnormal liver function tests may be the first, and often the only indication of existing liver disease. Alcohol excess or previous infection by any one of the viruses that can cause hepatitis are the common causes.
- A high neutrophil count associated with an infection which persists after the infection subsides requires investigation to exclude a chronic granulocytic leukemia.
- A report of dysplastic changes noted on a pap smear is often the first indication of disease in a seemingly normal cervix.
- Metastatic preterminal malignancy may be symptomless till death is imminent. The following are two examples.
  - A previously symptomless patient woke up one morning, looked in the mirror and saw that her face looked yellow. Investigations showed disseminated pancreatic malignancy. She died a month later.
  - A 55 year old male patient came to see me complaining of lassitude and work-related back pain. Chest, lumbar and dorsal spine X-rays were normal. Routine blood studies showed a significant number of nucleated red cells in the peripheral circulation and an alkaline phosphatase in excess of 1000U/L (normal values for the testing laboratory were 40-122 U/L). The results were highly suggestive of bone metastases and the diagnosis was confirmed by a bone marrow aspirate and a nuclear bone scan (but not by routine X-rays or a CT scan). This failure of standard X-rays, and even CT scans to demonstrate metastatic disease is not uncommon but unfortunately, not widely known. MRIs are usually diagnostic. No primary was ever identified and the patient died soon after. The wife refused permission for an autopsy.

Global and focal organ dysfunction syndromes.

Syndromes of dysfunction may be global or focal. These are terms commonly used by pathologists to indicate generalized (global) or localized disease (focal). They are frequently used when the nervous systems is involved by disease. An infarct is an example of focal disease while the dementias and encephalopathies are usually global dysfunctions.

Disease could be systemic from the beginning.

The following are three common examples:

Infections. Acute, subacute or chronic infections may be, and often are systemic at one time or another during the course of the disease. The dissemination of organisms and/or their toxic products throughout the body can have serious and varied consequences. Examples are fever, bacteremia, septicemia, metastatic abscesses, vascular occlusions and disruptions of blood vessels (an often diagnostic feature of meningococcal septicemia), septic shock, microangiopathic anemia, disseminated intravascular coagulation and, at times, dcath or chronic invalidism.

Atheromatous disease of the arteries is another common example of a disease which is often systemic from the beginning. It can affect any or all arteries of the body and cause vascular insufficiency of one or more organs: the heart, the brain, the extremities, the kidneys and/or the intestines. Hence when dealing with a dysfunction caused by vascular disease, e.g., myocardial infarction, it is essential to evaluate the function of other organ systems which can be affected in a similar way.

Autoimmune disease is a systemic disease which is less common than the above two. Even if only one organ or organ system appears to be affected, the whole body must be thoroughly examined and appropriate ancillary tests done. For example, lung function tests, studies of cardiac, and esophageal and renal function. The object is to identify or exclude clinical or sub-clinical involvement of other organ systems.

Disease which is not systemic at the beginning but has the potential for systemic spread.

In the poorer parts of the world the commonest cause of metastatic disease is infection, usually untreated or untreatable infection. The causes are many; pyogenic infections, granulomatous disease, especially tuberculosis, and parasitic disease such as malaria. Metastatic infections favor location in the spleen and the muscles. Strangely, metastatic malignancies in the muscle and spleen are uncommon. They favor location in the bones, lungs, brain and liver. Metastatic malignant disease in the spleen or muscles is almost anecdotal.

A common disease which has the potential for systemic spread is malignancy. When a malignancy is first identified a full physical examination and appropriate ancillary investigations are requisites. The object is to ensure that the tumor is not a metastatic lesion, and if it is a genuine primary, to exclude or identify metastatic disease before therapy begins. The existence of metastatic lesions will usually require modification of proposed therapy.

Some possible effects of tumors.

Tumors can also cause local and/or systemic effects. Accidental complications include hemorrahges, torsion, strangulation, rupture, infection, necrosis and the pressure effects of benign as well as malignant tumors, and any one or more of their metastases.

Systemic effects due to the tumor are production of excess hormone or suppressions of hormone production. These can occur with benign as well as malignant tumors. Finally, this paragraph would not be complete without mention of the uncommon paraneoplastic syndromes which tumors occasionally produce: vascular occlusions, especially deep vein thromboses in the legs, endocrine dysfunctions and bizarre neurological syndromes.

Other relevant factors in clinical assessments.

The following additional topics are now discussed: **pain, the role of language in clinical assessments, the effects of aging, the etiologies of disease and the categorization of medical problems.**

Pain.

Pain is probably the most frequent complaint of sick people. It could be the principal complaint or one which is incidental to others. At times the patient does not have any pain. The first indication of malignant disease could be a palpable but painless lump or clinical features resulting from metastases. Often, patients with chronic cardiac dysfunctions do not have pain but only consult physicians because of shortness of breath, or swollen legs.

On the other hand pain is the usual presenting symptom when an individual has a myocardial infarction or an acute abdomen. Chest pain due to lung disease only appears when the parietal pleura is inflamed. The pain results from the rubbing of painless visceral pleura against pain-sensitive inflamed parietal pleura during inspiration. Of course these patients often also have pains because of sore throats and tracheitis.

Pain facilitates localization and identification of dysfunctions. It does so because pain has different qualities and different modes of onset depending on the nature of the dysfunction. Is it superficial type pain, deep pain or referred pain? What is its intensity? What was its mode of onset (sudden or gradual)? Was it maximum at the onset or did it gradually worsen? Is it continuous or discontinuous? Is it increasing or decreasing in intensity? The responses to these questions are needed for making accurate clinical assessments.

Pain sensations are transmitted to the CNS by afferent somatic and sympathetic nerves. Pain is probably perceived in subcortical structures such as the thalamus as electrical stimulation of the cortex does not produce pain. But pain-related information reaching the cortex has the potential for exciting reflexes which are mediated by the cortex.

There are two types of pain fibers: A-delta fibers and C fibers. The former are myelinated nerves which transmit fast and account for the immediate sharp and localized pain which immediately follows a painful stimulus. The latter account for the dull diffuse and unpleasant sensations which follow. Pain fibers enter the cord by the dorsal nerve roots. Their subsequent course are any one or more of the following:

- To the thalamus and then the sensory cortex via the spinothalamic tracts. These tracts begin after an initial synapse of pain information in the dorsal horn. The postsynaptic nerve crosses over to the opposite side of the cord and ascends to the thalamus and sensory cortex in the spinothalamic tract which is located in the ventral white matter. In the mid brain it incorporates fibers from the contralateral trigeminothalamic tract. Autonomic afferents transmitting sensations of visceral pain have similar courses.
- Some pain afferents course along the ipsilateral posterior columns to reach the thalamus.
- Finally, many pain fibers have posterior and anterior horn synapses for rapid segmental reflexes.

Superficial pain, deep pain and referred pain.

There are three types of pain: superficial pain, deep pain and referred pain.

Superficial pain.

Dermal pain is typical of superficial pain. It results from dermal trauma of many sorts: pricks, cuts, bruises, heat, cold and crush injuries. Superficial pain precisely localizes the affected area. It is sharp at first and is then followed by a dull diffuse and unpleasant component.

Superficial type pain is not restricted to trauma affecting dermal structures. It also occurs when parietal (but not visceral) serous membranes are diseased: the meninges, the parietal pleura and pericardium and the parietal peritoneum. Pain is sharp, localized and aggravated by anything that suddenly separates the diseased membrane from adjacent structures or rubs them against an underlying structure. The former accounts for the rebound tenderness which precisely localizes an area where the underlying abdominal viscus and parietal peritoneum is inflamed. It results from the sudden separation of inflamed parietal peritoneum from the underlying inflamed viscus. Pleuritic superficial type pain results when an insensitive but inflamed visceral pleura rubs against the pain receptors of overlying inflamed parietal pleura during inhalation.

A similar type of pain characterizes the increased pain on neck flexion which accompanies meningeal inflammations and intracerebral bleeds involving the subarachnoid and subdural spaces. The pia mater, the arachnoid and the dura are insensitive to pain. However, the arteries of the pia-arachnoid and dura have pain sensitive nerve endings. It is postulated that the pain on neck flexion seen with patients having meningitis is due to stimulation of these pain-sensitive receptors. The brain is essentially insensitive to pain stimuli; encephalitis, infarcts, tumors and other brain pathologies do not cause pain unless the meninges are involved and/or intracranial pressure raised.

The capsules of solid organs such as the kidney and liver have receptors which can transmit pain. They respond when there is inflammation or distention by abscesses, tumors or intraorgan hemorrhages. Hence, the renal and hepatic tenderness on palpation when pathology affects these structures. Pyelonephritis and hepatitis both cause pain on palpation in the loins or the right hypochondrium, respectively.

Deep pain.

Deep pain results from pathology involving musculoskeletal structures or the viscera. The pain is usually aching in quality, poorly localized, and often associated with symptoms such as nausea, vomiting, sweating and blood pressure changes. The stimuli which cause deep pain vary with the structure affected. The four principal causes are ischemia, distention or spasm of a hollow viscus, inflammatory or degenerative disease affecting articular surfaces, or spasm of skeletal muscle. The intestines can be handled, burnt or cut without discomfort to the patient but ischemia, spasm or distention cause pain. When disease extends to and involves overlying parietal serous membranes the deep pain of visceral disease changes to a superficial type pain which is sharp and well localized.

Referred pain.

Another characteristic of deep pain is its perception in locales which are often distant from the site of origin of the pain. A paper by Ryle, written in 1926[2], detailed the facts well. The referral is usually to structures which developed from the same segmental dermatome as the affected tissue. Pain from structures which developed from midline mesoderm are perceived in the midline. Those which developed from lateral mesoderm (e.g., the urinary tract) are perceived laterally. For example, the typical referred pain of renal colic results from ureteric spasm and extends from loin to groin, usually along the distribution of somatic nerve L1.

The sensations of deep pain and referred pain are transmitted to the spinal cord by autonomic afferents. Frequent accompaniments are autonomic reflexes such as sweating, changes in blood pressure, vasomotor changes and occasionally, reflex emptying of rectum, bladder and seminal vesicles.

The pains of cardiac ischemia and intermittent claudication are examples of deep pains resulting from ischemia. Cardiac pain is typically felt as referred pain. The pains of gastrointestinal colic, of intestinal obstruction, torsion or volvulus, of ureteric obstructions and colic, and of bladder spasms, are examples of deep pain of referred type resulting from the distentions or spasms of hollow viscera.

Chest pain, abdominal pain and head pain merit additional text. They are often difficult to assess, and the consequences may be dangerous if they are erroneously interpreted.

Chest pain.

A common cause of chest pain is a sprain or inflammation (Tietze's disease) of a costochondral junction. There is local tenderness on palpation and perhaps some swelling. The only treatment needed is a pain reliever and lots of reassurance that the symptoms do not result from cardiac disease.

A serious cause of chest pain results from ischemia of cardiac muscle. The manifestations range from mild angina of effort to a severe, catastrophic, devastating and often fatal pain.

The pain of angina of effort is typically felt in the substernum and is often accompanied by a sensation which the patient describes as a squeezing or constriction of the chest. It ceases when the patient rests. The pain of unstable angina is similar but unrelated to exertion and usually relieved by sublingual nitrates. It is usually of shorter duration than the pain of a myocardial infarction. The pain of infarction is usually more severe and usually not relieved by rest. Sublingual nitrates often provide some relief but the relief is usually only temporary.

The localization of pain due to myocardial ischemia is a consequence of referral to developmental dermatomes T1-5; the chest from first rib to the xiphoid process and along the ulnar aspect of the upper limb (T1). The pain can spread or, at times, be confined to other locales; the shoulder and outer aspect of the upper limbs (C5-6), the neck (C3), or the epigastrium (T6). This localization of pain in the C3, C6 and T6 areas probably represent abnormalities in dermatome differentiation or fringe summation effects in the neural pools.

Chest pain of undetermined cause.

At times patients with pains typical of angina, or even myocardial infarction have normal electrocardiograms, normal blood biochemistry and chest X-rays which show no abnormality. Many of these patients have normal treadmill exercise tests and even normal coronary angiograms. The term "Cardiologic Syndrome X" was used by Kemp[3] to describe patients with exertional angina, normal coronary arteriograms and positive or negative ECG responses to treadmill exercise testing. Later the term "Microvascular angina" was used by Canon and Epstein[4] to describe similar conditions appearing at rest. Features which help to distinguish it from exertional angina and unstable angina are angina at rest, (though this is also a feature of unstable angina), pain which is prolonged, and a poor response to sublingual nitrates[5]. A common characteristic is that the pain is not as severe as that of myocardial ischemia and is not relieved by rest nor nitroglycerin. So-called, microvascular angina is not common but is detailed here because of the diagnostic difficulties it can cause.

The non-Q wave infarct and the subendocardial infarct are identified by the symptoms and signs of an infarct without the characteristic ECG Q waves. The distinction from unstable angina is based on biochemical studies. Non-Q wave infarcts and subendocardial infarcts have raised Troponin T and CK-MB levels. Unstable angina does not.

An aortic dissection or an acute pulmonary embolus must always enter the differential diagnosis of acute chest pain or the sudden onset of dyspnea. The pain of a dissecting aneurysm is usually excruciating, described as tearing sensation and located centrally. Often there is downward extension of the pain along the spine. The pain is worse when combined with coronary stenoses caused by the dissection extending proximally. The chest X-ray often shows widening of the aortic shadow and an ultrasound and CT scan are usually diagnostic. The pain is usually central and associated with different blood pressures in the arms. This is a major emergency because it can, at times, be surgically remedied so that early diagnosis is essential,

A report in 1978[6] applied the label: "Chest pain, cause undetermined." to some 20% of patients initially thought to have angina. The literature to date presents comparable figures in other studies. Over half of these patients have symptoms due to acid regurgitation into the esophagus or esophageal spasm. This is understandable in view of the comparable innervations of heart and esophagus and their development from comparable segmental dermatomes. If microvascular angina is a real clinical syndrome it must enter into the differential diagnosis of "Chest pain, cause undetermined". The troponin-T and CK-MB levels will be normal.

Distinction of esophageal pain from cardiac pain can be difficult because sublingual nitroglycerin often relieves both types of pain. A distinguishing feature indicating that the pain is of esophageal origin is the often rapid relief which follows swallowing of a 50ml mixture of an antacid such as Maalox and viscous xylocaine in a 2:1 ratio! Of the rest, biliary and musculoskeletal pain account for some and the remainder will have a diagnosis of microvascular angina, a diagnosis difficult, if not impossible to substantiate.

Acute pulmonary embolism only results in pain when infarcted lung tissue is inflamed with extension of the inflammation to the overlying parietal pleura. The typical onset is an episode of acute breathlessness for no obvious reason. A myocardial infarct can present in the same way and enters the differential diagnosis and the requirement for appropriate investigations.

Abdominal pain.

The parietal peritoneum is exquisitely sensitive to pain. When it is inflamed the pain has the typical characteristics of superficial pain. It is sharp and precisely localized and the overlying muscle is rigid or, at least, tense. In contrast, little, if any, pain results when any of the abdominal viscera and their covering visceral peritoneum are cut, handled, or even burned. However, stretching, distention or spasm does result in pain which has the characteristics of deep pain; it is dull, aching, poorly localized, and often referred.

Referred pain from the abdominal viscera.

Transmission of visceral pain is by afferent autonomic nerves. Pain afferents from the intestine follow the main blood vessels and pass through prevertebral celiac, superior mesenteric, aortico-renal and inferior mesenteric ganglia prior to reaching their cell bodies in the dorsal roots. They then travel in the spinothalamic tracts and thalamic radiations with fibers conveying somatic sensations. Their final terminations are the somatosensory cortex where they mingle with the other pain transmissions. Referred pain is pain which is not felt in the area producing the pain but in areas developed from the same segmental dermatome as the affected viscus.

1. **Referred pain from tissues supplied by the celiac artery.** The celiac artery supplies the esophagogastric junction, the duodenum up to the entrance of the common bile duct, the gall bladder, the bile ducts, the pancreas and liver. Pain afferents enter the spinal cord between segments T5-9 and pain is referred to the surfaces of the segmental dermatomes from which these structures developed. Segments T5-9 correspond to the mid epigastrium and supraumbilical areas. Because of the involvement of T6 and sometimes T5 during development, abdominal pain is occasionally referred to the lower chest. The pain of myocardial disease is sometimes referred to dermatome segments T5-6 alone, resulting in a misdiagnosis that it is pain coming from an abdominal viscus such as the gall bladder.

   The parietal peritoneum and somatic structures are close to each other in many areas; especially over the stomach, the pancreas, the liver and gall bladder. All these viscera develop from midline tissue. Initially, gall bladder colic is referred to the epigastrium. When inflammation develops with extension to the overlying parietal peritoneum pain, palpable tenderness, rebound tenderness and muscle guarding is demonstrable over the gall bladder in the right upper quadrant of the abdomen. As mentioned previously, pain receptors exist in the covering of the liver and kidneys and local palpation will usually elicit non-referred deep pain over the gall bladder in the right upper quadrant of the abdomen. As mentioned previously, pain receptors exist in the covering of the liver and kidneys and local palpation will usually elicit non-referred deep pain if these structures are inflamed.

2. **Referred pain from tissues supplied by the superior mesenteric artery.** This artery and its branches supplies the intestine from the point at which the bile duct enters the duodenum to the right half to two-thirds of the transverse colon; the middle colic branch of the superior mesenteric artery ceases to vascularize at about this point and vascularization by the superior mesenteric artery ends there.

   Pain afferents from tissues vascularized by the superior mesenteric artery pass through the retroperitoneal superior mesenteric ganglia and enter the cord in the T8-L1 segments. The intestines develop from midline tissues and the referred pain from the distribution of the superior mesenteric artery is typically felt in the umbilical and periumbilical areas.

3. **Referred pain from tissues supplied by the renal and suprarenal arteries.** As mentioned above, there are pain receptors in the coverings of the kidneys and liver. Hence, renal and hepatic pain from inflammations and other pathology often result in local tenderness. However, when there is spasm due to renal colic or some comparable pathology pain is of referred type - autonomic afferents from the kidney and ureter enter the cord between T12-L2 levels resulting in the characteristic loin to groin referred pain; lateral because the involved structures develop from lateral embryonic tissue.

4. **Referred pain from tissues supplied by the inferior mesenteric artery.** The inferior mesenteric artery supplies the left half or one-third of the transverse colon, the descending and sigmoid colons, the upper part of the anal canal, the bladder, the urethra and in females the uterus and fallopian tubes. In males it supplies the prostate and seminal vesicles. Pain afferents pass through the retroperitoneal inferior mesenteric ganglia. Sympathetic afferents enter the cord from segments T11-L1 and the parasympathetic afferents pass through pelvic ganglia and enter the cord between segments S2-S4. The structures mentioned develop from midline tissue and pain is correspondingly referred to midline somatic segments; the perineum and the areas between the umbilicus and pubis.

Acute appendicitis.

Acute appendicitis demonstrates well the features of deep referred pain and its evolution to somatic superficial type pain.

Stage 1:. The lumen of the appendix is blocked for any one of many reasons; impaction of a fecolith, lymphoid hyperplasia, etc. Intestinal secretions accumulate in and distend the viscus which then contracts to expel the trapped fluids. There is colicky central abdominal pain; an example of deep referred pain from an abdominal viscus.

Stage 2. Inflammation develops in the wall of the appendix and the viscus becomes more sensitive to stimuli such as distention and abortive contractions. The colicky central abdominal referred pain increases in intensity, fever and leukocytosis develop, and nausea and vomiting result from autonomic reflexes. At this stage it is uncommon to elicit much tenderness when the right iliac fossa or pouch of Douglas is palpated.

Stage 3. Inflammation extends to the visceral peritoneum covering the appendix and then to the overlying parietal peritoneum. Involvement of the latter results in pain of superficial type; pain which is sharp and well localized. Palpation elicits sharp pain in the right iliac fossa, or in the pelvis if that is where the appendix is located. A mass may or may not be palpable but a characteristic finding is rebound tenderness. When the palpating hand is suddenly lifted off the area of tenderness there is a momentary exacerbation of pain as the visceral and parietal peritoneal layers part. In addition there is reflex abdominal rigidity ("guarding") over the area of tenderness.

Stage 4. The next stage depends on the intensity of inflammation and the resistance of the individual to infection. The following are some possibilities:

- Complete resolution with or without the aid of antibiotics. This is not common.
- Localization of inflammation by coils of intestine and adjacent omentum. The signs and symptoms are the

antibiotics. Alternatively, it could increase in size and, if not drained and emptied, rupture through the abdominal or rectal wall. Alternatively it could rupture into the peritoneal cavity. This last eventuality will result in generalized sharp abdominal pain with extensive muscular rigidity and rebound tenderness. Usually there are also various combinations of systemic toxemia, bacteremia, septicemia and septic shock, and rarely, development of pyemic metastatic abscesses. If untreated death eventually ensues.

Head pain.

There are innumerable causes for head pains. Usually the cause cannot be identified for most headaches have no obvious cause and are normally self-curing.

Identifiable pains include tension headaches, the pains of migraine and cluster headaches, the pains of sinusitis, the headaches of uncontrolled hypertension and of cerebrovascular hemorrhages. An ominous cause is increased intracranial pressure caused by expanding space occupying lesions such as tumors, collections of blood, the bleeding and edema which often results from trauma, and the fluid collections of meningeal inflammations.

Tension headaches They are related to perceived or unrecognized stress. The pain is typically bitemporal and occipito-nuchal. Muscle spasms probably cause most of the symptoms.

Migraine. Migraine affects some 5-10% of the population. "Classic migraine" is usually preceded by an aura which lasts for 15-60 minutes. Typical aura are neurological deficits such as unilateral loss of vision, a homonymous hemianopia and even speech, sensory and/or motor deficits. At times the prodrome is some unusual feeling such as excitability, tiredness, cravings for certain foods and yawning. Often, sufferers from classic migraine have a family history. The prodrome is followed by the headache which is typically unilateral and accompanied by nausea, vomiting, diarrhea, photophobia and increased sensitivity to noise and smells. The headache is intense and can last for three days; a duration of 4-8 hours is more usual.

"Common migraine" has a similar headache but an aura is unusual and there is rarely any family history.

Cluster headaches. As the name implies these headaches occur in clusters, each headache lasting 15 minutes to about three hours, with a frequency of one or many daily occurrences. Remissions with no headaches may last for weeks, months or even years.

The typical pain is severe, localized to one orbit or periorbital area and accompanied by one or more of the following: conjunctival injection, lacrimation, ptosis, miosis and local sweating. The clinical picture is unmistakable. **Chronic paroxysmal hemicrania** is a variant with similar clinical features but with headaches which are shorter but more frequent. Relief by indomethacin is said to be diagnostic of this variation of cluster headaches.

Subarachnoid bleeds. The usual cause of these bleeds are trauma, or a ruptured intracranial aneurysm or arterio-venous malformation. Typically, the headache is severe, devastating, and of sudden onset. It is usually maximum at the onset of the bleed or shortly after. Consciousness is often lost and symptoms resulting from increased intracranial pressure soon follow. It is a grave and often fatal emergency.

Head injuries. Unpleasant and often severe, continuous or intermittent headaches are frequent late sequelae of head trauma. Headaches in the immediate aftermath of a head injury may result from space-occupying intracranial or subdural blood and blood clots.

Hypertension. Hypertensive headaches are fairly common when diastolic pressures exceed 100mg mercury. Typically, hypertensive headaches are occipital in location and are present when the individual wakens in the morning. As the day passes the headache usually disappears.

Space-occupying lesions. Primary brain tumors do occur but the commonest brain tumors are single or multiple metastases. The headache has no special features and probably results from the increased intracranial pressure of a space-occupying lesion. Space-occupying lesions include tuberculomas, brain abscesses and parasitic granulomas. The pain of space-occupying lesions is deep and may be throbbing, episodic or continuous, or, at times, mild and tolerable. As the lesion or lesions progress the symptoms and signs of increased intracranial pressure develop: increasing head pains, neurological deficits, confusion, coma, and finally, death.

Increased intracranial pressure. The subject of raised intracranial pressure is detailed in Chapter 6 which is a discussion of the central nervous system and its dysfunctions. Increased intracranial pressure is common in many neurological conditions and an important cause of headaches.

The causes of increased intracranial pressure include edema and hemorrhage within and around traumatized brain tissue, an infarct or an intracerebral hemorrhage. Other causes include extradural space occupying lesions such as subdural hematomas, the inflammatory exudate and cerebral edema of infections, progressively growing intracranial tumors (benign tumors or primary or metastatic malignant tumors) and hemorrhages from aneurysms or arterio-venous malformations.

The rigid skull confines the underlying expanding mass. Clinically there is headache, defective mentation, vomiting, occasionally convulsions, torpor, inability to comprehend, inability to respond intelligently to questions or comments, and finally, if uncorrected, coma and death. Papilledema, when present, is fairly diagnostic of increased intracranial pressure but it is also a feature of advanced malignant hypertension. The various pupillary changes which result from increased intracranial pressure are detailed in Chapter 6.

Language.

It is impossible to over-emphasize the importance of language for assessments of clinical problems. Language is the vehicle for interactive communication between patient and physician. It includes verbal, gestural and prosodic language.

A diversion is merited to detail some of the facets of language. Knowledge of the facts will help the physician when assessing symptoms and signs. It will also help formulation of appropriate questions when the patient is unable to clearly state what ails. This inability can result from normal or pathological difficulties of expression or because of any one of the rather uncommon syndromes of speech dysfunction.

Verbal and written language.

Our knowledge about the physiology of language still has many deficiencies and it is in the frame of this caveat that one describes the processes involved. This section should more correctly be placed in the chapter detailing central nervous system dysfunctions. It is incorporated in this chapter because of its relevance to an important component of the clinical assessment - the recording and interpretation of the clinical history. Chart 3-8 on the next page summarizes the anatomy and physiology of speech as, at present, generally acceptable to most.

The principal organs involved in speech are the lungs which function as bellows blowing air. Many structures modify the velocity and turbulence of the air stream: the glottis, pharynx and larynx; the vocal cords; the mouth and nose acting as resonators; the uvula; the soft and hard palate and the tongue, the teeth and the lips. Sounds result from changes in the velocity and turbulence of air blown out by the lungs. Differences of pitch are produced by variations in the lengths of the vocal cords; the higher-pitched voices of women result from vocal cords which are shorter than those of men. Changes in air turbulence and velocity result in differing frequencies of air waves striking the basilar membrane of the cochlea. As a result many different nerve impulse patterns are generated, each characteristic for the sound transmitted (the process is really much more complicated but for the purposes of the present discussion does not need consideration in additional detail). These nerve impulse patterns reach the brain and after many synapses the final interpretation of the sound probably takes place in the part of the tempero-parietal heteromodal area known as "Wernicke's area[7]".

A link is established between visual information and auditory information by tracts which connect the occipital visual cortex with Wernicke's area and the angular gyrus (located immediately beyond Wernicke's area). Newly integrated information passes from Wernicke's area and the angular gyrus to Broca's area via the arcuate fasciculus. Broca's[8] area is located immediately anterior to the face area of the Rolandic precentral cortex. Here there is development and storage of programs for conversion of multimodal auditory information into motor programs for spoken, gestural and prosodic language. The proximity of Broca's area to the motor cortex facilitates their interactions.

The left cerebral hemisphere controls verbal speech. It is said to be dominant in over 90% of right-handed individuals and in about 50% of those who use the left hand for writing and other activities[9]. In the others the

Chart 3-8: LANGUAGE: LATERAL ASPECT OF THE CEREBRAL HEMISPHERE SHOWING THE INTERCONNECTIONS AND FUNCTIONS OF THE TEMPERO-PARIETAL HETEROMODAL ASSOCIATION AREA [1,2]

Broca's area.

Programs for execution of the motor activity needed for verbal, gestural and prosodic speech are developed and stored in Broca's area.

The proximity of Broca's area to the motor cortex facilitates the muscular activities needed for speech.

The angular gyrus.

An important function of the angular gyrus is integration of auditory sounds and visual images by many to and fro interconnections with the occipital visual areas.

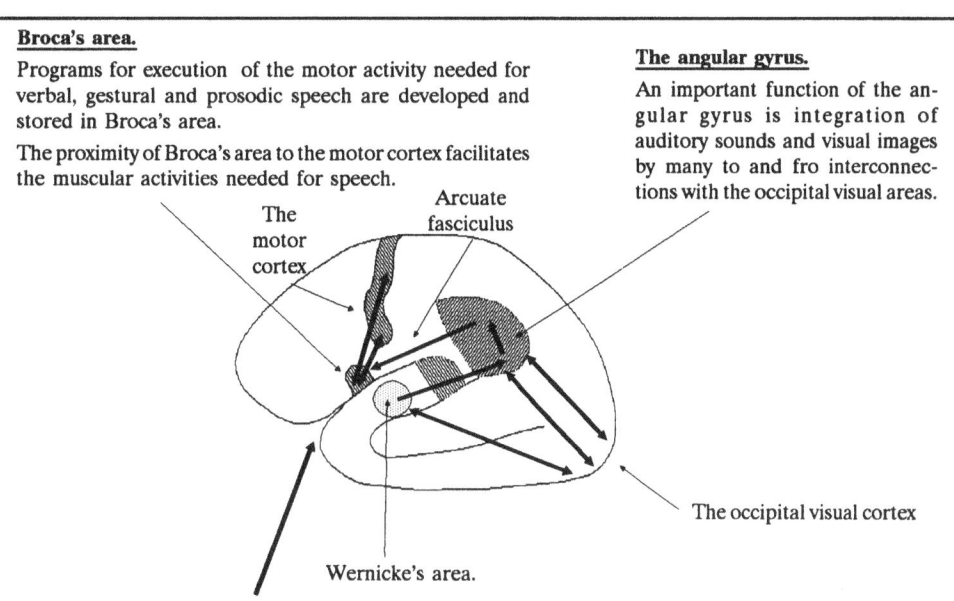

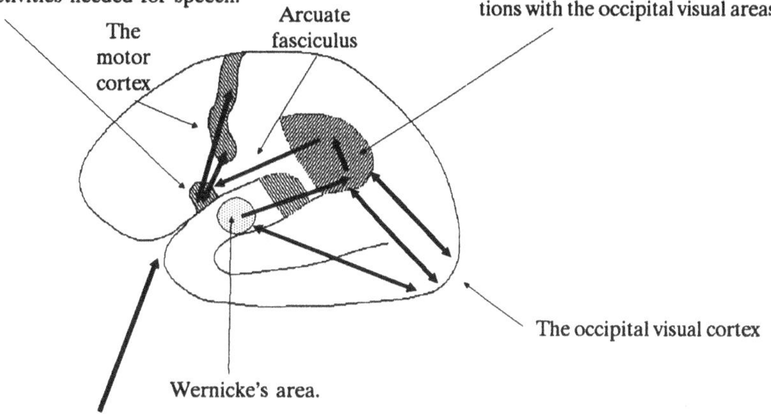
The motor cortex
Arcuate fasciculus
The occipital visual cortex
Wernicke's area.

Auditory nerve transmitting auditory nerve impulses from the inner ear.

The Organ of Corti is located in the inner ear. Here sounds are converted to different nerve impulse patterns. These patterns pass along the auditory (VIIIth.) nerve to the primary auditory cortex in the floor of the lateral fissure for simple auditory recognitions. The next relay is to Wernicke's area on the lateral surface of the superior temporal gyrus. In this area there is multimodal integration and recognition of sounds.

[1] Lesions of Wernicke's area or of the tracts leading to it result in loss of comprehension of language, both of the spoken and the written word. The ability to speak and to express oneself is retained if Broca's area is unaffected but responses to questions and comments are usually nonsensical.

[2] Damage to Broca's area or of the tracts leading to it results in speech which is inarticulate. There is retention of auditory comprehension if Wernicke's area is unaffected. A lesion of Broca's area is usually accompanied by a left hemiplegia due to an associated vascular lesion affecting the right hemisphere (the left hemisphere is dominant for speech in 90% of right-handed and 50% of left-handed people).

right hemisphere dominates. The right hemisphere is dominant for the paralinguistic components of speech: gesture and prosody. Communications between the right and left areas is by tracts which traverse the corpus callosum.

Clinicians are often faced with patients whose language is nonsensical or incomprehensible. This usually results from pathology affecting the brain. Hence, some knowledge of the syndromes of speech disorders is desirable. Numerous types of speech, reading, writing and calculating defects have been described[10], depending on the anatomical area affected by disease. The commonest are lesions which directly or indirectly involve Broca's or Wernicke's areas. A lesion involving Broca's area results in an aphasia characterized by inarticulate speech but with unaffected auditory and intellectual comprehension because of an intact Wernicke's area. A lesion of this type is usually associated with and caused by a common cause of stroke; occlusion of the middle cerebral artery. Often there is an accompanying hemiplegia.

A lesion of Wernicke's area results in loss of auditory comprehension and comprehension of the written word. The ability to speak remains intact and speech may be fluent but is usually nonsensical. The same happens if there is damage to any of the tracts or nuclei which act as relay stations for impulses arriving at Wernicke's area. Many other types of aphasia have been described, e.g., conduction aphasia resulting from a lesion of the arcuate fasciculus, and other related structures. A detailed discussion of this subject would not be appropriate given the context of this book.

Finally, listening to a person often reveals speech dysfunctions due to benign and malignant neoplasms. The hoarseness of acute laryngitis is, of course, unmistakable but persistence of hoarseness does need a laryngoscopy to exclude polyps and tumors.

How is language learnt?

The majority of humans learn language by associating visual images with spoken words. The association probably takes place in the angular gyrus. It has many connections with the occipital visual areas and this enables the linkage of auditory and visual information needed for learning.

A **"nativist" theory** tries to explain how children acquire language. The Nativists hypothesize that pre-existing biologically determined abilities enable an individual to structure sounds into words and words into comprehensible sentences. As time passes there is progressive improvement towards adult patterns of speech. Prominent initial members of this school were the psycholinguists Chomsky and Lenneberg[11]. Chomsky[12] has hypothesized that each child has a language acquisition device (LAD) which permits processing of language heard in the environment. He postulates that words and grammar are learnt because of this hypothetical LAD. The literature on verbal language is large but the preceding suffices for the purposes of this book. One suspects that terms such as LAD are merely scientific jargon for those who reject the fact that some observations are currently inexplicable and probably extend into the metaphysical.

Language used by children.

These musings on the controversies about language learning precede some important facts about the learning of language by children[13,14,15]. The child normally begins to speak between the eighteenth and twenty-eighth month, and language development is virtually complete by the end of the fourth year. A number of refinements are added between the ages of 5 and 10 but most children have completed the greater part of the basic language acquisition process by the age of 5.

Children will be frequent patients. When they speak it is appropriate to recognize that after the age of 5, and at times earlier, any history given and any symptoms complained about should be accepted at face value, assuming that there has been no brain-washing by well-meaning or abusive adults. Incorrect grammar and pragmatics should not be cause for disregarding what is said for these will change and correct with time.

The uses of verbal and written language.

In spoken or written form language is the indispensable vehicle for human interaction and intellectual activity. It is a process which reduces a multiplicity of observed phenomena to the shorthand code needed for human interaction. Medicine could not be practiced, except in a limited way, without the use of language for interactions between patients and physicians, between physicians and other physicians and/or other individuals involved in health care such as nurses, technicians, and operators of ancillary services.

Language is a code that transforms many observations into a few sounds. Thus, the words "woman" or "man" and the differences between the two, are well known by all but if one were required to detail them it would require a lot of words and time. The same applies to most other objects: books, tables, houses, etc.

There are two types of written languages. Those which are pictorial and ideographic and those which use an alphabet. The former goes back to antiquity, to the first written records of human thought. From about 4000 B.C. to the time of Christ, the peoples of Mesopotamia (Sumerians, Assyrians, Babylonians and Persians) used cuneiform tablets. These were representations of pictures and ideas produced on wet clay tablets by engraving with wedges. Later ideo-pictorial languages include modern Chinese and Japanese. The representation of ideas, facts and concepts by pictorial forms is not as restrictive as those who do not use such forms might think. It has been stated that some forty thousand compound words can be formed by pictorial forms. An additional sophistication is the formation of words compounded of two parts, one for meaning and the other for pronunciation.

Alphabetic languages derive from the one brought by the Central Asian invaders of the world some 3,000-5,000 years ago. All the Indo-European languages derive from this basic language. They begin with the Sanskrit Vedic hymns (2000 B.C.) followed by Greek (1500 B.C.) and Latin (500 B.C.).

A phonetic alphabet probably has a wider range of expressions, probably because more permutations and combinations are possible. An alphabet of 26 letters could theoretically be combined in millions of ways. They are not and this is probably because words containing more than ten letters are difficult to use. The English vocabulary only consists of some million words and few know a fifth of these; an estimate is that the average English-speaking person seldom uses more than 1000-1500 words of the language. As a rule many more are known but most are rarely used. Of course, the environment and social and educational factors are important in determining the volume of an individual's vocabulary.

Gestural language.

The spoken word is not the only component of language. Language is used by individuals to think, to make decisions and to communicate with each other. This is why language includes gestures (gestural language), the written language, the read language, and the way in which language is spoken (prosodic language). It also includes pictorial and symbolic systems of communications. The systems of communication that have been devised by humans since the beginning of time are innumerable but the visually demonstrable word, whether written, typed, word processed, faxed or otherwise transmitted, remains the most enduring means of communication. A Latin quotation correctly justifies this: "Verba volant, scripta manent." (What is spoken flies away, what is written endures).

Gestural language or so-called "body language" is produced by subtle, and sometimes not so subtle, movements of muscles: facial, limb, spinal, etc. Various combinations of different intensities and locations of muscular contractions of facial, truncal and limb muscles can result in many different implied verbalizations. For the clinician, just watching a patient while interacting can often yield more information than the history itself. The process requires self-training and will improve over the years.

The existence and importance of gestural language was recognized by Hughlings Jackson[16] who defined it as those movements which were employed for emphasizing and giving hidden meaning to speech. He described such movements as "pantomine". Prior to that the importance of gestural language, albeit in another context, was recognized a century or two earlier by William Shakespeare[17]

> "I think there's never a man in Christendom
> an lesser hide his love or hate than he,
> For by his face shall you know his heart."

Prosody.

Prosody is a para-linguistic component of language. It conveys emotions and attitudes in many different ways: by varying vocal pitch (e.g., in questioning); by introducing pauses into speech, either in mid-sentence or at the end of sentences; by varying the melody of spoken words; by emphases and diminuendos; by variations in tone; by the use of sounds which are not part of language (e.g., grunts, sighs, etc.); and by many other ways, some tangible, others not.

Prosody adds emotion to speech by conveying feelings, passions, likes, dislikes, agreements and disagreements, contempt and respect and many other emotions. Without prosody language is wooden and unfeeling. An example is the often expressionless speech and faces of individuals with the akinetic muscles of Parkinson's disease.

The verbal history consists of words. Without prosody these words do not quantify degree or intensity, acceptance or rejection, they do not indicate stoicism or low symptom thresholds for items such as pain. All these factors need determination during the clinical assessment and most must be done by judgments of the patient's gestural and prosodic responses.

Prosody has been intensively studied by many, in particular, by Monrad-Kohn[18] and by Crystal[19]. Some of the literature even suggests that the basic units of language acquisition by infants are prosodic and not verbal. Monrad-Kohn's studies of prosody were detailed. He proposed that prosody came in four different forms: intrinsic, intellectual, emotional and inarticulate. It is difficult to clearly understand the natures of these differences but he did describe clearly various clinical disorders characterized by deficits of prosody. The details need not concern us in the present context except in a general way.

Gesture and prosody can convey wealths of meanings with few words. Both are important components of the clinical decision-making process for without them clinical histories and the reactions during the proddings of a clinical examination are difficult to assess. In the absence of gesture and prosody there is little addition of meaning and emotion to words and sentences. One of the obstacles to the use of the computer for making clinical decisions is its inability to recognize and interpret language which is not written or spoken, i.e., gesture and prosody.

Aging.

Aging is not a disease but a process which results in decreased functional reserve in most organs. A consequence is a decreased resistance to almost any disease process. The decrease in functional reserve with aging always needs recognition when evaluating a clinical dysfunction. The following are some of the physiological changes seen in aging:

The nervous system: Throughout life there is a continual death and loss of neurons - one estimate is that some 50,000 neurons are lost each day. This sounds like an alarmingly large figure but is only 0.5×10^9 neurons for an individual aged 80 losing 50,000 neurons a day from the age of 50. The brain has between $10\text{-}100 \times 10^9$ neurons so that the loss during this period will not exceed 5-10% of the total neuron population. Ample numbers of neurons remain. Certainly enough for normal or almost normal mentation. Of course, functional reserve can be greatly reduced if there is additional neuron loss from degenerative disease, multiple minute infarcts or other global or focal brain disorders.

The loss of neurons with aging could cause some decrease in attention, in alertness, in cognition, and in memory. In these individuals confusional states are common when they get sick for any one of many reasons (for example fever, infections, trauma, metabolic disturbances, drugs, and congestive heart failure). Of course, when there is associated neurological disease of any sort the increased reduction in the pool of functionally usable reserve neurons can result in major deficits: deficits of memory, of cognition, of understanding, of reasoning, of motor function and of sensory perception, with eventual dementia.

The heart and blood vessels: With aging, myocardial tissue stiffens because of replacement of elastin with connective tissue. One consequence is that peak tension takes longer to develop. Another is the decreased functional reserve when an ischemic event occurs.

In medium-sized and small blood vessels somewhat similar changes occur. An important consequence is that the peripheral resistance increases, both, at rest and during exercise because there is a decrease in the capacity of vascular smooth muscle to dilate.

Similar changes in the larger arteries decrease their ability to distend. One consequence is a rise in arterial blood pressure, partially countered by aortic dilation which increases aortic volume and may progress to the formation of aneurysms. The age-related changes in the large arteries, together with the increase in peripheral resistance which results from changes in the medium-sized and small arteries, combine to increase cardiac afterload and consequently, reduce stroke volume. At rest these changes usually result in little or no disability. However, when the aged individual exercises significant changes are often demonstrable. The expected increases in heart rate, stroke volume, and cardiac output are all less than the expected increases in younger individuals.

The kidney: Glomerular filtration rates fall throughout life. The average value in the mid seventies is only half that of a healthy counterpart in the mid twenties. Again, as with the heart, there is a decreased functional reserve if renal disease develops.

The lungs: With advancing years there is also a decrease in normal lung function reserve. There is a linear fall of arterial oxygen tension levels (pO_2) from about 95mm Hg at age 15 to approximately 75mm Hg at age 80[20].

The bones and joints: Dysfunctions associated with advancing years include degenerative joint disease (osteoarthritis) - a condition that is not life-threatening but can cause much joint pain and limitation of movement. Osteoarthritis can also result from previous joint or bone disease such as septic arthritis or old healed tuberculosis, or from fractures involving cartilaginous joint surfaces and torn menisci. However, osteoarthritis is usually age related or the result of a life doing manual labor. The affected joints of osteoarthritis are stiff and swollen and movement is usually limited. Joint stiffness in the morning is common. Characteristically it only lasts for less than half an hour in contrast to the morning stiffness of rheumatoid arthritis which usually lasts much longer. The only treatment for osteoarthritis are analgesics to relieve pain and in extreme situations, surgery to replace joints with artificial prostheses. It is an often distressing malady of advancing years.

Equally distressing is the osteoporosis that often accompanies aging. Pain is common as well as deformities due to collapse of vertebral bodies. Particularly dangerous is the liability of bones to fracture when subjected to strains and trauma that would leave younger individuals unaffected. Fracture of the femoral neck and wrist (Colle's fractures) are not uncommon. If surgery is needed the eventual outcome is not without hazard.

The etiologies of disease.

Unknown etiology.

Often etiology cannot be identified with certainty or without unnecessary, unpleasant and, at times, potentially hazardous investigations. This does not preclude optimum therapy based on a "most likely" presumption of etiology. For example, on many occasions the cause of congestive heart failure cannot be determined with certainty; the usual assumption in elderly patients is that the cause is myocardial insufficiency from a combination of coronary artery disease and the anatomical myocardial changes that accompany aging. Despite the inability to precisely identify the cause of failure perfectly adequate therapy can be provided to control and stabilize.

Multi-organ disease.

Any of the causes of disease can, and often do affect any one or more organs or organ systems. Hence, a complete physical examination and appropriate ancillary investigations are essential when a patient consults a physician with a clinical problem of any complexity. This is particularly important if there is any suspicion of malignancy. Favorite sites of clinical or occult metastatic disease are the liver, the lungs, the bones and the brain. They are easily missed if the clinical assessment is not thorough.

Multiple etiology.

The simultaneous existence of more than one cause of disease in any one individual is not uncommon, especially in the elderly. A frequent consequence is multi-organ disease with multiple organ and systems dysfunctions of varying degree and often, puzzling complexity.

The causes of disease.

The following summarizes the principal causes of disease:

Congenital causes:

- **Disease due to inherited chromosomal abnormalities:** Mendelian type inheritance of abnormal dominant or recessive genes, and fortuitous gene mutations and/or abnormalities. Examples are the thalassemias and other abnormalities of the blood, lysosomal diseases such as Tay-Sacks disease, Huntington's dementia and many other comparable disabilities.
- **Fortuitous, unknown and unpredictable chromosomal abnormalities.** Examples are the many neurological retardations associated with such abnormalities - Down's syndrome is an example.
- **Disease due to abnormal fetal development because of** infections (e.g., rubella or AIDS), drugs, alcohol (the fetal alcohol syndrome is described on page 362) and/or other toxins.

Acquired disease:

- **Trauma.** Examples are accidents in the home, automobile accidents, assault or homicide, suicide, injury from exposure to toxic chemicals, injury due to burns and to extremes of heat or cold, injury due to extreme changes in environmental pressure, and injury from exposure to excessive radiation.

— **Infections.** By bacteria, viruses, rickettsiae, protozoa, helminths, and fungi. The consequences could be acute, subacute or chronic disease.

— **New growths.** Benign tumors and primary or metastatic malignancies. Any combination is possible.

— **Neurological.** Central or peripheral, focal (i.e., localized) or global (i.e., generalized lesions.). The possibilities are numerous. Chapter 6 is a summary of the more common afflictions that affect the nervous system.

— **Arterial disease.** Cardiovascular dysfunctions. Cerebrovascular disease, carotid artery disease and disease affecting peripheral limb, renal, mesenteric and retinal vessels in different combinations. The causes are many and are detailed in Chapters 6 and 11.

— **Diseases of the veins and lymphatics.** Thrombophlebitis, phlebothrombosis and its embolic complications, varicose veins and lymphatic diseases. The disfiguring and disabling edemas from lymphatic occlusions by Filaria Bancrofti are major problems in the poorer parts of the world. In all countries lymphatic occlusions from radiation given for control of malignant disease often result in unpleasant, painful and frequently disfiguring post-radiation edema and fibrosis.

— **Musculoskeletal disease.** The various monoarticular and multiarticular arthropathies, osteoporosis and osteomalacia and the primary muscular dysfunctions.

— **Endocrine disease.** Hypofunction or hyperfunction syndromes affecting any one or more endocrine systems. Commonest are those causing dysfunctions of the pancreas and/or the thyroid. Less common causes are pituitary microadenomas. Another cause of endocrine dysfunction is of iatrogenic origin, i.e., long-term corticosteroid administration.

— **Immunological dysfunctions.** A few are congenital. The remainder are acquired. The subject of immunological dysfunctions is detailed in Chapter 8.

— **Disease of the blood.** There are four principal groups of blood diseases with frequent overlaps - diseases involving the red cells, the white cells, the platelets, and the clotting mechanisms. Recognition is usually not difficult. Blood counts are frequent and almost routine ingredients of almost any clinical examination and hemorrhagic disorders are readily identified by abnormally long bleeding after minor wounds and/or by purpura. Once the existence of an abnormality is identified, determination of the nature of dysfunction is usually not too difficult as, in this group of diseases, many useful laboratory tests are available for diagnosis.

Transfusion reactions are components of this group. Incompatible transfusions can result in serious hematologic and renal dysfunctions and transfusions of infected blood can result in acute or lifelong chronic infections with hepatitis B, and/or C, and/or AIDS.

— **Nutritional and metabolic.** Subnutrition, malnutrition, obesity and various deficiencies of specific foods and vitamins. Some of these dysfunctions may be genetically acquired but most are not. They are all summarized in Chapter 15 which details therapy that prevents disease.

— **Diseases that result from recreational drugs.** Some of these are legal in most countries (e.g., alcohol and tobacco), others are not (e.g., marijuana, opiates and cocaine).

— **Iatrogenic disease.** Common examples are unexpected adverse reactions to drugs and to immunizations, to erroneous medication, to inappropriate doses of drugs, intolerance of necessary medications, unavoidable adverse effects of drugs given as cancer chemotherapy, and anticipated or unexpected post-surgical disabilities and complications.

Some claim that the administration of unnecessary, inappropriate or otherwise incorrect administration of drugs is a major cause of in-hospital mortality. One suspects that this is somewhat alarmist. Most drugs given in this way in hospitals are administered as last-hope remedies or as palliatives for the pain and suffering of preterminal disease.

— **Miscellaneous.** Some diseases do not easily fall into any one of the above groups. Important examples are many of the nephropathies and the nephrotic syndrome, Crohn's disease and ulcerative colitis. Etiologies are unknown at present but often assumed. Correct information will almost certainly eventuate with time.

This summarizes the causes of disease. It is only a summary for the actual numbers of etiologies are many more and would take many pages to even just identify by name.

Categorization of the clinical problem

This is the final step in a clinical assessment. It sorts clinical problems into those which are easily resolved and a few into a small category of problems which are complex, need analyses and are not easily resolved.

The three categories of clinical dysfunction.

There are three broad categories of clinical problems. Diagnosis and decision-making is made easier if the clinical problem is placed in one of these categories at an early stage of the assessment.

Category 1. The problem is simple and the therapeutic decision is obvious.

Clinical problems that fall into this category may be as simple as the common cold. Alternatively, this category can include complex acute medical emergencies or multi-system trauma where the immediate therapeutic decision is obvious or, at least, should be. For example, after major multi-organ and multi-system trauma the first priority is to ensure that the brain has sufficient oxygen and glucose for immediate needs. An airway must be established and CPR started and continued till oxygen and artificial cardio-respiratory equipment is available. Once the initial resuscitation is effected the clinical problem falls into the third category detailed below. It is now a complex multi-system clinical problem

Another example is a patient, often elderly, who develops a viral respiratory infection that can, at first, be categorized as a simple clinical problem with an obvious therapeutic decision. The subsequent development of a secondary bacterial pneumonia and any one or more of its possible complications (pleural effusions, empyema, septicemia, metastatic infections, confusional states bordering on dementia, and respiratory, cardiac, renal, or any other type of organ failure) requires that the clinical problem be placed in the third category detailed below. Now it is a complex and perhaps preterminal condition. A simple viral infection has become a serious clinical problem and therapy and management need care, analysis and reflection.

Category 2. The problem is probably psychiatric or psychosomatic.

Features that suggest that the clinical problem is psychiatric or psychosomatic appear during the initial to-and-fro verbal, gestural and prosodic interactions between patient and physician. At one extreme are patients, usually easily identified, with psychoses or dementias. Their bizarre ideation, nonsensical speech, detachment from reality, paranoias, and generally abnormal, and often violent and antisocial behavior are diagnostic.

The other extreme is symptomatology due to simple situational stress, or at least the inability to cope with such stress. In between are the combinations of symptoms and signs typical of many psychiatric syndromes such as situational and endogenous depressions, panic attacks, psychosomatic conditions, conversion reactions, and suicidal threats (not to be disregarded as they may eventually change from play-acting to a true performances). Additional features that suggest psychiatric disease include irrational conduct and speech and symptom-combinations not compatible with any known syndrome of dysfunction. These symptoms are often related with florid gestural and prosodic accompaniments. Other features suggesting psychiatric or psychosomatic disease are labile emotions, weeping for no apparent reasons or for reasons that are trivial, irritability for no obvious cause, inability to sleep, and weight loss for which no cause is demonstrable.

Even if one suspects that the patient's clinical problem is psychiatric disease it is always necessary to exclude organic disease as the cause before providing therapy for psychiatric disease. Organic cerebral disease can cause psychiatric dysfunction and it is always desirable to use all available ancillary services to exclude this possibility before assuming that the problem is not due to organic disease. Once an initial general physical examination, routine laboratory investigations and possibly, a CT scan have excluded organic disease it only remains to treat the psychiatric problem by means that may be within the competence of the attending physician, or, if not, by referral to one who specializes in psychiatry.

Category 3. The problem is not simple nor psychiatric, but complex.

The physician may not be able to make an immediate decision based on accumulated knowledge, judgment and experience. Reflection and analysis of the diagnostic and therapeutic possibilities are needed as well as evaluations of risk-benefit ratios. It may be necessary to consult books and journals and to seek the aid of colleagues, teachers, mentors and specialists. No physician should ever feel that this is an admission of incompetence for none can know all there is to know about medicine. When a doctor does not know, seeking advice from others is an obligation. As time passes the physician will find that increasing experience, judgment and knowledge will reduce the numbers of patients in this category.

In these patients rigorous systems analysis can be helpful. Chapter 5 details the processes and requirements for systems analyses of biological systems.

Chapter 3 References

1. Ryle, J.A. The natural history of disease. Oxford. Oxford University press, 1948.
2. Ryle, J.A. Visceral pain and referred pain. Lancet 1926; 1:895.
3. Kemp, H.G. Left ventricular function in patients with the anginal syndrome and normal coronary arteriograms. Am. J. Cardiol. 1973; 32:375.
2. Wernicke, K. Der aphasische Symptomencomplex. Breslau, Germany. Cohn and Weigert, 1874.
4. Canon, R.O., Epstein, S.E. Microvascular angina as a cause of chest pain with angiographically normal coronary arteries. Am. J. Cardiol. 1988; 61:1338.
5. Kaski, J.C., Rosano, G.M.C. et al. Syndrome X - clinical characteristics and left ventricular function - a long-term follow-up study. J. Am. Coll. Cardiol. 1995; 25:807.
6. Marchandise, B., Bourassa, M.G. et al. Angiographic evaluation of the natural history of normal coronary arteries and mild coronary atherosclerosis. Am. J. Cardiol. 1978; 41:216.
7. Wernicke, K. Der aphasische Symptomencomplex. Breslau, Germany. Cohn and Weigert, 1874.
8. Broca, P. Sur la faculté du langage articulé, Bull. Soc. Anthropolog. (Paris) 1861; 6:337.
9. Subirana, A. The relationship between handedness and language function. Int. J. Neurol. 1964; 5:125.
10. Brown, J.W. Aphasia, apraxia and agnosia. Springfield, Ill. Charles C. Thomas, 1972.
11. Lenneberg, E. The Biological Foundations Of Language. New York. Wiley, 1967.
12. Chomsky, N. Review of B.F. Skinner: "Verbal Behavior". Language 1959: 35:26.
13. Brown, R. Psycholinguistics. New York. Free Press, 1970.
14. Brown, R. A. First Language: The Early Stages. Cambridge, Mass. Harvard University Press, 1973.
15. McNeill, D. The Acquisition Of Language: The Study Of Developmental Psycholinguistics. New York. Harper and Row, 1970.
16. Hughlings Jackson, J.J. Words and other symbols. In Taylor, J. (Ed.): Selected writings of John Hughlings Jackson. London. Hodder and Stoughton, 1932.
17. William Shakespeare in "The Tragedy of King Richard III".
18. Monrad-Kohn, G.H. The third element of speech: Prosody and its disorders. In Halpern, L. (Ed.): Problems of Dynamic Neurology. Jerusalem. Hebrew University Press, 1963.
19. Crystal, D. Prosodic Systems and Intonation in English, Cambridge, England, University Press, 1969.
20. Murray, J.F. The Normal Lung. Philadelphia. W.B.Saunders, 1976.

4

Clinical Decision-Making: Some Basics
4. Energy - its Vital Role in Biology

Table of Contents

Notation.

The notation ~P denotes phosphorous with a high energy bond. Depending on the context in which the term is used, ~P may also denote the energy liberated when a high energy phosphate bond detaches from ATP or ADP.

The importance of energy in biology.

This is a short chapter but it is the most important chapter in the book. It details the role of energy in biology. **Energy in the form of energy contained in high energy phosphate bonds (denoted as ~P) is the foundation that supports the whole edifice of functioning biological systems. Without energy that is usable for biochemical synthesis and other biological activities life would end. Oxidative catabolism of food or, when necessary, intracellular stores of fats, carbohydrates and proteins provides the ~P needed for biological activities. Energy is the fundamental, essential and seminal basis of all biology.**

Solar photons provide the energy for synthesis of energy substrate from the environment, i.e., vegetable food which may be eaten by animals and converted to meat. The energy in this food substrate cannot be used for biological activities till first converted by oxidative catabolism to the energy in high energy phosphate bonds, i.e., ~P. This energy is stored in adenosine triphosphate (ATP) or (ADP) till needed. Oxygen, water, vitamins and minerals are also needed for production of ~P. Biologically usable ~P can also come from intracellular catabolism of stored fats, carbohydrates and proteins. Alternatively, the catabolic products of fat, glycogen and protein metabolism are transported by the cardiovascular complex and the blood to cells where there are energy deficits. Intracellular oxidative catabolism in those cells produce ~P for biochemical reactions, as and when needed.

The energy in one ~P is freed when ATP or ADP loses a terminal phosphorous.

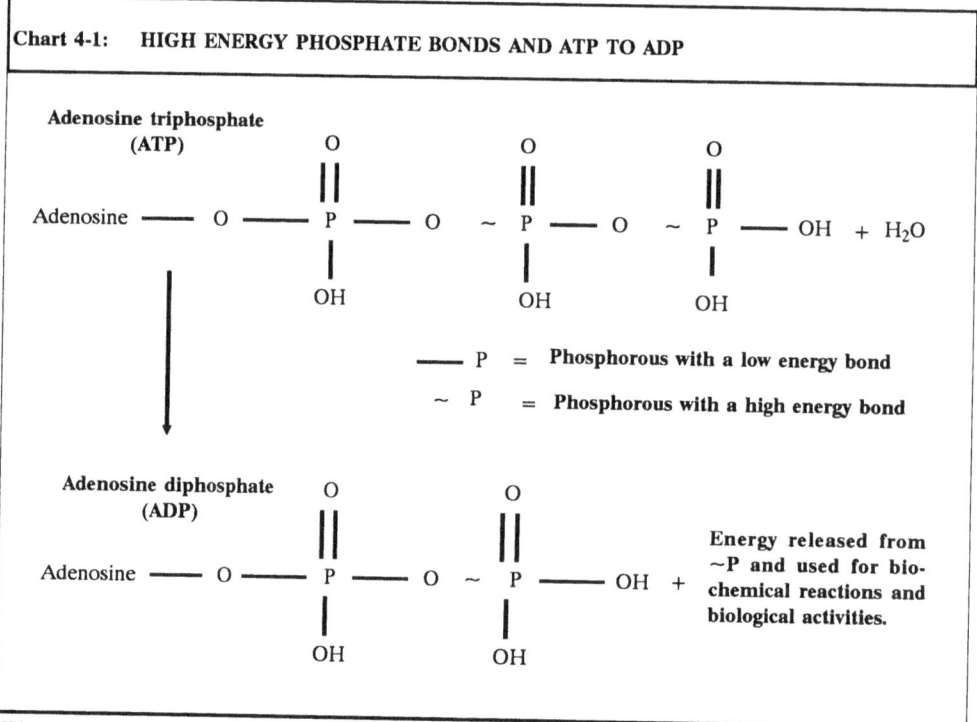

Chart 4-1: HIGH ENERGY PHOSPHATE BONDS AND ATP TO ADP

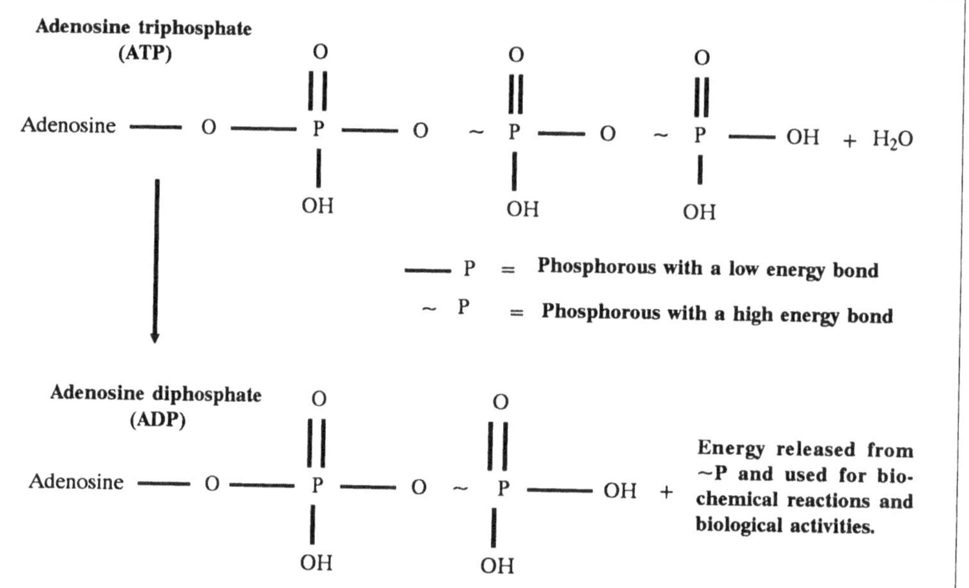
Adenosine triphosphate (ATP)
Adenosine — O — P — O ~ P — O ~ P — OH + H_2O
— P = Phosphorous with a low energy bond
~ P = Phosphorous with a high energy bond
Adenosine diphosphate (ADP)
Adenosine — O — P — O ~ P — OH +
Energy released from ~P and used for biochemical reactions and biological activities.

When energy is needed for a biochemical reaction or biological activities an enzyme which acts as an ATPase (e.g., Na^+-K^+ATPase or myosin ATPase or some other hydrolytic enzyme) hydrolyzes ATP. The terminal P_i breaks off and releases its contained energy (~P). This energy is an obligatory requirement for the energy needed for biochemical reactions and biological activities. If energy is insufficient and there is no more ATP available the enzyme hydrolyzes ADP to get more energy.

ATP + ATPase → ADP + ~P → energy for a biological activity or biochemical reaction.

ADP + ATPase → AMP + ~P → energy for a biological activity or biochemical reaction.

The central nervous system (CNS) is a voracious consumer of ~P. Glucose is the obligatory substrate but after a period of starvation some ketones are usable for production [f ~P. The CNS is the principal controller of biology and when it ceases to function death ensues. Without ~P, deficits in brain function appear in 20-40sec and death follows if deficits arenot restored to normal levels in approximately four minutes. Earlier restoration of energy deficits could avoid a fatal outcome but usually with a recovery marred by decreased intellectual and motor functions. Central nervous system deficits of ~P which are not acute or complete result in slow deterioration of brain function. These are characteristic of dementias due to multi-infarct dementias, Alzheimer's disease and prion infections. Chart 4-1 summarizes the biochemistry of ATP, ADP and ~P.

In addition to the absorbed products of food digestion production of ~P needs the intestinal absorption of water, minerals and vitamins, and the transfer of environmental oxygen to the blood by the lungs. All meet inside cells where there is production of ~P, mediated by cytoplasmic and mitochondrial enzymes.

What is energy?

Energy is the capacity for doing work. Examples are mechanical work, heat transfer from one system to another, generation of electricity, and chemical synthesis (anabolism). Catabolism breaks bonds and releases energy.

High energy phosphate bonds.

Compounds with high energy phosphate bonds (i.e.,~P) release about 7.3KCal of energy each time phosphorous breaks off at ATP or ADP terminals.

The following are equations for energy release from ATP, ADP and adenosine monophosphate (AMP):

1. ATP + water → ADP + inorganic phosphorous + 7.3KCal\mole
2. ADP + water → AMP + inorganic phosphorous + 7.3KCal\mole
3. AMP + water → Adenosine + inorganic phosphorous + 3.4KCal\mole

The average human cell contains more than 3000 enzymes. All use ~P for their synthesis from nuclear DNA, and for their synthetic activities. Catabolism releases ~P which is stored in ATP or ADP till needed. Hence, the central, seminal, and essential role of ~P in biology. As previously mentioned, glucose is an obligatory substrate for creation of ~P in the central nervous system (CNS). So also is oxygen. Ketones can be used as a source of some energy for CNS use after a few days of starvation.

Other compounds with high energy phosphate bonds.

High energy phosphate bonds are also present in compounds other than ATP and ADP:

Guanosine triphosphate (GTP). This compound is important for protein synthesis and for the transfer of extracellular messages to the interiors of cells.

Phosphocreatine. Creatine is synthesized in the liver and phosphorylated in skeletal muscle to phosphocreatine. Normally, the neuromuscular impulse eventuates in activation of myosin ATPase which detaches ~P from intracellular ATP. The released energy is used for ratcheting thin filaments over thick filaments. The result is muscle contraction. Phosphocreatine is a reserve source of ~P for muscle contraction during exercise. It provides the additional ~P needed when energy needs exceed the ~P available from local ATP and ADP. When even this does not suffice because of local oxygen deficits some additional energy is obtained from anaerobic glycolysis (see later for a description). Lactic acid enters the blood but is removed soon after the exercise ceases. When the need for additional energy ends the creatine reverts to phosphocreatine. Both the catabolic and the anabolic reactions are catalyzed by the enzyme, phosphocreatine kinase.

Acylphosphates such as 3-phosphoglyceryl-1-phosphate, acylthioesters and acetyl coA. Acetyl coA is particularly important because it is a key intermediate in metabolism and can be derived from glucose via pyruvic acid and also from the oxidation of fatty acids and amino acids.

Why are high energy phosphate bonds used as energy banks?

Compounds containing ~P are energy banks. The currency unit of biology is ~P. The cell uses many enzyme catalyzed reactions that use inhaled oxygen to convert the products of intestinal absorption to ~P. This energy is stored in ATP and ADP. Subsequent release of ~P from ATP and ADP provides biological systems with usable energy, as and when needed.

The body needs lots of energy to drive its systems. This is why the binding and subsequent release of ~P from ATP and ADP is continuous. Typically, an ATP molecule may exist as such for only a few seconds before breaking down to ADP. The cell uses the energy in ~P to effect a biological activity such as muscle contraction.

An obvious disadvantage is that many complex chemical reactions must take place before biochemical reactions in the body can use the energy in ingested food, or in intracellular stores of fat and protein. The mechanisms for transformation of energy derived from the environment to energy that is usable for biochemical reactions and biological activities require complex and sequential intracellular reactions and viable enzymes. Normal cells are not immortal. The inevitable and progressive degeneration and death of cells from aging, from disease, or from a combination of both, eventually reduces the intracellular activity required to produce ~P and, as a corollary, to sustain life.

Certainly, there are advantages. It is more economical to store energy as ~P (7.3KCal per chemical bond) than as low energy bonds (3.4KCal per bond). In addition, the needs for energy may not, and often do not temporally coincide with available energy. Storage of energy as ~P in ATP or ADP conserves it until needed. Otherwise, whatever was not immediately needed would release as heat. The excess heat liberated could compromise the heat regulating mechanisms of the body with failure of body temperature control and eventual death. In addition, the use of energy substrate without initial conversion and conservation as ~P could result in energy deficits when energy substrate was not available. The conversion and storage of environmental energy as ~P permits energy to be supplied on an economical as-needed basis. It also conserves energy that exceeds immediate needs.

The process is similar to the mechanics of gasoline stations where gasoline is always available (not always but usually) and stored in tanks. Similarly energy usable for biology is stored as high energy phosphate bonds in cells. When more gasoline is needed we go to the pump and fill up. Similarly, when more energy is needed the cell goes to stored ~P and fills up with energy. Both systems are efficient and easy to use and wastage is minimal. Gasoline is a commodity for execution of a purpose and so are the high energy phosphate bonds. Without gasoline the car will not function and neither will the body if energy usable for biological activities is not available.

How is energy quantified?

Biological energy is quantified as calories. One calorie is the heat needed to warm one gram of water from 14.5°C to 15.5°C at a pressure of 1 atmosphere. The kilocalorie (KCal) is the usual measure employed for expressing the energy content of food and the energy needs of the body. It is equal to 1000 calories. Energy is measurable in other ways, depending on its nature; electron volts measure electricity and joules measure work.

The law of energy conservation.

This law is one of the fundamental laws of our planet. It states that one can never create energy. It can only be transformed from one type to another. The law of energy conservation applies to all biological reactions, regardless of whether the reaction is enzyme-catalyzed or not. In biology the changes in mass during chemical reactions is so small that corrections for this can be ignored. Chart 4-2 summarizes the mechanisms of biological energy interconversions and the different potential functions of intracellular energy. There is some over-simplification in the chart but it does depict the basic principles of the interconversions of energy.

Every substance has an amount of energy which is intrinsic to its physical and chemical state. However, some heat is usually produced and often lost when one form of energy converts to another. An example is the conversion of the chemical energy in muscle to the mechanical energy needed for muscle contraction. There is always some heat produced and lost in the process. Some of this heat is used to maintain body temperature and to warm ingested food to temperatures that are optimal for activity of digestive system enzymes. Heat in excess of needs dissipates into the environment. The amount of energy used in the conversions remains unchanged.

Where does biological energy originate?

I have obtained the information in this paragraph from the Encylopedia Britannica which probably confers on the information a qualified imprimatur for accuracy. Biological energy originates in the sun which is some 93 million miles distant from our planet. Deep in the core of the sun hydrogen atoms fuse to form helium. The process generates a temperature of some 27 million degrees fahrenheit. The energy generated gradually works its way to the surface of the sun over a period of millions of years. It then radiates into space as photons. The earth only intercepts about 1 part in 2,200,000,000 of this energy but this is optimal for development of complex life forms; more would roast us while less would freeze.

Environmental energy substrate to high energy phosphate bonds (~P)

Many processes are required. Each is considered in sequence.

Photosynthesis.

Photosynthesis is the process that converts light energy to energy substrate which the body uses to make energy that is usable for biological activities. Chlorophyll in green plants soak up the light **(Contd. on page 84.)**

Chart 4-2: INTRACELLULAR PRODUCTION AND INTERCONVERSIONS OF ENERGY USABLE FOR BIOLOGICAL NEEDS

When energy is needed for biochemical reactions and other biological activities ATP is catabolized to ADP, ~P separates and the energy in its high energy phosphate bonds is released. If this does not provide enough energy ADP is catabolized to AMP with release of more energy. Each time ~P separates from a mole of ATP or ADP 7.3KCal energy is released and used for any or more of the activities listed below.

Intracellular energy from:

1. Energy substrate is inhaled environmental oxygen and the absorbed products of food digestion (glucose, galactose, fructose, fat microbodies, fatty acids, glycerol, glycerides and amino acids) and absorbed water, minerals and vitamins.
   Intracellular oxidative catabolism converts the substrate to energy usable for biological needs and stored in high energy phosphate bonds (~P) which, in turn are stored in ATP and ADP. As and when needed, the terminal bonds binding inorganic phosphorous to ATP or ADP are broken and the ~P released is used for biological needs.
2. Energy for biological needs can also be produced by similar catabolisms which use oxygen and the intracellular breakdown products of stored glycogen, fat and protein to produce ~P. Glucose is produced by gluconeogenesis from protein and is used during periods of low glucose intake for production of ~P.
3. Alternatively, the breakdown products could be transferred by the blood stream to distant cells where energy deficits exist. There, intracellular catabolism can convert them to the energy in ~P.

1.

Energy usable for biochemical reactions and biological activities, packaged as high energy phosphate bonds (~P) and stored in ATP and ADP till needed.

When energy is needed enzymes detach the terminal phosphorous bond of ATP or ADP and ~P is released. The energy in ~P is used to produce ATP from ADP.

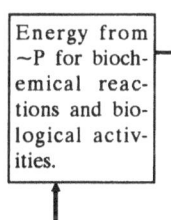

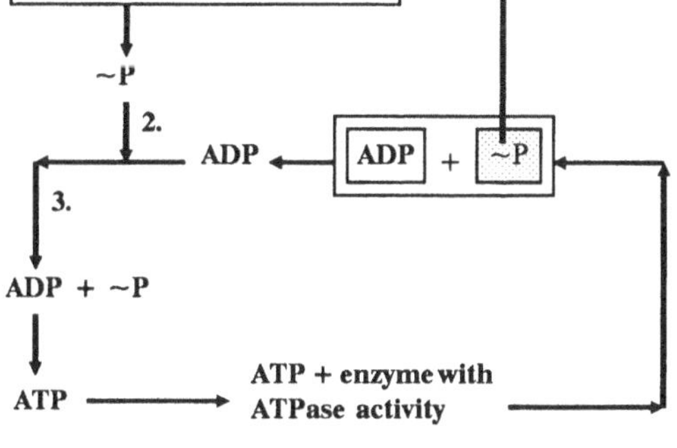
~P
2.
ADP
ADP + ~P
3.
ADP + ~P
ATP
ATP + enzyme with ATPase activity
4.

Energy from ~P for biochemical reactions and biological activities.

5.

CHEMICAL WORK.

1. Energy for biochemical syntheses.
   Examples of synthetic activities are:
   a. Synthesis of enzymes and other proteins from the intracellular DNA.
   b. Synthesis of fats, carbohydrates and proteins, of enzymes, of neurotransmitters, of endocrine, and exocrine secretions, of cell wall receptors and pump systems, and many other items.
   c. Synthesis of systems which perform intracellular housekeeping (e.g., the Golgi apparatus), and detoxifications.
2. Energy for other biological activities such as activations of cell membrane pump systems and muscle contraction.
   One estimate is that the sodium pump systems use about 30% of the energy released when ATP catabolism results in release of ~P in cells. In muscle and nerves the estimated figure has been as high as 60-70%. Most of this energy is used by the sodium pumps to extrude Na^+ ions and thus restore intracellular negativity.

ELECTRICAL WORK.

Energy for the generation and propagation of nerve and muscle action potentials.

MECHANICAL WORK.

Energy for:

1. Contraction of striated muscle for volitional activity and for maintenance of muscle tone and resistance against the stresses of gravity.
2 Contraction of cardiac muscle.
3. Contraction of non-striated smooth muscle (vascular, gastro intestinal, etc.).

HEAT PRODUCTION.

1. Used to maintain body temperature. It also heats ingested food and water to body temperature for optimum processing.
2. Heat in excess of needs is dissipated into the environment or used to convert more ADP to ATP or to participate in anabolic reactions and other biological activities..

(Contd. from page 82
)energy in photons. Plant enzymes use this energy to produce food. The principal products of photosynthesis are carbohydrates. Amino acids, proteins, lipids and other organic compounds may also form during photosynthesis. Nitrogen, phosphorous, sulfur and other elements provide the raw materials for these syntheses. The amounts produced are small.

The general equation of photosynthesis is:

$nCO_2 + nH_2O$ + the energy in solar photons + chlorophyll → $(CH_2O)_n + nO_2$

The oxygen used for carbohydrate production comes from the water in the equation. $(CH_2O)_n$ could be a simple carbohydrate such as glucose ($C_6H_{12}O_6$) or more complex conjugated carbohydrates such as starch. Most of the glucose units produced do usually convert to starch.

Humans eat the products of photosynthesis, either as vegetables or grains, or after its processing to meat by animals. The intestines digest food into energy-containing components that are absorbed and enter a blood stream containing oxygen derived from inhaled atmospheric air. These substances, and absorbed water, vitamins and minerals, are the substrates for production of ~P within cells. Charts 4-3, 4-4 and 4-5 depict the intracellular enzyme-mediated reactions that effect these conversions.

A lot of water is needed for the reactions of photosynthesis. Where does it come from? Water is abundant on the surfaces of the earth. It constitutes some 70% of the earth's surfaces. Their depths vary from 0 at sea levels to maximums of 10,924m in the Challenger Deep in the Pacific ocean Mariana Trench and 8,605m in the Milwaukee Deep of the Puerto Rico Trench in the Atlantic ocean. Continual convection currents exchange water between those at different depths. Many computer program claim to determine the currents and convections in these oceans. The cynic wonders if many are not written to confirm the preconceived ideas of their originators as the conclusions and programs often differ from one to the other. The task of determining convections in large oceans seem daunting and beyond the current capabilities of humans. All that is sure is that when surface hot water evaporates deeper cold water must move to the vacated area.

Light energy from the sun heats ocean and other waters. Surface water evaporates and enters the atmosphere as water vapor. Water vapor then travels long distances because atmospheric temperature and pressure changes generate winds. Eventually water vapor re-condenses into rain or snow. They fall on, and are used in areas where there are new plant and animal lives developing. Unused water drains into rivers that in turn drain into seas and oceans. This cycle repeats again and again. It is a cycle well known and described in antiquity:

> "Southward goes the wind, then turns to the north; it turns and turns again; back then to its circling goes the wind. Into the sea all the rivers go and yet the sea is never filled and still to their goal the rivers go." (Ecclesiastes 1:6).

The oxygen produced during photosynthesis.

Photosynthesis produces oxygen which radiates into the atmosphere. Living organisms inhale it, transfer it to their blood streams and then to their intracellular environments. Intracellular enzyme systems use oxygen to catabolize the products of intestinal digestion and absorption to ~P which binds to AMP or ADP to form ADP and ATP respectively. Our basic need for oxygen is about 250ml/min at rest. Obviously this requirement will increase with activity.

The brain uses about 20% of this oxygen. When oxygen is in short supply because of disease or because of life at high altitudes, the needs of the brain overrides those of other tissues. Normally, every 100gm of brain tissue must have about 5.5mg of glucose and 3.5ml of oxygen each minute. The consequences of oxygen and glucose insufficiency were previously described. They directly result from insufficient ~P for normal cerebral function as glucose is the only substrate the brain can use for production of ~P (ketone metabolism can provide the CNS with some energy after a period of starvation).

Anaerobic and aerobic metabolism.

Energy substrate (i.e., oxygen, the absorbed products of food digestion and absorbed water, minerals and vitamins) enters the blood and the heart pumps it through the ramifications of the vascular system. They enter cells by a variety of methods: diffusion, facilitated transport and carrier-mediated transport. **Once in the cells three sequential processes convert them to the high energy bonds that bind inorganic phosphorous to AMP or ADP to form ADP and ATP respectively. These three processes are:**

- **Anaerobic metabolism.**
- **Aerobic metabolism and**
- **The Electron Transport System.**

Anaerobic metabolism.

The process is depicted in Chart 4-3. It does not require oxygen and is the only form of metabolism available for production of ~P when mitochondria are absent (e.g., in the red cells), or when not enough oxygen is available. Oxygen needs increase during vigorous muscular exercise. When not enough oxygen is available for intracellular aerobic production of ATP aerobic metabolism of muscle phosphocreatine provides ~P. If even this is not enough anaerobic metabolism provides additional ~P. The lactic acid end-product of anaerobic metabolism enters the blood. Eventually respiratory and hepatic adjustments restore the previous status quo.

Aerobic metabolism in the Kreb's cycle.

The basic processes are summarized in Chart 4-4. It is the next step in the production of high energy phosphate bonds. The chart depicts the essentials in enough detail for the purposes of this monograph and additional text is not needed.

The Electron Transport System.

In the Electron Transport system the products of Kreb's cycle metabolism sequentially transfer to compounds with increasing affinities for electrons. Each time a compound takes up hydrogen there is a simultaneous release of energy that binds inorganic phosphorous to AMP or ADP to form high energy phosphate bonds. Energy release occurs at four points in the Electron Transport system. Oxygen is the recipient of the final transfer of electrons and the final equation for this system is:

$\frac{1}{2}O_2 + 2H^+ + 2e^- = H_20$

The electron transport chain is essentially a continuation of aerobic metabolism and is depicted as such in Chart 4-4.

Energy balance sheets for glucose and tristearins.

The oxidative catabolism of 1mole glucose yields 38moles ATP. Chart 4-5 summarizes the energy balance sheet for glucose and tristearin metabolism. Tristearins are first metabolized in the beta-oxidation system to acetyl-Coenzyme A. Oxidative catabolism in the Kreb's cycle and Electron Transport chain converts this acetyl coenzyme A to ~P.

Gluconeogenesis.

When blood glucose levels are critically low because glucose is not being ingested mechanisms must exist for glucose production from other sources. They are glycogenolysis of liver glycogen and gluconeogenesis (Chart 4-6).

Protein is the main source of gluconeogenesis when starvation is prolonged as only odd-chain fatty acids can convert to glucose (they only constitute about 5% of the body's fatty acid content).Enzymes for conversion of even-chain fatty acids to glucose do not exist in the body. Hence, the principal substrates of gluconeogenesis are amino acids (especially alanine) released from peripheral stores of protein. Other sources are glycerol and odd-chain fatty acids. Amino acids and these other sources of glucose are first converted to pyruvate or oxaloacetate, and glucose is then synthesized from them. The liver and, to a lesser extent, the kidney are the principal sites of gluconeogenesis. The process of amino acid gluconeogesis is shown in Chart 4-6.

When there is prolonged and continuous gluconeogenesis, as in starvation or a hunger strike there is continuous loss of body protein. When this loss approximates 30-50% of body stores of protein death from respiratory failure is imminent. Most 100% hunger strikers die within 60 days of beginning **(Contd. on page 88)**

Chart 4-3: **1. THE ANAEROBIC CATABOLISM OF GLUCOSE (~P DENOTES ENERGY IN A HIGH ENERGY PHOSPHATE BOND)[1]**

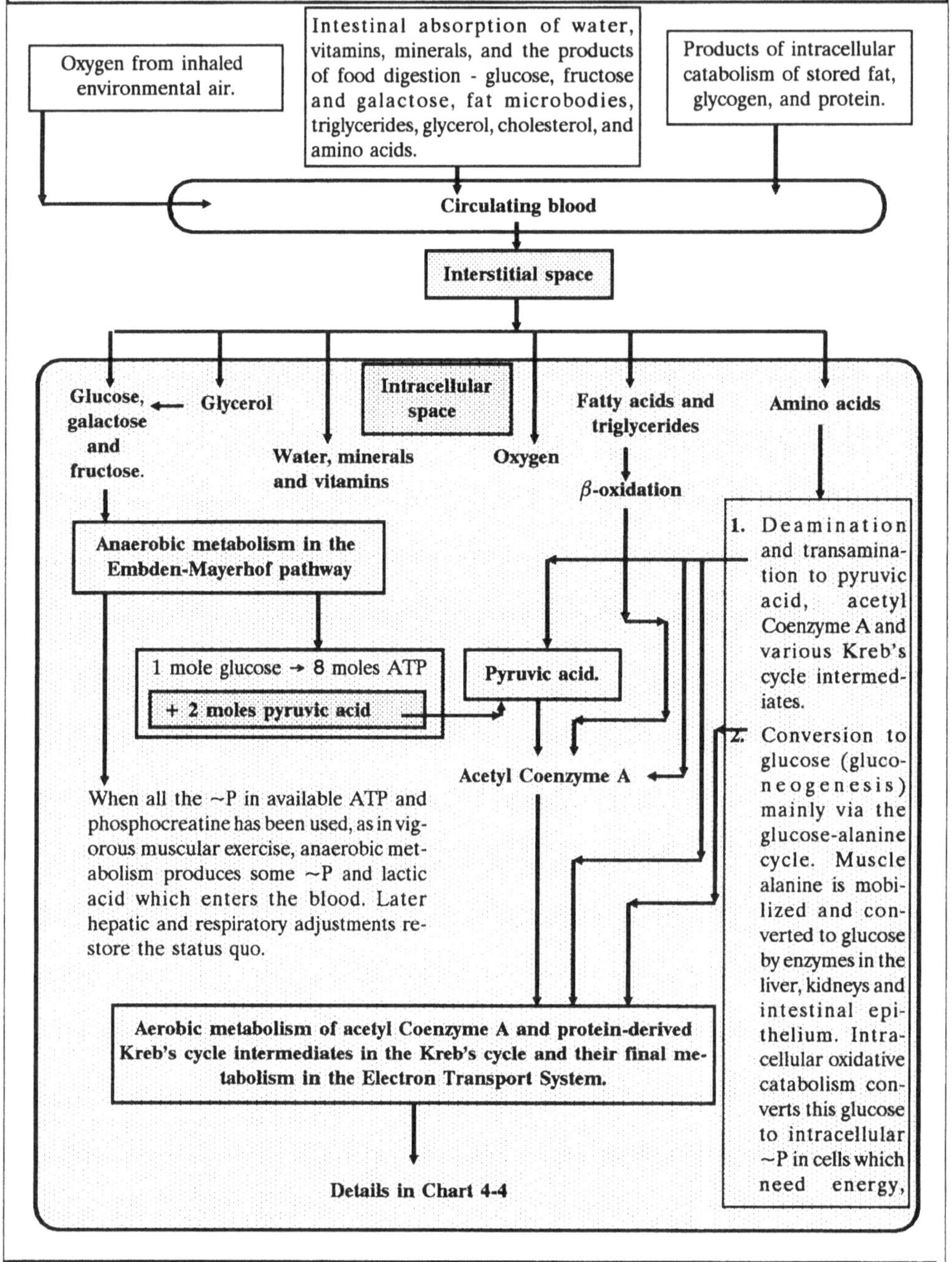
Oxygen from inhaled environmental air.
Intestinal absorption of water, vitamins, minerals, and the products of food digestion - glucose, fructose and galactose, fat microbodies, triglycerides, glycerol, cholesterol, and amino acids.
Products of intracellular catabolism of stored fat, glycogen, and protein.
Circulating blood
Interstitial space
Intracellular space
Glucose, galactose and fructose.
Glycerol
Water, minerals and vitamins
Oxygen
Fatty acids and triglycerides
Amino acids
β-oxidation
Anaerobic metabolism in the Embden-Mayerhof pathway
1 mole glucose → 8 moles ATP
+ 2 moles pyruvic acid
Pyruvic acid.
Acetyl Coenzyme A
When all the ~P in available ATP and phosphocreatine has been used, as in vigorous muscular exercise, anaerobic metabolism produces some ~P and lactic acid which enters the blood. Later hepatic and respiratory adjustments restore the status quo.
1. Deamination and transamination to pyruvic acid, acetyl Coenzyme A and various Kreb's cycle intermediates.
2. Conversion to glucose (gluconeogenesis) mainly via the glucose-alanine cycle. Muscle alanine is mobilized and converted to glucose by enzymes in the liver, kidneys and intestinal epithelium. Intracellular oxidative catabolism converts this glucose to intracellular ~P in cells which need energy,
Aerobic metabolism of acetyl Coenzyme A and protein-derived Kreb's cycle intermediates in the Kreb's cycle and their final metabolism in the Electron Transport System.
Details in Chart 4-4

[1] **Anaerobic metabolism balance sheet:** 1mole glucose → 2moles pyruvic acid + 2moles ATP + 2 pairs of hydrogen atoms which are metabolized in the Electron Transport Chain to 6moles of ATP. Therefore the anaerobic metabolism of 1mole glucose yields 8moles ATP.

Chart 4-4: 2. OXIDATIVE CATABOLISM IN THE KREB'S CYCLE AND ELECTRON TRANSPORT SYSTEM (~P DENOTES HIGH ENERGY PHOSPHATE BONDS)

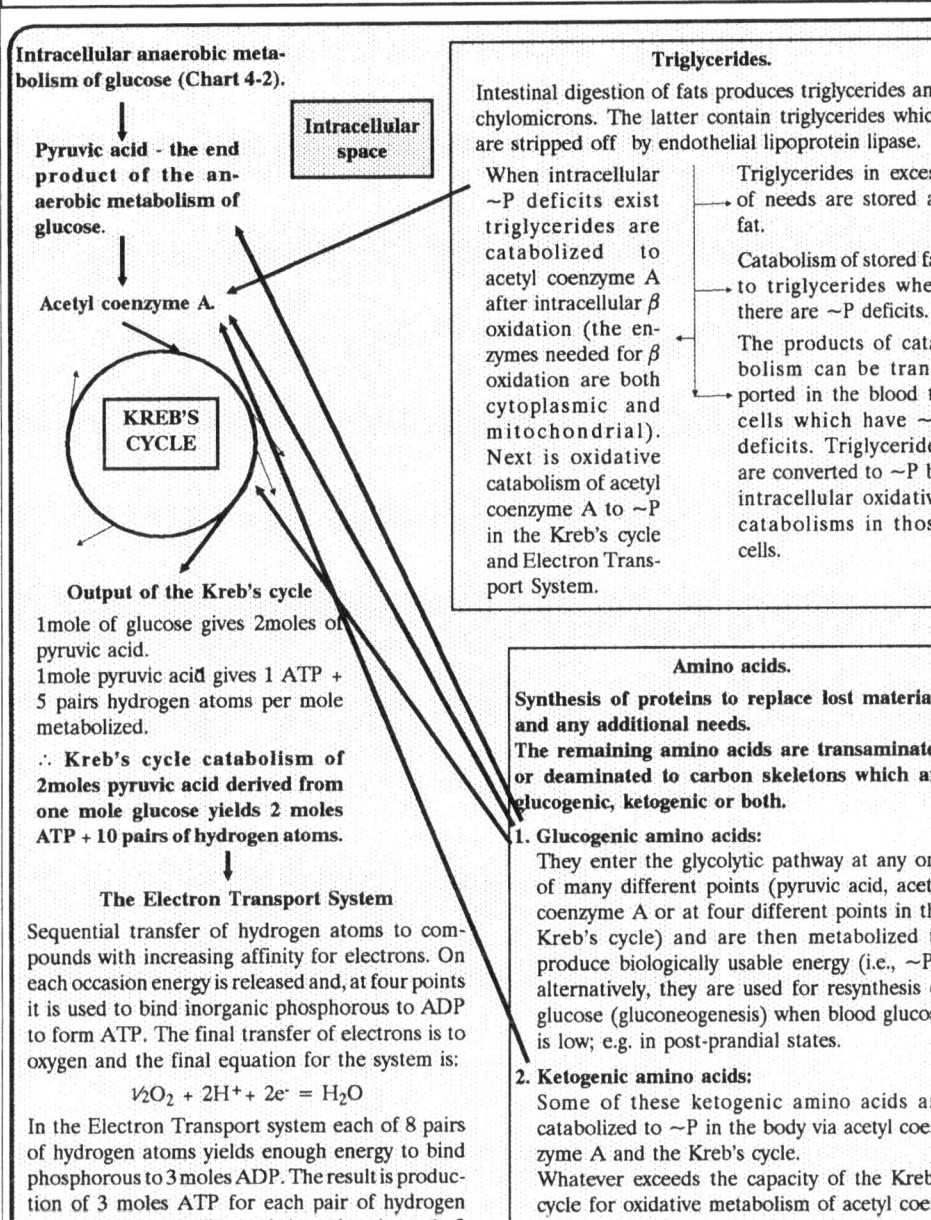

Intracellular anaerobic metabolism of glucose (Chart 4-2).

↓

Pyruvic acid - the end product of the anaerobic metabolism of glucose.

↓

Acetyl coenzyme A.

Intracellular space

KREB'S
CYCLE

Output of the Kreb's cycle

1mole of glucose gives 2moles of pyruvic acid.
1mole pyruvic acid gives 1 ATP + 5 pairs hydrogen atoms per mole metabolized.

∴ Kreb's cycle catabolism of 2moles pyruvic acid derived from one mole glucose yields 2 moles ATP + 10 pairs of hydrogen atoms.

↓

The Electron Transport System

Sequential transfer of hydrogen atoms to compounds with increasing affinity for electrons. On each occasion energy is released and, at four points it is used to bind inorganic phosphorous to ADP to form ATP. The final transfer of electrons is to oxygen and the final equation for the system is:

$$\tfrac{1}{2}O_2 + 2H^+ + 2e^- = H_2O$$

In the Electron Transport system each of 8 pairs of hydrogen atoms yields enough energy to bind phosphorous to 3 moles ADP. The result is production of 3 moles ATP for each pair of hydrogen atoms transferred. Two of the pairs give only 2 moles ATP each. ∴ the 10 pairs of hydrogen atoms from aerobic metabolism of 1mole glucose yields 28 moles ATP ((8 x 3) + 4)[1].

Triglycerides.

Intestinal digestion of fats produces triglycerides and chylomicrons. The latter contain triglycerides which are stripped off by endothelial lipoprotein lipase.

When intracellular ~P deficits exist triglycerides are catabolized to acetyl coenzyme A after intracellular β oxidation (the enzymes needed for β oxidation are both cytoplasmic and mitochondrial). Next is oxidative catabolism of acetyl coenzyme A to ~P in the Kreb's cycle and Electron Transport System.

→ Triglycerides in excess of needs are stored as fat.

→ Catabolism of stored fat to triglycerides when there are ~P deficits.

→ The products of catabolism can be transported in the blood to cells which have ~P deficits. Triglycerides are converted to ~P by intracellular oxidative catabolisms in those cells.

Amino acids.

Synthesis of proteins to replace lost materials and any additional needs.

The remaining amino acids are transaminated or deaminated to carbon skeletons which are glucogenic, ketogenic or both.

1. Glucogenic amino acids:

They enter the glycolytic pathway at any one of many different points (pyruvic acid, acetyl coenzyme A or at four different points in the Kreb's cycle) and are then metabolized to produce biologically usable energy (i.e., ~P); alternatively, they are used for resynthesis of glucose (gluconeogenesis) when blood glucose is low; e.g. in post-prandial states.

2. Ketogenic amino acids:

Some of these ketogenic amino acids are catabolized to ~P in the body via acetyl coenzyme A and the Kreb's cycle.
Whatever exceeds the capacity of the Kreb's cycle for oxidative metabolism of acetyl coenzyme A to ~P is converted to ketone bodies (acetoacetic acid and then acetone and β-hydroxybutyric acid) and excreted in the urine.

[1] The aerobic metabolism in the Kreb's cycle of 2moles pyruvic acid derived from 1mole of glucose yields 2moles ATP and 10 pairs of hydrogen atoms. Metabolism of the hydrogen atoms in the Electron Transport chain yields 28moles ATP. ∴ aerobic metabolism of 1mole glucose in the Kreb's cycle and subsequent metabolism in the Electron Transport System yields 30moles ATP.

(Contd. from page 85)

Chart 4-5: GLUCOSE AND TRISTEARIN METABOLISM BALANCE SHEET SUMMARIZED

1. Anaerobic metabolism of 1 mole glucose → 2 moles pyruvic acid	⟶	8moles ATP
2. Aerobic metabolism of 2moles pyruvic acid in the Kreb's cycle and then in the Electron Transport System	⟶	30moles ATP
∴ Total yield from metabolism of 1mole glucose	=	38moles ATP
Each mole ATP can yield 7.3KCal energy. ∴ total energy output from metabolism of 1 mole glucose is 38 x 7.3KCal energy	=	277KCal/mole of glucose metabolized
Energy from in vivo metabolism of 1mole of a tristearin = 463moles ATP. ∴ total energy output is 463 x 7.3KCal/mole[1]	=	3380KCal/mole of tristearin

[1] Before conversion to acetyl coenzyme A tristearins are first catabolized by β oxidation.

the fast, provided water is available and drunk. As mentioned above, death is usually the result of respiratory failure secondary to respiratory muscle failure because of protein loss.

Fat stores provide some 80% of the body's stores of energy - enough to provide basic calories for about two months. It can provide energy for all body systems except the CNS. Admittedly, after some days of starvation the brain begins to use ketones for some of its energy needs.

Energy homeostasis.

An instructive way to study energy homeostasis is to compare the biochemical changes in the immediate and the late post-absorption phases after eating a meal.

The immediate post-absorption phase.

The products of intestinal food digestion and absorption are glucose, galactose and fructose from carbohydrates; amino acids from proteins, and fatty acids, glycerol and chylomicrons from fat digestion. Chylomicrons are complexes of triglycerides and some cholesterol with coatings of protein and phospholipids. Lipoprotein lipase in capillary endothelia extract the triglycerides which are catabolized locally to provide ~P. The cholesterol remnant goes to the liver. There is also intestinal absorption of water, vitamins and minerals. Immediately after consumption of a meal glucose is the main source of energy for body cells and especially the cells of the central nervous system. At this stage protein and fat only provide a small portion of the energy the body needs.

Some of the absorbed amino acids and fat products synthesize the protein and fat needed to replace intracellular stores that are being continually broken down. Most of the absorbed products of fat and carbohydrate digestion that exceed immediate energy needs are stored as fat. Fat is ideal for storage of energy substrate. One gram of fat can store 9 calories of energy compared with the 4 calories per gram that can be stored as carbohydrate or protein. In addition, fat storage does not need intracellular water. One estimate is that storage of energy as carbohydrate rather than fat would result in a body mass six to eight times greater (Metabolism and Nutrition. In Smith, L.H., Thier, S.O. (Ed.): Pathophysiology. The Biological Principles of Disease. Philadelphia: W.B. Saunders Company, 1981, p. 501.)

The late post-absorption phase.

No glucose is being absorbed but maintenance of blood glucose within a normal physiologically desirable range is essential for continued normal brain function. This is effected by liver and muscle glycogen catabolism to glucose which enters the circulation. About 700KCal/day can be obtained by these reactions. About 75% of the glucose used during and at the end of an overnight fast derives from glycogen breakdown. The importance

Chart 4-6: ALANINE AMINO ACID GLUCONEOGENESIS [1]

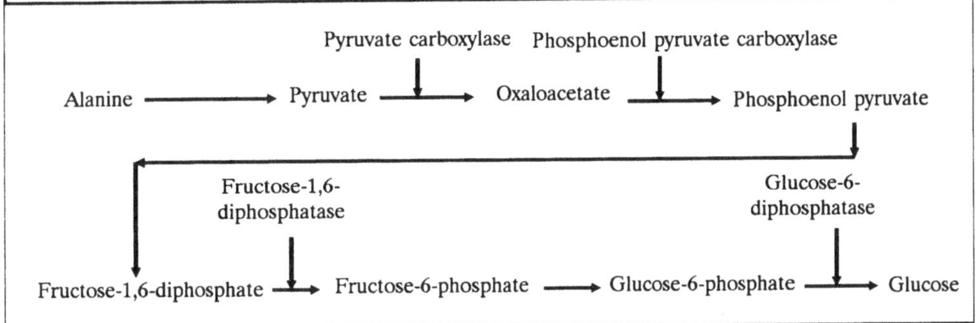
Pyruvate carboxylase
Phosphoenol pyruvate carboxylase
Alanine
Pyruvate
Oxaloacetate
Phosphoenol pyruvate
Fructose-1,6-diphosphatase
Glucose-6-diphosphatase
Fructose-1,6-diphosphate
Fructose-6-phosphate
Glucose-6-phosphate
Glucose

[1] The four enzymes pyruvate carboxylase, phosphoenol pyruvate carboxylase, fructose-1,6-diphosphatase and glucose-6-diphosphatase are all present in liver, kidney and intestinal epithelium.

of liver glycogenolysis as a source of blood glucose is seen in the rare Type 1 glycogen storage disease (von Gierke's disease). A deficiency of the enzyme glucose-6-phosphatase prevents the breakdown of glycogen to glucose and the result is hypoglycemia during a short fast.

The source of additional blood glucose is gluconeogenesis from protein, especially alanine (Chart 4-6). A glucose-alanine cycle has been described. Fats can provide energy to all tissues but not to the brain though some ketones can be used by the brain after a period of starvation. Fats are a negligible source of glucose for only odd-chain fatty acids can effect this conversion. As previously mentioned, such fatty acids only constitute about 5% of total body fatty acids.

In the post-absorptive phase most of the intracellular energy requirements (excluding the requirements of the brain) are met by intracellular oxidation of stored fat; intracellular catabolism liberates fatty acids which, after beta oxidation, enter the Kreb's cycle and Electron Transport Systems. The products are ~P stored in ATP or ADP.

Alternatively, the fatty acids released by intracellular catabolism of fat enter the blood for transfer to cells (but not brain cells) in which there are energy deficits. If fasting continues there is depletion of liver glycogen, lipolysis and gluconeogenesis from protein to provide for energy needs, especially those of the brain.

Control mechanisms for production of ~P during biological activities.

At three points in the Kreb's cycle ATP itself acts by negative feedback mechanisms to control energy production. The facts are graphically depicted in Chart 4-7.

Hormone interactions during energy homeostasis.

two principal hormones involved in glucose homeostasis are insulin and glucagon (Chart 4-8). Blood glucose levels are controlled by these two pancreatic hormones; insulin produced by the β cells and glucagon produced by the α cells. Control is by simple positive and negative feedback reactions between blood glucose levels and the islet cell receptors of the pancreas. An important and possibly, principal effect of insulin is to promote entry of glucose into cells. When the blood sugar is high insulin production increases, more glucose enters cells and blood glucose falls (this is an over-simplification of what happens but summarizes the basic facts). When blood glucose levels fall below physiologically desirable levels glucagon secretion increases. The blood sugar rises because of increased conversion of liver glycogen to glucose and increased gluconeogenesis (but not glycogenolysis) in muscle. There is a continual fluctuation in insulin-glucagon ratios. This fluctuation keeps blood glucose within physiologically permissible and desirable levels.

Diabetic and starvation ketoacidosis and the ketone bodies.

When starvation is prolonged or diabetes is severe and untreated intracellular deficits of glucose develop. This

Chart 4-7: ATP AND ADP AS REGULATORS OF ENERGY PRODUCTION. [1]

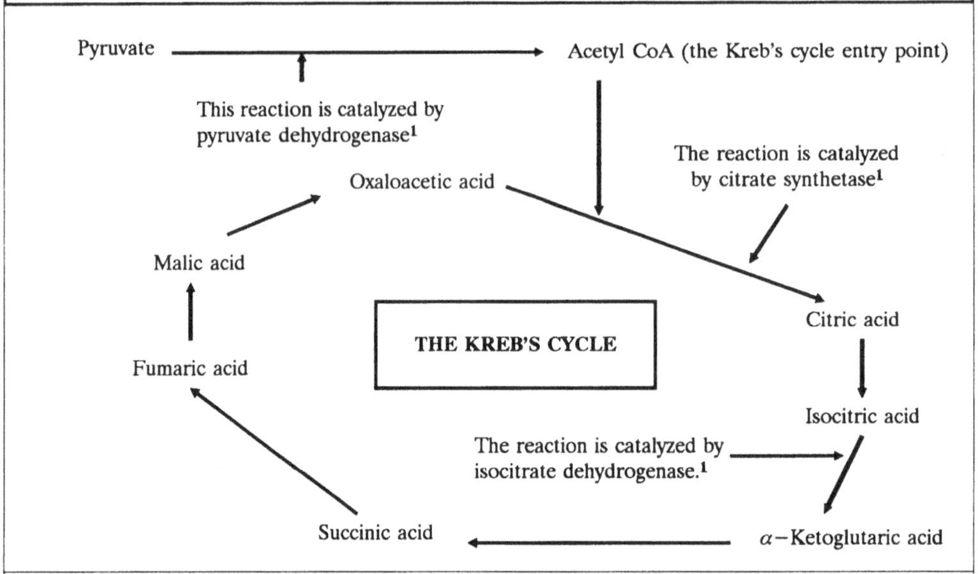
Pyruvate
Acetyl CoA (the Kreb's cycle entry point)
This reaction is catalyzed by pyruvate dehydrogenase[1]
The reaction is catalyzed by citrate synthetase[1]
Oxaloacetic acid
Malic acid
Citric acid
THE KREB'S CYCLE
Fumaric acid
Isocitric acid
The reaction is catalyzed by isocitrate dehydrogenase.[1]
Succinic acid
α−Ketoglutaric acid

[1] The three enzymes, pyruvate dehydrogenase, citrate synthetase and isocitrate dehydrogenase are regulators of ATP production. They are inhibited by high or adequate local concentrations of ATP. The enzymes are activated when insufficient ATP is present or local concentrations of ADP are high.

Chart 4-8: THE INSULIN-GLUCAGON COMPLEX FOR CONTROL OF BODY GLUCOSE

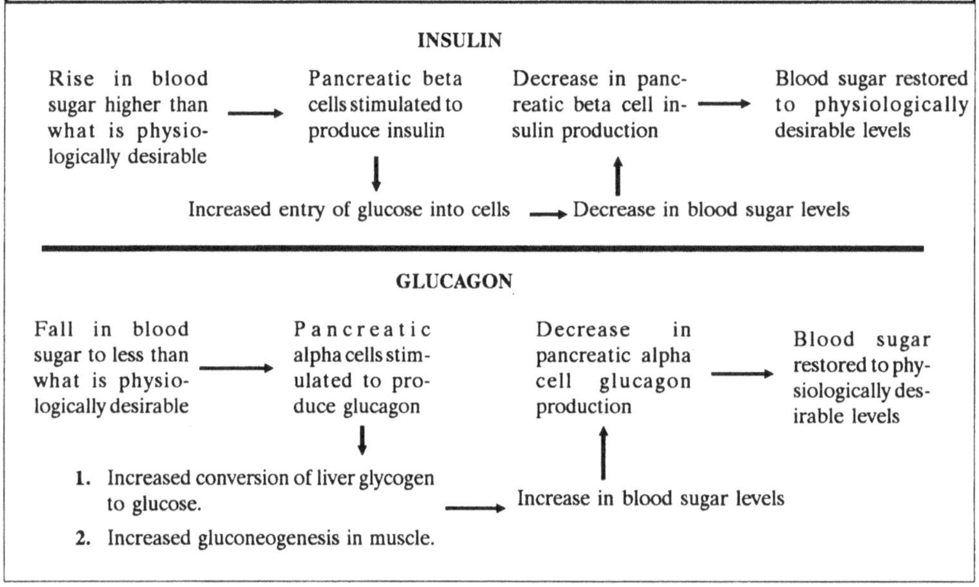
INSULIN
Rise in blood sugar higher than what is physiologically desirable
Pancreatic beta cells stimulated to produce insulin
Decrease in pancreatic beta cell insulin production
Blood sugar restored to physiologically desirable levels
Increased entry of glucose into cells
Decrease in blood sugar levels
GLUCAGON
Fall in blood sugar to less than what is physiologically desirable
Pancreatic alpha cells stimulated to produce glucagon
Decrease in pancreatic alpha cell glucagon production
Blood sugar restored to physiologically desirable levels
1. Increased conversion of liver glycogen to glucose.
2. Increased gluconeogenesis in muscle.
Increase in blood sugar levels

is because insulin promotes entry of glucose into cells and when the amount of circulating insulin is insufficient intracellular glucose decreases. Increased fatty acid oxidation can provide for energy needs in cells other than those in the CNS. An early step in fatty acid oxidation is formation of acetyl CoA (Chart 4-9). The acetyl coA which exceeds the rate of its oxidation in the Kreb's cycle is converted to ketone bodies; acetoacetic acid and then β- hydroxybutyric acid and acetone. These three substances enter the blood. The first two result in a metabolic acidosis, the third to the characteristic fruit-like odor of diabetic ketoacidosis. After a period of

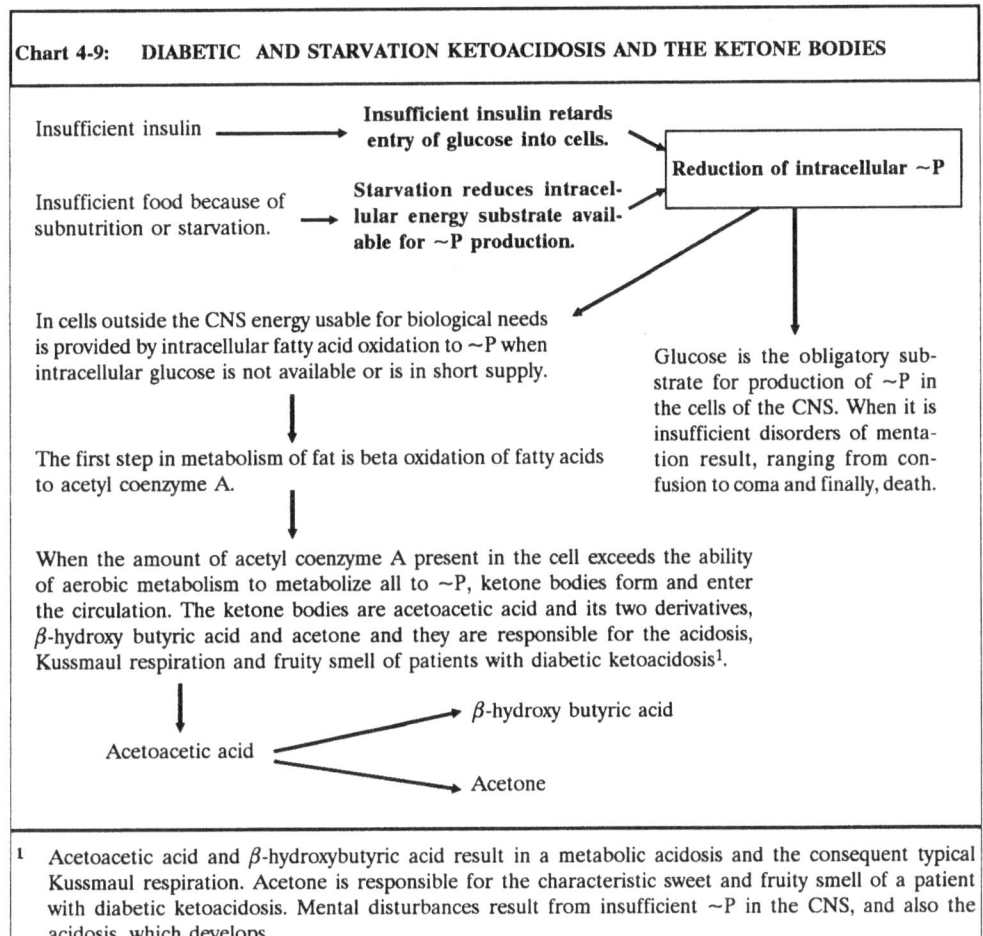

Chart 4-9: DIABETIC AND STARVATION KETOACIDOSIS AND THE KETONE BODIES

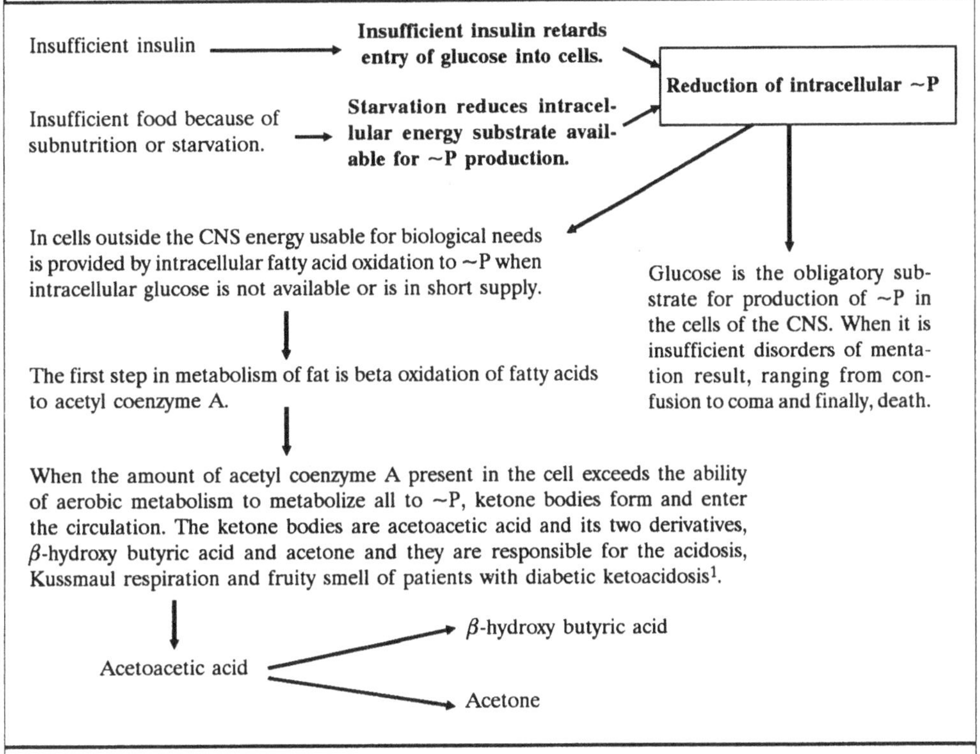
Insufficient insulin
Insufficient insulin retards entry of glucose into cells.
Reduction of intracellular ~P
Insufficient food because of subnutrition or starvation.
Starvation reduces intracellular energy substrate available for ~P production.
In cells outside the CNS energy usable for biological needs is provided by intracellular fatty acid oxidation to ~P when intracellular glucose is not available or is in short supply.
Glucose is the obligatory substrate for production of ~P in the cells of the CNS. When it is insufficient disorders of mentation result, ranging from confusion to coma and finally, death.
The first step in metabolism of fat is beta oxidation of fatty acids to acetyl coenzyme A.
When the amount of acetyl coenzyme A present in the cell exceeds the ability of aerobic metabolism to metabolize all to ~P, ketone bodies form and enter the circulation. The ketone bodies are acetoacetic acid and its two derivatives, β-hydroxy butyric acid and acetone and they are responsible for the acidosis, Kussmaul respiration and fruity smell of patients with diabetic ketoacidosis1.
β-hydroxy butyric acid
Acetoacetic acid
Acetone

1 Acetoacetic acid and β-hydroxybutyric acid result in a metabolic acidosis and the consequent typical Kussmaul respiration. Acetone is responsible for the characteristic sweet and fruity smell of a patient with diabetic ketoacidosis. Mental disturbances result from insufficient ~P in the CNS, and also the acidosis. which develops.

prolonged starvation the brain can use ketone bodies for some of its metabolic needs when glucose is in short supply. This also spares gluconeogenesis from protein, thus delaying respiratory muscle failure and death.

The role of energy in clinical decision-making

This chapter is not meant to be an irrelevant intellectual exercise. The topic of energy is very relevant to every aspect of clinical decision-making because the consequences of dysfunctions are the result of insufficient local energy, i.e., ~P, which is usable for biological needs.

As a rule the deficits are focal. Very frequently they have systemic consequences. Thus an infarct of the heart results in cardiac dysfunction because of a decrease in cardiac muscle blood supply. The decrease in blood supply reduces the availability of substrate, especially oxygen, for ~P production. The force of heart muscle contraction decreases and less blood is pumped into the peripheral vasculature which results in diffuse ~P deficits throughout the body.

It helps when physicians analyzing complex medical problems start with basic concepts. The most basic of all are questions relating the the availability of energy usable for biochemical reactions and biological activities, i.e. ~P. Some questions that need an answer are:

- Is the diet providing enough energy substrate?
- Is there pollution which reduces available oxygen?
- Is the individual unable to live in the low pO_2 levels which exist in a mountainous area? Many individuals have great difficulty in living in the high towns of Tibet or the Andes. Usually there is eventual acclimatization.
- Is there enough potable water for daily needs? Drought and famine go hand in hand in the decimations of populations.
- Are foods being digested and absorbed normally? Specifically, are there any gastrointestinal dysfunctions present?
- Where are the deficits of biologically usable energy located?
- Is delivery of insufficient oxygen to cells impaired because of lung dysfunctions or anemias which decrease the amount of oxygen that hemoglobin can carry to cells? Alternatively and/or additionally, are there any abnormal hemoglobins which have dysfunctional carrying, delivering and anatomical abnormalities? These are topics extensively detailed in Chapter 12.
- Is there any inadequate perfusion of tissues with energy substrate? Common systemic causes are cardiac dysfunctions and hypovolemic syndromes. Other causes include small (e.g., in the renal arterioles) and large (e.g., in limb vessels) vascular stenoses and occlusions. These are topics detailed in Chapter 11.
- Is tissue damage so extensive that even if ample amounts of substrate and oxygen are supplied the tissues cannot produce enough ~P? An extensive myocardial infarct is an example. When it approximates 40% of myocardial muscle acute cardiogenic shock and eventual death are probable.
- How effective are compensatory mechanisms in responding to any deficits?
- Are there any deficits of ~P production in other organs or systems?
- What, if any, are its consequences in other body structures?
- What can be done to improve the performance of cells which are not yet dead but are performing subnormally? Medications chosen should assist these responses. When the heart is involved they include medications to reduce afterload and preload by controlling hyprertension, reducing fluid retention and decreasing the normal tonic contractions of the arteriolar bed. Tissues damaged by infections can be helped by appropriate antibiotics and "good care". Respiratoery dysfunctions may require antibiotics, and possibly, corticosteroids and supplemental oxygen. Endocrine dysfunctions are often ameliorated by appropriate replacement or suppressive therapy. Many other therapies exist to assist physiological mechanisms to produce more ~P. A bleak area is the treatment of neurological dysfunctions where available therapies for control or cure are limited. Alas, a final demise is inevitable however effective the therapy given..

This chapter concludes with the repeated suggestion that biological dysfunctions be analyzed from first principles. Start with localization and treatment of ~P deficits. The next chapter shows how energy which is usable for biological needs, i.e., ~P, knits together all biological systems into an edifice of coordinated interaction.

5

Clinical Decision-Making: Some Basics

5. Enzymes, Homeostasis and Biological Systems

Table of Contents

Notation.

The notation ~P denotes phosphorous with a high energy bond. Depending on the context in which the term is used, ~P may also denote the energy liberated when a high energy phosphate bond detaches from ATP or ADP.

Four topics are detailed in this chapter:

- **Enzymes and their role in biology.**
- **Homeostasis.**
- **The enumeration and classification of biological systems and**
- **The principles of systems analysis of biological systems.**

The object is to establish a frame that shows how biological systems coordinate and integrate as a single unit that functions with purpose, smoothness, precision and coordination. This is not an intellectual exercise. The object of therapy should not be limited to only treating the specific disease. Equally important is the elimination of factors adversely affecting the integration and coordination of all body systems. Alternatively, if complete elimination of these factors is not possible, the objective should be the prevention of additional deterioration. Achievement of these objectives needs a frame that is logical and orderly and shows how biological systems interact and coordinate to act as a single smoothly functioning unit. Physicians who treat patients need a frame of this type to systematically study all systems of the body, in addition to those obviously diseased. The object is to determine which, if any, need functional amplifications or reductions to attain or retain the integrated coordinations of systems which are essentials for the satisfactory functional performances of all animates.

Enzymes.

Enzymes are the control units of in vivo biochemical reactions. They are catalysts that accelerate chemical reactions. An enzyme-catalyzed reaction does not change the amount or nature of the enzyme, nor does it change the final equilibrium constant of the reaction. Over 1500 enzymes are known. They are proteins with differing molecular weights (15,000 to greater than one million). Enzymes originate within cells by transcription and translation from DNA templates. All cells of an individual have similar DNA and hence, the capacity to produce any enzyme which exists in the body. They do not because most of the synthetic mechanisms are initially repressed. During life, each cell derepresses the DNA operons for synthesis of the enzymes that it needs. The remaining DNA operons remain repressed.

Control of enzyme synthesis.

Many questions remain about the process that selects which fragments of DNA are derepressed to produce the necessary enzymes. The basic model remains based on the one originally proposed by Jacob and Monod in 1961 to explain the functioning of the lac operon which synthesizes lactase. Subsequent findings have modified this original model but the basic propositions remain.

The sequence of genes needed for production of a protein is called an operon. The operon has an I gene at its beginning. The I gene is not repressed. It produces an I repressor protein that binds to the beginning of the operon and prevents synthesis of its enzyme protein. When substrate, in this instance lactose, is present, the substrate binds to the I protein and changes its shape so that it cannot bind to the starting point of the operon. A complex of catabolite activator protein (CAP) and c-AMP-receptor protein forms in the presence of substrate. The complex binds to the beginning of the operon and allows adjacent RNA polymerase to start lactase synthesis by the operon. The CAP-cAMP complex is a regulator of operon derepression. For example, when glucose or glycerol are present the amount of CAP-cAMP decreases and there is a corresponding reduction in lactase synthesis by the lac operon.

The above explanation of DNA derepression assumes cell walls with controlled passive or active transport mechanisms for intracellular introductions of specific substrates which deactivate corresponding I repressor proteins. Most studies on gene derepression have been done on bacteria. Whether or not similar processes determine gene derepressions in multicellular organisms certain incontrovertible facts remain. All cells have identical nuclear DNA and this DNA can produce any enzyme that exists in the body. It does not because of DNA repression by intracellular I gene products. Each cell derepresses DNA fragments that can synthesize enzymes which it requires. Some of these are common to all cells. Examples are the enzymes needed for the biochemical reactions that produce ~P, items needed for general housekeeping and transport, for degradation and elimination of undesirable endogenous or exogenous materials, for maintenance of cell wall integrities and transport systems, for replacement of deteriorated pump mechanisms and for many other activities.

In addition, each cell derepresses the DNA fragments that synthesize the enzymes needed for its specific functions. For example, thyroid cells derepress DNA fragments that transcribe the enzymes needed for thyroid hormone production but not those needed for production of gonadal hormones. Similarly, the cells of the adrenal cortex derepress the DNA fragments that synthesize enzymes for adrenal hormone production but not those required for synthesis of thyroid hormones. In addition, if the Monod-Jacob model is correct a feedback system between substrate and operon controls the amount of enzyme produced

One additional fact is important. The synthesis of an enzyme requires energy, i.e., **intracellular ~P.**

The basic qualities of enzymes.

Enzymes accelerate biological reactions.

- They do not change the amounts or natures of the products formed but only accelerate the reactions of synthesis or catabolism.
- Enzymes do not alter energy used or released in the reaction. How then does it accelerate reactions?

  The input of energy that is needed for chemical reactions to begin is the **"energy of activation"** of the reaction. Reactants which have the energy of activation are said to be in the **"transition state"** (a theoretical concept as the transition state cannot be isolated). The transition state can revert to reactants or proceed to formation of products. In either case the energy of activation is lost as thermodynamic stability is regained.

  The energy content of reactants and products are the same in enzyme-catalyzed reactions and in reactions not catalyzed by enzymes. **Enzymes accelerate reactions by reducing the amounts of energy needed by the reactants to reach their transition state.** Their ability to do this is substantial. Some enzymes can increase reaction rates of non-catalyzed reactions by as much as 10^{12}.
- Enzymes are not consumed in the reactions they catalyze. The amounts of enzyme at the beginning and end of a reaction are unchanged
- Enzymes work fast and this quality is measured in terms of "turnover numbers". The turnover number is the number of moles of substrate which are catalyzed by one mole of enzyme in one minute. It allows one to compare the catalytic effectiveness of different enzymes. For example, the turnover number for catalase is $5x10^6$ while for carbonic anhydrase it is $56x10^6$. Carbonic anhydrase is the enzyme needed for combination of CO_2 and H_2O to form H_2CO_3. It has one of the highest turnover number of known enzymes.

Enzyme specificity.

Reaction specificity is specificity that indicates the nature of reaction catalyzed. The principal ones are hydrolases, oxidoreductases, transferases, lysases, isomerases and ligases.

Substrate specificity. Substrate specificity is not as absolute as reaction specificity. For example alcohol dehydrogenase catalyzes oxidation-reduction reactions of different alcohols such as ethanol and methanol, up to butanol. However, in general, functionally specific enzymes prefer one substrate over others. Thus, even though alcohol dehydrogenase can catalyze different alcohols its preferred target is ethanol.

Reaction and substrate specificity lets enzymes choose reactants and respond to feedbacks from products. Cells contain many different chemicals. Normally the choice and speeds of biochemical reactions are determined by the concentrations of the available reactants and the physicochemical conditions in the milieu. If intracellular reactions were solely determined by physicochemical conditions a consequence could be the chaotic production of many unnecessary, biologically useless, and potentially toxic compounds.

Enzyme specificity bypasses biochemical reactions solely determined by intracellular physicochemical considerations. If enzyme is not available substrate derepresses the DNA operon which synthesizes the needed enzyme and so it goes from one reaction to the next. The net result is biochemical reactions that produce compounds needed for biologically effective cell function. Compounds that are not immediately needed are not produced.

Enzyme structure.

Each enzyme has two sites; a substrate binding site and an active site. Most have an additional site, the allosteric binding site.

The substrate binding site. As its name implies, the substrate binding site is the place where enzyme binds to substrate. The specificity of an enzyme derives from the chemical structure and composition at this site. There are two theories as to the mechanism of enzyme activation by binding of substrate. One is **the "lock-and-key" model"** which proposes that enzyme activation results from an exact and rigid fit between enzyme and substrate at the binding site. The other is **the "induced fit" model** which proposes that the initial fit between substrate and enzyme at the binding site is loose. After the interaction between enzyme and substrate a change in conformation takes place at the enzyme binding site, a change that makes the fit tight and results in enzyme activation. Those who accept this latter hypothesis also feel that allosteric controllers activate or inhibit enzyme activity by changing the conformation at the binding site, thus inducing a functional change in enzyme activity.

The "active site". The chemical groups needed for enzyme activation are located at the **"active site".** This site could be in the substrate binding site, be located adjacent to it, or be sited at some distance from the substrate binding site and edge to it after formation of tertiary structural folds.

The allosteric binding site. An allosteric binding site exists in most enzymes. It is needed for feedback controls of enzyme activity. As a rule the allosteric site is located at a distance from the active and substrate binding sites. Allosteric regulators can be substrate, products, products of other reactions, hormones, metabolites and ions. They bind at the allosteric sites and induce deformations that can inhibit or stimulate enzyme-mediated reactions.

Biological control by enzymes.

Enzymes are the basic units of biological activity and are essential for maintenance of homeostasis.

An increase in available enzyme does not increase the amount of product. It only increases the rate of the reaction. The amount of substrate determines the amount of product.

Most control of enzyme activity is the result of **feedbacks**. There are many forms of feedback control. Most involve the binding at the allosteric binding site of allosteric activators or inhibitors. Feedback mechanisms are essential for the biochemical controls of all cells.

The following are some examples of the ways that feedback control works:

Feedback inhibition. The end product of the reaction inhibits the enzyme responsible for its production.

Feedback activation. The enzyme is activated by a product of its reaction.

Sequential activation. This occurs when a number of different enzymes are required for a necessary biochemical change. An example is seen in Chart 4-5 on page 88. It shows the sequence of enzymes needed for gluconeogenesis from an amino acid. Another example is the synthesis of steroid and sex hormones from cholesterol (Chart 7-5 on page 166).

Parallel activation. The initial enzyme of a metabolic sequence is activated or inhibited by the metabolite of an independent but parallel sequence. This is a process often used to maintain a balance between metabolites that will be assembled in a group of macromolecular compounds.

Activation through a precursor. This can increase precise control of enzyme action. It is frequently seen in the activation of gastrointestinal enzymes.

Activation of the enzyme by the substrate itself. The substrate functions as an activator and also as an allosteric effector.

It is unusual for an enzyme to be limited to one form of control. The usual pattern is for the existence of many controls; end-product inhibition, substrate activation, sequential activation, parallel activation and complex interactions between the products and metabolites of several related reactions.

Dysfunctions due to defective enzymes.

Most dysfunctions resulting from abnormal enzymes are the result of Mendelian type inheritance or chance intrauterine chromosomal aberrations. A few are common but most are not. Texts on medical genetics are the best source of information about inherited enzyme dysfunctions. The chapter on the Gastrointestinal Tract (Chapter 9) describes three relatively common genetically determined dysfunctions of the gastrointestinal system: lactase deficiency, cystic fibrosis and celiac disease. The chapter on the Blood (Chapter 12) references many dysfunctions due to abnormal enzymes and describes a few such as the thalassemia syndromes, other hemoglobinopathies such as sickle cell anemia and various inherited deficits of the coagulation system. Huntington's disease is an inherited CNS disease that results in eventual dementia.

Homeostasis

Homeostasis.

Homeostasis is effected by intracellular and extracellular organs and organ systems. It ensures optimal intracellular conditions for the biochemical reactions and the enzymes that catabolize environmental energy substrate (absorbed products of digested food, water, minerals, vitamins and inhaled oxygen) to energy that is usable for biological reactions, i.e., ~P which is stored in ATP or ADP till needed for biochemical reactions and biological activities (Chart 4-1, page 83). **Catabolism releases energy and anabolism needs it.**

The concept of homeostasis.

The concept of homeostasis derives from observations made by Claude Bernard in the latter half of the nineteenth century[1,2]. He postulated that the "fixity of the milieu intérieur" was a requirement for "free and independent life". This original proposition of Claude Bernard was amplified and extended by Cannon[3] in the early part of the last century. He coined the word "homeostasis" to describe the coordinated physiological processes that maintain intracellular conditions within physiologically desirable and permissible levels. Four principles of homeostasis were postulated and detailed by him in the book, "The Way of an Investigator"[4]. He wrote:

1. "Our bodies constitute open systems engaged in continuous exchanges with our external environment. They are compounded of highly unstable material. They are subjected to highly disturbing conditions. The maintenance of a steady state within them is in itself evidence that agencies are acting or are ready to act to maintain this constancy."
2. "If a steady state remains steady it does so because any tendency towards change is automatically met by increased effectiveness of the factor or factors which resist the change."
3. "The regulating system which determines homeostasis of a particular feature may comprise a number of cooperating factors brought into action at the same time or successively."
4. "When a factor is known which can shift a homeostatic state in one direction it is reasonable to look for automatic control of that factor or factors which act in the opposite direction."

The observations of Claude Bernard and of Cannon were made when much less was known about the complexities of biological interactions than is recognized today, especially the complex biochemical reactions required for conversion of environmental energy to ~P which is the energy needed for in vivo biochemical reactions and biological activities.

Homeostasis - why is it needed?

In an industrial or laboratory setting reactions can be accelerated by heating. In vivo this is not possible for life cannot continue if body temperature varies by more than a few degrees above or below a mean of 37°C - excess heat denatures proteins (enzymes are proteins) and excessive cooling retards their activities. Numerous biochemical reactions are needed for the oxidative catabolism of environmental energy (i.e., the absorbed products of food digestion and of water, minerals and vitamins, and inhaled oxygen) to ~P. The enzymes and the reactions they catalyze have stringent and specific physicochemical requirements for optimal performance Indeed all intracellular enzymes have similar stringent requirements. These requirements have limited tolerances for transgressions beyond physiologically permissible and desirable levels of osmotic pressures, the electrolyte and chemical compositions and electrical neutralities of body fluids, and their pH and temperatures. Homeostasis provides intracellular conditions which are optimal for the activities of these enzymes.

Enzyme regulation needs ~P for derepression of the DNA operons that synthesize them. As detailed at the beginning of this chapter intracellular substrate is needed for the derepression and this determines the rates and quantities of enzyme synthesized. Presumably in a sequential biochemical process such as anaerobic and aerobic metabolism there are corresponding derepressions of DNA operons as each new intracellular substrate

Chart 5-1: THE SYSTEMS WHICH MAINTAIN HOMEOSTASIS [1]

Systems providing the cell with environmental oxygen and energy substrate from ingested food for catabolism of the latter to energy usable for biochemical reactions and biological activities, i.e., ~P.

a. **The gastrointestinal tract and its appendages** (the liver, gall bladder and pancreas) for ingestion and digestion of food and the subsequent absorption of the products of food digestion, and of ingested water, minerals, and vitamins.

b. **The respiratory complex** for oxygenation of blood, removal of CO_2 and pH control.

c. **The cardiovascular complex** for pumping and transport of environmental energy substrate to cells.

d. **The blood** which transports the products of gastrointestinal absorption and inhaled oxygen to cells, removes intracellular carbon dioxide, other undesirable products of intracellular housekeeping, and the products of detoxification and degradation of endogenous and exogenous toxins. It also conveys hormones to the cells and generates and disseminates protective immune responses.

e. **Intracellular cytoplasmic and mitochondrial enzyme complexes** for using inhaled oxygen to catabolize absorbed products of digested food and water, minerals and vitamins to ~P which is stored in ATP or ADP till needed for biochemical reactions and other biological activities. The metabolic sequence for production of ~P from energy substrate is anaerobic intracellular metabolism, then intracellular oxidative catabolism in the Kreb's cycle and finally, metabolism in the Electron Transport System to energy (**~P**) stored in ATP or ADP.

The cell

Homeostasis: Maintenance of intracellular physicochemical conditions which are optimal for the biochemical reactions and the activities of the enzymes which convert energy substrate (i.e. inhaled oxygen and the absorbed products of food digestion, and of absorbed water, minerals, and vitamins) to ~P for use in biochemical reactions and biological activities. ~P is stored in ADP or ATP till needed.

Extracellular systems which maintain intracellular physicochemical conditions which are optimal for the biochemical reactions and enzymes which use oxygen to catabolize energy substrate to ~P.

a. **Renal, pulmonary and other mechanisms** for osmotic pressure, water, electrolyte, and pH regulation.

b. **The liver, the kidneys and the lungs** for detoxification, degradation and elimination of noxious materials.

c. **Systems which maintain intracellular temperatures** within physiologically permissible levels.

d. **Systems which protect:** natural barriers and chemicals, innate and generated immunity, and protective pathology (hypertrophy and hyperplasia, functional changes, and inflammation and repair).

e. **A musculoskeletal system** to obtain food, to masticate, to provide a rigid bony rib cage for normal respiration and to maintain the frame needed for orderly positioning of anatomical structures.

[1] **The functional performance of all biological systems** are recorded continuously by the CNS and the endocrine control systems. Information is transmitted via peripheral receptors, or directly by autonomic and somatic (e.g. from the respiratory muscles) nerves. If the CNS and/or the autonomous peripheral endocrine control systems deem that there are needs for changes in the functional performances of one or more systems commands are transmitted to effect these changes. Transmission of commands is by autonomic or somatic nerves, and/or by quantitative changes in levels of circulating hormones controlled directly by the hypothalamus (e.g., ADH), or indirectly by hypothalamic releasing factors. These factors vary production of pituitary hormones which have peripheral hormone-producing target cells, e.g., the thyroid, the adrenals and the male and female gonads. Alternatively, and often additionally, changes are effected by quantitative changes in hormones produced by the main autonomous peripheral endocrine control systems.

Intracellular and extracellular microenvironmental systems provide optimal responses to control center commands by modifying them in concord with local conditions in the microenvironment.

appears. Intracellular proteolytic activity also degrades enzymes so that the requirement for de novo synthesis is continuous when substrate remains in the cell.

Unless asleep, we think, speak, feel and move in many different ways, as a rule, with intelligence, logic, purpose, smoothness and precision. This is because homeostasis ensures an abundance of ~P. Admittedly, it is rapidly used but equally rapidly replenished throughout life. The availability of abundant ~P lets us function as humans

Chart 5-2: A HYPOTHESIS ON THE ROLE OF HOMEOSTASIS IN MAINTENANCE OF BIOLOGICAL PERFORMANCE AND INTEGRATION

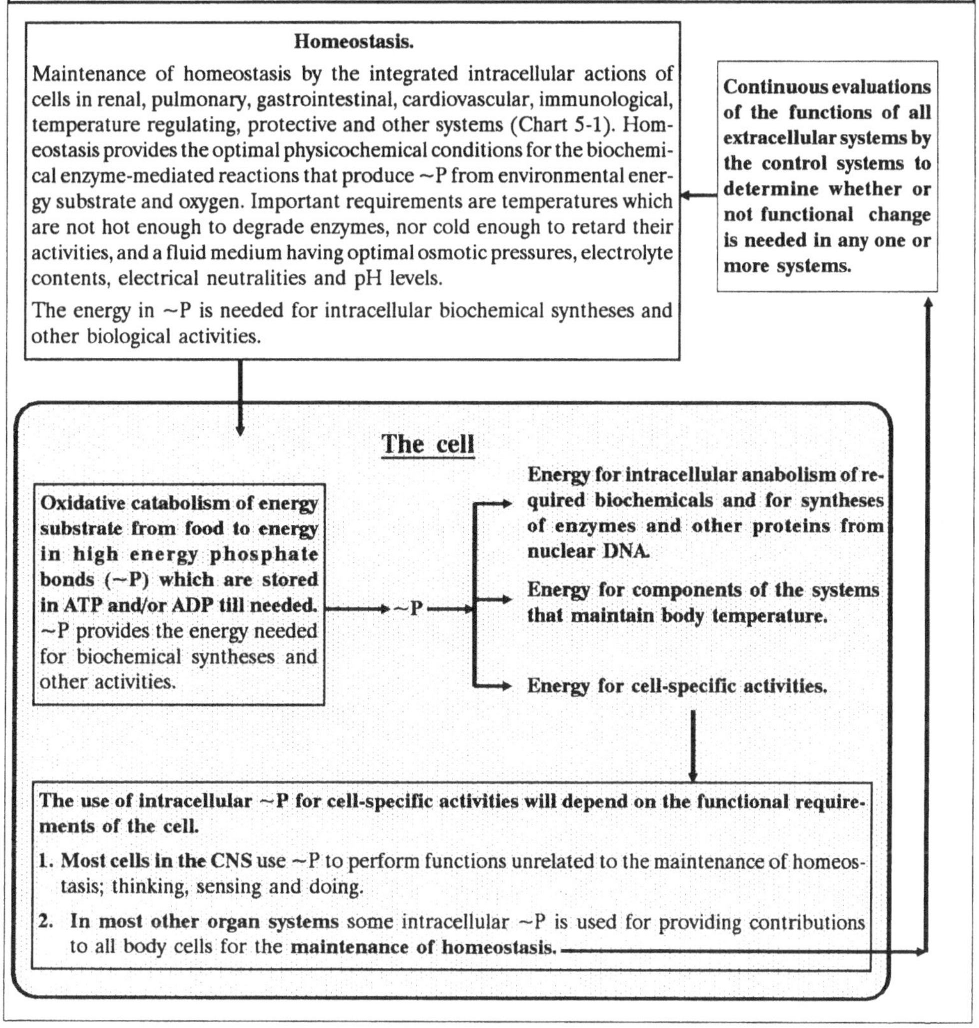
Homeostasis.
Maintenance of homeostasis by the integrated intracellular actions of cells in renal, pulmonary, gastrointestinal, cardiovascular, immunological, temperature regulating, protective and other systems (Chart 5-1). Homeostasis provides the optimal physicochemical conditions for the biochemical enzyme-mediated reactions that produce ~P from environmental energy substrate and oxygen. Important requirements are temperatures which are not hot enough to degrade enzymes, nor cold enough to retard their activities, and a fluid medium having optimal osmotic pressures, electrolyte contents, electrical neutralities and pH levels.
The energy in ~P is needed for intracellular biochemical syntheses and other biological activities.
Continuous evaluations of the functions of all extracellular systems by the control systems to determine whether or not functional change is needed in any one or more systems.
The cell
Oxidative catabolism of energy substrate from food to energy in high energy phosphate bonds (~P) which are stored in ATP and/or ADP till needed.
~P provides the energy needed for biochemical syntheses and other activities.
~P
Energy for intracellular anabolism of required biochemicals and for syntheses of enzymes and other proteins from nuclear DNA.
Energy for components of the systems that maintain body temperature.
Energy for cell-specific activities.
The use of intracellular ~P for cell-specific activities will depend on the functional requirements of the cell.
1. Most cells in the CNS use ~P to perform functions unrelated to the maintenance of homeostasis; thinking, sensing and doing.
2. In most other organ systems some intracellular ~P is used for providing contributions to all body cells for the maintenance of homeostasis.

and not as status quo vegetables waiting for the day of death. This sufficiency of energy usable for biochemical reactions and biological activities continues as long as enough environmental energy substrate is available and as long as there is enough intracellular ~P for accurate transcription and translation of the necessary enzymes from derepressed DNA fragments. Death is an inevitable and invariable sequel to life so that available ~P will eventually decrease to the point of insufficiency as aging and disease result in cellular degeneration and death.

How is "fixity of the milieu intérieur" maintained?

Chart 5-1 summarizes the requirements for maintenance of homeostasis and Chart 5-2 is a hypothetical depiction of the ways in which homeostasis contributes to biological function. Two groups of systems are needed for maintenance of homeostasis.

One supplies energy substrate from the environment and **the other** provides intracellular conditions that are optimal for the biochemical reactions and the enzyme complexes that catabolize energy substrate to ~P. As previously mentioned, the biochemical reactions and enzymes needed for oxidative catabolism of substrate to ~P have stringent physicochemical requirements for optimal function. These are provided by this second group of systems.

All biological systems must interact and coordinate in order to attain the above objectives. They include systems that control intracellular osmotic pressures, volumes, electrolyte compositions, electrical neutralities, pH and temperatures. Others that detoxify, degrade and eliminate toxic materials. Some of these toxins are of endogenous origin (e.g., the products of red cell breakdown) while others are exogenous to the body. Examples of the latter are therapeutic drugs, environmental toxins, and "recreational" drugs. Finally, the body has systems that protect and others that provide compensations and protective pathology for functional deficits.

The central nervous system and the autonomous peripheral endocrine systems continuously monitor and control the functions of all systems, including themselves. Autonomous microenvironmental control systems ensure optimal execution of commands from control systems in concord with conditions existing in the microenvironment.

One concludes by proposing that the reason for maintaining the "fixity of the milieu intérieur" is provision of optimal intracellular conditions for conversion of environmental energy substrate to ~P. This proposition does not unintentionally or intentionally dispute the original contention of Claude Bernard that "the fixity of the milieu intérieur" is the condition of "free and independent life". It merely extends and amplifies this most fundamental and important proposition of biology.

The systems of biology

Biological integration - some general comments.

The task of formulating a frame that depicts the totality of physiological and pathophysiological integration is not simple. Many authors have recognized this problem. Thus, Porter in his book, "Cybernetics Simplified"[5] wrote:

> "It must be emphasized and re-emphasized that the most complex control process known to man is man himself. Man is controlled by a vast coordinated network of neurons, nerves and muscles, which carry out his thought processes and activate his behavior with almost negligible power requirements, and in a manner which is far beyond our comprehension at present. As a decision-making system man is supreme."

Not quite. Porter correctly described the central nervous system (CNS) as the principal controller of most biological complexes. But its power requirements are not negligible. Blood flow to the brain is about 750ml/min which is 10-15% of the resting cardiac output of a 70Kg man. The CNS needs about 50ml/min oxygen which is about 20% of oxygen needs of the whole body at rest. Normally, glucose is the principal and only substrate for production of ~P in the brain (after a period of starvation ketones can satisfy a part of its energy needs). On a normal diet the brain needs about 75mg glucose/min. As previously detailed, insufficient oxygen and/or glucose result in neurological dysfunctions ranging from tremors and confusion to coma and finally death if satisfactory perfusion is not restored in four minutes or so. As a corollary, a blood glucose estimation is essential when an individual is found unconscious for no obvious reason. Accidental or deliberate insulin overdosage is not uncommon in insulin dependent diabetics.

Later in the same book Porter wrote:

> "Of all control the fantastic network of interconnected neurons in the brain, the communicating nerve fibers, the countless chemical reactions, and the vast array of human muscles all together constitute by many orders of magnitude the most complex system with which man is confronted. How this system manages to be self-stabilizing in the presence of a multiplicity of disturbances of all kinds, including severe brain damage, is far beyond the present status of control theory to explain."

Additional knowledge generated since Porter wrote the above facilitates the task but difficulties remain. However, despite difficulties of portrayal, the facts of our daily existence are incontrovertible proof that the body does exist as a superbly functioning and self-stabilizing unit, at least until old age, disease, or both intervene with consequent destabilization, malfunction and finally, death.

Note: I have made repeated attempts to get permission from the "English Universities Press" to quote Porter's comments but without any response. They were the publishers of his book. The quotes are therefore made regardless and without permission as they are important for understanding the frustrations of those who have attempted systems analysis of biology and its systems.

Biological systems classified.

There are two main groups of biological systems. **The first is a group of control systems** and the **second is a group of "slave systems".** Chart 5-3 itemizes the main systems of human biology.

What are "slave systems".

At the outset one defines the terms **"slave systems"** and **"control systems"**. These are two concepts used in this and subsequent chapters to establish a frame which shows how biological coordination and integration are attained. A frame of this type is a necessity for the orderly and sequential evaluation of all biological systems. As mentioned earlier in this book it is not enough to just treat the presenting disease. Equally important is preservation or restoration of the integrated coordination of systems. The normal function of every animate depends on this. Assessment of every biological system is needed as this alone enables the physician to identify systems which might need functional amplifications or dampenings.

The phrase, "slave systems", is not nor meant to be, a derogatory term. It merely denotes the fact that many important biological systems are systems subordinate to control systems, especially the CNS, for their optimal and desired functional attainments. Most of the slave systems are the systems that maintain homeostasis. They maintain optimal intracellular conditions for the enzymes of oxidative catabolism which produce ~P.

The concept of "slave systems" and "control systems" derives from a comment in "Humans use of Human Beings" published by Wiener in 1954[6]. He wrote:

> "Control in other words, is nothing but the sending of messages which effectively change the behavior of the recipient."

Hence, the recipients are slaves of the systems that control. It is a useful concept for analyzing clinical dysfunctions.

There is an analogy between the actions and interactions of biological systems and a model used by Wiener[7] to introduce the science of cybernetics, the discipline that deals with control and communications. He wrote:

> "We have decided to call the entire field of control and communication theory, whether in the machine or the animal, by the name cybernetics ...."

He derived the word cybernetics from the Greek word, κυβερνητηζ, which translates as "steersman", because:

> "The steersman of a ship has to be sure that a ship goes to its prescribed destination with accuracy and within the prescribed time. The ship's resources (machine and men) have certain performance characteristics and its environment is continually changing. The captain institutes various kinds of information systems throughout the ship to inform him about deviations which might have occurred, to evaluate the performance of the ship and to change his plans from time to time based on the information obtained. This is called the cybernetic loop."

Analogies with human biology are easily derived. The ship has controllers, the captain and his executive staff. Its objectives are to travel undamaged and with celerity and precision to a designated point. It has resources; oil and coal for propulsion energy, and a crew which is supposed to optimize propulsion, and to use a compass, a rudder or other more modern tools to navigate with precision. The objective is precise movement to a predetermined point. All resources of the ship interact, usually, in seemingly automatic, effortless and effective ways to attain the desired objective or objectives. If at any time the captain or an executive of his staff deems that function is not optimal and that functional change is required in one or more of the resources, appropriate

Chart 5-3: THE SYSTEMS OF HUMAN BIOLOGY

The control systems

1. The central nervous system.
2. The peripheral autonomous endocrine control systems.
3. The autonomous pericellular and intracellular micronenvironmental control systems.
4. Systems for protection, compensation and protective pathology. They include body surface fluids and anatomical barriers, innate and generated immunity, hypertrophy, hyperplasia, inflammation and repair. These systems often begin and are restricted to the microenvironment. Others are systemic ab initio.

The slave systems

Most of the slave systems are the systems that maintain homeostasis.

1. **Systems which provide cells with energy substrate from the environment for oxidative catabolism to the energy in high energy phosphate bonds (~P) which are stored in ADP or ATP till needed:**
   - — The system complex which provides the intracellular compartments with energy substrate from the absorbed products of food digestion and absorbed water, minerals and vitamins.
   - — The respiratory complex for oxygenation of blood and removal of carbon dioxide.
   - — A heart and a vascular complex for delivery of energy substrate and oxygen to every vascularized cell.
   - — The blood for transfer of materials to and from cells.
2. **Systems which maintain intracellular homeostasis, i.e., provision of optimal conditions for the intracellular enzymes which use oxygen for oxidative catabolism of ingested energy substrate to ~P:**
   - — Hormones (especially ADH, angiotensin and aldosterone), and renal and pulmonary systems which maintain within physiologically permissible and desirable levels the osmotic pressures, electrolyte concentrations, electrical neutralities, volumes and pH levels of fluids in the different body compartments. The lungs also exhale volatile toxins such as gases used in anaesthesia.
   - — Hepatic and renal function for detoxification, degradation and elimination of undesirable endogenous (e.g., the products of red cell breakdown) and exogenous materials (e.g., therapeutic drugs, environmental toxins and "recreational drugs").
   - — Systems for maintenance of body temperature within physiologically desirable levels.
   - — Systems which control sexual activity, maturation, pregnancy and the menopause.
   - — Intracellular cytoplasmic and mitochondrial enzymes for oxidative catabolism of energy substrate to energy (~P) usable for biochemical syntheses, construction of membrane pumps, structures such as the Golgi apparatus, the lysosomes that digest and extrude unwanted materials, the ion channels and a variety of other syntheses and activities. ~P is stored in ATP or ADP till needed.

commands are issued and optimal function is regained (hopefully).

The interrelations of biological control systems and the systems that maintain homeostasis are comparable. Each slave system has one or more resources and each resource attains it objectives by many intrinsic minor systems (all described in detail later). The slave systems are always subordinate to commands from the control systems. This is why they are termed "slave systems" in this text. The control systems determine and effect any necessary functional changes in the slave systems. Presently one explains how this conceptual division of biological systems into control systems and slave systems helps classifying systems and their inter-relationships for integration and coordination.

The systems for control and command have their own objectives and their own internal controls, in addition to their control of the slave systems. For example, the CNS is responsible for the initiation and execution of intellectual activities, and of sensing and doing. The autonomous peripheral endocrine systems ensure CNS function and also control some slave systems. Finally, the microenvironmental control systems ensure optimal responses of slave systems to commands from the other two control systems in concord with local microen-

Chart 5-4: INTERACTIONS OF THE MAIN SYSTEMS OF BIOLOGY

Autonomous peripheral endocrine systems for control.

The insulin-glucagon system, the renin-angiotensin-aldosterone complex, the parathyroid hormone-serum ionized calcium mechanisms, the erythropoietin-red cell maturation system and the atrial natriuretic peptide-angiotensin interaction are the most important of these systems. These five systems are autonomous of CNS control, probably because they are needed to ensure normal brain function and the normal transmission of nerve impulses. They also control and command the slave systems together with the CNS and its extensions. Many other autonomous hormone control systems exist, especially systems which control gastrointestinal secretions. They have little general effect on overall biological controls.

↓

The control systems.

1. The central nervous system (the brain and spinal cord). This is the most important control system.
2. The autonomous (of CNS control) peripheral endocrine control systems (see above).
3. Systems for compensation and pathology. Some are microenvironmental in origin while others are systemic from the beginning, e.g., generated immunity.

↕

The slave systems (systems for maintenance of homeostasis).

Each system has intrinsic resource systems and each resource system has many minor system components. Hypofunctions or hyperfunctions of the performances of all body systems are continuously sensed by the CNS and the autonomous endocrine control systems. When necessary, commands to effect functional changest are transmitted to one or more resources systems. Commands are transmitted by somatic or autonomic nerve discharges and/or by quantitative changes in circulating hormones.

↕

Another control system.

4. **Microenvironmental intracellular and pericellular control systems.**
   These systems use local axon reflexes and locally produced chemicals such as histamine, the kinins and prostaglandins to vary vascular diameters and permeabilities and to activate cell wall receptors. The objective is optimization of responses to control systems commands in concord with local microenvironmental conditions.

vironmental conditions. Chart 5-4 is a hypothetical overview of the interactions of the different main biological system complexes of the body. The control systems, and especially the central nervous system (CNS) have their own internal mechanisms for control and correction.

The anatomy of biological integration

The following is a summary of the complexities of biological interactions:

■ **The principal systems.**

Chart 5-5 depicts the anatomy of systems integrations. All animates are composites of many principal biological systems, all integrated to provide smooth, coordinated, purposeful and precise activities. **Each system has an objective.** Chart 5-6 depicts a system which is probably the most complex of body systems and has a single objective: the conversion of environmental energy substrate to energy which can be used for biological activities. The substrate is food, water, vitamins, minerals and oxygen and the end product is the energy in high energy phosphate bonds (~P). The control systems have their own intrinsic controls and also control the functional performances of all slave systems.

In general the principal systems do not communicate with each other. If the principal systems communicated

with each other on an ad hoc basis to determine what functional changes were needed the result would be chaos. There must only be one or two (the CNS and the autonomous endocrine control systems) systems that integrate information from all systems of the body. This ensures unitary non-chaotic control.

■ **The resource systems.**

The objective or objectives of a system are partitioned between resource systems. I have not called them "major systems" rather than "resource systems" because the word "resource" better denotes the functions of these systems. Examples of the many resource systems a complex principal system might need are listed below the main depiction in Chart 5-6. In contrast a system could have only a few resource systems. An example is the heart where there are only two resource systems: heart muscle contraction and a resource which preserves normal rate or adequately compensates for any dysrrhythmia. When resource systems of a principal system are multiple they interact and integrate with each other to attain the objective or objectives of the main system.

■ **The minor systems**

Each resource system has many minor system components. The components of these minor systems interact to attain the objectives of the parent resource system. The interactions are rapid, frequent, and probably, for these reasons, autonomous and automatic. Chart 5-7 is a hypothetical depiction of the ways in which these minor systems could interact. The interactions are probably mediated by biochemical reactions which use allosteric enzymes with set-points and continue till all allosteric set-points are reached, or no more substrate for the reaction or for production of ~P is available. Alternatively, till more ~P cannot be produced by cells which are diseased, or have little functional reserve because of aging.

■ **Mechanisms for control.**

The totality of the functional effects of all systems are continuously recognized and sensed by the control systems. Information is transmitted by neural impulses, either directly or via peripheral receptors and also by changes in blood hormone levels, blood pressure, pCO_2, pO_2 and the osmotic pressures, volumes, electrolyte contents, pH and temperatures of body fluids. If the control systems feel that the function of any one or more systems needs amplification or dampening commands are transmitted to the resource systems as neural discharges and hormonal changes. The neural discharges are transmitted by autonomic and somatic nerves. Their effects are mediated by neuromediators; norepinephrine and acetylcholine at endings in visceral organs and glands and acetylcholine at neuromuscular endings. The control systems have intrinsic control systems of similar type. Neuromediators exist in the CNS though dissimilar to those in extracerebral tissues. **Note that commands are transmitted to the resource systems of the principal system, not to the minor systems. The resources are given objectives and the minor systems attempt to attain them.**

Summary.

Every principal biological system has one or more resource systems. Each resource has many minor system components. These interact with each other automatically and probably, autonomously. The interactions are rapid and designed to attain the specified objective of the resource.

The resources also interact with each other but in a more directed and structured way. The principal systems do not interact. Any functional dysfunction of a principal system is recognized by the control systems which receive information about the total functional effects of all systems. Afferent transmission of information is by autonomic and somatic nerves, either directly or after initial recording by receptors, by osmotic and other changes in the blood, and by quantitative changes in levels of hormones in the blood. The control systems compute and decide whether change is needed. Commands for change are not transmitted to the principal system but to one or more of its resources.

If interactions of the minor systems cannot attain the desired performance of the resource help is provided by the control systems as mentioned above. Help is in the form of neural discharges and quantitative changes in hormone production. If and when functional change is needed in one or more systems commands are transmitted to one or more resources, not to the principal system. Transmission is by autonomic sympathetic and/or parasympathetic nerves, by somatic nerves (e.g., to the respiratory muscles) and by quantitative and/or qualitative

(Contd. on page 107)

Chart 5-5: THE ANATOMY OF A COMPLEX SYSTEM. THE EXAMPLE IS THE SYSTEM WHICH TRANSPORTS ENVIRONMENTAL ENERGY SUBSTRATE TO THE CELLS FOR OXIDATIVE CATABOLISM TO ~P.

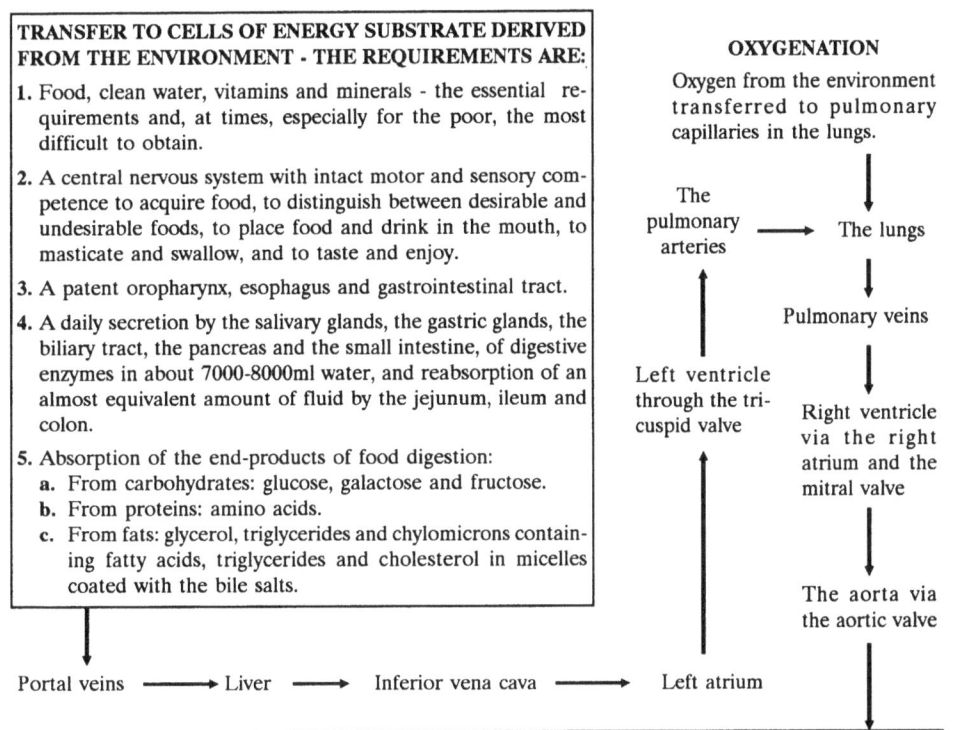

TRANSFER TO CELLS OF ENERGY SUBSTRATE DERIVED FROM THE ENVIRONMENT - THE REQUIREMENTS ARE:

1. Food, clean water, vitamins and minerals - the essential requirements and, at times, especially for the poor, the most difficult to obtain.
2. A central nervous system with intact motor and sensory competence to acquire food, to distinguish between desirable and undesirable foods, to place food and drink in the mouth, to masticate and swallow, and to taste and enjoy.
3. A patent oropharynx, esophagus and gastrointestinal tract.
4. A daily secretion by the salivary glands, the gastric glands, the biliary tract, the pancreas and the small intestine, of digestive enzymes in about 7000-8000ml water, and reabsorption of an almost equivalent amount of fluid by the jejunum, ileum and colon.
5. Absorption of the end-products of food digestion:
   - **a.** From carbohydrates: glucose, galactose and fructose.
   - **b.** From proteins: amino acids.
   - **c.** From fats: glycerol, triglycerides and chylomicrons containing fatty acids, triglycerides and cholesterol in micelles coated with the bile salts.

↓

Portal veins → Liver → Inferior vena cava → Left atrium

↑

Left ventricle through the tricuspid valve

↑

The pulmonary arteries → The lungs

OXYGENATION

Oxygen from the environment transferred to pulmonary capillaries in the lungs.

↓

The lungs

↓

Pulmonary veins

↓

Right ventricle via the right atrium and the mitral valve

↓

The aorta via the aortic valve

↓

The terminal ramifications of the vascular system reach the immediate vicinity of almost every body cell. Energy substrate from the environment enters cells. Intracellular metabolism by anaerobic, aerobic, and electron transport systems converts the energy in substrate to energy usable for biochemical reactions, i.e., high energy phosphate bonds (~P) which are stored in ATP and ADP till needed.

The chart shows that a single system usually needs many other systems to attain its objectives. The following summarizes the requirements.

1. **Control systems:** Undamaged and functionally effective systems for control and command: the central nervous system, the autonomous peripheral endocrine systems and the autonomous microenvironmental control mechanisms.
2. **Slave systems::**

a. The gastrointestinal complex for ingestion, digestion and absorption into the blood of the products of food digestion, and ingested water, minerals and vitamins.

b. The respiratory complex for transport of environmental oxygen to hemoglobin and then to the cells.

c. The heart, the vasculature and the blood for transport of all materials to and between cells.

d. Normal cell membrane structures, receptors, and miscellaneous transport mechanisms. Insulin and glucagon are the main hormones that determine whether or not circulating glucose enters the cell. Glucose is an important component of energy substrate, especially for the brain. The brain can only use glucose for production of ~P though some ketones can be used for its energy needs after a few days of starvation.

e. Renal and hepatic systems and other mechanisms for intracellular housekeeping and maintenance of physiologically permissible levels of osmotic pressures, electrolyte contents, electrical equivalences and pH of fluids in the different body compartments.

f. Systems which maintain body and intracellular temperatures within physiologically permissible levels.

Chart 5-6: THE INTERACTIONS OF THE MINOR SYSTEM COMPONENTS OF A RESOURCE SYSTEM OF THE CARDIOVASCULAR COMPLEX. I.E. THE HEART

The heart is a system of the cardiovascular complex. It pumps blood into the conduits of the vascular complex.

The objective:

Propulsion of blood sufficient to satisfy tissue needs in the prevailing circumstances (i.e. at rest or during moderate or severe exercise). The objective requires optimization of the heart rate and the contractile force of the left ventricular muscle because **output per minute = Beats per min x Stroke volume (i.e., output in ml/left ventricular contraction).**

The heart rate at rest is about 70 beats per minute and the stroke volume is about 70-90ml/ventricular contraction in a 70Kg man at rest. Hence, the output at rest of such an individual is about 5-6.5L/min

The main resources.

1. **The contractile force of the left ventricle.**
2 **An intrinsic electrical system for normal rhythm or well compensated rate and rhythm of an arrhythmia.**
3. **A valve system which ensures unidirectional flow.**
4. **A coronary circulation which provides substrate for production of energy (~P) for heart muscle.**

Each resource system has many minor systems components which rapidly interact by automatic and autonomous to-and-fro interactions and repeated iterations till all the allosteric set-points of the enzymes involved in the reactions are reached or substrate is finished or not responsive and/or more ~P is not available. At all times **the microenvironmental control mechanisms** are intimately involved in interacting with any one or more of the resources to obtain an optimal result in concord with conditions in the microenvironment.

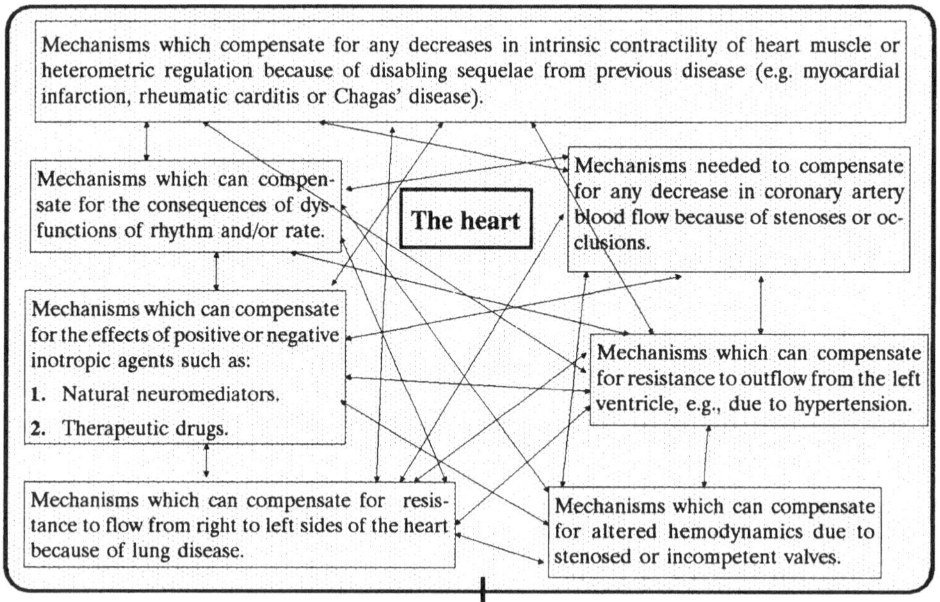
Mechanisms which compensate for any decreases in intrinsic contractility of heart muscle or heterometric regulation because of disabling sequelae from previous disease (e.g. myocardial infarction, rheumatic carditis or Chagas' disease).
Mechanisms which can compensate for the consequences of dysfunctions of rhythm and/or rate.
The heart
Mechanisms needed to compensate for any decrease in coronary artery blood flow because of stenoses or occlusions.
Mechanisms which can compensate for the effects of positive or negative inotropic agents such as:
1. Natural neuromediators.
2. Therapeutic drugs.
Mechanisms which can compensate for resistance to outflow from the left ventricle, e.g., due to hypertension.
Mechanisms which can compensate for resistance to flow from right to left sides of the heart because of lung disease.
Mechanisms which can compensate for altered hemodynamics due to stenosed or incompetent valves.

Information about the functional performance of all systems of the body is transmitted continuously to the hypothalamus and to the medullary cardiac, vasomotor and respiratory centers. If function is deemed inadequate the CNS sends appropriate commands to the resource system or systems of one or more principal systems. For example, when cardiac performance is suboptimal, medullary centers send coordinated and integrated commands to the cardiac beta receptors, the peripheral vasculature and the respiratory apparatus. Transmission is by autonomic and somatic (to the respiratory muscles) efferents and by quantitative changes in hormones produced in the hypothalamus (e.g., ADH) or hormones controlled by hypothalamic releasing factors via the pituitary.

In addition, hypotension is sensed by the JG apparatus, renin production is stimulated with eventual production of angiotensin II and III. Both are potent vasoconstrictors.

(Contd. from page 104)
changes in blood levels of hormones produced in the hypothalamus (e.g., ADH) or controlled by the hypothalamus via the pituitary or by the pituitary alone.

Chart 5-6 depicts the most complex and most important of biological systems. It is a principal system. The Chart is a flow sheet and the resources needed by the system are depicted below the flow chart. Chart 5-7 hypothesizes on the mechanics of the interactions of the minor system components of a resource, in this instance the heart.

The control systems

The following are the systems which control:

- **The central nervous system (CNS).** This is the most important control system. Its capabilities and the ways in which it commands are depicted in Chart 5-8.

Chart 5-7: A SUMMARY OVERVIEW OF THE CAPABILITIES AND OBJECTIVES OF THE CENTRAL NERVOUS SYSTEM

The capabilities of the CNS:

1. **Capacity for intellectual activity:** logical reasoning and decision-making, abstract thought, memorization and recall of information, likes and dislikes, love and hate, knowledge of moral and legislated law, and many other items.
2. **Capacity for volitional activity**: movement in precise, coordinated and purposeful ways, maintenance of different static postures and of balance during movements, and verbal, gestural and prosodic language.
3. **Capacity to receive, perceive and recognize sensory stimuli which enter consciousness:** perception and recognition of cutaneous and visceral pain, visual, auditory, olfactory, and gustatory information, cutaneous touch, and changes in surface temperatures and pressures. Multimodal integrations of received information are effected in the heteromodal areas, especially the tempero-parietal heteromodal area.
   Changes in the internal environment are sensed by baroreceptors, chemoreceptors, osmoreceptors, pain receptors and thermoreceptors, or transmitted directly to the CNS by somatic (e.g., from the muscles of respiration) and/or autonomic nerves.
   Responses to information from the interval environment are usually mediated by involuntary reflexes from medullary and hypothalamic control centers. Higher centers have the abilities to modify these involuntary responses and to initiate reflexes to pain sensed in subcortical areas.
4. **Knowledge of the objectives and functions of every biological system** (including itself) and the ability to integrate all information and then decide if functional changes are needed in one or more systems. Commands for change are transmitted by autonomic and somatic nerves and by qualitative and/or quantitative changes in hormone secretions controlled by the CNS.

The other three important control systems are

- **The autonomous (i.e., from CNS control) peripheral endocrine control systems.**
- **The system complexes for compensation and protection and**
- **The microenvironmental complex of autonomous control systems.**

1. The central nervous system (CNS).

The capabilities of the CNS.

Chart 5-7 summarized the capabilities of the CNS and Chart 5-8 shows how it controls and commands. It is the most important of the control systems and Chart 5-9 hypothesizes on the interactions of the CNS with

(Contd. on page 110)

Chart 5-8: CONTROL AND COMMAND BY THE CENTRAL NERVOUS SYSTEM

The unit of command is the nerve impulse.

The central nervous system

- Somatic nerves → Skeletal muscle
- Autonomic nerves → Cardiac muscle, smooth muscle and secreting glands
- The hypothalamus

Neural communications to the hypothalamus result in quantitive and qualitative variations in production of hypothalamic hormones (e.g., ADH) and releasing factors. The latter vary the amounts of pituitary hormones synthesized and in the products of their peripheral targets, i.e., the thyroid, the adrenals and the gonads.

Regulation of peripheral hormone production depends on feedback control reflexes between the hypothalamus and pituitary on the one hand and the products of pituitary targets on the other.

Chart 5-9: A HYPOTHETICAL MODEL OF CNS CONTROL

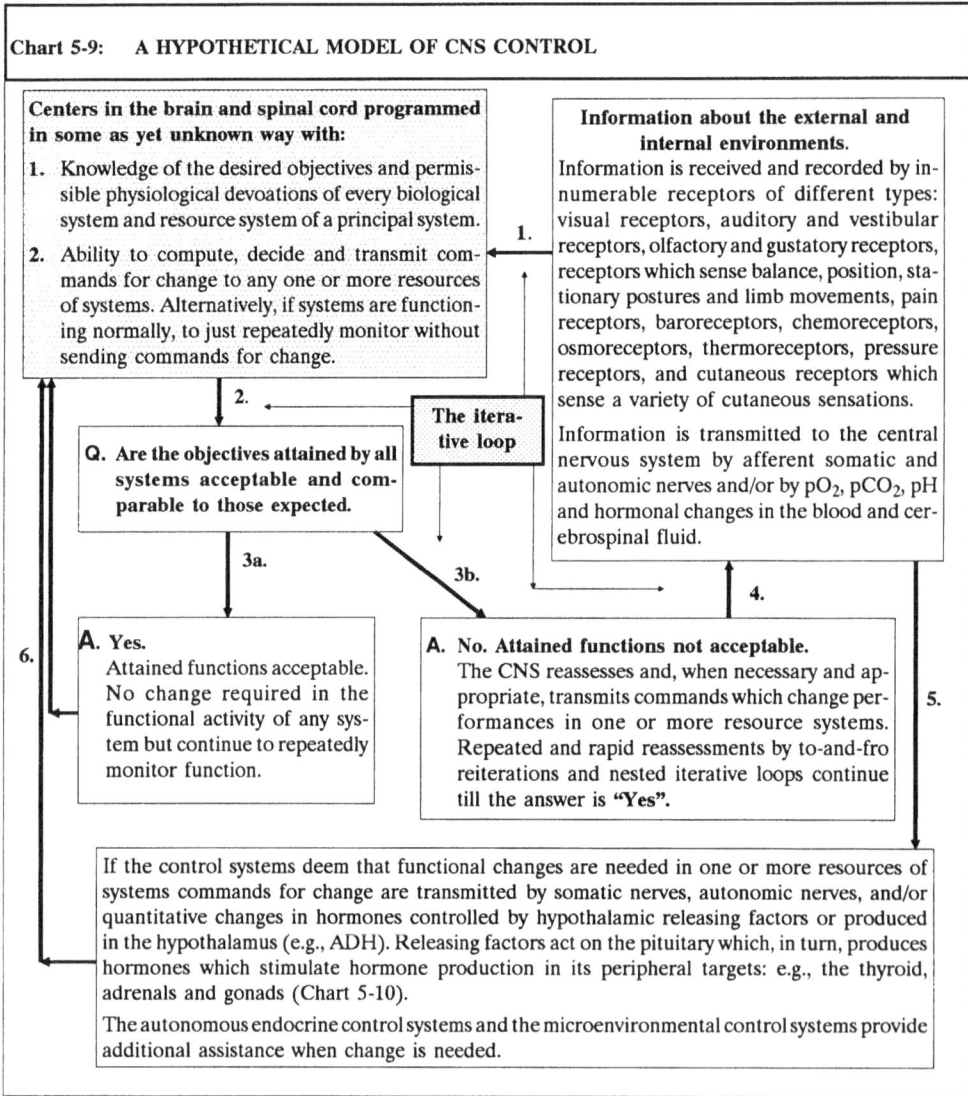

Centers in the brain and spinal cord programmed in some as yet unknown way with:

1. Knowledge of the desired objectives and permissible physiological devoations of every biological system and resource system of a principal system.
2. Ability to compute, decide and transmit commands for change to any one or more resources of systems. Alternatively, if systems are functioning normally, to just repeatedly monitor without sending commands for change.

Information about the external and internal environments.

Information is received and recorded by innumerable receptors of different types: visual receptors, auditory and vestibular receptors, olfactory and gustatory receptors, receptors which sense balance, position, stationary postures and limb movements, pain receptors, baroreceptors, chemoreceptors, osmoreceptors, thermoreceptors, pressure receptors, and cutaneous receptors which sense a variety of cutaneous sensations.

Information is transmitted to the central nervous system by afferent somatic and autonomic nerves and/or by pO_2, pCO_2, pH and hormonal changes in the blood and cerebrospinal fluid.

[1. Information → Centers]

The iterative loop

[2.] **Q. Are the objectives attained by all systems acceptable and comparable to those expected.**

[3a.] **A. Yes.** Attained functions acceptable. No change required in the functional activity of any system but continue to repeatedly monitor function.

[3b.] **A. No. Attained functions not acceptable.** The CNS reassesses and, when necessary and appropriate, transmits commands which change performances in one or more resource systems. Repeated and rapid reassessments by to-and-fro reiterations and nested iterative loops continue till the answer is **"Yes"**.

[4.] [5.]

If the control systems deem that functional changes are needed in one or more resources of systems commands for change are transmitted by somatic nerves, autonomic nerves, and/or quantitative changes in hormones controlled by hypothalamic releasing factors or produced in the hypothalamus (e.g., ADH). Releasing factors act on the pituitary which, in turn, produces hormones which stimulate hormone production in its peripheral targets: e.g., the thyroid, adrenals and gonads (Chart 5-10).

The autonomous endocrine control systems and the microenvironmental control systems provide additional assistance when change is needed.

[6.]

Chart 5-10: HYPOTHALAMIC HORMONES AND RELEASING FACTORS, PITUITARY HORMONES AND THE PRODUCTS OF THEIR TARGETS - THYROXINE, ADRENAL HORMONES AND GONADAL HORMONES.

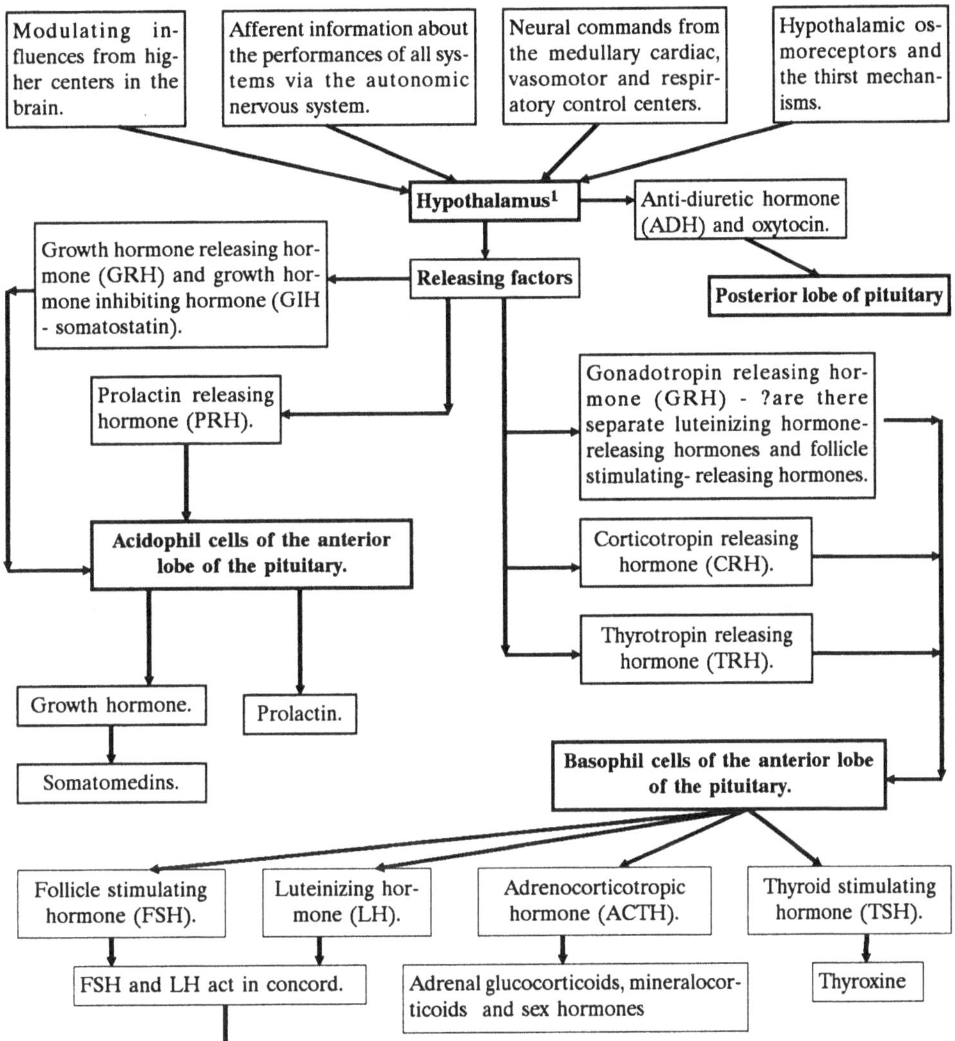
Modulating influences from higher centers in the brain.
Afferent information about the performances of all systems via the autonomic nervous system.
Neural commands from the medullary cardiac, vasomotor and respiratory control centers.
Hypothalamic osmoreceptors and the thirst mechanisms.
Hypothalamus¹
Anti-diuretic hormone (ADH) and oxytocin.
Posterior lobe of pituitary
Releasing factors
Growth hormone releasing hormone (GRH) and growth hormone inhibiting hormone (GIH - somatostatin).
Prolactin releasing hormone (PRH).
Gonadotropin releasing hormone (GRH) - ?are there separate luteinizing hormone-releasing hormones and follicle stimulating- releasing hormones.
Corticotropin releasing hormone (CRH).
Thyrotropin releasing hormone (TRH).
Acidophil cells of the anterior lobe of the pituitary.
Growth hormone.
Prolactin.
Somatomedins.
Basophil cells of the anterior lobe of the pituitary.
Follicle stimulating hormone (FSH).
Luteinizing hormone (LH).
Adrenocorticotropic hormone (ACTH).
Thyroid stimulating hormone (TSH).
FSH and LH act in concord.
Adrenal glucocorticoids, mineralocorticoids and sex hormones
Thyroxine

1 **In females:** FSH and LH act sequentially on the ovary during the menstrual cycle. FSH promotes estrogen secretion and development of the ovarian follicle. After ovulation estrogen secretion decreases and LH secretion increases with promotion of progesterone production and development of the corpus luteum. If pregnancy results the placenta secretes human chorionic gonadotropin (measured as β-HCG) as well as estrogen and progesterone.

2 **In males:** LH promotes secretion of testosterone by the interstitial Leydig cells of the testis. Testosterone is required for normal spermatogenesis and for maintenance of the secondary sex characteristics of males. FSH maintains the seminiferous tubules and promotes spermatogenesis by converting the primary spermatocytes to secondary spermatocytes. Testosterone is a requisite for the final maturation of sperms and also stimulates seminiferous tubule growth.

1 There is continual feedback control of as-needed hormone production by the final target cell products (thyroxine, corticosteroids, FSH, LH, and ADH) on the one hand and the hypothalamic releasing factors, pituitary hormones, and hypothalamic osmoreceptors on the other.

(Contd. from page 107)
other systems. Chart 5-11 summarizes the mechanisms it uses to control by variations in hormone production. It does so by its action on the hypothalamus which produces its own hormones (e.g., ADH) and many releasing factors which control pituitary hormone production. Controls are also exercised by feedback mechanisms between the hypothalamus and pituitary on the one hand and blood levels of hormones on the other. The processes involved are depicted in Chart 7-3, page 162.

Almost nothing is known about how the CNS performs all these functions. The facts of day-to-day living are immutable confirmations that it does what is detailed in Chart 5-7. One should treat the problem in the same way as one who has little or no knowledge of computer electronics uses the machine to perform complex tasks with rapidity. The basic physiology of nerve impulse initiation and transmission is well known. But this does not help too much. The complexities of CNS interactions remain largely unexplained.

CNS control of systems function.

As a rule information about systems function is not consciously perceived. The main receptors are in the medulla where there are centers for vasomotor control, respiration and cardiac function. The efferent discharges from the hypothalamus and the medullary vasomotor, respiratory and cardiac centers are distributed by the autonomic nervous system. They go to the reticular nuclei, then to the intermedio-lateral segments of the spinal cord and eventually, to their final destinations in gland or muscles (the autonomic nervous system is described in detail on pages 130-134). The afferent inputs are mainly autonomic nerve impulses and somatic impulses from the respiratory muscles. They follow paths that are the reverse of those traversed by the efferent fibers. Autonomic pain afferents are the exception. They synapse in the dorsal root ganglia and most of the post-synaptic fibers ascend with somatic pain fibers in the contralateral spino-thalamic tracts to reach the thalamus and the sensory cortex. Pain is probably perceived and recognized in the region of the thalamus as the cortex is insensitive to stimuli such as cutting or burning. The sensory cortex probably mediates the reflex responses to pain recognized in the thalamic region. Many of the autonomic afferents convey information already recorded by peripheral receptors such as the carotid and aortic bodies.

Cortical control of systems.

Cerebral activity can amplify or decrease control center commands. This is uncommon but can occur in urgent situations. Examples are sudden fear or danger, and rage or pain.

Most decisions to override control center commands depend on rapid recognitions and responses to multimodal information about the external environment. There is an initial requirement for unimodal and heteromodal recognition, a subsequent one for integration with previously stored information and final requirements for appropriate intellectual, sensory and motor reactions in different combinations. The response to a situation not previously encountered could be slow. Once learnt, future responses would be progressively faster. I write from personal experience. My first response to a mugging was slow and ineffectual. The responses on two subsequent occasions were rapid, effective and personally satisfying.

2. Control by autonomous peripheral endocrine systems.

Autonomous endocrine control systems are numerous, especially in the gastrointestinal tract. However, the most important ones are those that nourish the CNS and ensure accurate transmission of nerve impulses. Five such systems are depicted in Chart 5-11 on the next page. Their principal objectives seem to be the autonomous maintenance of neurological function by appropriate perfusion with blood (the angiotensin effect), and by providing the cells of the CNS with a sufficiency of glucose (the insulin effect). Glucose is essential for production of ~P in the brain though some ketones can be used after a period of starvation. The parathyroid hormone-plasma ionized calcium system controls serum-ionized calcium levels to ensure normal orderly nerve transmission and muscle contraction. The erythropoietin-red cell maturation system ensures the long-term adequacy of red cells for oxygen transport to the brain.

Chart 5-10: FIVE PERIPHERAL ENDOCRINE SYSTEMS NOT CONTROLLED BY THE CNS

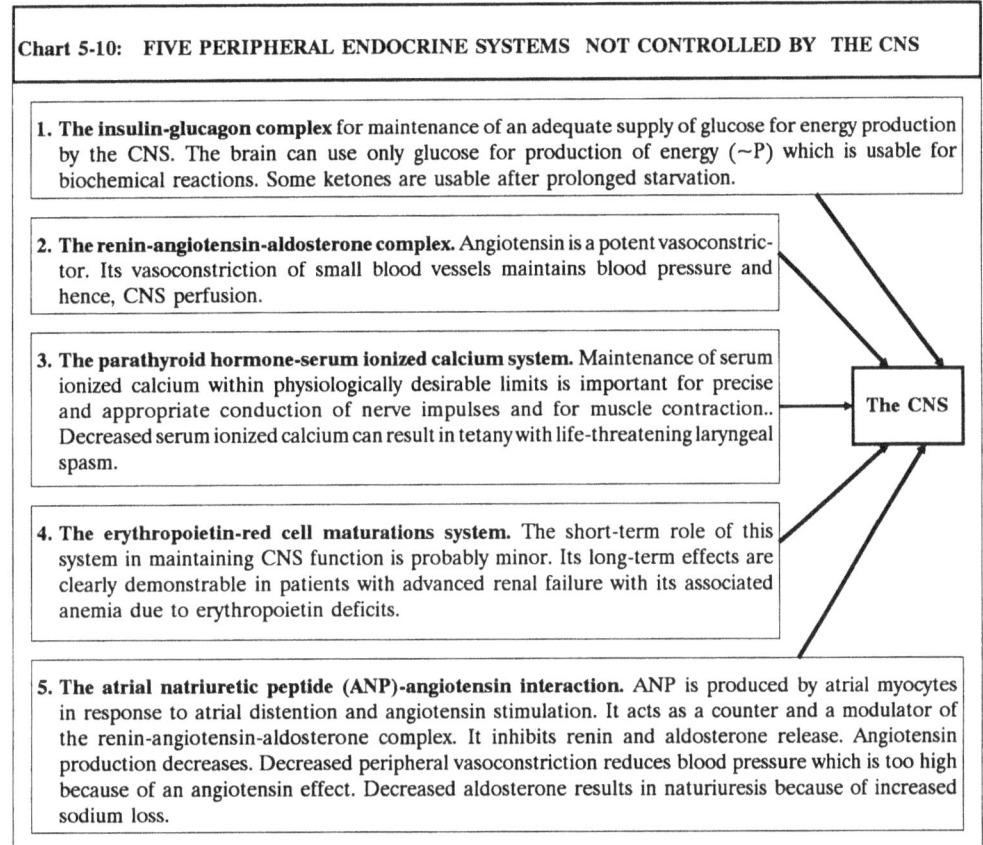

1. **The insulin-glucagon complex** for maintenance of an adequate supply of glucose for energy production by the CNS. The brain can use only glucose for production of energy (~P) which is usable for biochemical reactions. Some ketones are usable after prolonged starvation.

2. **The renin-angiotensin-aldosterone complex.** Angiotensin is a potent vasoconstrictor. Its vasoconstriction of small blood vessels maintains blood pressure and hence, CNS perfusion.

3. **The parathyroid hormone-serum ionized calcium system.** Maintenance of serum ionized calcium within physiologically desirable limits is important for precise and appropriate conduction of nerve impulses and for muscle contraction.. Decreased serum ionized calcium can result in tetany with life-threatening laryngeal spasm.

4. **The erythropoietin-red cell maturations system.** The short-term role of this system in maintaining CNS function is probably minor. Its long-term effects are clearly demonstrable in patients with advanced renal failure with its associated anemia due to erythropoietin deficits.

5. **The atrial natriuretic peptide (ANP)-angiotensin interaction.** ANP is produced by atrial myocytes in response to atrial distention and angiotensin stimulation. It acts as a counter and a modulator of the renin-angiotensin-aldosterone complex. It inhibits renin and aldosterone release. Angiotensin production decreases. Decreased peripheral vasoconstriction reduces blood pressure which is too high because of an angiotensin effect. Decreased aldosterone results in naturiuresis because of increased sodium loss.

The CNS

3. Systems for compensation and protection.

This is a complex of many systems: epithelial barriers, body fluids, natural and generated immunity and protective pathology which includes hyperplasia, hypertrophy, inflammation and repair. Their detailing merits a separate chapter. All are described in the next chapter (Chapter 8).

4. The microenvironmental control systems.

These are a complex of intracellular and the extracellular autonomous systems that maximize the responses to commands from the CNS and the autonomous endocrine control systems in concord with conditions in the local microenvironments of target cells. They include many systems.

Microenvironmental intracellular control systems.

The following are some examples:

- The important and essential cytoplasmic and mitochondrial enzyme complexes that convert energy substrate from the environment to ~P which is stored in ATP or ADP till needed.
- Accurate derepressions of DNA fragments needed to produce enzymes and other proteins needed by the cell.
- Accurate protein synthesis from DNA templates, and effective mechanisms for the repair or deletion of errors of transcription and/or translation.
- Transport systems for moving products of intracellular housekeeping to the exterior. Most of these mechanisms use lysosomes and vesicles derived from the Golgi system. They prevent intracellular accumula-

tions of undesirable materials.

— Quantitative and qualitative production of cell surface receptors, transport systems and cell membrane pumps.

The microenvironmental extracellular control systems.

These systems act in one or both of two ways:

Firstly, by changing the diameters and permeabilities of vessels in the microenvironment, and

Secondly, by directly affecting cell membrane permeabilities and receptors.

The principal effectors are local changes in pH, pCO_2 and pO_2, local axon reflexes and a variety of autacoids (a word used by Schäfer[8] to describe locally produced hormone-like substances). The autacoids include histamine, angiotensin, the prostaglandins the kinins and locally produced adenosine. Vascular and cell wall changes vary the quantity of substrate available to the cell for production of ~P.

Blood flow into capillaries depends on arteriolar diameter and pressure. In general arteriolar diameter is increased by a raised pCO_2, a decreased pO_2 and pH and by the prostaglandins and bradykinin. Histamine increases capillary permeability by causing the swelling and consequent separations of endothelial cells from each other.

The slave systems

A classification of the slave systems

There are two main groups of slave systems.

1. **The first is the group of slave systems required for conversion of energy in environmental energy substrate to energy usable for biochemical reactions and biological activities (i.e., ~P).**

   A least seven principal slave systems are required:

   — **A gastrointestinal system** for ingestion, digestion and absorption into the blood of the products of intestinal digestion and of ingested water, vitamins and minerals.

   — **A respiratory complex** which delivers oxygen from the environment to the intracellular compartments of body cells and removes CO_2.

   — **A cardiovascular complex** that provides the pump and the conduits to ensure that energy substrate reaches all cells.

   — **The blood** which is the fluid medium that transports energy substrate, oxygen and other essentials to, from and between cells. It is also the vehicle for removal of undesirable cellular materials such as CO_2 and the intracellular breakdown products of biological debris, drugs, and other toxins, some of endogenous origin (e.g., heme) and others from the environment (therapeutic drugs, toxins and recreational drugs).

   — **The systems that maintain homeostasis.** These systems provide the optimal intracelluar conditions needed for the activity of intracellular enzymes. They regulate the contents of the different compartments of body fluids by controlling osmotic pressures, volumes, electrolyte contents and electrical neutralities, pH and temperatures. All are detailed in Chapter 13.

   — **Intracellular metabolic systems for conversion of energy substrate,vitamins, minerals, oxygen and water to the energy in high energy phosphate bonds** (~P). This is the energy required for almost all biological activities. These systems were described in Chapter 4.

   — **A musculoskeletal system** to provide for mobility, for balance during kinesthetic activity and static postures, for the orderly placement of organs, for maintenance of the erect posture of bipeds, and perhaps most important of all, the mobile strong frame of bone that is essential for normal respiration.

2. **The second are systems within the CNS. The CNS initiates, control and executes these activities.**

- **Systems that initiate and control neuromuscular activity.** These are systems scattered throughout the central nervous system They are described in detail in Chapter 6 which describes normal neuromuscular contraction and details some of the pathological dysfunctions of movements. They are slave systems of the CNS and their controls are also intrinsic to the CNS
- **Systems for sensing.** They include the eyes, the ears, olfactory and gustatory receptors and cutaneous receptors that sense touch pain, pressure and other cutaneous sensations. The brain perceives, recognizes and selects material for storage in long-term memory. It imparts to this information a variety of emotional additions in the limbic system. Finally, it can recall required information from memory and use it for reasoning, logical and abstract thinking and decision-making. The brain also senses and reacts to neural impulses from pain receptors. All are slave systems of the CNS and all are controlled by systems intrinsic to the CNS.
- **Systems for intellectual activity, mentation, reasoning and decision-making.** Little information is available on the locations and modes of action of these centers. We know what they can do but not how things get done. For the moment accept that these are imponderables which might be explained one day but are without explanation today.
- **Systems that control sexual activity, maturation, pregnancy, parturition and the menopause.** The principal effects of these systems were summarized in Chart 5-10.

Every system, regardless of whether it is a control system or slave system, requires many resources to attain its objectives. In turn, each resource uses many intrinsic and interacting, automatic and autonomous minor systems to attain its specific objective or objectives.

Disease results when any one or more of these systems are dysfunctional and the efforts of the control systems cannot provide compensation which suffices to avert clinically demonstrable dysfunction.

Systems analysis in biology.

Some clinical problems are too complex to be rapidly assessed and decided on. They require systems analysis and assessment to determine, if possible, their natures and etiologies, to identify optimal therapy, and to monitor the clinical response to the therapy. Only a small proportion of clinical problems will need this type of analysis and the numbers will decrease as experience increases. Detailed analysis is rarely needed when the problem is simple and the decision obvious or when the clinical problem is a psychiatric dysfunction. It is necessary when the clinical problem is complex and unresolved and the therapeutic decision not obvious.

Biological systems analysis of a difficult clinical problem is designed to identify the nature of a dysfunction, to prognosticate on its probable course and to decide on optimal therapy. It also helps to monitor the response to therapy and to determine when continued or additional therapy will be of no avail. At that point, either the therapy provided is wrong for any one of the many reasons detailed in Chapter 16, or the clinical problem is preterminal. If the latter, medications and other measures for relief of pain and suffering should replace unnecessary, useless and uncomfortable investigations and treatments.

The basis of systems analysis of biological systems is information about the permissible deviations of normal physiology from a mean. Dysfunctions can only be evaluated by their degrees of deviations from these norms. Some deviations are acceptable while others may be life-threatening.

The systems analysis of biological systems differs in one important way from systems analysis used in disciplines such as engineering or business management. The methodologies are similar but the variables in biology are usually not quantifiable with precision whereas in the other disciplines they often are. Most biological differences are qualitative and any analysis must recognize and make allowances for this uncomfortable fact.

Maxim.

The analysis of a clinical problem begins with identification of the disease or syndrome of dysfunction. Next is an attempt to identify etiology. If a specific etiology is not identifiable therapy needs to be based on a "most

likely etiology" basis. Next are determinations of the qualitatives of the dysfunctions. The choice of therapy and monitoring of the response to therapy depend on a knowledge of the permissible deviations from biological norms. The extent of deviations from these norms by the clinical and other features of the disease or dysfunction is a guide to the qualitatives of these deviations. The effectiveness or otherwise of therapy is determined by the extent of returns of abnormals to these desired norms. Animates are not immortal and the day will always come when no return eventuates.

The normal biology of each control and slave system is detailed in subsequent chapters. Clinical conditions are only mentioned to show how identification of deviations from desired and acceptable norms is possible and desirable for good clinical decision-making and for assessing and monitoring the responses to therapy.

As previously mentioned in Chapter 2, few of these deviations can be expressed in precise quantitative terms. Most are qualitative and determinations of their degrees of deviations from desirable norms are subjective and frequently vary from one physician to another. This is why the medical practice is too difficult to be called a science. It is an art and in all arts there are the avant-garde, the tradionalists, the masters, the geniuses, the individuals with average competence and others who do not merit classification in any of the above groups.

The tools of systems analysis are algorithms, flow charts, statistical analyses and block diagrams. These show how systems are controlled, how they interact, and how they are interrelated. Algorithms are useful when quantitative values and relationships are identifiable. In clinical medicine most variables can only be expressed as qualitatives and for such variables the ideal tools are statistical analyses, Bayesian analysis, block diagrams and flow charts.

Flow charts of normal physiology and biology are especially useful as aids to clear thinking about dysfunctions. Each requires precise sequential depiction of events that take place when the system is not dysfunctional. It should sequentially depict the events that take place in a system from its initiation till the attainment of its objective or objectives.

The sequential steps of systems analysis in biology.

1. **Precise definition of the objective or objectives of the dysfunctional system. Also needed is a listing of their resource systems and the minor system components of each resource.**

   This first requirement of biological systems analysis is of primary importance. It permits evaluations of the qualitatives of the existing dysfunction. It also facilitates the choice of therapy and determination of the effectiveness of any therapy. If the qualitatives of the dysfunction are returning to desired functional norms the therapy is appropriate and the patient's response is the one desired. If they are not therapy is incorrect for any one of the reasons detailed in Chapter 16 or the dysfunction is probably preterminal.

   To give a dysfunction a name is not difficult. The name given to a dysfunctional syndrome may change from time to time but not the symptoms and signs. Occasionally a new syndrome is described but most of the dysfunctions we deal with each day have symptoms and signs comparable to those described for the same dysfunctions a century ago. The differences between then and now are the investigations and therapies currently available and their interpretations. In Osler's time there were no antibiotics, no cardiac medications except for digitalis and relatively ineffective mercurial diuretics, no chemotherapy for malignant disease, no CT scans or MRIs and only unsophisticated laboratory studies. Therapy was almost non-existent.

   The difficult part of any clinical assessment is evaluation of the patient's gesture and prosody in statements and in responses to questions. At times similar difficulties attend the assessments of clinical findings, ancillary investigations and non-clinical information that is relevant for identifying optimum therapy. The practice of clinical medicine is not a science but an art and the tools are knowledge, common sense, objective reasoning, judgment and experience.

   Many factors can increase the difficulties of any analysis. The following are some examples:

   — **Complex multisystem disease** with one or more pathologies affecting one or more organ systems, and often caused by one or more etiologies. The result could be a multisystem dysfunction with each dysfunctional complex contributing some or all of its clinical features to the pool of signs and symptoms.

a) At times identification of objectives can complicate the clinical assessment and therapy because the system might have components with different objectives which are not equally affected by the disease. The following are some examples:

Single organs with dissimilar systems for different objectives.

— **The kidney is a single organ with two objectives.**

b) The principal ones are effected by a single complex of interrelated systems that control water retention and excretion, electrolyte excretions and retentions and the hydrogen ion concentrations of body fluids.

— The second is vasomotor control and control of sodium excretion by renin produced when the JG apparatus is stimulated by a lowering of blood pressure and/or the macula densa senses a low sodium concentration in tubular fluid. Renin is converted to a potent vasoconstrictor, angiotensin and angiotensin promotes aldosterone production and thus increases sodium and water retention.

Organs with a single system which performs different tasks.

— **The lung** which transfers environmental oxygen to the blood and exhales carbon dioxide to preserve the pH levels of body fluids.

— **The hepatocyte** is another example. It maintains blood glucose levels; synthesizes proteins and clotting factors; detoxifies, degrades and removes endogenous and exogenous undesirable materials; produces cholesterol and also excretes it in the bile; metabolizes ammonia to urea (the Kreb's-Henseleit cycle) and stores vitamins. Dysfunctions of the hepatic cell frequently decrease its different functions in dissimilar degrees. This suggests that each of the above functions of the hepatocyte might require its own separate enzyme complex and that these complexes might not be equally affected by a disease.

Diffuse systems with diffuse objectives.

Examples are the blood and the mechanisms for protection and compensation.

— **The blood** has four component systems; the red cells, the white cells, the platelets and plasma. Each has many dissimilar and complex functions as detailed in a later chapter. They are infrequently affected in similar ways or degrees by disease.

— **The systems for protection and compensation are complex and have the potential for systemic dissemination.** They include systems for natural protection and innate immunity, systems for generated immunity, for hypertrophy and hyperplasia and for protective pathology (e.g., inflammation and repair). Each of these diffuse systems have many dissimilar intrinsic objectives and any analysis requires that each be precisely defined and separately analyzed.

The following summarizes the other sequential steps needed for analyzing biological systems:

2. **Identification of the resources available to the system to achieve its objectives.**

   How does the system work and what are its resource systems? Which ones of the resources are dysfunctional? Are they hyperfunction or hypofunction dysfunctions? What is the appropriate therapy for the functional abnormalities of one or more resources? Resource systems are intrinsic to the system. Together with the microenvironmental control systems, they interact to attain the objective of the resource without assistance from extrinsic extracellular mechanisms.

   Control systems (the CNS and the endocrine control systems) are extrinsic systems. continuously monitor the performances of all body systems.

   When the function of any system requires change commands are transmitted to appropriate resource systems by autonomic and somatic efferents and/or by qualitative and/or quantitative changes in blood hormone levels.

3. **Identify the clinical features (both, symptoms and signs) which should be present if the diagnosis is correct.**

These comparisons allow for the qualitative assessments needed for diagnosis, the choice of therapy and monitoring of the response to therapy. They are subjective judgments which are often disputed by others, and often with justification.

4. **Protective, adaptive and compensatory mechanisms.**

   Does the dysfunction result form failure of mechanisms that normally protect and compensate for functional deficits?

   All relevant protective, adaptive and compensatory mechanisms require identification and assessment when analyzing a syndrome of dysfunction.

5. **The temporal phase of the dysfunction.**

   Is it acute, subacute or chronic. Is it progressive, stable or will recovery eventuate. There are other possibilities as depicted in Chart 3-6 on page 59.

6. **Evaluate the "hierarchical importance" of any dysfunctional system or systems.**

   The phrase "hierarchical importance" was introduced by von Bertalanffy[9] in recognition of the fact that some systems are more important to an organism than are others. Evaluation of the "hierarchical importance" of systems in relation to each other, is a frequent requisite for problem solving and decision-making.

   First, a physician is often confronted with a clinical problem in which multiple pathologies are present. The following is an extreme example. The victim of an automobile accident may present with multiple fractures, severe hypotension, a head injury which has resulted in exposure of the underlying brain, an abdominal injury that has resulted in suspected lacerations of the liver and spleen, significant hypotension, and a facial injury which has resulted in the mouth and pharynx filling with blood. In what order are these injuries to be dealt with? A hierarchical classification of the systems of the body helps to decide.

   The primary consideration must be maintenance or restoration of brain function by perfusion with oxygen and energy substrate (i.e., glucose). The mouth and pharynx must be cleared of blood and other obstructing materials, establish an adequate airway, start manual CPR and continue till mechanical equipment for ventilation and cardiac monitoring arrives. These measures provide the brain with blood that is sufficient in amount, and in oxygen and glucose. Cross-match blood for transfusion and start an intravenous transfusion of saline or plasma. The first and most important objective is preservation of brain function. Of slightly, very slightly, less hierarchical importance is immediate surgery for the rapid control of bleeding from abdominal organs. Protection of the exposed brain from trauma and/or infection is next on the list. Fractures can be dealt with as a final measure.

   Secondly, classification of the systems of the body in terms of their hierarchical interrelationships often helps a clinician to anticipate the natural history of a disease. When physiological resources are stretched to the limit available resources are diverted to systems in descending order of their hierarchical importance to each other. Failure begins in those systems that are starved of energy substrate, oxygen or both.

Disease without demonstrable dysfunction.

A final comment is that disease can exist without demonstrable dysfunction. A common example is atheromatous disease of the coronary vessels. Many studies have shown that narrowing of coronary vessels can exist without any clinical symptoms and signs. A startling fact is that about a third of patients with evolving myocardial infarctions die before hospitalization, presumably from massive infarctions or lethal arrhythmias such as ventricular fibrillation. Many die without any premonitory symptoms of myocardial insufficiency[10].

Another example is malignant disease. Numerous studies have shown that the development of most malignancies is a slow and gradual process. A common sequence is the slow alteration of normal cells to cells that are dysplastic and finally express the malignant phenotype. As a rule a number of years elapse before normal cells become malignant and an additional number of years usually precede the development of clinically diagnosable malignancy. At times, even when malignant lesions are palpable and/or radiographically demonstrable symptoms may be absent. Needle aspiration biopsies, studies of the cytologies of sputum and other body fluids and the

Papanicolau cytological studies of cervical and endocervical smears detect dysplastic changes before expression of malignant phenotypes.

The final assessment before therapy

In this book, each chapter on diagnosis as it affects different systems has an initial summary of the basic biology of the dysfunctional system or diseased tissue or organ. The principal features of the clinical disorders are deliberately listed in summary form. The absence of a single piece of information which is essential for correctness of the diagnosis is enough to warrant the reassessment, deletion or modification of the clinical assessment. It is acceptable to disregard the absence of symptoms or signs which are not essential for confirmation of the validity of the diagnosis. It is never acceptable to disregard those which are. The summarized descriptions of clinical dysfunctions in subsequent chapters itemize these essentials for they are the ones that need comparisons with the desired norms of physiology and biochemistry to determine the qualitatives of the dysfunction and the choices and responses to therapy. In addition, these deviations often confirm the validity or otherwise of a diagnosis.

The amount of available clinical information is very large. No matter. Most clinical problems can be resolved by comparing the clinical features with the desired norms of biology to obtain some assessment of the qualitatives of the dysfunction. It is not difficult to provide a summary of reasonable size that encompasses the facts of normal physiology, biochemistry and protective pathology that are relevant to the practice of clinical medicine, especially facts which are essential for concluding that a diagnostic assessment is correct. The word "relevant" is not used to derogate the writers of texts on physiology or biochemistry or pathology. Each is mandated to provide comprehensive texts about their subject. Thus, a text on physiology meets the needs of physiologists but only a small portion is needed for the day-to-day practice of clinical medicine. It is these small but relevant facts of physiology, biochemistry and protective pathology that provide the bases for comparisons between clinical features and the permissible and desirable limits of systems functions. These comparisons provide the bases for assessments of the qualitatives of any disease or syndrome of dysfunction, for deciding on optimal therapy and for monitoring the response to therapy.

Equally important is that they provide information about the absence of presence of factors which are essential if the diagnostic assessment is correct. **As mentioned above, the absence of a single factor which must be present if the diagnosis is correct requires a reassesment of the facts and modification or deletion of the diagnostic assessment in favor of another.**

Identification of etiology is always desirable, especially if treatment for the etiology is available. It is not always possible to determine etiology but often, treatment on the basis of "most likely etiology" provides acceptable control. I have a number of patients in their eighties who have congestive heart failure. The presumption has been that failure resulted from a combination of coronary insufficiency and the changes of aging. A few have died with the passage of time but the others remain well controlled on various therapeutic cocktails which need modification from time to time.

This ends a large chapter on biological systems and their associated biologies.

Chapter 5 References.

1. Bernard, C. English translation by H.C. Green in 1957 of "Introduction a la medecine experimentale." 1865.

2. Bernard, C. Lecons sur les Phenomenes de la Vie Communs aux animaux et aux Vegetaux." 1878.

3. Cannon, W.B. Organization for physiological homeostasis. Physiol. Rev. 1939; 9:399.

4. Cannon, W.B. The Way of an Investigator. New York. Hafner Publishing Co., 1965.

5 Porter, A. Cybernetics simplified. London. The English Universities Press Ltd., 1969.

6. Wiener, N. Human use of human beings. New York. Avon Books, 1986.

7. Wiener, N. Cybernetics. New York:. John Wiley and Sons, 1948.

8. Schäfer, E.A. The Endocrine Organs: An Introduction to the Study of Internal Secretion. New York. Longmans, Green & Co, 1916.

9. Bertalanffy, L. Von. An outline of general systems theory. J. Phil. Sci.; 1, 1950.

10. Huikuri, H.V., Castellanos, A. et al. Sudden deaths due to cardiac arrhythmias. N. Engl. J. Med. 2001; 345:1473.

6

Diagnosis: The Control Systems

1. The Central Nervous System (CNS)

Table of Contents

Notation.

The notation ~P denotes phosphorous with a high energy bond. Depending on the context in which the term is used, ~P may also denote the energy liberated when a high energy phosphate bond detaches from ATP or ADP.

A general comment on the methodology of clinical assessments.

Clinical assessments of the qualitatives of a dysfunction or dysfunctions, and the choice and monitoring of the responses to therapy must be based on assessments of the deviations of the clinical picture from the accepted and acceptable norms of human biology. If etiology can be identified well and good, especially if it is etiology for which there is available therapy. If etiology cannot be identified treatment should be on a "most likely etiology" basis or as supportive or palliative therapy.

Equally important is that clinical assessments provide information about the absence or presence of factors which are essential if the diagnostic assessment is correct. The absence of a single clinical feature which must be present if the diagnosis is correct requires a reassesment of the facts and the modification or deletion of the diagnostic assessment in favor of another. The absence of clinical features which are not essential for confirmation that the diagnosis is correct can be disregarded. Many will probably appear later. It is never acceptable to disregard those which are essential if the diagnosis is correct. These paragraphs are not repeated in subsequent chapters but recommendations to read them are.

The objectives and capabilities of the CNS.

The objectives and capabilities of the CNS were summarized in Charts 5-7 on page 107. For convenience of the reader a copy is reproduced here (Chart 6-1).

The human body is a centralized system. One system, the central nervous system (the brain and spinal cord, collectively called the CNS), has a dominant role in controlling biological systems. The CNS is analogous to the seat of government of a far-flung empire. Sensors continuously provide information about the external and internal environments of the body. Afferent information is transmitted by somatic and autonomic nerves, either directly or after reception in peripheral receptors such as the carotid baroreceptors and chemoreceptors.

The hypothalamus has osmoreceptors which sense osmotic pressure changes in perfusing blood. These receptors determine the amounts of ADH produced and released into the circulation. Hypothalamic releasing factors control pituitary hormone production. These hormones stimulate peripheral targets in the thyroid, adrenals and gonads to produce hormones which have many different biological effects. Control of peripheral hormone production is by long-arm reflexes between the levels of circulating hormones on the one hand and hypothalamic and pituitary receptors on the other. The hypothalamus also receives neural impulses from medullary control centers and the cortex for hypothalamic integrations with vasomotor, cardiac and respiratory centers and the cortex (Charts 7-3 and 7-4 on pages 162 and 163).

Chart 6-1: A SUMMARY OVERVIEW OF THE CAPABILITIES AND OBJECTIVES OF THE CENTRAL NERVOUS SYSTEM

The capabilities of the CNS:

1. **Capacity for intellectual activity:** logical reasoning and decision-making, abstract thought, memorization and recall of information, likes and dislikes, love and hate, knowledge of moral and legislated law, and many other items.
2. **Capacity for volitional activity**: movement in precise, coordinated and purposeful ways, maintenance of different static postures and of balance during movements, and verbal, gestural and prosodic language.
3. **Capacity to receive, perceive and recognize sensory stimuli which enter consciousness:** perception and recognition of cutaneous and visceral pain, visual, auditory, olfactory, and gustatory information, cutaneous touch, and changes in surface temperatures and pressures. Multimodal integrations of received information are effected in the heteromodal areas, especially the tempero-parietal heteromodal area.
   Changes in the internal environment are sensed by baroreceptors, chemoreceptors, osmoreceptors, pain receptors and thermoreceptors, or transmitted directly to the CNS by somatic (e.g., from the muscles of respiration) and/or autonomic nerves.
   Responses to information from the interval environment are usually mediated by involuntary reflexes from medullary and hypothalamic control centers. Higher centers have the abilities to modify these involuntary responses and to initiate reflexes to pain sensed in subcortical areas.
4. **Knowledge of the objectives and functions of every biological system** (including itself) and the ability to integrate all information and then decide if functional changes are needed in one or more systems. Commands for change are transmitted by autonomic and somatic nerves and by qualitative and/or quantitative changes in hormone secretions controlled by the CNS.

Central control centers receive and process afferent information and decide if functional changes are needed in any one or more systems. If they are, commands for change are transmitted by somatic and autonomic nerve impulses, and/or by quantitative changes in hormones controlled by the hypothalamus and/or the pituitary.

Everything is done to protect the CNS. It is enclosed in a hard bony covering, cushioned in fluid, wrapped in membranes and abundantly supplied with blood which is replete with oxygen and glucose. The CNS can only use glucose as a substrate for production of energy (~P) which is usable for biological activities. After a period of starvation some ketone bodies are usable. The CNS needs abundant glucose and oxygen: about 50ml oxygen and 75mg glucose each minute. These requirements are met by perfusion of the brain with about 750ml/min of blood (approximately 15-20% of total cardiac output at rest). Any reduction in available oxygen or glucose, or both, results in neurological dysfunctions ranging from tremors and confusion to coma and finally, death after about four minutes of hypoglycemia or acute and total anoxia.

There are many possible causes for decreased energy production in the CNS. Acute and total ~P deficits are rapidly fatal in about four minutes. The usual causes are strangulation (judicial or criminal) or a large dose of intravenous insulin. Slower lapses into confusion, coma and death result from increased intracranial pressure, acute or chronic and progressive circulatory failure, or advanced pulmonary dysfunction. As a corollary, a blood glucose estimation is essential when an individual is unconscious for no obvious reason.

To ensure survival of the CNS, a whole system complex of autonomous endocrine systems has developed to maintain adequate cerebral perfusion with glucose and oxygen and the orderly transmission of nerve impulses. All were detailed in the previous chapter.

The objectives.

The objectives and capabilities of the CNS are listed in Chart 6-1. It needs no additional textual amplifications

The resource systems of the CNS.

The CNS has two principal resource systems:

- **The nerve impulse.** The nerve impulse is the basic functional unit of neurological function.
- **The neuron.** Most are located in aggregates, each with specific functions (e.g., the aggregates for memory and motor activity). Each aggregate usually has many components. Most components of an aggregate are separated by distance (Chart 6-8). Neural interactions, communications and integrations are frequent..

The nerve impulse - the first resource system of the CNS

The basics of initiation and transmission of nerve impulses were well described by seminal works by Hodgkin and Huxley (**Hodgkin, A & Huxley, A.** A quantitative description of membrane current and its application to conductions and excitation in nerve. J. Physiol. (London) 1952; 117:500. **Hodgkin, A.L.** Conduction of the Nervous Impulse. Springfield, Ill, Thomas, 1964.). The facts were extensively detailed in Chapter 1, page 24 et seq. It was necessary to do so there because a comparison of the capabilities of the human brain versus the computer would not have been possible without an accompanying description of CNS neural capabilities..

- Estimates of the numbers of neurons in the cerebrum vary from 10 billion to two hundred billion and of synapses from 10^{11} to 10^{15}. Information comes to the neuron by many synaptic contacts between its body, its dendrites and its axon terminals with the same structures in other neurons.
- Intracellular electrical negativity in relation to the extracellular space is the basis for transmission of nerve impulses. It is maintained by cell membrane sodium pumps which use the enzyme, Na^+/K^+-ATPase to extract ~P from cell membrane ATP. The pump uses this energy to extrude Na^+ ions which have entered the cells through ion channels or by diffusion along concentration gradients. Each time, for every $3Na^+$ ions extruded $2K^+$ions are retained. Thus intracellular negativity with respect to the interstitium is preserved.
- As a rule, many axon terminals and dendrites end at synapses on the surfaces of many neurons. Eccles estimates[1] that each pyramidal cell receives some 10,000 synapses while Ito[2] has estimated that many of the cerebellar Purkinje cells communicate with cerebellar climbing and parallel fibers at more than 100,000 synapses each. These assessments suggest that there are 10^{11} to 10^{15} synapses in the CNS.
- A small space at each axon terminal separates it from the next dendrite, soma or axon body. When stimulated the axon terminal secretes a neurotransmitter into this terminal. Some neurotransmitters excite and contribute to the generation of a nerve impulse. Others inhibit and dampen the postsynaptic response. The former result in excitatory post-synaptic potentials (EPSPs) and the latter in inhibitory post-synaptic potentials (IPSPs).
- Each axon has many terminals which end on the soma, dendrites or axons of other neurons. One estimate is that a single neuron can communicate with some 10,000 other neurons by synaptic relays.

Excitatory and inhibitory postsynaptic potentials.

The cell membrane of the neuron has ion channels for sodium, potassium and chloride ions. They are not the same as the sodium pump channels. The sodium, potassium and chloride channels are closed by charged "gating particles". Neurotransmitters change the potential differences at these gated channels and alter their permeabilities. Neurotransmitters that stimulate (those that produce excitatory post-synaptic potentials or EPSPs for short) open the sodium channels. Na^+ flows in and the internal surface of the cell membrane becomes less negative. Neurotransmitters that inhibit (the inhibitory post-synaptic potentials or IPSPs for short) open the potassium channels and potassium moves out of the neuron, thus increasing intracellular negativity. The changes produced by an EPSP or IPSP at a single postsynaptic locus is small - about 1mV or less[3]. The algebraic sum of EPSPs and IPSPs must approximate a change of about +25mV at the axon hillock before the neuron can generate an action potential with a decreased negative charge. The axon has the same intracellular negativity as its parent neuron. Once generated the action potential is an electrical current which flows down the nerve as each point successively becomes positive with respect to the next; dissimilar electric charges attract each other while similar charges repel. **This is the nerve impulse.** The action potential can initiate another action potential in a postsynaptic neuron. Alternatively, it can initiate contraction in striated, smooth or cardiac muscle by a neurotransmitter discharged into the small space between an axon terminal and its target. The action potential can also induce glandular secretion, also via a neuro-transmitter which terminates on a receptor in the gland. Peripheral receptors of information transmit information along afferent nerves by essentially similar processes.

An almost infinite numbers of neural discharge patterns are theoretically possible.

The intervals between discharges vary as the algebraic sum of EPSPs and IPSPs acting on the neuron via thousands of synapses. At times the algebraic sum of EPSPs and IPSPs reaching the neuron will exceed the +25mv change needed at the axon hillock for generation of a nerve impulse. At other times it might not or it might persist at the +25mv levels. In the first instance the neural discharge will be irregular because of variations in frequency and this will result in irregularities of transmission. The second will result in a strong continuous discharge of impulses. The refractory period and the rate of transmission along a specific nerve determines the maximum rates of discharges.

Variations because of different speeds of nerve transmission can be significant. They range from 120m/sec in the $A\alpha$ motor activity and proprioception fibers to 1m/sec in the slow C fibers of the postganglionic sympathetic fibers and some fibers in the dorsal roots. Most small nerves do not transmit faster than 100 nerve impulses/sec. Neurons in the central nervous system can fire at 500-1000 times per second. Rates of nerve discharge can vary from nil to high rates, especially in interneuron systems. In the Renshaw cell interneuron system discharge rates can exceed 1600 per second.

A single neuron could receive information from any one or more of these different nerves. Only the final algebraic sum of the EPSPs and IPSPs determine whether or not an action potential develops. The integrations of these patterns of nerve discharges for information recording, transfer and recall are currently unknown. The end result is predictable. It is the smooth, precise and coordinated activities of all animates. At present we do not know how this coordination is effected but the features of daily living are immutable proof that it is done.

Long-term synaptic potentiation and depression.

A topic of much current interest is long-term synaptic potentiation (LTP). It may provide the basis for development of preprogrammed movements which only require small as-and-when needed modifications by the motor complex.

It was Ramón y Cajal who first suggested that learning resulted from synaptic strengthening following intense activity. Hebb pursued this concept in his book, "The Organization of Behavior"[4] but seemingly not with much enthusiasm. It was not till 1973 that the subject was revitalized by a publication from Bliss and Lomo[5]. A revue by Martinez and Derrick[6] provides an excellent introduction to the subject of long-term synaptic potentiation and depression (LTP and LTD) and so does a review by Martin and Grimwood (Ann. Revu. of Neurosciences, 23:659). Subsequent publications on these topics run in the hundreds and dozens are added each year.

Long-term potentiation and depression are phenomena which can be expressed at any of the many synapses. The proposed mechanisms are complex and neither space nor the objectives of this book permit any additional detailing of these topics. They have been proposed as mechanisms for many cerebral activities such as learning, memorizing and the preprogramming of movements. The concepts are reasonable and exciting but, for ethical reasons, their importance in human cerebration can only be assumed by the deductions of physiologists and experimental psychologists who correlate clinical findings with the results of trauma, disease or therapeutic surgical ablations. Long-term synaptic depressions have also been described and together with the potentiation mechanisms could provide a satisfactory explanation about the mechanisms of preprogramming and learning.

Myelin.

In myelinated nerves an insulating material, myelin, is wrapped around nerves except at certain points known as the nodes of Ranvier. In the CNS myelin is produced by the oligodendrocytes and in the peripheral nerves by Schwann cells. Voltage-gated sodium channels are plentiful at the non-myelinated nodes. Increased local positive charge bolsters the nerve impulse each time it passes a node. The result is rapid and reinforced propagation of the nerve impulse. This type of conduction is called saltatory conduction because it jumps like a rabbit from one node to the next (in Latin, "saltatio" means a leap). Conduction is much faster in myelinated nerves than in those which lack myelin - in the former it increases directly with axon diameter, in the latter with the square root of axon diameter. The consequences of demyelination are disturbances of previously programmed pathways. Consequences are uncoordinated movements and eventual paralyses. Multiple sclerosis is a devastating and common example. The demyelinating dysfunctions are summarized in a later chapter.

Reflexes.

Reflexes are involuntary reactions to any one of a variety of stimuli. Descartes must receive credit for the initial clear description of a reflex. The example used was the rapid removal of a foot suddenly placed near a fire and equally suddenly withdrawn - in modern parlance, "the flexor withdrawal reflex".

Hundreds of different reflexes control biological activities. Many were detailed in previous chapters on homeostasis and biological systems. They range from monosynaptic reflexes to those of much complexity. Credit is due to Sherrington[7] for an initial classification of many different types of reflexes. Examples of both types are detailed below:

Monosynaptic reflexes.

The knee jerk or stretch reflex is a typical example. When the patella is tapped the quadriceps are stretched and the leg extends. This is because impulses from the stretched muscle travel via the dorsal root of the spinal cord to anterior horn cells which send neural impulses for extension of the leg - the knee jerk. Of course the activity of the anterior horn cell which mediates extension of the leg can be modified by central and local neural impulses. Thus, a lesion of the upper motor neuron will amplify the response while one affecting the lower motor neuron or the afferent and efferent paths in the peripheral nerves will decrease it.

Complex reflexes.

Two examples are detailed. Both are of clinical importance.

The Babinski reflex.

This is a complex reflex using a number of different synaptic connections. Normally, when one gently strokes the lateral aspect of the bottom of the foot there is a downward movement of the big toe. If the Babinski reflex is present the big toe moves upwards. If the response is vigorous the foot is everted from the site of stimulation and the limb may be withdrawn. A positive Babinski reflex is usually a concomitant of an upper motor neuron lesion.

The pupillary reflexes and their associated accommodation and light reflexes.

These are complex reflexes of clinical importance because increased intracranial pressure is often characterized by a fixed and dilated pupil. A finding such as this merits urgent investigation when an unconscious individual is found without obvious cause for the comatose state. Chart 6-2 is a summarized depiction of the pupillary reflexes.

The iris is a circular structure surrounding the pupil. It controls the size of the pupil and hence, the amount of light entering the eye. Two muscles are used; a concentric sphincter muscle at its periphery and radial dilator muscles. Chart 6-2 shows the innervation of these muscles and the mechanisms of the pupillary reflexes.

Nerve impulses for pupillary reactions are generated by light which travels along the optic nerves to the lateral geniculate bodies and superior corpora quadrigemina. Efferent parasympathetic constrictor fibers traverse the third cranial nerve to reach the constrictor muscle. They are derived from connections between the corpora quadrigemina and the third nerve nucleus. Increased intracranial pressure decreases the function of the third nerve. The result is partial or complete paralysis of constrictor muscle of the iris with a pupil which is fixed in dilation. The anatomical cause is pressure on the third nerve between a herniation of the temporal lobe on the affected side and the adjacent medial petroclinoid ligament.

Chart 6-2: THE PUPILLARY REFLEXES [1] (post-numeral: a = parasympathetic, b = sympathetic)

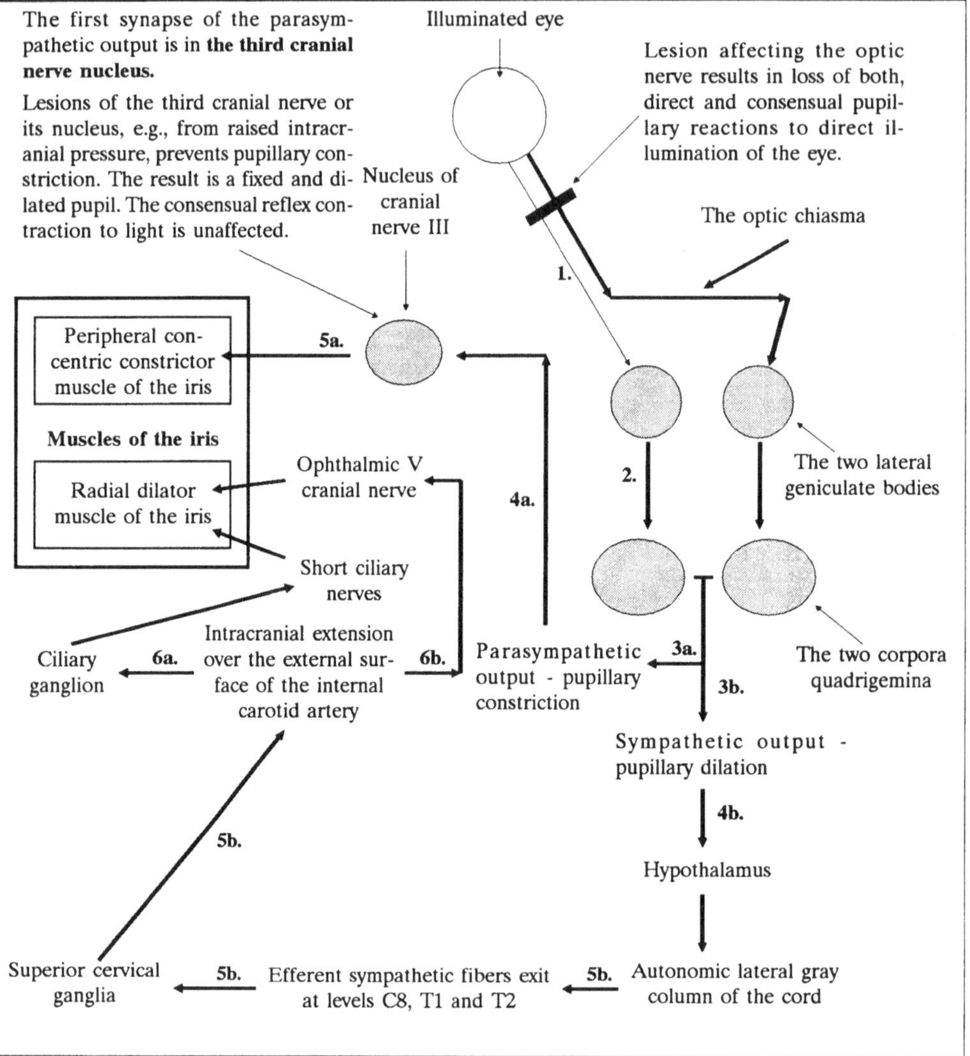
The first synapse of the parasympathetic output is in **the third cranial nerve nucleus.**
Lesions of the third cranial nerve or its nucleus, e.g., from raised intracranial pressure, prevents pupillary constriction. The result is a fixed and dilated pupil. The consensual reflex contraction to light is unaffected.
Illuminated eye
Lesion affecting the optic nerve results in loss of both, direct and consensual pupillary reactions to direct illumination of the eye.
Nucleus of cranial nerve III
The optic chiasma
1.
Peripheral concentric constrictor muscle of the iris
5a.
Muscles of the iris
Radial dilator muscle of the iris
Ophthalmic V cranial nerve
Short ciliary nerves
4a.
2.
The two lateral geniculate bodies
Intracranial extension over the external surface of the internal carotid artery
Ciliary ganglion
6a.
6b.
Parasympathetic output - pupillary constriction
3a.
3b.
The two corpora quadrigemina
Sympathetic output - pupillary dilation
4b.
5b.
Hypothalamus
Superior cervical ganglia
5b.
Efferent sympathetic fibers exit at levels C8, T1 and T2
5b.
Autonomic lateral gray column of the cord

[1] When light illuminates one eye the pupil contracts (the direct reaction) and so does the opposite non-illuminated pupil (the consensual reaction). The anatomical connections between the retina and lateral geniculate bodies of the non-illuminated eye are not shown in order to introduce a little clarity to the depiction. They are the same as those of the illuminated eye as are all subsequent connections. Fibers from the illuminated eye which cross over at the chiasma are probably responsible for the consensual pupillary reaction which is preserved even when the parasympathetic output on the other side is impaired. as in compression of Cranial Nerve III by increased intracranial pressure.

The sympathetic dilators have a more complicated course. They pass from the corpora quadrigemina to the hypothalamus and then to the lateral gray horn of the cord in segments C8, T1 and T2. Next they pass to the superior cervical ganglion. They then enter the skull along the internal carotid artery. Those which have synapsed in the superior cervical ganglion enter the ophthalmic division of the fifth cranial nerve. The rest go to the ciliary ganglion where they synapse and innervate the dilator muscles by the short ciliary nerves. Innervation is of the radial dilator muscle of the iris.

The light reflexes. Both pupils constrict when the amount of entering light increases. Constriction of the illuminated eye is called the **direct reflex** and that of the opposite eye, the **consensual reflex.** Both reflexes are absent when there are interruptions of the optic nerve of the illuminated eye. The direct reflex is lost but the consensual preserved when the lesion affects the fibers of the third cranial nerve innervating the constrictor muscle. The pupil is fixed and dilated on the affected side. An ominous cause of bilateral fixed and dilated pupils is increased intracranial pressure. A single fixed and dilated pupil indicates an unilateral lesion; an ipsilateral extradural or intracerebral bleed after trauma, or pressure on Cranial Nerve III by tumors or aneurysms.

The accommodation reflexes. The pupil constricts and oculomotor nerve contractions result in convergence of the eyes when they focus on a near object. Both, the direct light reflex and the accommodation reflexes are impaired when the third cranial nerve is damaged. Loss of the accommodation reflex with preservation of the light reflex is rare but may occur when mid brain lesions exist.

Argyll Robertson pupil. This type of pupillary abnormality is characteristic of tabes dorsalis. The pupils are small, irregular and dissimilar in size. The light reflex is lost but the response to accommodation is retained Blood studies are usually positive for syphilis.

Horner's syndrome. The syndrome results from damage to the sympathetic fibers going to the eye. Responsible lesions may lie adjacent to the superior cervical ganglion (e.g., infiltration by malignant lymph nodes), or destructive lesions involving the internal carotid artery. Characteristic of the full-blown syndrome are pupillary contraction, ptosis, enophthalamos, and absence of sweating on the face of the affected side.

Adie's syndrome. This is a benign condition though alarming when first identified. The pupil is dilated and the reactions to light and accommodation are sluggish. Its etiology is unknown but investigations are needed before the diagnosis is made. A suggestive feature is weak or absent tendon reflexes.

The neuron - the second resource system of the CNS

Most of the needs of the CNS are met by aggregates of neurons each with a specific overall function. These aggregates are often separated from each other by distance. For example the motor cortex which initiates movement is at a distance from the cerebellum and basal ganglia which modulate motor activity. Easy and rapid access between neuronal aggregates results from neural and synaptic communications which transmit signals with the speeds of neural transmissions. As mentioned previously, it is estimated that at any one time a single neuron can provide information to some 10,000 others by repeated relays of information along different synaptic communications and by simultaneous parallel processings.

Another example is the requirements for recognition and processing of sensory information. Most of the needed neuronal aggregates are located in anatomically separate areas: the primary reception areas, the unimodal and heteromodal areas, the limbic cortex and their attention filters (it is assumed that these filters are located in that area), short-term memory and the memory banks of long-term memory. All these neuronal aggregates have a single function: the processing of sensed information. They are anatomically separated by cortical tissues but accurate interactions and coordinations are assured by the speed of the nerve impulse and the interactions of neurons. The locales and functions of these neuronal aggregates were detailed in Chapter 2, pages 45-53.

The functions of the CNS were previously depicted in Chart 6-1. **Sensory processing** and the use of information were discussed in detail in Chapter 2, pages 45-53. The processes involved in **intellectual activity** are essentially unknown. It is not further discussed in this text. Just accept that it happens, don't ask how? A knowledge of what is required of intellectual activity is the basis for the identification and diagnoses of the dementias and other disorders of mentation.

Two topics remain. One is **motor activity** and the other is **maintenance of homeostasis.**

Homeostasis was a topic detailed in Chapter 5, pages 97-100. The main conduits of information and commands which maintain homeostasis are components of the **autonomic nervous system.** The anatomic and physiological attributes of this latter system are detailed after the next section which is a summary detailing of the mechanisms of motor activity. Systems which maintain homeostasis get extensive coverage in Chapter 13, page 290 et seq. and only the anatomy and physiology of its autonomic controls are detailed in this chapter.

Volitional motor activity and maintenance of static postures and balance

The normal physiology of movement and maintenance of balance and posture involves the interaction of many complex component systems as shown in Chart 6-3. The motor cortex is located just in front of the Rolandic sulcus. When areas of the motor cortex are stimulated there are contractions of localized groups of muscles. Starting in the midline and progressing down over the lateral surface of the cerebral hemisphere are the areas for toes, feet, legs, thighs, body, shoulder, arms, hand, fingers, thumb, neck, head, face and tongue. Areas involved in fine skilled movements such as thumb, tongue, lip and larynx are represented by proportionately larger areas than those needed for movements needing less skill and precision. Representation is of movements, not the contractions of individual muscles.

The objectives of the system are smooth, precise and coordinated volitional movements.

The resource systems are shown in Chart 6-3. They are and have to be numerous. Each resource attains its

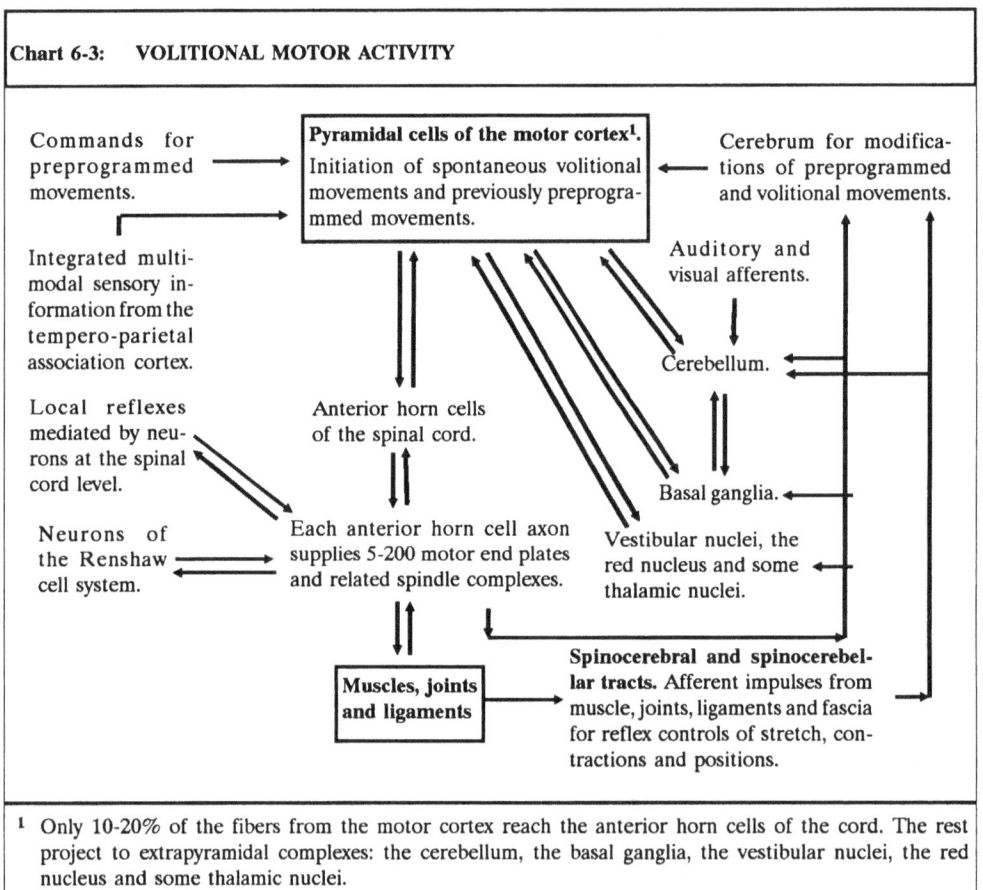

Chart 6-3: VOLITIONAL MOTOR ACTIVITY

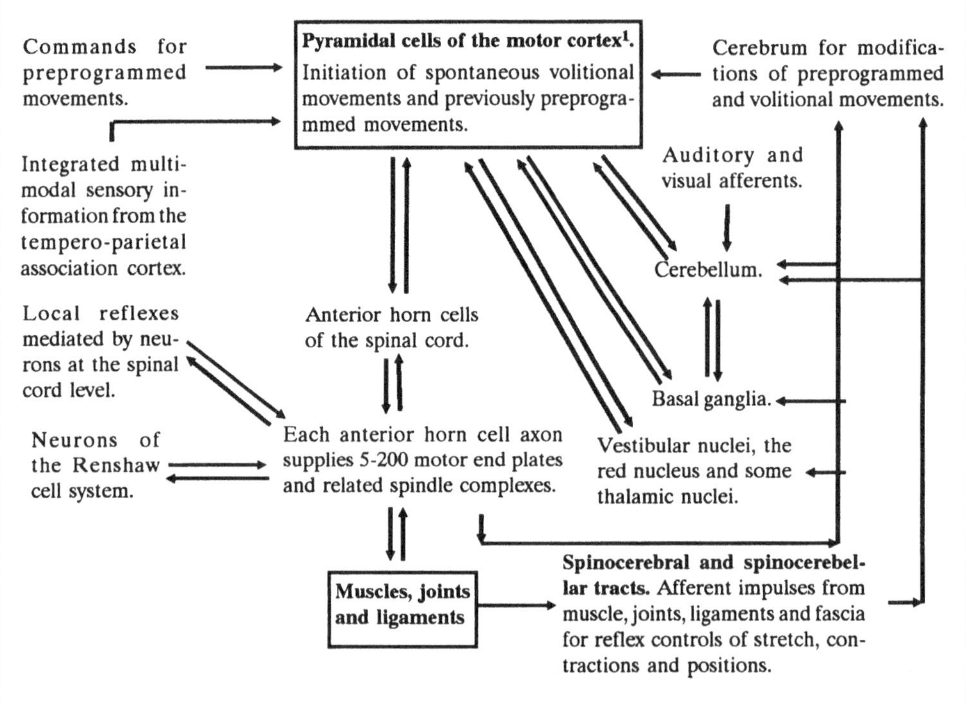
Commands for preprogrammed movements.
Pyramidal cells of the motor cortex[1]. Initiation of spontaneous volitional movements and previously preprogrammed movements.
Cerebrum for modifications of preprogrammed and volitional movements.
Integrated multimodal sensory information from the tempero-parietal association cortex.
Auditory and visual afferents.
Cerebellum.
Local reflexes mediated by neurons at the spinal cord level.
Anterior horn cells of the spinal cord.
Basal ganglia.
Neurons of the Renshaw cell system.
Each anterior horn cell axon supplies 5-200 motor end plates and related spindle complexes.
Vestibular nuclei, the red nucleus and some thalamic nuclei.
Muscles, joints and ligaments
Spinocerebral and spinocerebellar tracts. Afferent impulses from muscle, joints, ligaments and fascia for reflex controls of stretch, contractions and positions.

[1] Only 10-20% of the fibers from the motor cortex reach the anterior horn cells of the cord. The rest project to extrapyramidal complexes: the cerebellum, the basal ganglia, the vestibular nuclei, the red nucleus and some thalamic nuclei.

objective by automatic and autonomous interactions of many minor system neuron components.

The functional effector unit of motor function is an anatomically related group of motor neurons in the spinal cord which receive their input from cortical motor neurons. The spinal cord complex probably innervates all the muscles acting around one joint. Coordinated movements result from variable activations of many such units lying adjacent to each other.

Nerve fibers responsible for motor activity originate from the pyramidal cells of the motor cortex. They descend in the pyramidal tracts and innervate the contralateral cranial nerve nuclei by connections which cross the midline. The pyramidal tracts decussate in the lower medulla to innervate the contralateral motor nuclei of the spinal cord. Of the fibers which comprise the pyramidal tract only a minor proportion (about 10-20%) continue in these tracts. The remaining 80% project to extrapyramidal complexes; the cerebellum, the basal ganglia, the vestibular nuclei, the red nucleus, and some thalamic nuclei. The cerebellum also receives auditory and visual afferents. **These neural aggregates are all resource systems of the main cortical motor system.**

In some unknown way there are multiple integrations of motor activity with new and previously stored sensory information, with resident cerebellar and basal ganglia information, and with information brought to the cerebellum and cerebrum by spinocerebellar and spinocerebral tracts respectively. Eccles[1] has estimated that each pyramidal cell has approximately 10,000 synaptic communications with other neurons.

In the region of the anterior horn cells of the spinal cord the contraction impulses are modulated by neural impulses from the Renshaw cell system, and by the simple local spinal reflexes originally described by Sherrington[6] and associates. The end result is the smooth, precise, purposeful and coordinated contractions of the muscle groups required for the desired movement. All these corrections occur continuously, millisecond after millisecond, throughout the movement. Chart 6-3 shows the complexities of the motor cortex interactions with the cerebellum, the basal ganglia, the sensory association cortices, and the spinal motor neurons. **When a clinical neurological dysfunction is present it is necessary to check the performance of each of these neuronal aggregates before arriving at any conclusions about diagnosis.**

Cerebellar and basal ganglia interactions and afferent information from the spinal neurons are all essential for smooth, coordinated and precise movements. When cells of the motor cortex fire impulses down the pyramidal tract collaterals transmit the patterns of this discharge to the cerebellum. After computation in the cerebellar cortex the output is rapidly returned to the motor cortex in about 10-20msec of the initial command. This input provides a continuous correction and modification of the motor commands. In addition, when the motor command brings about a movement, receptors from muscles, skin, and joints, send afferents along the spino-cerebellar tracts to the same regions of the cerebellar cortex as were involved in the more direct loop, and to the cerebrum by the spinocerebral tract. These inputs additionally modify the motor response. Modifications of this sort are of special importance in walking, standing, balancing, and in the postural adjustments required for maintenance of stability during voluntary movements.

The caudate nucleus, the putamen and the globus pallidus constitute the basal ganglia. Another closed loop circuit exists between the basal ganglia and motor cortex which modulates motor activity for precise action. There is continual variation of the motor cortex discharge as the result of cerebellar and basal ganglia modulations. These impulses rapidly pass to the spinal centers to provide immediate correction and to the association and motor cortex to re-program[9]. Clinical manifestations of dysfunctions in any one or more of these systems are detailed later in the chapter.

The Renshaw cell system.

The Renshaw cell system lies adjacent to the anterior horn cells and provides an important system for precise and forceful muscle action. After it originates from the anterior horn cell but before it leaves the cord the motor neuron impulse synapses via collaterals with adjacent inhibitory Renshaw cells. Renshaw cell collaterals form inhibitory synapses on adjacent as well as the originating motor neurons. When a group of motor neurons are discharging strongly the Renshaw system inhibits all motor neurons in the adjacent area. As a consequence, weak discharges are suppressed. The strongly excited neurons continue to fire. This increases the precision of motor performance by negating the effects of weakly responding motor neurons which could cause disorder and imprecision in movement. The whole process is an automatic fast control reflex system located at the anterior horn cell and designed to deliver precise, purposeful, and appropriately powered movement.

Are movements preprogrammed?

The answer is a qualified yes. It seems probable that most common movements have a preprogrammed basis which is continually modified, as and when necessary, by cerebellar, basal ganglia, and various other inputs. However, it is possible that with rapid movements we rely almost completely on preprogrammed movements as there is no time for correction during performance once a fast movement such as speech has begun. Preprogramming is difficult for musicians who need to simultaneously coordinate intellectual perception and interpretation with vision, hearing and motor activity. Basic preprogramming is probably possible but difficulty in preprogramming more than this probably explains the need these artists have for daily repetition and practice of their repertoire.

In learning a movement we first execute it slowly because it is not preprogrammed. After repeated cerebral concentrations and interactions with the cerebellum and basal ganglia most of the movement can be preprogrammed and executed more rapidly. In sum, exploratory movements are imperfectly programmed while trained movements are largely preprogrammed. The above is hypothesis as we do not know exactly how movements are preprogrammed. Long term potentiation (LTP) and long-term depressions (LDP) were discussed previously. They could provide the basis for preprogramming of movements. Correlations between pathology and clinical findings suggests that at least the preprogrammed movements needed for speech are stored in Broca's area which is located adjacent to the lower end of the motor cortex (Chart 3-8 on page 71).

The initiation of a preprogrammed movement utilizes learnt information and results in appropriate discharges to groups of motor neurons. There are repeated and continuous modifications of the firing patterns of the motor cortex which depend on sensory information derived from stored and new information in the cerebellum, the basal ganglia, and afferent spinocerebral and spinocerebellar afferents from joints, skin, fascia, tendons and muscles. These afferents inform the cortex of items such as progression of movement, position of the limb, load and resistance. This allows the cortex to perceive any mismatch between intended and actual movement and to make appropriate corrections. Also to make corrections for unexpected events such as a stumble over a stone.

Neuromuscular activation and muscle contraction.

The total number of motor neurons in the human spinal cord is about 20,000 (this does not include motor neurons for the head). Transmission from nerve impulse to muscle is by a chemical mediator, acetylcholine. Each axon innervates 5-200 muscle fibers by its terminal branches. Usually each muscle fiber only receives one axon terminal branch. The higher the frequency of discharge the stronger the resulting contraction. At about 20 discharges per second the contractions tend to fuse and at about 80 per second there is a strong smooth contraction.

The myelin sheath ends just before the motor end plate. The axoplasm ends in little buttons which indent the surface of the muscle fiber but are separated from it by intervals of about 400 angstroms. Numerous vesicles, each about 500 angstroms in diameter are located in the axon at the region of the synaptic cleft. Each vesicle contains about 5000 molecules of acetylcholine and their discharge is in these quanta. The termination of the nerve impulse depolarizes the presynaptic membrane of the axon terminal. Calcium enters the axoplasm and the vesicles discharge their contents into the synaptic junction. Whether or not a muscle potential is generated depends on the amount of acetylcholine released because this determines whether the end-plate potential is large enough to generate a muscle action potential. If one is generated it is an all or nothing impulse, just the same as nerve impulses generated in the CNS.

Muscle contraction.

There are three types of muscle: striated skeletal muscle, smooth muscle and cardiac muscle.

Striated muscle contraction.

The facts are summarized in Chart 6-4. Striated muscles are the muscles of the musculoskeletal system. They usually begin and end in tendons attached to bones. Their coordinated contractions and relaxations move the rigid bone levers at joints to effect the characteristic smooth and coordinated movements of animates.

A muscle has many individual muscle fibers. Each is a single multinucleated cell. Each fiber contains many myofibrils, each surrounded by a sarcotubular system. Microscopically, the fibrils shows cross-striations because of the different refractive indices of their components. The unit of contraction is the sarcomere which is the

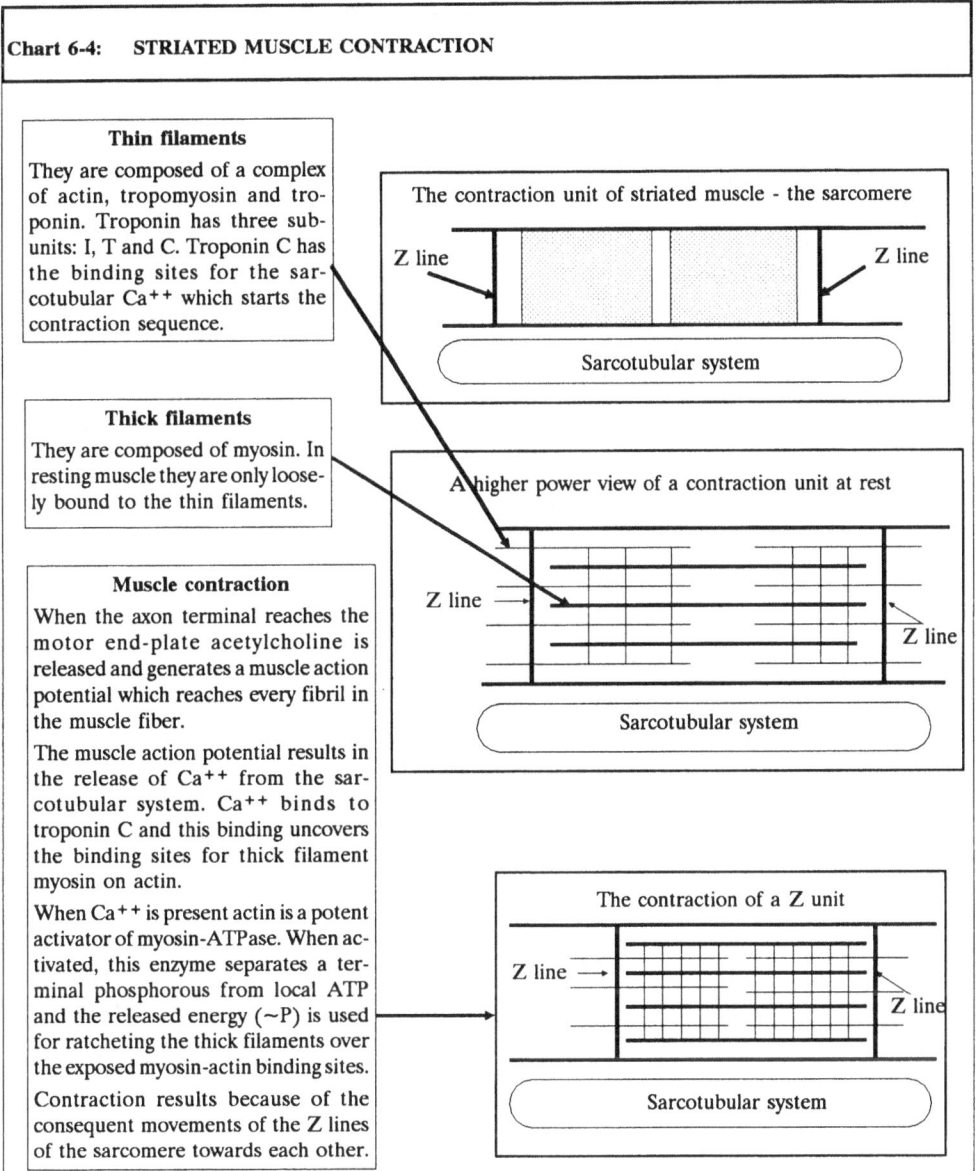

Chart 6-4: STRIATED MUSCLE CONTRACTION

Thin filaments

They are composed of a complex of actin, tropomyosin and troponin. Troponin has three subunits: I, T and C. Troponin C has the binding sites for the sarcotubular Ca^{++} which starts the contraction sequence.

Thick filaments

They are composed of myosin. In resting muscle they are only loosely bound to the thin filaments.

Muscle contraction

When the axon terminal reaches the motor end-plate acetylcholine is released and generates a muscle action potential which reaches every fibril in the muscle fiber.

The muscle action potential results in the release of Ca^{++} from the sarcotubular system. Ca^{++} binds to troponin C and this binding uncovers the binding sites for thick filament myosin on actin.

When Ca^{++} is present actin is a potent activator of myosin-ATPase. When activated, this enzyme separates a terminal phosphorous from local ATP and the released energy (~P) is used for ratcheting the thick filaments over the exposed myosin-actin binding sites.

Contraction results because of the consequent movements of the Z lines of the sarcomere towards each other.

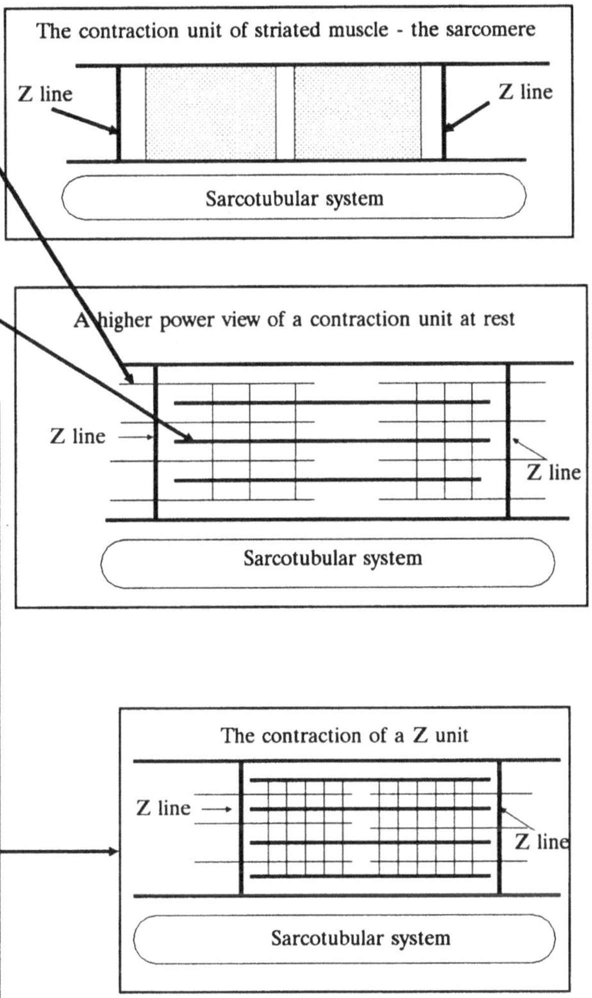
The contraction unit of striated muscle - the sarcomere
Z line
Z line
Sarcotubular system
A higher power view of a contraction unit at rest
Z line
Z line
Sarcotubular system
The contraction of a Z unit
Z line
Z line
Sarcotubular system

area between two dark striations - the Z lines. Chart 6-4 depicts the structure of a sarcomere and summarizes the processes of striated and cardiac muscle contraction.

The end-plate potential depolarizes the muscle fiber and results in a muscle action potential which reaches every fibril in the fiber. It initiates release of Ca^{++} from the terminal cisterns of the sarcoplasmic reticulum. Ca^{++} binds to troponin C and this interaction uncovers myosin binding sites on actin. In the presence of Ca^{++} actin is a potent activator of myosin-ATPase. This enzyme detaches the terminal phosphorous from ATP and the energy released (i.e. ~P) is used to increase myosin-actin binding so that the thick filaments ratchet over the thin filaments. Contraction results because the Z lines of each sarcomere move towards each other.

Cardiac and smooth muscle contraction.

The mechanisms of **cardiac muscle contraction** are similar to those of striated muscle. This is of clinical importance as calcium channel blockers are medications usable for treatment of hypertension and coronary artery insufficiency. Preventing the efflux of calcium from the sarcotubular system reduces intrinsic vascular tone and the continuous vasoconstrictor effects of the medullary control centers. The results are decreased cardiac afterload and a decreased peripheral resistance with a consequent reduction in blood pressure. Calcium channel blockers are cardiac muscle negative inotropes because of their modes of action. The therapeutic value of calcium channel blockers in the individual patient depends on whether or not the effects on the peripheral resistance and on coronary flow are sufficient to counteract their negative inotropic effects on cardiac contractility. In certain circumstances these negative inotropic effects of the calcium channel blockers can increase the clinical features and, at times, the mortality from congestive heart failure[8].

Smooth muscle is different. After entry of Ca^{++} from the ECF a complex biochemical sequence results in phosphorylation of myosin. Myosin-ATPase is activated, ~P is released from local ATP and provides the energy for myosin thick filaments to ratchet over the thin filament complexes. Muscle contraction results. Smooth muscle has intrinsic tone and it contracts when stretched or distended. Neural control is exercised by the medullary vasoconstrictor center which imparts to smooth muscle a continuous background of vasoconstriction which is modulated by local axon reflexes and changes in local pH, pCO_2, pO_2, kinins, histamine, prostaglandins, angiotensin, adenosine and circulating norepinephrine and epinephrine.

The autonomic nervous system

Homeostasis was considered in detail in Chapter 5, pages 97-100. The autonomic nervous system is an important and principal mediator of the neural impulses needed for maintenance of homeostasis. The anatomy and functions of autonomic nerves are detailed in the text that follows. Maintenance of homeostasis also requires endocrine and microenvironmental control systems. The next chapter (Chapter 7) is a detailed discussion of these two topics and Chapter 13 (page 290) summarizes the requirements for maintenance of homeostasis.

The autonomic nervous system begins in the hypothalamus but also has many connections to the cerebrum. The hypothalamus integrates and sets the level of autonomic activity in the body. It is responsible for regulation of body temperature, for modulations of blood pressure and respiration, for regulation of many, if not all metabolic activities, for regulation of body weight, for sleep, and for sexual reflexes and the seminal vesicle discharge of sperms. The hypothalamus also receives neural inputs from the vasomotor, cardiac and respiratory control centers in the medulla. Some are commands for hormonal change and these end in the hypothalamus. Others continue with hypothalamic efferents to the spinal cord autonomic nervous systems.

Hypothalamic connections to the spinal cord are by axons which pass from the hypothalamus to the the reticular system of the cord and then to the autonomic nervous system in the intermedio-lateral column of the cord. Connections are also made with the oculomotor, facial, glossopharyngeal and vagus nerves for parasympathetic control. The autonomic nerves innervate smooth muscle, cardiac muscle and glands that secrete, but not striated muscle. There are two systems in the autonomic nervous system, and each system has afferent and efferent components. The two main systems are the sympathetic and the parasympathetic systems.

The efferents of the autonomic nervous system.

The efferents exit from the intermedio-lateral column of the cord between segments T1-L3 and S2-4. All synapse once with another neuron before ending at a postganglionic terminal. Sympathetic efferents usually synapse at some distance from their targets. The many terminal postsynaptic branches of each axon end at widely dispersed synapses. The result is a fairly diffuse innervation. In contrast, the first synapse of parasympathetic nerves is near or in their targets. The postganglionic fiber is usually short and its innervation is localized to its target.

Because most of sympathetic synapses are in ganglia distant from the target organ a sympathetic preganglionic

Chart 6-5: SYMPATHETIC EFFERENTS

<table>
<tr><th>Output from spinal cord inter-medio-lateral column segment.</th><th>Sympathetic ganglia where the first synapse takes place.</th><th colspan="2">Innervation by sympathetic efferents</th></tr>
<tr><td rowspan="2">Segments T1-T4</td><td>1. Superior, middle and inferior cervical ganglia (by fibers which ascend in the paravertebral chain).</td><td colspan="2">Efferents to the head and neck. Presynaptic fibers enter the paravertebral chain from T1-4 and pass upwards to the inferior, middle and superior cervical ganglia which are upward extensions of the paravertebral sympathetic chain. The first synapse is in one of these ganglia. Postsynaptic fibers ascend in a plexus surrounding the carotid vessels. They innervate the radial dilator muscles of the iris and the lacrimal, buccal and salivary glands.</td></tr>
<tr><td>2. In paravertebral ganglia T1-T4.</td><td colspan="2">Efferents to the heart and respiratory complex (the larynx, trachea, bronchi and lungs). The efferents synapse in adjacent T1-T4 paravertebral ganglia and the postganglionic fibers pass to the structures detailed above.</td></tr>
<tr><td rowspan="4">Segments T5-L3</td><td colspan="3">These efferents do not synapse in the paravertebral sympathetic chain. They pass through the chain into the greater and lesser splanchnic nerves to end in the ganglia at the roots of the main intestinal vessels. Their first synapses occur in ganglionic plexuses surrounding the origins of these vessels from the aorta. The postganglionic fibers are distributed as follows:</td></tr>
<tr><td>Segment</td><td>First synapse</td><td>Postsynaptic innervation</td></tr>
<tr><td>T5-T12</td><td>Celiac ganglion and superior mesenteric and aortico-renal ganglia which they reach via the splanchnic nerves. The plexuses are located at the origins of the vessels from the aorta.</td><td>Stomach, small intestine and colon to the junction between transverse and descending colons. Also, the liver, biliary tracts, gall bladder, pancreas, kidneys and adrenal medulla.</td></tr>
<tr><td>L1-L3</td><td>Inferior mesenteric ganglion. Innervation is by fibers which pass directly from the cord through the paravertebral chain and then, via the splanchnic nerves, to the neural plexus surrounding the origin of the inferior mesenteric artery where they synapse.</td><td>Descending colon, rectum, upper part of anal canal, bladder, ovaries, uterus, prostate and seminal vesicles.</td></tr>
</table>

fiber usually ends in many postganglionic fibers. A ratio of 1:15 is common. This permits diffuse discharges and summations of innervation. The parasympathetic system differs in that the synapse is usually close to the target so that the ration of presynaptic to postsynaptic fibers is often only 1:1.

Presynaptic sympathetic efferents originate from the thoraco-lumbar intermedio-lateral cell column of the spinal cord (the lateral gray horn located between the anterior and posterior gray horns of the cord) from T1-L3 levels. They exit via the ventral root of the cord and travel to the paravertebral sympathetic chain via the white rami communicantes. The subsequent courses of these efferents are detailed in Chart 6-5. The principal ganglia of the sympathetic nervous system (Chart 6-5) are the superior, middle and inferior cervical ganglia, the paravertebral thoracic ganglia and the ganglia at the roots of the main vessels of the abdominal aorta (celiac, superior and inferior mesenteric and hypogastric plexuses). As mentioned previously, the first synapses take place in these ganglia. **These locales are distant from their targets and this permits diffuse innervations by postsynaptic fibers.**

The presynaptic parasympathetic efferents (Chart 6-6) originate in cranial and sacral outflows. The cranial component arises from the mid-brain (the Edinger-Westphal nuclei), the ponto-medullary junction (the superior and inferior salivary nuclei), and the medulla (the dorsal nucleus of the vagus). The sacral outflow is from the intermedio-lateral cell column located in the S2-4 segments of the cord. The efferents terminate in synapses

Chart 6-6: PARASYMPATHETIC EFFERENTS

The cerebral outflow

Origin in medulla and midbrain	First synapse	Postsynaptic innervations
N. III	Nucleus of cranial nerve III.	Peripheral concentric constrictor muscle of the iris.
N. VII	Sphenopalatine ganglion.	Innervation of the lacrimal gland and, of the buccal, submaxillary and sublingual glands via the chorda tympani.
N. IX	Otic ganglion.	The parotid gland.
N. X	In visceral ganglia near its terminations.	The heart and respiratory complex, the small intestine and colon up to the junction of transverse and descending colons, the liver, biliary tract, gall bladder, pancreas, and kidneys.

The sacral outflow

N. S2-4	In visceral ganglia near its terminations.	Descending colon, rectum, upper part of anal canal, and bladder. In females the uterus, fallopian tubes and clitoris. In males the prostate, seminal vesicles, testes and penis.

close to their target organs so that the postsynaptic efferents end close to a single target organ or group of target organs.

The afferents of the autonomic nervous system.

The afferents traverse the same paths as the efferent fibers but in reverse direction. Most autonomic activity is the result of reflexes which do not involve centers located above the midbrain. The exception is visceral pain afferents which synapse in dorsal root ganglia and pass to the thalamus in the contralateral spinothalamic tracts. Even though most autonomic activity is reflex the brain does have the capacity to exert overriding control over autonomic activity for reasons previously detailed (Chapter 5).

The afferents mediate various reflexes and sensations. Examples are visceral sensation and pain, and the many cardio-respiratory and vasomotor reflexes mediated in the hypothalamus and the medullary centers. With the exception of visceral pain little autonomic information is consciously recognized. Additionally, many reflexes are mediated at the level of the spinal cord. Examples are reflex emptying of the bladder and colon, sweating, and vasomotor changes in response to alterations in temperature. Autonomic innervation of the adrenal medulla is not preceded by an initial presynaptic connection.

Autonomic neurotransmitters.

The neurotransmitter at the first synapses of both, sympathetic and parasympathetic preganglionic synapses is acetylcholine. Most postsynaptic sympathetic fibers stimulate end-organs by norepinephrine production. Exceptions are sweat glands and muscle blood vessels where the sympathetic end-organ stimulator is acetylcholine. The adrenal medulla is part of the sympathetic system but the presynaptic fiber ends there with production of epinephrine at its axonal terminations. The neurotransmitter at parasympathetic end-organs is acetylcholine.

Norepinephrine and acetylcholine have antagonistic effects as summarized in Chart 6-7. In addition, the sympathetic effectors can act at different receptor sites: e.g., α_1, α_2, β_1 and β_2.The beta receptors are of clinical importance. Norepinephrine stimulates cardiac β_1 receptors which are the receptors of the S-A node, the atria, the A-V node, the Purkinje system and the ventricles. The lungs are innervated by β_2 receptors. However, there is usually some overlap so that an inhibitor at a β_1 receptor could also produce some inhibition at a β_2 receptor. Many cardiac medications claim cardio-selectivity by only blocking β_1 receptors. However, the selectivity is often not absolute. Hence the importance of not giving β_1 blockers to individuals with lung disease because of the possibility of overlap and simultaneous blocking of β_2 receptors with deleterious effects on any existing lung dysfunction. Similarly, an agonist of β_2 receptors (e.g., salbutamol), given to produce bronchodilation, can have adverse cardiac effects by stimulating cardiac β_1 receptors, especially in patients with coronary insufficiency, arrhythmias and/or hypertension.

The destruction of autonomic effectors.

For accurate, rapid and precise reactions the autonomic effectors must be rapidly removed and regenerated immediately after producing their effects.

The destruction and regeneration of acetylcholine.

There are about 2000-5000 acetylcholine vesicles in the axon near the end plate. This is only enough for a few minutes supply. Acetylcholine liberated is broken down by local choline esterase which is attached to receptors on the postsynaptic membrane, close to the acetylcholine receptor. Part of the liberated acetylcholine goes to these receptors and is immediately inactivated. The remainder goes to the acetylcholine receptor of the muscle fiber. Within 1-2ms after reaching its receptor and generating an end plate potential the acetylcholine leaves

Chart 6-7: THE NEUROMEDIATORS OF THE AUTONOMIC NERVOUS SYSTEM AND THEIR EFFECTS.

	Acetylcholine	Norepinephrine
Eye	Pupillary constriction because of contraction of the peripheral sphincter muscle of the iris.	Dilation of pupil from contraction of radial dilator muscles of the pupil.
Heart	Decrease in rate, conduction velocity and atrial contractility.	Increase in atrial and ventricular muscle contractility, in heart rate, and in intracardiac conduction velocity.
Blood vessels	Dilation of arterioles.	Contraction of arterioles.
Lungs	Bronchial muscle contraction and stimulation of bronchial gland secretion.	Bronchial muscle relaxation and reduction of bronchial gland secretion.
Intestinal tract	Increased motility and tone, relaxation of sphincters and stimulation of secretions.	Decreased motility and tone, contraction of sphincters and reduction of secretions.
Genitourinary tract	Contraction of bladder muscle and relaxation of sphincter.	Relaxation of bladder muscle and contraction of sphincter.
Skin	Sweating.	Pilomotor contraction and sweating in a few areas: e.g., the palms of the hands.

its receptor and is destroyed by local choline esterase. Local new production of acetylcholine is essential because transport from distant sites would be too slow. This is effected by combining liberated choline with local acetic acid to form acetylcholine which then re-enters the vesicle. The reaction is mediated by the enzyme, choline acetyl transferase.

The re-use of norepinephrine and destruction of material which escapes re-use.

After producing its effect, norepinephrine at nerve terminals is rapidly taken up by the nerve terminal and re-used. Some is degraded by mitochondrial monoamine oxidases to inactive substances. Some catecholamines remain in the circulation and are inactivated by complex mechanisms. Most of the catabolism is hepatic and two enzymes are involved: catechol-O-methyltransferase (COMT) and monoamine oxidase (MAO). The processes that inactivate circulating norepinephrine and epinephrine are depicted in Chart 6-8.

MAO (monoamine oxidase) inhibitors.

A comment is necessary on the use of MAO inhibitors - psychiatric medications used for treatment of some patients with depression not amenable to other drugs. MAO inhibitors increase the concentration of circulating adrenergic agents because they block the metabolic breakdown of circulating amines such as epinephrine, norepinephrine and serotonin. They are also said to be adrenergic agonists. Catecholamines remain in the neurons of patients receiving MAO inhibitors because they cannot be catabolized because of decreased monoamine oxidase activity. Tyramine potentiates the discharge of these stored catecholamines. Frequent results are hypertensive crises and other effects which can be fatal. Patients must avoid foods with high concentrations of tyramine or dopamine. Examples are cheese, wine and beer, smoked, pickled, fermented or aged foods, dried meats (salami, pepperoni and bologna), soy sauce, broad beans, avocados, raisins, figs and bananas.

Chart 6-8: **CATABOLISM OF <u>CIRCULATING</u> NOREPINEPHRINE AND EPINEPHRINE** [1]

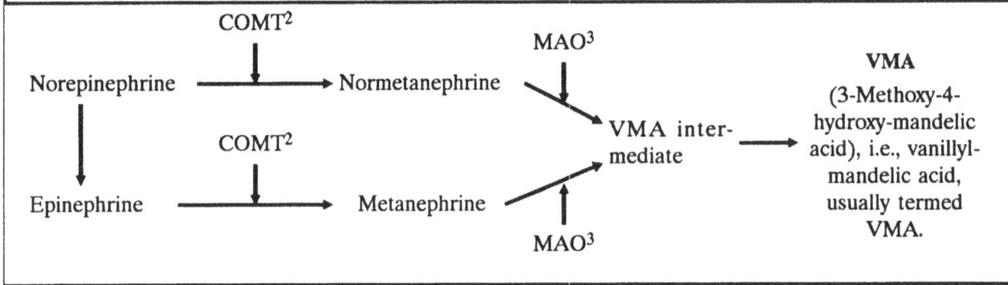
COMT[2]
MAO[3]
VMA
Norepinephrine
Normetanephrine
(3-Methoxy-4-hydroxy-mandelic acid), i.e., vanillylmandelic acid, usually termed VMA.
VMA inter-mediate
COMT[2]
Epinephrine
Metanephrine
MAO[3]

[1] The end products of catecholamine catabolism include epinephrine, norepinephrine, metanephrine, normetanephrine and VMA (vanillylmandelic acid). VMA is usually the most plentiful catabolic end-product in the 24 hour urine specimen of an individual with a pheochromocytoma.

[2] COMT is the enzyme, catechol-O-methyltransferase.

[3] MAO is the enzyme, monoamine oxidase.

A decreased intake of alcohol, coffee and chocolate is also necessary. Good therapy for those made obese by other anti-depressants?

Similar hypertensive crises can result if patients on monoamine oxidases inhale or ingest the sympathomimetic amines in many nasal sprays and drops and pills which claim to cure the common cold. MAO inhibitors also interact with opiates, especially demerol, and are potentially fatal if combined with SSRIs such as Prozac.

Pheochromocytomas.

This is another opportunity to show the value of seemingly unimportant physiological knowledge for identifying uncommon conditions. The measurement of the metabolic end-products of circulating norepinephrine and epinephrine are a requisite for investigating individuals with hypertension which cannot be controlled by routine therapy. On rare occasions the resistant hypertension is due to a pheochromocytoma (a tumor of chromaffin tissue). Half of these tumors develop in the adrenals and the rest in chromaffin cell collections, usually subdiaphragmatic. Some of these uncommon tumors are predominantly norepinephrine-producing, others epinephrine-producing and the rest produce both hormones. The diagnosis requires measurement of epinephrine, norepinephrine and the metabolic end-products of their catabolism (free catecholamines, metanephrine, normetanephrine, and vanillylmandelic acid) in a 24 hour specimen of urine.

Hormonal control systems

The CNS effects some changes by quantitative variations in production of releasing factors and hormones (e.g., anti-diuretic hormone) produced in the hypothalamus. Releasing factors affect the amounts and qualities of hormones produced by the pituitary and its target organs, i.e., the thyroid, the adrenals the gonads and systems which affect growth and lactation. There are many interneural communications between the hypothalamus and the medullary control centers. Control of the secretion of hypothalamic hormones and releasing factors, and of pituitary hormones is regulated by feedback mechanisms involving the pituitary and hypothalamus on the one hand and blood levels of circulating hormones on the other (Chart 7-3 and 7-4, pages 162-163).

Common neurological dysfunctions and diseases

Symptoms and signs of neurological dysfunction.

Symptoms and signs which suggest dysfunction of the central or peripheral nervous systems, or both, include any one or more of the following:

- Pain - headaches, neck pain and stiffness, and pain due to any one or more of many other causes (examples are the pains of migraine, cluster headaches, and sympathetic dysfunctional syndromes).
- Any combination of intellectual, motor and sensory deficits.
- Hyperactivity syndromes such as seizures.
- Abnormal movements are seen in basal ganglia dysfunctions such as Parkinson's disease, chorea and athetosis.
- The unsteadiness, disturbances of balance and clumsy movements of cerebellar disease.
- Disorders of mentation, speech and comprehension.
- Sensory and motor deficits affecting peripheral nerves and muscle: e.g., peripheral neuropathies, muscular dystrophy, other myopathies and myoneural disorders such as myasthenia gravis.

CNS dysfunctions may be focal or global, and multimodal or unimodal. Those which are initially focal may later acquire the features of a global dysfunction and those which initially seem to be global may eventuate to a focal lesion. Focal lesions are usually caused by vascular occlusions or by space occupying lesions such as tumors, granulomas, tuberculomas and collections of blood from a hemorrhage. Global lesions result from degenerative lesions, the demyelinations, basal ganglia and cerebellar dysfunctions, seizure syndromes and the various encephalopathies.

The possible causes of neurological dysfunction.

Any one or more of the causes of disease listed in a previous section (pages 75-77) can also affect the CNS: for example, congenital dysfunction, trauma, tumor, inflammations, vascular occlusions, and degenerations. There are a few etiologies which are specific to the CNS. Notable examples are the demyelinating diseases, the amnesia and dementia syndromes, some degenerations (e.g., amyotrophic lateral sclerosis and basal ganglia dysfunctions such as Parkinson's disease), and the seizure syndromes. Focal vascular occlusions are common in most infections but when they occur in the CNS, as for example in some meningeal infections, the consequences can be calamitous and occasionally fatal. The usual causes of death in CNS dysfunctions are extensive destruction of neural tissue, increased intracranial pressure, concurrent and progressive infections, and severe infections of other tissues, especially the lungs and the urinary tract.

Increased intracranial pressure (ICP)

This is an example of a dysfunction initially caused by a focal lesion but often progressing to one which is global and potentially fatal.

Normal production and removal of cerebrospinal fluid.

The cerebrospinal fluid is formed by the plexuses in the lateral ventricle. It passes through the third ventricle and then through its foramina (the foramina of Luschka and Magendie) to reach the subarachnoid space where it forms a cushion of fluid surrounding the brain. Outside the body the brain weighs about 1500gm. It is said that in its CSF cushion the effective weight is only some 50gm so that its flimsy vascular attachments can suspend it in the cranium without hazard. After bathing the brain and spinal cord the cerebrospinal fluid enters the blood in the intracranial venous sinuses via the arachnoid villi. These are minute projections of the sub-arachnoid membranes into the intracranial venous sinuses.

The volume of CSF produced each day is about 500ml. The subarachnoid space contains about 150ml at any one time. The turnover is approximately 3-4 times a day. The normal CSF pressure is 70-200mm of water. The cell content is mainly a small number of lymphocytes. The glucose CSF/plasma ratio is about 0.65. Blood glucose should be measured at the same time as CSF glucose because it equilibrates with blood glucose. The usual CSF/plasma glucose ratio is an average of 0.65 and protein in normal CSF should be less than 50mg/100ml. When there are untreated bacterial infections the cell content rises, at times as high as 100,000 polymorphonuclear leukocytes/mm^3, glucose is low and protein increased. Bacteria are usually demonstrable. In viral infections there may be significant increases in the cell population, at first mostly polymorhonuclear leukocytes but lymphocytes later. Glucose and protein levels and CSF/plasma glucose ratios are usually unchanged.

Pathophysiology of raised intracranial pressure.

An intracranial pressure which does not transgress physiologically desirable and permissible levels is an essential for normal neurological function. Most neurological deaths are due to extensive brain damage or the effects of increased intracranial pressure or to a combination of the two.

The brain is protected by a rigid cranium but, in certain circumstances this anatomical protection can be counter-productive because it does not allow much expansion of the underlying contents. A raised intracranial pressure can result from many different neurological pathologies. Progressively increasing intracranial pressure results in death if it remains uncorrected or is not correctable.

The causes of increased intracranial pressure include edema and hemorrhage within and around traumatized brain tissue, or an infarct or intracranial hemorrhage and hemorrhages from aneurysms or arterio-venous malformations. Other causes include extradural space occupying lesions such as subdural hematomas, and intracerebral lesions such as the inflammatory exudate and cerebral edema of infections and progressively growing intracranial space occupying lesions caused by tumors (primary or metastatic malignant tumors and benign tumors), cysts and granulomas.

The rigid skull confines the underlying expanding mass. Clinically there is headache, defective mentation, vomiting, occasionally convulsions, torpor, inability to comprehend and inability to respond intelligently to questions or comments, and finally, if uncorrected, coma and death. A fixed dilated pupil on one or both sides are fairly diagnostic. Papilledema, when present, is also diagnostic of increased intracranial pressure. The normal ICP is 1-15mm Hg.

An ICP which exceeds 20mm Hg is life-threatening and needs immediate therapy. The therapy, the methods of estimating ICP and its treatment are detailed on page 153 as part of the section which details decision-making and therapy for neurological disease.

The pathophysiological lesions are herniations of cerebral tissue into every available intracranial space:

- The cingulate or supracallosal gyrus herniates under the free edge of the falx cerebri.
- The hippocampal gyrus herniates through the tentorial notch between the brain stem and the free edge of the tentorium cerebelli. The consequences are serious and eventually fatal if raised intracranial pressure is not corrected. Compression of vessels results in infarction of tissue in the distribution of the posterior cerebral artery and/or the brain stem, compression paralysis of the third and sixth cranial nerves, and compression of the third ventricle and aqueduct. Third nerve compression results in the typical fixed and dilated

pupil or pupils.

- Finally, the cerebellar tonsils herniate into the foramen magnum, compress the medulla and result in death.
- An additional factor is the generalized cerebral ischemia which results from increased intracranial pressure. A vicious cycle is established of increasing pressure and increasing ischemia till there is total CNS failure from deficient perfusion with blood.

CNS dysfunctions due to trauma

Head injuries.

Head injuries result from blunt trauma and/or from injuries which result in acceleration-deceleration forces and the forces of rotation. Typical causes are motor vehicle accidents involving frontal or rear collisions. There is injury opposite the site of impact (the coup injury) because the moving brain is pulled against the rigid skull at a point opposite to that of impact. The contrecoup injury follows as it is flung back to the opposite point. Injuries of this type often include intracerebral tears from the forces of rotation. When injuries result from being struck by blunt instruments there is also brain injury at the point of impact.

The focal areas of trauma are often accompanied by many small and often microscopic intracerebral tears and hemorrhages. These are probably responsible for the long-term headaches and deficits of memory and learning which follow many head injuries which often seem trivial.

Concussion is a loss of consciousness following a head injury. It is associated with loss of memory prior to trauma and the duration of unconsciousness and memory loss have been used to determine the severity of concussion. Because of the complete recoveries from concussions there is no verifiable information on the pathophysiological lesions in concussed humans.

Brain injury. Head injuries can also result in a variety of brain injuries. They range from small focal hemorrhages and neuron destructions to large areas of contusion, laceration and bleeding. Increased intracranial pressure is often present together with its associated clinical features, as previously described. The symptoms of head imjuries are obvious concomitants: prolonged unconsciousness, neurological deficits and severe headache if the patient is conscious. Other pathology includes internal hydrocephalus and cerebral edema.

Even if there is recovery significant neurological deficits often persist. Some 20-40% of patients who have had cerebral lacerations have a life-long tendency to get seizures. Most of them need prolonged control by anti-seizure drugs. Other long-term complications include post-traumatic hydrocephalus. Recovery may also leave significant intellectual deficits and psychiatric syndromes which can resemble the symptoms of a bipolar disease. Examples are bizarre behavior, depressions, outbursts of mania, violent temper, and homicidal and/or suicidal tendencies.

Complications of head injury include subdural hematoma - usually in association with a fracture of the temporal or parietal bone somewhere along the course of the middle meningeal artery. Other complications are brain infections from compound fractures of the skull, and fractures of the base of the skull with rhinorrhea which is often associated with ascending infections.

Cord compression syndromes.

Compression of the spinal cord and/or one or more of its afferent and efferent nerves within the spinal canal can be due to any one or more different causes. The cord only extends to the L1-2 level. The usual, but not invariable cause of neurological deficits above this level is a fracture dislocation of the spine. The nature and intensity of the neurological deficits depend on the location of the injury and the force of delivery. At times transverse myelitis due to any one or more different causes results in neurological deficits below the lesion. Sudden shearing injuries to the spinal cord can result in major neurological deficits without bony injury.

Case history.

Male patient age 56 was tugging at a door leading to a cellar. It was at floor level, had been unopened for years and was jammed. The door suddenly gave. The patient who was bending was suddenly flung back. When I saw him he had most unusual findings - a typical Brown-Sequard syndrome. Muscular paresis of the legs on the right and decreased perception of pain and temperature on the left. Presumably, a shearing injury had injured the cord in the dorsal region. A CT scan did not show any abnormality but an MRI did show scattered spinal cord dehiscences extending from T4-6 on the right. No treatment was possible. He has adapted well enough to his disabilities to return to heavy manual work.

As mentioned previously, the cord ends at L1-2 level. The nerves of the spinal cord are bunched together below L2. Common causes of neurological dysfunctions below L2 are pressures from intervertebral disc protrusions and spinal stenoses. Typically, pain is felt along the course of compressed nerves and there may be associated motor deficits and/or sensory deficits. A common physical finding is pain on straight leg raising, made worse by dorsiflexion of the ankle.

Incidentally, the spinal cord and associated nerves can also be affected by any one or more of the causes of cerebral pathology. Some examples are congenital abnormalities, vascular occlusions, inflammations, tumors, demyelinating diseases, and the fibrotic sequelae of hemorrhages and inflammations which could compress the cord or any one of its afferent or efferent nerve roots. When a cord compression syndrome exists and a CT scan does not show unequivocal confirmation of a spinal stenosis or an intervertebral disc protrusion these possibilities must be kept in mind.

CNS dysfunctions due to infections

Infections of the meninges.

There are two forms of infections that can affect the meninges: acute meningitis (e.g., meningitis due to infection by meningococci, streptococci, staphylococci, pneumococci, hemophilus or any one or more of many viruses) and chronic meningitis (usually tuberculous or syphilitic).

Acute meningitis.

The patient has a fever, headache, neck stiffness and a positive Kernig's sign. Meningeal pain and the pain of neck flexion and the Kernig's sign are probably due to stimulation of pain-sensitive receptors in meningeal arteries. The pia mater, the arachnoid and the dura are essentially insensitive. The brain is also insensitive to pain. It can be cut or burnt without any pain. Conditions such as encephalitis, infarcts, tumors, seizures and other comparable brain pathologies do not cause pain unless the meninges are involved and/or intracranial pressure raised.

In meningitis any confusional symptoms are the result of fever and infection because the disease does not usually affect the brain. If it does it does so by thrombosing meningeal veins and thus producing focal cerebral deficits. These may result in convulsions and focal neurological deficits.

Examination of the CSF is diagnostic. The pressure is raised, there are many polymorphonuclear leukocytes, bacteria are often seen, glucose is decreased and protein elevated. The meningitis of fungal infections has CSF values comparable to those of bacterial infections except that the predominant cells are lymphocytes and not polymorphonuclear leukocytes. In viral meningitis the initial examination may show polymorphonuclear leukocytes. Later they are replaced by lymphocytes, bacteria are not seen, and glucose levels remain unchanged. Protein levels may increase in viral meningitis but rarely exceed 100mg/dl.

With appropriate treatment the prognosis for acute meningitis is good. However subsequent problems do occasionally result: from post-infection fibrosis; from cerebral damage due to focal infarcts; from fibrosis resulting in hydrocephalus; from various cranial and spinal nerve deficits due to fibrosis round their roots; and from residual cerebral damage resulting in occasional deficits of intellect and/or function.

Meningococcal septicemia.

Meningococcal septicemia is an ominous feature of meningococcal meningitis. It results from systemic dissemination of meningococcal endotoxin. Many children with viral or bacterial infections develop rashes. Most disappear when pressure is applied to the rash. In meningococcal septicemia the rash is due to bleeding into the skin and will not fade on pressure. The "tumbler test" is diagnostic - the rash does not fade when pressure is exerted with the end of a tumbler. Parents should be advised to use this test on any child with a fever and a rash. The meningococcal endotoxin affects all blood vessels, plasma leaks out and shock develops. The incidence of meningococcal septicemia in children with meningococcal meningitis is about 20%. The mortality of those affected is high. When meningococcal septicemia develops the death rate is 40-60% of those affected. In contrast less than 5% of children with meningococcal meningitis die if septicemia has not developed.

Subarachnoid bleeds.

The neck stiffness of a **subarachnoid bleed** is dissimilar in evolution and symptoms. As a rule it is of sudden onset and pain and symptoms are often maximum at the onset, or within a few hours of the onset. There is severe headache and frequently a rapid loss of consciousness. The bleed may be from a ruptured aneurysm or a vessel in an arterio-venous malformation. The unconsciousness is probably due to the sudden pouring of blood into the subarachnoid space with obstruction of CSF flow, acute hydrocephalus and unconsciousness. The last results from cerebral ischemia due to the sudden appearance of a large intracranial accumulation of blood acting as a space occupying lesion causing increased intracranial pressure.

Chronic meningitis.

The two most common causes are tuberculosis and syphilis.

Tuberculous meningitis. The meninges over the base of the brain are covered with small tubercles. The disease is usually seen in poorly nourished young children because of bacterial dissemination from a primary Ghon focus, or in older adults because of reactivation of dormant bacteria. The patients complain of headache, loss of weight, fever, night sweats and neck stiffness. Diagnosis is by lumbar puncture. The CSF shows an increased protein content, reduced glucose levels and up to 1000 white blood cells, about 90% of which are lymphocytes. Organisms may be demonstrable by special stains and positive cultures are diagnostic. A low sugar content distinguishes the CSF of tuberculous meningitis from a viral meningitis.

The fibrosis which is part of the active and of the quiescent disease can result in hydrocephalus and cranial nerve deficits. In addition, arterial lesions are frequently seen with underlying foci of cerebral ischemic necrosis. In the third world this is a common and devastating disease, accompanied as it is by malnutrition, as well as unavailable and unaffordable drugs. In both, developed and under-developed countries tuberculous meningitis is an increasingly common and often fatal opportunistic infection in individuals with AIDS.

Syphilitic meningitis. Only few individuals with secondary syphilis are affected by a meningitis. The usual cause is tertiary syphilis and the lesions are meningovascular lesions characterized by areas of endarteritis obliterans. They may be focal or widespread. The latter is probably responsible for the dementia syndrome termed "general paralysis of the insane" (tabes dorsalis and general paralysis of the insane are often called quarternary syphilis).

Infections of the brain.

Encephalitis can be acute or chronic.

Acute encephalitis.

Three types are described:

Primary encephalitis which is an encephalitis caused by viruses and results from transmission of virus from animals to man. Examples are rabies and the arthropod-borne encephalopathies. There is fever, headache, convulsions in children, and disturbances of mentation ranging from mild confusion to deep coma. Neurological deficits are common. In rabies, brain stem dysfunction appears soon after the onset of the disease and death ensues in the next 1-3 weeks. In the other viral infections of the brain the prognosis is better and recovery is not uncommon, usually after 1-2 weeks unless irreversible neurological changes have occurred.

Secondary encephalitis is an inconstant accompaniment of various systemic diseases caused by bacteria, spirochetes (e.g., tertiary syphilis and relapsing fever), parasites (e.g., malaria and trypanosomiasis), rickettsiae (e.g., typhus) and viruses (e.g., mumps, yellow fever, herpes viruses, etc.).

Post-infectious encephalomyelitis is usually a demyelinating disease and is best considered in the section which deals with CNS dysfunctions due to demyelinations.

Chronic encephalitis.

These diseases are usually due to slow viruses or prions and eventually result in dementia and death. They are considered in detail in the section on "The confusion-dementia syndromes".

CNS dysfunctions due to tumors

Metastatic brain tumors are far more common than primary tumors. Primary brain tumors are well described in standard texts and no detailed description is provided in this monograph. They are common causes of sensory, motor and intellectual deficits of CNS function. Pain usually results from increased intracranial pressure. Before deciding that referral for a biopsy is needed be sure it is not a metastatic lesion from another site.

Intracranial but extracerebral tumors are the meningiomas which are benign tumors arising from arachnoid cells. They cause local pressure symptoms and pain due to intracranial pressure but are potentially curable by excision.

Most primary brain tumors arise from glial tissue (the astrocytomas and glioblastomas). The medulloblastoma is a tumor of childhood and is of neural origin. The treatments of brain tumors are specialized and evolving. Based on the few that I diagnosed and followed up after therapy by oncologists the outlook seems bleak.

CNS dysfunctions due to vascular lesions

After middle age stroke is the third most common cause of death; heart disease is first and a combination of all cases of cancer is the second. Stroke is not a dysfunction predominantly confined to affluent societies - Murray and Lopez[9] have reported that ⅔ of deaths from stroke occur in under-developed countries.

Strokes due to cerebrovascular occlusions.

Vascular occlusions result in focal or global CNS deficits of glucose and oxygen. These deficits result in dysfunctions with sequelae which range from complete recovery, through recovery with residual functional deficits, to coma and death. After the age of 55 stroke is the commonest cause of CNS dysfunction; automobile accidents, assault, trauma and suicide are the common causes in younger age groups. Intracerebral vascular occlusions may present as dementia due to small multiple infarcts, as transient ischemic attacks or as stroke syndromes. A transient ischemic attack (TIA) has been arbitrarily defined as a stroke-like syndrome with complete recovery in the 24 hour period following onset. Hence, the differentiation between a TIA and a stroke is almost impossible in the first 24 hours after onset of neurological deficits.

Strokes are the result of vascular occlusions in the brain. Common causes are emboli from atheroma in the carotid arteries, local thrombosis superimposed on an atheromatous cerebrovascular lesion and emboli from the heart, especially if atrial fibrillation is present. Other cardiac causes include emboli from diseased and/or infected heart valves or from vegetations on a congenital abnormality such as a patent interventricular or interatrial foramen. Vascular occlusions from parasitic, tuberculous or syphilitic infections, or from the vascular lesions of collagen diseases, do occur but are uncommon.

Hemorrhagic strokes.

Strokes also occur because of intracranial hemorrhage. Uncontrolled hypertension is a major risk factor for such an event. Increased levels of blood cholesterol are associated with coronary artery atheroma but do not seem to increase the chances of having a stroke[10]. As a rule the functional deficit resulting from intracerebral hemorrhage is greater than that which results from simple vascular occlusion. A stroke due to intracranial hemorrhage is often a cataclysmic event with immediate death or death after prolonged unconsciousness.

The diagnosis of stroke.

Diagnosis by clinical assessment is important. CT scans are useful in distinguishing hemorrhagic infarcts from those due to occlusions and in demonstrating the presence of underlying pathology causing the stroke: e.g., a tumor. A normal CT scan does not exclude a non-hemorrhagic stroke as the cause of the presenting symptom-sign complex. About 30-50% of non-hemorrhagic infarcts are never demonstrable on a CT scan[11], especially the smaller ones. In fact few non-hemorrhagic infarcts are demonstrable on CT scans done in the initial few hours after onset of an embolic stroke[12]. Those which do become demonstrable on a CT scan only appear some time in the week following infarction. Current thrombolytic therapy relies on early clinical diagnosis and exclusion of a hemorrhagic stroke by a CT scan.

Characteristic of stroke is the sudden onset of focal neurological deficits, with or without varying degrees of dysfunctional mentation ranging from a mild confusional state to loss of consciousness. The neurological deficits depend on the location of the area perfused by the occluded blood vessel.

The clinical consequences of intracerebral vascular occlusions or hemorrhages are determined by any one or more of the following:

— **Was the occlusion acute or gradual?**

Many thrombotic lesions result from the slow multiplications of small vascular occlusions and symptoms are often few. In fact the only evidence that there had been previous infarcts could be the gradual evolution of a dementia (multi-infarct dementia).

In contrast, major embolic lesions are usually acute events with the immediate development of neurological deficits. A variety of deficits are seen depending on the vessel occluded: motor, sensory, visual and auditory deficits, postural deficits when one or other cerebellar or vertebrobasilar vessel is occluded, and any one or more of the many syndromes of dysfunctional speech and comprehension. Post-stroke depressions, other psychiatric manifestations, and deficits of memory are common during the recovery period. The motor, sensory and intellectual deficits which result from a stroke are usually delineated by the area supplied by the occluded vessel or the hemorrhage. The deficits may indicate a partial or complete loss of function in the affected area of distribution but they are not randomly distributed in time, space, or form as are the symptoms and signs of a demyelinating disease such as multiple sclerosis.

Hemorrhagic strokes often result in acute and devastating neurological deficits. The area of infarction is usually greater than those which result from embolic strokes. Sudden loss of consciousness or sudden death are not uncommon. The residual deficits are usually more disabling than those which result from embolic occlusions. As long as the EEG does not show brain death artificial mechanical technology and intravenous infusions are often needed to maintain life

— **Are the effects of the embolic stroke short-lived or prolonged?**

The syndrome of "transient ischemic attacks (TIAs)" is used to describe the former. A neurological deficit develops and disappears within 24 hours. Study of the carotid vessels show that a significant number of these patients have atheromatous lesions in the carotids which are the source of emboli which occlude cerebral vessels.

All TIAs are best treated as strokes if neurological deficits are seen soon after onset; it is impossible to predict that there will be complete resolution of symptoms and signs in the next 24 hours. TIAs need thorough investigation and assessment as they are frequent harbingers of more severe occlusions. If carotid atheromas are demonstrable an estimate of the degree of stenosis is a requisite for determining whether surgery is indicated. This topic gets more detailed attention at the end of this chapter.

— **Are there enough anastomotic vessels to restore blood to the infarcted areas?**

Nervous system deficits which appear disastrous at the onset often ameliorate in a short time. A possible cause is restoration of some blood supply to the area of vascular occlusion by an existing anastomotic circulation. The functional plasticity of brain tissue could also account for the almost complete recovery occasionally seen after devastating hemiplegias.

— **Are there any clinical features which suggest increased intracranial pressure?**

Increased intracranial pressure from edema often results from and coexists with cerebrovascular occlusions.

The possible causes and consequences of a raised intracranial pressure were detailed at the beginning of this chapter.

— **Are there any deficits of intellect and mentation?**

These are common after strokes, during its evolution or as a sequel in the recovery phase. Memory deficits are common as are confusional states, hallucinations and inability to comprehend or to respond intelligently. Extensive cerebrovascular occlusions, especially hemorrhagic strokes, can result in delirium, coma and even death. Post-stroke depressions are real entities and usually require medication.

It is of clinical importance to remember that **confusional states are often associated with medical problems which are not neurological.** Hypoglycemia must always be excluded as a cause of neurological deficits of mentation, especially if the individual is confused or comatose for no obvious reason. Infections, especially those affecting the lungs or kidneys of the elderly often result in confusional states and other intellectual deficits.

Two common stroke syndromes - middle and posterior cerebral artery occlusions.

Occlusion of the middle cerebral artery.

This is the vessel most frequently occluded in strokes. It has a wide distribution: the motor cortex, the adjacent sensory areas, the motor speech area of the dominant hemisphere, and the optic radiation deep in the temporal lobe. The extent of the deficits will depend on the location of the occlusion - whether the main artery is occluded or only one of its minor branches. When the main artery is occluded the deficits include motor and sensory deficits in the contralateral face, arm and leg. In the brain motor efferents cross to innervate the cranial nerve nuclei on the opposite side. The fibers going to the spinal motor neurons decussate in the lower medulla to innervate the musculature of the opposite side.

Other deficits from middle cerebral artery occlusion include motor aphasia if the dominant hemisphere is involved. Comprehension of spoken and written language is usually unaffected as infarcts of the middle cerebral artery usually leave Wernicke's area unaffected. Affected patients may also have a homonymous hemianopia, often only affecting the inferior quadrants. Chart 6-9 depicts the visual tracts and the possible dysfunctions that can result from vascular occlusions which might affect their functions. Deficits of intellect are common. They range from a confusional state with some memory loss to complete loss of consciousness.

Occlusion of the posterior cerebral artery.

This is another fairly common site of occlusion. It supplies the medial and inferior surfaces of the occipital lobes and the inferior surface of the temporal lobe. Before it reaches the cerebrum the posterior cerebral artery supplies important branches to the midbrain and cerebral peduncles. Occlusion of vessels supplying the midbrain often results in coma, bilateral pyramidal signs, deep coma and a decerebrate rigidity. The artery at its terminal gives branches to the thalamus and adjacent areas. A variety of eponymous syndromes describe the various permutations and combinations of deficits when there are one or more occlusions of the different branches of the posterior cerebral artery and the basilar artery. Occlusions of the posterior cerebral artery frequently result in visual disturbances (Chart 6-9) which range from a minor upper quadrant homonymous hemianopia to bilateral homonymous hemianopia. The chart also summarizes the visual deficits which result when the visual tracts are compressed or transected at other levels.

The pupillary reflexes (Chart 6-2) are a useful guide to the degree of increased intracranial pressure that exists after any stroke.

Speech deficits after strokes.

The physiology of speech and the pathology of speech deficits have been discussed comprehensively in a previous chapter (pages 70-74).

Other causes of stroke syndromes.

Even though vascular occlusions are the most common cause of stroke syndromes one needs to remember that the neurological deficits of stroke syndromes can result from other causes. Examples are trauma, infection (acute encephalitis or one of the chronic slow virus encephalopathies), demyelinating diseases, focal vascular

Chart 6-9: THE VISUAL TRACTS AND DEFICITS FROM LESIONS AT A, B, AND C

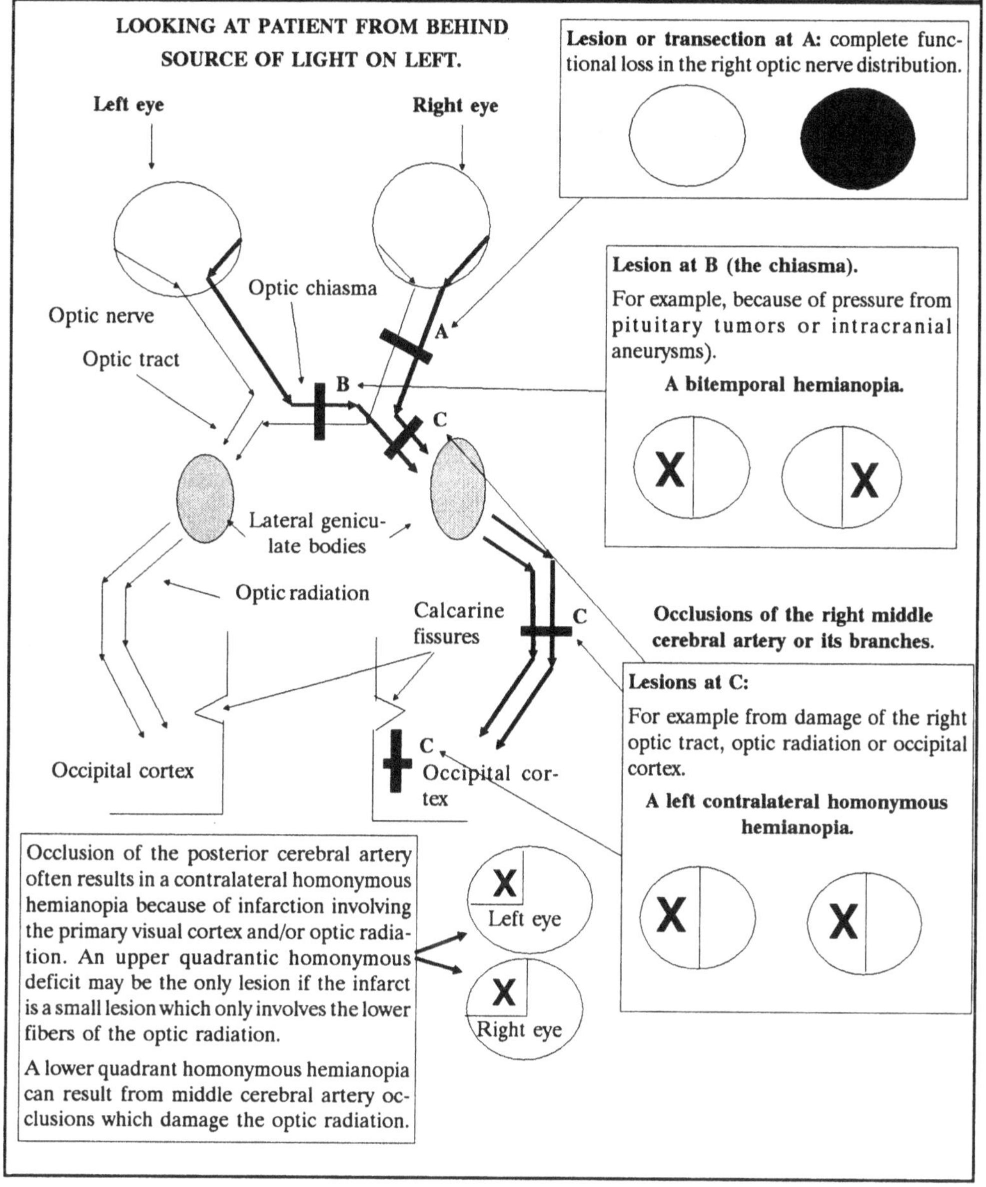
LOOKING AT PATIENT FROM BEHIND
SOURCE OF LIGHT ON LEFT.
Left eye
Right eye
Optic chiasma
Optic nerve
Optic tract
A
B
C
Lateral genicu-
late bodies
Optic radiation
Calcarine
fissures
C
Occipital cortex
C
Occipital cor-
tex
Lesion or transection at A: complete functional loss in the right optic nerve distribution.
Lesion at B (the chiasma).
For example, because of pressure from pituitary tumors or intracranial aneurysms).
A bitemporal hemianopia.
X
X
Occlusions of the right middle cerebral artery or its branches.
Lesions at C:
For example from damage of the right optic tract, optic radiation or occipital cortex.
A left contralateral homonymous hemianopia.
X
X
Occlusion of the posterior cerebral artery often results in a contralateral homonymous hemianopia because of infarction involving the primary visual cortex and/or optic radiation. An upper quadrantic homonymous deficit may be the only lesion if the infarct is a small lesion which only involves the lower fibers of the optic radiation.
A lower quadrant homonymous hemianopia can result from middle cerebral artery occlusions which damage the optic radiation.
X
Left eye
X
Right eye

thromboses in acute meningeal infections, benign or malignant neoplasms of the brain or of adjacent meninges or bone, degenerative diseases (e.g., Alzheimer's disease and multiple infarct dementias), and any of the immunological (presumed) vascular dysfunctions.

CNS dysfunctions due to cerebellar and basal ganglia disease

Cerebellar and basal ganglia dysfunctions are common causes of motor dysfunctions. They often present with symptoms and signs affecting the whole body. Most descriptions of cerebellar and basal ganglia dysfunctions are based on correlations between premortem or post-surgical findings with pre-existing or previous clinical symptoms and signs.

Cerebellar lesions.

Cerebellar lesions are frequent concomitants of cerebrovascular occlusions affecting the vertebro-basilar vasculature and the posterior cerebral arteries. They are also frequent targets of degenerations and the demyelination syndromes so that the symptomatology of dysfunctions are often of global distribution. Cerebellar dysfunctions are characterized by:

Unsteadiness and other disturbances of balance, and movements which are clumsy and uncoordinated. The following are some features that suggest cerebellar dysfunction:

- **Hypotonia** is common.
- **Dysmetria.** A movement cannot be stopped at any given point. For example, when the patient reaches out to a point the hand either over-reaches or stops before arriving at the target. It results from correction movements which are inappropriately large and badly timed due to dysfunctional feedback mechanisms.
- **Intention tremor.** When the patient tries to reach an object the individual overshoots it and then overcompensates again and again, trying to access the desired position till it is finally reached.
- **Decomposition of movements.** Movements which require interactions of different joints and muscles get broken down into their component movements.
- **Dysdiadochokinesis.** Rapid change from one movement to another is slowed. Thus, for example, rapid pronation-supination movements of the wrist are slower than expected.
- **Nystagmus.** This results from dysfunctions affecting the connections between the cerebellum and the vestibular nuclei.
- **Decreased ability to perform smooth and appropriately timed sequential and relatively skilled movements.** Lesions of the lateral lobes are the usual cause and the clinical features affect the ipsilateral extremities, especially those controlled by vision.

Motor dysfunctions due to basal ganglia dysfunctions.

The basal ganglia can be affected by a variety of pathological conditions similar to those which can result in cerebellar dysfunctions. In addition there are some unusual pathologies which only affect the basal ganglia. The following are some examples:

Huntington's chorea. This is a genetically predetermined degeneration. It is an autosomal dominant inherited disorder. More description is detailed below.

Depositions of copper (Wilson's disease), mercury and other metals.

Parkinson's disease. Probably due to an accelerated aging of the cells of the substantia nigra.

The following are some clinical features of basal ganglia disease:

The basal ganglia control movements by amplifications and reductions which result in precise and well-timed movements. The dysfunctions of basal ganglia disease reflect the decrease or loss of these capabilities. They include the following:

- **Bradykinesia** which is a slowing down of some voluntary movements. The probable cause is a reduction of the normal basal ganglia amplifications of motor activity. The bradykinesia of basal ganglia disease is slowness in initiating and executing voluntary movements. It is often a presenting symptom appearing long before other symptoms. The patient finds it difficult to smile or to stretch out a hand to shake another.
- **Hypertonia, involuntary movements and tremors.** These features probably result from release symptoms due to decreases in the basal ganglia activity which inhibits and controls. They are probably responsible for many of the symptoms of chorea and athetosis.
- **Muscle weakness.** The face is like a mask and emotions do not register with typical facial manifestations, movements are started slowly and stop with difficulty, and the swinging of arms during walking is decreased

or absent,

- **Rigidity.** Two types of rigidity are demonstrable. Plastic rigidity where resistance to passive movements exist but are smooth, and cogwheel rigidity where passive movement is resisted by repeated jerks.
- **Tremor.** Alternating tremors result from alternating contractions of opposing muscles. It is involuntary and one manifestation is the "pill-rolling" phenomenon seen in the hands. This type of tremor disappears during voluntary activity.

  Another form of basal ganglia tremor is **the intention tremor** which is seen when voluntary movement is attempted. It increases as the act proceeds and can be a major problem when the patient attempts to drink from a glass or place food in the mouth.
- **Involuntary movements.** These range from the slow twisting, involuntary movements of athetosis and the sudden jerky movements of Sydenham's (post rheumatic fever) chorea, to the violent bizarre flinging involuntary movements of ballism.

Chorea.

In **chorea** there are series of rapid, random and uncontrolled movements of muscles all over the body. In the past the usual cause was a post-streptococcal infection. At present, in societies where streptococcal infections are promptly treated with antibiotics, the commonest cause is probably Huntington's disease which is an inherited autosomal dominant basal ganglia degeneration which appears in the 40s and progresses to incapacity, imbecility and death.

Parkinson's disease.

The symptomatology of Parkinson's disease is the triad of **hypertonia, bradykinesia and tremor.** Hypertonia results in rigidity of the limbs without significant disturbance of posture. The rigidity is described as of "lead-pipe" type. The limb is difficult to move but once moved does not spring back to its original position. Often, "cog-wheel" rigidity is also present in Parkinson's disease - when the hypertonic muscle is passively stretched the resistance to stretch is rhythmically jerky. The hypertonia and related disturbance of balance is probably responsible for the characteristic gait; small shuffling steps which progressively speed-up as if the patient is chasing a center of gravity (the festinating gait).

The tremor of Parkinson's disease is an alternating contraction of agonist and antagonist muscles which occur at intervals of about 10 seconds. In the hand this takes the form of pill rolling; alternate flexion of fingers and repeated appositions of thumb to fingers. Other manifestations of this phenomenon are the head or the trunk moving up and down or from side to side at irregular frequencies. Initially, the tremor stops during voluntary movements. The tremor of Parkinson's disease is slower than that of the normal physiological tremor which everyone exhibits to greater or lesser degree as they age.

CNS dysfunctions due to neuromuscular disease

Motor neuron disease.

The usual causes are degenerations of the anterior horn cells, the cranial nerve nuclei and the Betz cells of the motor cortex. The etiologies of these conditions are not known. Clinically, there are progressive muscle weaknesses, fasciculations, and atrophy. Three types are described but any one or more combinations are frequent; progressive bulbar palsy when the cranial motor nuclei are involved, progressive muscular atrophy when degenerative changes affect the anterior horn cells of the cord, and amyotrophic lateral sclerosis when Betz cell degeneration results in degeneration of the pyramidal tracts.

Myasthenia gravis.

Myasthenia gravis is considered by many to be an autoimmune disease with antibodies directed against the acetylcholine receptors of muscle. The disease characteristically affects bulbar muscles. Involvement of limb muscles is uncommon. There is weakness and the affected muscles are easily tired. Typical initial complaints are ptosis due to weakness of palpebral muscles and diploplia resulting from weakness of bulbar muscles. Later there is facial weakness and weakness on chewing, difficulty in swallowing and a nasal or dysarthric quality to speech. Limb weakness usually affects only proximal muscles with delayed arm abduction times. The antibody to acetylcholine receptors is demonstrable in most patients and often there are one or more associated autoimmune diseases such as rheumatoid arthritis and/or disseminated systemic lupus erythematosus.

Treatment with anticholinesterase drugs helps but complete relief is unusual. The role of thymectomy is controversial. Exacerbations of myasthenia gravis can be precipitated by intercurrent infections and endocrine disease (e.g., hyperthyroid disease). A myasthenic crisis can be a real emergency, often precipitated by an excess of medication (the "cholinergic crisis").

CNS dysfunctions due to demyelinations

Neurological dysfunctions due to demyelinations present as acute or chronic dysfunctions.

Acute demyelinating diseases.

Post-infectious encephalomyelitis results from an inconstant immune response to any one of a number of viral diseases or to immunizations. The viral diseases which might result in this syndrome include measles, smallpox, chickenpox and rubella. The demyelination syndrome appears concurrent with or shortly after the exanthem, typically 2-4 days after the rash first appears. Symptoms result from multiple areas of demyelination in the white matter. The process is thought to result from some type of immuno-allergic reaction. Typically the disease begins with headache, fever and vomiting. Convulsions are not uncommon. Delirium and coma are frequently seen as is spinal cord involvement. This is followed by neurological deficits involving the brain and spinal cord.

There is a substantial mortality and even if there is recovery, significant neurological deficits can persist. On the other hand, in occasional cases there is recovery of consciousness and little residuum.

Fortunately the post-vaccination syndrome has significantly decreased in numbers since the eradication of smallpox, immunization against measles, mumps, rubella and chicken pox and the development of new and safer anti-rabies vaccines.

Chronic demyelinating diseases.

Many exist. Examples, apart from multiple sclerosis, are the demyelinations of vitamin B_{12} deficiency, Schilder's disease and the various leukodystrophies. Only multiple sclerosis and the neurological features of vitamin B_{12} deficiency are considered in this section. The others are rarely encountered by anyone other than specialist neurologists.

Multiple sclerosis.

This is a neurological disease of unknown etiology. It is rare in tropical countries but common in temperate climes. The disease is of unknown etiology and usually presents at the age of 30 ± 10 years. The lesions of multiple sclerosis may be focal or global.

The pathological lesions are plaques of demyelination in the white matter of the brain and spinal cord. The plaques vary in size from minute lesions to ones that exceed many centimeters in diameter. They frequently encroach on gray matter but do not destroy nerve cells. They are readily detected on an MRI scan.

The effects of demyelination are many. Impulses are conducted at reduced velocities so that preprogrammed movements become dysfunctional because they depend on the precise and coordinated interaction of several nerves, each conducting impulses at previously recognized and preprogrammed rates. Typically, there are disturbances which affect the coordinated movements of the eyes, the limbs, the trunk, and the bulbar muscles. In addition to dysfunctions of movements, sensory perceptions, and autonomic functions, demyelination in the spinal cord can also result in distressing dysfunctions affecting bladder and bowel evacuations.

Demyelinated axons can discharge spontaneously giving flashes of light when the eyes move (phosphenes). Demyelination also results in cross-talk between demyelinated axons with bizarre fleeting symptoms lasting one or two minutes. Examples are tetanic posturing of limb muscles and fleeting dysarthria and ataxia.

The clinical features. The first symptom in about a third of patients is an optic neuritis - loss of vision in one, but almost never, both eyes at the same time. About a third recover completely, another third partially, and the rest not at all. Others will present with diplopia or disturbances of spinal cord or central nervous system function. The classical description of the symptoms is that they are dissimilar in space and in time. The deficits can occur, remit and recur for over 30 years. Common features are visual disturbances, ataxia, intention tremors, motor and/or sensory deficits (the former can result in eventual paraplegia), disturbances of bladder and bowel function, and impotence in males. Depression and emotional reactions are common (and with good reason) and contrary to what is widely believed cognitive disabilities do develop in some patients (**Lynch, S.G., Parmenter, G.A. et al.** The association between cognitive impairment and physical disability in multiple sclerosis. Mult. Scler, 2005; 11:469.)

Initially, the disease is characterized by frequent episodes of dysfunction with complete or partial recovery. Later, recovery becomes progressively less complete until finally fixed deformities and disabilities develop, and often progress. The course is unpredictable; the average life span of a patient is about 25 years from onset of the disease. Frequent terminal events are respiratory and urinary tract infections, or progressive neurological deficits affecting the bulbar muscles or those of respiration.

Vitamin B_{12} and folic acid deficiencies.

Vitamin B_{12} ("extrinsic factor") is present in meat and dairy products. It is absorbed in the terminal ileum after an initial and essential complexing with gastric "intrinsic factor". An inadequate diet is an uncommon cause of deficiency as only 1-5μg is the daily requirement and the vitamin is widely distributed in dairy products and meat. The total body stores are 2000-5000μg and only 0.1% is lost each day. Common causes of deficiency syndromes are lack of gastric intrinsic factor (due to pernicious anemia or total gastrectomies) and bacterial overgrowth and destruction or utilization of B_{12} in intestinal blind loops and diverticula.

The neurological complications result from posterior and lateral column demyelinations in the spinal cord ("subacute combined degeneration") as well as peripheral neuropathies. The following are some of the clinical features: spastic and uncoordinated gait, peripheral and often symmetric paresthesiae, muscle weakness and loss of vibration sense. Mental changes are not uncommon and can range from trivial irritability to dementia (megaloblastic madness). B_{12} deficiency is discussed in greater detail in Chapter 12.

Deficiencies of B_{12} or folates can result in megaloblastic anemias which are readily reversed by replacement therapy. A caveat is that folic acid alone can reverse the anemia of B_{12} deficiency but worsen the neurological deficits.

CNS dysfunctions of peripheral nerves

The symptoms and signs of peripheral neuropathies are those of lower motor neuron deficits. Varying degrees of sensory loss, motor deficits, decreased knee and ankle jerks, and occasionally, deformities due to the unequal pull of unaffected muscle groups. An example is the pes cavus of Charcot-Marie-Tooth disease. The sensory deficits may present as paresthesiae, hypesthesiae, or traumatic and often infected lesions caused by the patient's inability to sense and hence, to avoid harmful situations such as those caused by excessive heat or insensitivity to trauma.

The mononeuropathies.

The mononeuropathies are usually the result of trauma or compression. Examples of the latter are the carpal tunnel syndrome (admittedly, often bilateral), and ulna nerve entrapments and the palpable lateral peroneal nerve thickenings caused by leprosy; a common syndrome is weakness of the foot combined with thickening of the lateral popliteal nerve as it lies on the lateral aspect of the fibula.

The polyneuropathies.

The causes of peripheral polyneuropathies are numerous. Common ones are uncontrolled diabetes, alcoholism and deficiencies of B complex vitamins. The neuropathies which result from long-standing, and often inadequately controlled, diabetes are associated with vascular changes and are often painful. Less common causes of polyneuropathies are lead, mercury or arsenic poisonings, some drugs, the acute intermittent form of porphyria and inherited dysfunctions such as Charcot-Marie-Tooth disease.

At least two polyneuropathies are of special importance as they are potentially life-threatening. They are the Guillain-Barré syndrome and the polyneuropathies of diphtheria.

The Guillain-Barré syndrome.

The syndrome is usually a sequel to a viral infection, to any form of immunization, to pregnancy or to surgery. It often presents as an ascending motor neuropathy affecting respiratory and facial muscles (in my experience an early clue has been some blurring of vision). Respiratory failure is an ever-present danger and rapid hospitalization and monitoring is essential. A strange phenomenon is the association of a Guillain-Barré syndrome with Campylobacter intestinal infections. There are claims that some 40% of Guillain-Barré syndromes in the United States result from campylobacter infections.

The polyneuropathies of diphtheria.

They are of importance for two reasons. The first is that they can be life-threatening because of pharyngeal and laryngeal paralysis as well as paralysis of respiratory muscles. The second is that these paralyses frequently occur some three to four weeks after the infection so that regular monitoring of these patients is essential for the first month or two after the infection has resolved.

CNS dysfunctions - the seizure syndromes

A seizure is a motor, sensory, or psychic episode which occurs with speed, without warning and usually, with a return to normal. It probably results from an aberrant and uncalled for discharge of impulses from a group of neurons. Recruitment of adjacent neurons results in the seizure. Neural abnormalities are often demonstrable on an electroencephalogram, or presumed to be present if not demonstrable.

Four basic types of seizures are recognized: focal idiopathic seizures, focal seizures related to central nervous system pathology, generalized idiopathic seizures and generalized seizures resulting from central nervous system pathology.

An idiopathic seizure is one which occurs without demonstrable central nervous system pathology. Various theories have been proposed to account for such seizures - none seem to have general acceptance. Idiopathic seizures usually affect the younger age groups but a complete physical and especially, neurological, assessment is always needed to exclude pathology of the nervous system.

In older age groups seizures are often consequent on central nervous system pathology. When available, a CT scan is always necessary to exclude tumors and abscesses. The tumor is often a metastatic lesion from a primary tumor; common locations of the primary are the lungs, the colon, the prostate and the breast. There are many other causes for seizures secondary to central nervous system pathology. Examples are previous trauma, previous surgery, encephalitis and meningitis, sudden withdrawal of alcohol or drugs, ingested or inhaled toxins, and excessive alcohol drinking.

Focal seizures.

The typical focal seizure emanates from single or multiple foci in the gray matter. It is typically preceded by an aura of some sort such as numbness or tingling in a leg or hand or some psychic feeling. This is followed by tonic-clonic motor activity and finally, a postictal phase of headache, confusion, tiredness or focal weakness. The seizures may be focal from beginning to end or may spread from one muscle group to another - the "march of Jacksonian epilepsy".

Generalized seizures.

An aura is uncommon. There is a sudden loss of consciousness. The patient falls to the ground, often stops breathing and becomes blue. All muscles are tightly contracted in the initial tonic phase which lasts 30-60 seconds. Next is the clonic phase with rhythmic jerking of all parts of the body. The tongue may be bitten and there is often incontinence of urine and feces. Respiration is difficult, the patient may turn blue, and there is often frothing at the mouth. The third stage is one of complete flaccidity. Finally, there is a gradual return of consciousness, often with confusion and sleepiness of varying duration.

Variations in the form of seizures.

Temporal lobe epilepsy. These so-called psychomotor seizures may take many forms: dream states, automatism, bizarre emotional ideation and olfactory and auditory sensations, flashbacks, hallucinations, nausea, vomiting, epigastric discomfort and a variety of other symptoms. The focus for epilepsy is in some part of the temporal lobe and is usually demonstrable by electroencephalography.

Petit mal seizures (absence seizures). These seizures begin in childhood or adolescence. There is a sudden and short loss of contact with the surroundings. During the seizure phase the patient has a vacant expression, pauses in whatever is being done at the time or has a temporary arrest of speech. These attacks may be so frequent (at times more than 100 per day) that each day there may be long periods of confusion or deficient memory (petit mal status).

Status epilepticus. This is a life-threatening condition. Epileptic attacks occur one after another without any recovery between attacks. The repeated tonic-clonic phenomena may be seen but patients often present in coma. Many attacks are precipitated by sudden withdrawal of anticonvulsant medication or alcohol or by trauma or infections. Treatment is essentially symptomatic; appropriate sedation, maintenance of an airway, mechanical artificial respiration when necessary and possible, prevention of dehydration, and cardiac monitoring.

The therapy of seizures.

Many anti-convulsants are available. Each physicians has different views about treating first episodes and prevention. For this reason the topic is not discussed in detail. The principal danger relates to a prolonged tonic phase in a generalized seizure. Very little can be done about this as the tonically contracted muscles will resist any attempt at oxygenation. Wait and hope for the best. I had a patient whose son died in this phase. Hence, the need for effective and continued therapeutic prevention of seizures. Other dangers are injuries sustained if the patient has a seizure while standing on a ladder or otherwise precariously perched, or when driving a car. Swimming is another hazard.

Should therapy ever be discontinued and if so, when? Here again the opinions of neurologists differ. There are hazards to long-term therapy and it would be appropriate to get a second opinion if the recommendation is to stop therapy. As mentioned, status epilepticus is a medical emergency requiring immediate therapy and so is a prolonged tonic phase. The dangers of generalized seizures are death from respiratory failure or accidents. Life long control by good therapy is essential. Long-term anti-convulsants have some inherent hazards but the prevention of epileptic episodes is of over-riding importance. I have many patients who have been taking anti-convulsants for years. Some have no ill effects. Others have minor adverse reactions. A caveat is that regular monitoring of blood levels of the drug and blood and liver function tests are essentials.

Fever seizures.

Up to 5% of children between the ages of 6 months and five years will have seizures when fever rises above 102°F or so. The usual causes are respiratory tract infections, ear infections, or a viral infection such as measles or chicken pox. The seizure may be the first indication that fever and infection exists. Less than 1% are caused by meningitis but this possibility must always be excluded, especially in children younger than one year or those who remain ill even when the fever subsides.

Most fever seizures end after a few minutes and are usually generalized seizures. Seizures may recur up to the age of 5. Extensive investigations are usually not warranted if the child is mentally normal, the seizure was generalized and not focal, and did not last more than a few minutes. A seizure which is of focal type or lasts more than 10 minutes merits later investigation to exclude neurological disease. So do children who have more than one seizure in a 24 hour period or repeated seizures over a longer period.

Children with febrile infections often have rashes. Always advise parents about the tumbler test for exclusion of a meningococcal septicemia. A few children who have febrile seizures may proceed to true epilepsy. This is not because of the fever seizure but because those who would develop epilepsy anyway tend to have the first seizure during a fever.

During the seizure loosen clothing and turn the child on the side to avoid aspiration of vomit or saliva. Do not attempt to restrain movements. Place the child on a flat surface over a warm blanket. After the seizure try to bring down the fever as rapidly as possible by sponging with tepid water and insertion of an acetaminophen suppository if one is available.

CNS dysfunctions causing hydrocephalus

Hydrocephalus results from an excess of intracranial CSF. The three principal causes are:

- Obstruction of the exits from the third ventricle or from the arachnoid vill into the blood stream. Common causes include fibrosis and adhesions from previous infections or from previous trauma.
- Decreased absorption of CSF because of a superior vena cava syndrome or venous sinus thrombosis, and
- Excessive production of CSF by benign or malignant tumors of the choroid plexus.

Symptoms and signs of hydrocephalus.

In infants before fusion of the frontal bones the fontanelles bulge, the head circumference increases and dilated scalp veins are demonstrable. The child is irritable and head control is poor.

In adults the symptoms and signs are headaches, disturbances of gait, vomiting and visual changes. Papilledema is often present. If the hydrocephalus is progressive intracranial pressure will increase with eventual brain stem dysfunctions, coma and finally, death. In adults it is always necessary to exclude a tumor as the cause.

Normal pressure hydrocephalus.

This is a variant form of hydrocephalus which occurs in elderly patients. It is characterized by a bradykinetic, broad-based and shuffling gait which is similar to the gait of individuals with Parkinson's disease. True ataxia, rigidity, tremor and weakness are uncommon and this helps differentiation from Parkinson's disease. Other characteristics are dementia and memory loss with progression to a state similar to Alzheimer's disease. Incontinence of urine is frequent, even in the early stages.

The pathophysiology of the condition is unknown though many hypotheses have been proposed. Suggested etiologies include head injuries, meningeal infections and subarachnoid hemorrhages. Each of these conditions can cause true hydrocephalus but the way in which this could proceed to normal pressure hydrocephalus is not clear.

Distinction from Parkinson's disease is based on a CT or MRI pattern of ventricular enlargement and abnormally increased sulcal atrophy. Diagnosis is important for this is one of the few dementias that can respond to therapy. Surgical shunting of the CSF is the only available therapeutic modality. Proper selection for surgery is difficult, yet essential for a satisfactory outcome.

CNS dysfunctions of mentation - confusional states and the dementias

Confusional states.

These states are easier to recognize than to describe. The patient rambles about irrelevant matters, has difficulty in comprehension and expression, occasionally hallucinates and generally behaves in odd and inappropriate ways.

The possible neurological causes of confusional states are numerous and so are the non-neurological causes. The former includes responses to trauma, infections (meningitis as well as encephalitis), increased intracranial pressure from any cause, and confusional states in the period following a seizure. However, many causes of confusional states are not consequent on neurological pathology. The following are some examples: fever, unrecognized infections of the respiratory and urinary tracts, especially in the elderly; hypoglycemia from an excess of insulin or diabetic ketoacidosis from an insufficiency; an excess of alcohol, narcotics, hypnotics and tranquilizers or their sudden withdrawal; uremia; hepatic failure; hyponatremia (seizures may be the initial manifestation); water intoxication - usually the result of an excess of water ingestion during tube or intravenous feeding with consequent cerebral edema; ingestion of toxic elements such as lead, mercury and arsenic; hyperthyroid and hypothyroid disease; the vascular lesions of lupus erythematosus and polyarteritis; unsuspected head injuries; the electrolyte disturbances and the hypotension of untreated Addison's disease; Stokes-Adams attacks; ventricular arrhythmias; stenoses of the aortic valves; idiosyncratic or toxic reactions to therapeutic drugs; hypercalcemia; and lactic acidosis.

Recovery from confusional states is the rule when the apparent cause is remedied. Not so for recovery from dementia and this fact distinguishes the two.

The dementias.

Dementia is a term used to describe abnormal and progressive changes in intellectual function and ability. Initially there are impaired memory, dysfunctions of speech and comprehension, a general diminution of intellectual capabilities and decreased visuo-spatial skills.

Often the first change is a memory deficit, especially of short-term memory. Gradually the mood changes; the patient becomes more irritable, easily distracted, and unable to comprehend or to respond intelligently. A progressive loss of all mental faculties follows. Judgment is impaired, paranoid feelings may appear, and the patient begins to talk nonsense. Eventually the individual stops speaking, and fails to recognize partners and close relatives. Finally there is essentially a decortication; the patient lies in bed with eyes open but is completely unaware of events in the surroundings. The sphincters are incontinent and the facial and limb muscles are usually stiff and associated with other features of upper motor neuron failure - increased tendon jerks and positive Babinski signs.

The etiologies of the dementias.

The causes of dementia are numerous. They include any one or more different neurological diseases; some examples are vascular and degenerative disease, post-traumatic states, post-inflammatory states, viral and prion infections, acute syndromes of demyelination, neoplasms, and metabolic and toxic encephalopathies. Only the more common and important neurological dysfunctions are described here.

— **Alzheimer's disease.**

There is marked cerebral atrophy but a certain diagnosis is only possible at post-mortem examination of the brain. Confirmation of the diagnosis requires that an autopsy shows extensive loss of neurons, deposits of amorphous amyloid scattered throughout the cortex (called senile plaques), and fibrillary change due to masses of tangled and twisted microtubules within nerve cells.

— **Dementia due to vascular disease.**

Many types have been described depending on the location and size of the vascular occlusions or hemorrhages. Probably the most common causes are multiple small vascular occlusions and/or hemorrhages - multi-infarct dementia.

— **The dementia of Parkinson's disease.**

About 40% of patients with Parkinson's disease develop some degree of dementia and up to 70% will have some degree of intellectual deficit. From the clinical standpoint the importance of these facts is that such patients react adversely to drugs previously well tolerated. If the original medication and dosage continues the result could be hallucinations, delusions and various amplifications of existing dementia.

— **Dementia resulting from infections.**

Chronic meningitis, syphilis, AIDS and Creutzfeldt-Jakob disease are conditions which can result in dementia.

- **Dementia due to prions.**

  This is a topic of increasing interest because of the postulated link between bovine spongiform encephalopathy and Creutzfeldt-Jakob disease. It needs additional comment.

- **Other causes of dementia.**

  Most other causes are uncommon: Pick's disease; the dementia of Huntington's disease; Schilder's and other demyelinating diseases; the dementias caused by brain tumors; and the dementias caused by low pressure hydrocephalus, and by metabolic and toxic encephalopathies. Examples of toxic encephalopathies are hepatic disease, renal failure, occupational or environmental neurotoxic metals, chronic alcoholism, and addiction to so-called "recreational" psychotropic drugs).

Creutzfeldt-Jakob disease.

Current thinking ascribes the cause of this disease to abnormal protein molecules, the prions, first identified by Prusiner[14,15]. These diseases have long periods of latency, and cause progressive brain pathology. In Creutzfeldt-Jakob disease there is some loss of neurons but glial lesions predominate. Spongiosis is demonstrable throughout the cortex. The spongiosis consists of bullous cavities which are cytoplasmic cavitations in glial cells and neurons.

The clinical picture is fairly diagnostic and of particular importance at present because of the association thought to exist between bovine spongiform encephalopathy and human Creutzfeldt-Jakob disease. In the early stages disturbances of behavior, memory and reasoning, as well as hallucinations, confusional states and delirium coexist with visual disturbances. Later one sees sudden myoclonic contractions of muscles, at first in response to sudden sensory stimuli, but later of spontaneous origin; the twitching of individual fingers is one manifestation of this. Various neurological deficits are common; some examples are speech difficulties, convulsions, a masking of the face, generalized rigidity and ataxia. With progression there is a gradual deterioration of mentation with eventual coma and death, often in a year or less after onset of the disease, usually from an intercurrent infection. Many variations of this basic picture have been described.

Therapeutic options for neurological disease and dysfunctions

The scope for therapy is small but does exist. Therapeutic measures include any one or more of the following:

- Anticoagulants to reduce the incidence of carotid emboli or of cardiac emboli from blood clots in fibrillating heart chambers
- Rapid diagnosis and appropriate antibiotics for infections.
- Relief of pain.
- Immunizations against poliomyelitis, mumps, measles, rubella, tetanus, pertussis, diphtheria and hemophilus influenza have almost eliminated neurological disease caused by these agents if the individual was previously immunized. Unfortunately many remain unimmunized because vaccines ar often not available and many children are not immunized because of unreasonable doctrinaire reasons and beliefs of parents.
- Surgery for advanced carotid occlusions, for some tumors, and for evacuation of some hematomas (traumatic or cerebrovascular in origin).
- Surgical shunts for hydrocephalus. A recent innovation is third ventriculostomy for non-communicating hydrocephalus. A neuroendoscope is inserted into the third ventricle and a small hole is made in the base of the ventricle to allow fluid to bypass any aqueductal stenosis and drain into the CSF.
- Effective anticonvulsant control of individuals with histories of seizures.
- Attempts to reduce intracranial pressure by intravenous infusions of hyperosmotic solutions.

— Rehabilitation and appropriate physiotherapy.

— Medications to reduce post-stroke depressions.

— Tracheostomies and gastrostomies as and when indicated in some cases of advanced amyotrophic lateral sclerosis and in other dysfunctions involving cranial nerves such as the Guillain-Barré syndromes and the jugular foramen syndromes.

Case history.

The last is rare but I mention it because these rarities do occur and need recognition. At the age of 36 the patient had some difficulty in speaking and went to an ENT surgeon who said it was due to enlargement of a vocal cord lymph nodule. The lesion was removed and had some characteristics of lymphoid tissue. Difficulty in speaking continued and was followed by dysphagia. He consulted me for this. He had all the features of a jugular foramen syndrome - paresis of muscles supplied by nerves 9-12. An MRI showed a temporal bone lesion eroding the base of the skull. After many surgical excisions of tumor over a period of some twelve years infiltration outside the skull began. The tumor was designated a chondrosarcoma and the patient eventually died. Maintenance of nutrition and oxygenation were effectively maintained for 10 years by tracheostomy and gastrostomy.

— Hormone replacement therapies and therapies to reduce hormone over-production.

— Plasmapharesis. Occasionally used for Guillain-Barré respiratory failure or myasthenia gravis.

Regrettably, few other measures are available for prevention and treatment of neurological disease.

Therapy for raised intracranial pressure (ICP)

The normal ICP is 1-20mm Hg. It can be measured by insertion of a catheter into the lateral ventricle or by a subarachnoid screw which monitors the subarachnoid space. Alternatively, by a catheter which monitors the epidural space. An ICP >20mm Hg is life threatening and needs treatment. The giving of hyperosmotic solutions such as mannitol or other crystalloid solutions is common practice intended to reduce ICP. Mannitol acts as an osmotic diuretic and also draws out water in the brain along an osmotic gradient.

Therapy for cerebrovascular occlusions.

The surgical treatment of carotid artery stenoses is based on a study by Rothwell and associates[12] of pooled data from 6092 treated patients in Europe and North America. A clear benefit was demonstrable when the stenosis exceeded 70% of the caliber of the vessel. Borderline candidates for surgery were in the 50-79% category. The rest were best treated with ASA or some other anticoagulant preferred by the physician. The study of Rothwell and associates were confirmed in a later publication by Barnett and associates[16]. Many factors will determine therapy: previous stroke, its intensity and recovery from its effects, associated cardiac and other pathology, the experience of the surgeon and, perhaps most important of all, the wishes of a patient who has received information of all the pros, cons and consequences, especially the chances of paralysis because of anoxia during surgery.

With respect to stroke, very little can be done about hemorrhagic infarctions unless a localized collection of blood is suitable for neurosurgical evacuation. A CT scan is valuable because it almost always demonstrates a hemorrhagic infarct. A CT scan is usually not useful for assessing the presence or nature of an embolic stroke.

Therapeutic options are available for strokes which result from embolic occlusions or local thromboses. Aspirin provides some protection against recurrence and probably also decreases residual disability. Intravenous thrombolysis with streptokinase or intravenous recombinant tissue-plasminogen activator (Atelpase) is said to provide benefits such as a decrease in the extent of paralysis and a more rapid recovery. Of necessity the assessments are predictive and not always objective. It is therapy which has acceptance for general usage but with the caveats mentioned below. It is recommended that the injection not be given if the stroke exceeds three hours from inception. Even in simple occlusive infarcts thrombolysis is associated with 5% chance of fatal intracranial hemorrhage[17]. The 3 hour limit reduces the number of patients with occlusive stroke who are treatable - the average is about 10%, and that is only possible in metropolitan areas with efficient ambulance services.

There is a practical problem regarding thrombolytic therapy. A TIA is defined by neurologists as a neurological deficit which disappears within 24 hours of its onset. How does one clinically distinguish between a TIA and a stroke within three hours of the onset of symptoms? Spontaneous recovery from TIAs is expected. How then does one conclude that thrombolysis was responsible for recovery from a stroke if the lytic agent was given within three hours of the onset of symptoms?

Contraindications to thrombolysis include:

— **Refusal to give consent** by the patient or, if unconscious, by an authorized surrogate, spouse or offspring when told of the chances of a 5% mortality after injection.

— **Patients on anticoagulants.** If necessary, the effects of the anticoagulant can be rapidly reversed by an injection of vitamin K_1, but always recheck the INR before giving the thrombolytic.

— **Patients with a history of intracranial surgery or a recent head injury.**

— **Patients with intracranial pathologies** such as neoplasms, arteriovenous malformations and aneurysms.

— **Uncontrolled or poorly controlled hypertension.** A systolic pressure of 200mm Hg and/or a diastolic pressure which exceeds 110mm Hg are definite contraindications.

— **Patients with reticuloendothelial neoplasms** (especially uncontrolled leukemia).

— **A low platelet count,** whatever the reason.

The medical treatment of cerebrovascular occlusions.

Aspirin is the mainstay of treatment. ASA is a potent inhibitor of thromboxane A_2 production. The recommended dose is 50-325mg/day.

Ticlopidine (Ticlid) is another inhibitor of platelet aggregation. Adverse effects are common and the manufacturer recommends close monitoring of blood counts for at least the first three months of therapy.

Clopidogrel - (Plavix) irreversibly inhibits ADP-induced platelet aggregation. It has fewer side effects than ticlopidine but more than ASA. Comparison with ASA[18] suggests that there are no significant therapeutic differences between ASA and clopidogrel in patients with any one of the following: ischemic stroke, myocardial infarction and atheromatous peripheral vascular disease.

Therapeutic agents which affect autonomic neuromediators.

Acetylcholine receptors are either muscarinic or nicotinic. **The nicotinic receptors** are located at neuromuscular junctions. Their actions can be stimulated by acetylcholine or nicotine but negated by an excess of either and also by curare-like drugs such as D-tubocurarine and suxamethonium, agents routinely used in anaesthesia. Some nicotinic receptors are also present at synapses in parasympathetic and sympathetic ganglia. Botulinum toxin paralyses by preventing release of neurotransmitter. Anticholinestrase drugs such as physostigmine and prostigmin inhibit the breakdown of the neurotransmitter and are used in the treatment of myasthenia gravis.

The muscarinic receptors are present in effectors (mainly in glands) stimulated by acetylcholine and in symapthetic terminations which are cholinergic (muscle blood vessels and sweat glands). They are blocked by atropine.

In the central nervous system the main amines produced are the catecholamines. dopamine, serotonin norepinephrine and epinephrine. They or their antagonists are widely used in psychopharmacology. Gamma amino butyric acid (GABA) and glycine are amino acids produced in the brain. GABA and glycine seem to be the main inhibitory neurotransmitters in the CNS. It is said that the sedative effects of the benzodiazepines results from competition for glycine receptors where they have the same effect as glycine.

Conclusion.

This ends a summary of the features of common neurological dysfunctions. The central nervous system has many features which are unique and not shared with other systems. Hence, the length of this chapter.

I do recommend a re-reading of the "methodolgy of clinical assessments" on page 119 before proceeding to

subsequent chapters.

In subsequent chapters on diagnosis these comments will not be tediously repeated but the text will suggest that the reader once again read the comments made on page 119 of this chapter.

References for Chapter 6.

1. Eccles, J.C. Evolution of the brain: Creation of self. London & New York. Routledge, 1989.
2. Ito, M. The Cerebellum and Neural Control. New York. Raven press, 1984.
3. Spansky, B., Allen, D.J., et al. Review of Neuroscience. New York:. Macmillan Publishing Co., 1988.
4. Hebb, D.O. The Organization of Behavior. New York. Wiley, 1949.
5. Bliss, T.V.P. & Lomo, T. Long-lasting potentiation of synaptic transmission in the dentate area of the anaesthetized rabbit following stimulation of the perforant path. J. Physiol. (London) 1973; 232:331.
6. Martinez, J.L. & Derrick, B.E. Long term potentiation and learning. Annu. Rev. Psychol. 1996; 47:173.
7. Sherrington, C. The Integrative Action of the Nervous system. Cambridge, Eng. Cambridge University Press, 1906.
8. Goldstein, R.E., Boccuzzi, S.J., et al. Diltiazem increases late-onset congestive heart failure in postinfarction patients with early reduction in ejection fraction. The Adverse Experience Committee; and the Multicenter Diltiazem Postinfarction Research Group. Circulation 1991; 83:52.
9. Murray, C.J.L., Lopez, A.D. The Global Burden of Disease: a comprehensive assessment of mortality and disability from disease, injuries and risk factors in 1990 and projected to 2020. Boston, Mass. Harvard University Press, 1996.
10. Prospective Studies Collaboration. Cholesterol, diastolic blood pressure, and stroke: 13,000 strokes in 450,000 people in 45 cohorts. Lancet 1995; 346:1647.
11. Warlow, C., Sudlow, C., et al. Stroke. Lancet 2003; 362:1211.
12. Wardlaw, J.M., Lewis, S.C. et al. Is visible infarction on computed tomography associated with an adverse prognosis in acute ischemic stroke? Stroke 1998;29:1315.
13. Rothwell, P.M., Eliasziw, M. et al. Analysis of pooled data from randomized controlled trials of endarterectomy for symptomatic carotid stenosis. Lancet 2003; 361:107.
14. Prusiner, S.B. Novel proteinaceous infectious particles cause scrapie. Science 1982; 216:136.
15. Prusiner, S.B. Prion biology and diseases. Harvey lecture 1991; 87:85.
16. Barnett, H.J.M., Taylor, W., et al. Benefit of Carotid Endarterectomy in Patients with Symptomatic Moderate or Severe Stenosis. N. Engl. J. Med. 1998; 339:1415.
17. Albers, G.W. Easton, J.D. et al. Antithrombotic and thrombolytic therapy for ischemic stroke. Chest 1998; 114 (5suppl.):683S.
18. A randomised, blinded trial of clopidogrel versus aspirin in patients at risk of ischemic events (CARPRIE). Lancet 1996; 348:1329.

7

Diagnosis: The Control Systems

2. Endocrine and Microenvironmental Control Systems

Table of Contents

Notation.

The notation ~P denotes phosphorous with a high energy bond. Depending on the context in which the term is used, ~P may also denote the energy liberated when a high energy phosphate bond detaches from ATP or ADP.

A general comment on the methodology of clinical assessments.

The comments made **on page 119** about this topic are not repeated. They merit reading before proceeding with this chapter.

Endocrine biology: the normal physiology and the dysfunctions

The normal biology and the pathological physiology of endocrine dysfunctions are too closely linked for them to be considered as separate entities. In this chapter the two are described together.

The symptoms and signs of some common endocrine dysfunctions.

Diabetes is characterized by the symptom-complex of polyuria, thirst and weight loss. Confirmation of the diagnosis is readily made by estimations of the fasting blood sugar and effective control is possible with oral medications. If control remains unsatisfactory the disease is readily controlled by insulin injections.

Hyperthyroidism and hypothyroid disease have features that are fairly characteristic. They are described later in this chapter. Simple laboratory and radionuclear tests are diagnostic, and effective therapies are available.

Pituitary microadenomas are usually small - rarely bigger than 1cm. Extrasellar pressure effects on structures such as the optic chiasma are uncommon. Increased production of hormone by the microadenoma is possible. An example is the hyperprolactinemia of prolactin microadenomas. More common are endocrine deficits due to intrasellar pressure effects. Examples are the cortisol and gonadal hormone deficits due to pressure effects on pituitary structures producing adrenocorticotropic hormone and the gonadotropins. Often, if cortisol deficits exist there are inordinate responses to stresses of any sort, especially to fevers associated with relatively minor infections. A shock like syndrome can develop in such patients.

Long-term corticosteroids are usually given for chronic obstructive lung disease or for immunosuppression after allogeneic transplantation and one result is decreased endogenous corticosteroid production. Because of this failure of endogenous hormone production patients on prolonged oral corticosteroid therapy need additional oral or intravenous corticosteroids when there is stress: from infections or other diseases; from trauma; and before any surgery is performed. Unless this additional corticosteroid is given development of a hazardous shock-like syndrome is possible.

Deficits or over-productions of adrenal hormones, growth hormone , or ovarian or testicular hormones are uncommon. They present as hyperfunction or hypofunction syndromes of dysfunction.

The description of endocrine dysfunctions in this chapter is restricted to the more common ones. Given the limitations of space and the objectives of this book it would not be possible to do more. If the physician cannot identify or deal with the presenting problem it suffices to feel that an endocrine dysfunction probably exists. Help is readily available in standard texts, in CD-ROMs and the Internet, and especially, from colleagues and specialists.

There are two principal groups of endocrine control systems. One group is autonomous and not subject to CNS control. The other is controlled by the CNS.

The autonomous endocrine control systems.

There are five important autonomous endocrine control systems: **the insulin-glucagon system, the renin-angiotensin-aldosterone complex, the atrial naturiuretic hormone-angiotensin interaction, the parathyroid hormone-serum ionized calcium system, and the erythropoietin-red cell maturation interaction.** Usually these five systems are not affected by CNS commands, perhaps because they themselves are requisites for normal CNS activity and nerve impulse transmission. They ensure that blood sugar, blood pressure and serum ionized calcium levels are within physiologically desirable levels, and that the blood contains a sufficiency of hemoglobin-containing erythrocytes. Their roles were summarized in Chart 5-11 on page 110.

There are many additional minor autonomous endocrine control systems. Examples are the systems that control gastrin and other intestinal secretions. Even though these autonomous endocrine systems are not controlled by CNS centers their effects are perceived by these centers and, when necessary, the CNS can make appropriate functional modifications. Most are only of importance for the local secretory activities of glandular tissue, especially the enzymes secreted in the gastrointestinal tract.

Control of the functions of the autonomous peripheral endocrine systems is by simple positive and negative feedback control mechanisms. When there is an excess of product the catalyzing enzyme of the reaction is inhibited. If there is decrease in product the reverse occurs. Things can get complicated as many reactions can be linked to each other by different positive and negative feedback systems (Chart 7-3).

The insulin-glucagon system.

The insulin-glucagon interaction was depicted in Chart 4-7 on page 90. An important object of the system is to ensure that the brain will have sufficient glucose for its needs. Glucose is the only substrate that the brain can use to produce energy (~P) that is usable for its biochemical reactions and biological activities. Some ketones can be used after a period of starvation. Persistent insulin deficits result in diabetes mellitus. The blood sugar is raised, probably because an important and possibly principal effect of insulin is promotion of glucose transport into cells.

Conversely, when blood sugar is too low, (a frequent cause is injection of insulin in excess of needs) hypoglycemia develops. Initially there is sweating, dizziness, tremors and some confusion. If untreated by injections of glucose or glucagon there may be progression to seizures, coma and finally, death. Estimation of blood glucose is an immediate imperative in the clinical assessment of any comatose patient, especially if there is no obvious cause for the coma.

The renin-angiotensin-aldosterone complex.

The physiology of this system complex is depicted in Chart 7-1 on the next page. Products of renin release from the kidney are angiotensin II and III. Both are potent vasoconstrictors and stimulators of aldosterone synthesis. Angiotensin II is a more potent vasoconstrictor than angiotensin III. When intravascular volume decreases and blood pressure falls both angiotensin II and III supplement vasoconstriction mediated by the immediate neural response to hypovolemia and may substitute for it if brain function is compromised.

Inhibitors of angiotensin converting enzyme (ACE inhibitors) and blockers of the angiotensin receptor (Losartan potassium - Cozaar) are frequently used to control blood pressure. They are useful in treating hypertension and congestive heart failure because they reduce peripheral resistance and thus decrease cardiac preload and afterload. They are especially valuable in treating right heart failure in individuals with advanced chronic obstructive lung disease. Giving beta-blockers to these patients is hazardous. At times, beta blockers that are said to be cardio-selective blockers at β_1 receptors can have some blocking effects on β_2 lung receptors and worsen the effects of any existing lung pathology.

Atrial naturiuretic peptide (ANP).

It is difficult to evaluate the role of ANP in controlling this system. ANP (**de Bold, A.J., Borenstein, H.B. et al.** A rapid and potent naturiuretic response to intravenous injection of atrial myocardial extract in rats. Life Sci. 1981; 5:28) is produced by atrial myocytes in response to atrial distention and also blood angiotensin II. It inhibits release or actions of aldosterone, angiotensin II and renin. It also increases salt and water excretion. Thus ANP could be a feedback reflex control system that modulates the the productions and effects of the renin-angiotensin-aldosterone complex.

Parathyroid hormone and serum ionized calcium.

This system ensures that diffusible ionized calcium levels in the blood do not transgress the physiologically desirable levels needed for normal neural transmission and muscle contraction. Low levels of Ca^{++} increases excitation of nerve and muscle cells, for example, after intended or inadvertent parathyroidectomy. One consequence of lower than desirable blood levels of serum Ca^{++} is tetany, a condition characterized by diffuse contractions of skeletal muscle. Asphyxiation from laryngeal spasm is an ever present danger when tetany occurs.

Calcitonin has not been mentioned as part of this complex. Its role in human biology is controversial. The hormone may have a role in controlling osteoclast activity but there is controversy about its role in maintaining serum ionized Ca^{++} levels. Calcitonin is produced by the parafollicular cells of the thyroid but total thyroidec-

Chart 7-1: THE RENIN-ANGIOTENSIN-ALDOSTERONE COMPLEX

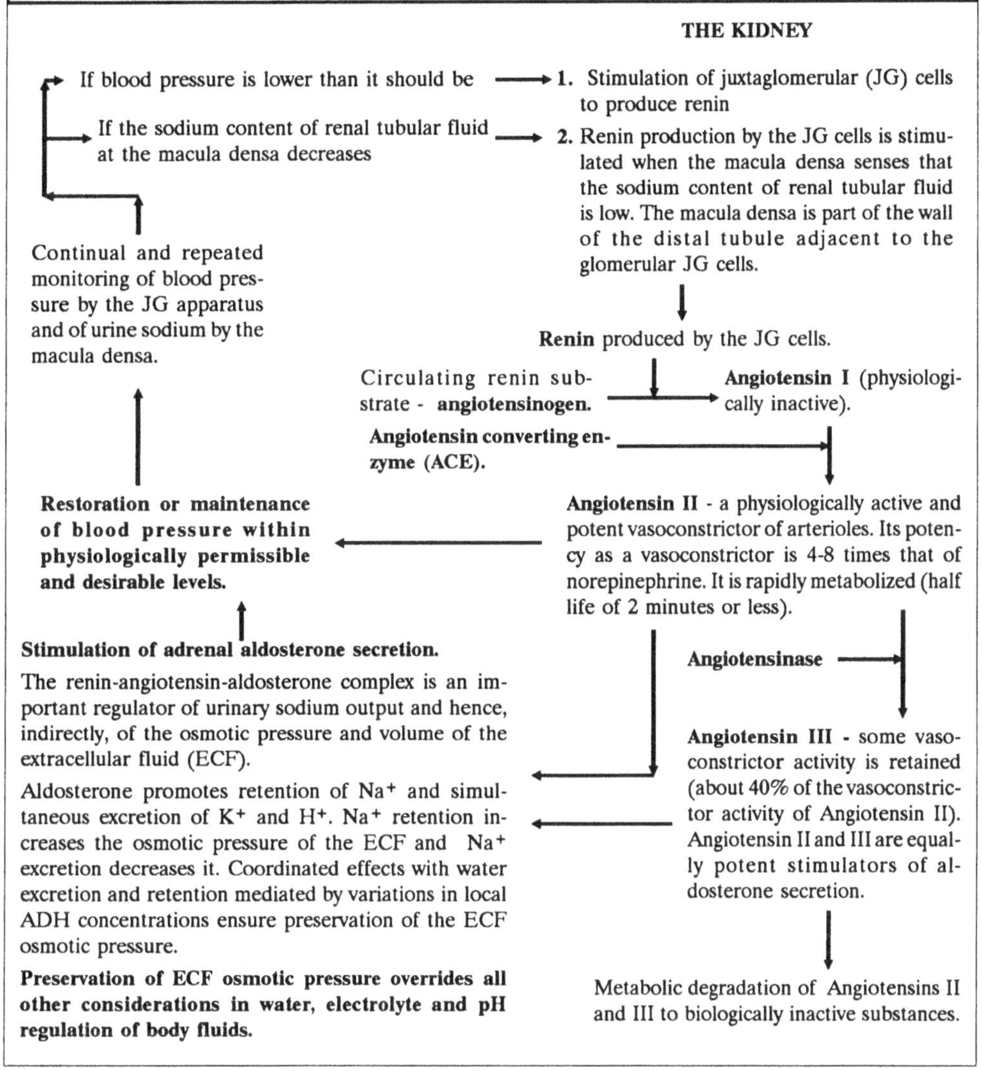
THE KIDNEY
If blood pressure is lower than it should be
1. Stimulation of juxtaglomerular (JG) cells to produce renin
If the sodium content of renal tubular fluid at the macula densa decreases
2. Renin production by the JG cells is stimulated when the macula densa senses that the sodium content of renal tubular fluid is low. The macula densa is part of the wall of the distal tubule adjacent to the glomerular JG cells.
Continual and repeated monitoring of blood pressure by the JG apparatus and of urine sodium by the macula densa.
Renin produced by the JG cells.
Circulating renin substrate - angiotensinogen.
Angiotensin I (physiologically inactive).
Angiotensin converting enzyme (ACE).
Restoration or maintenance of blood pressure within physiologically permissible and desirable levels.
Angiotensin II - a physiologically active and potent vasoconstrictor of arterioles. Its potency as a vasoconstrictor is 4-8 times that of norepinephrine. It is rapidly metabolized (half life of 2 minutes or less).
Stimulation of adrenal aldosterone secretion.
The renin-angiotensin-aldosterone complex is an important regulator of urinary sodium output and hence, indirectly, of the osmotic pressure and volume of the extracellular fluid (ECF).
Aldosterone promotes retention of Na+ and simultaneous excretion of K+ and H+. Na+ retention increases the osmotic pressure of the ECF and Na+ excretion decreases it. Coordinated effects with water excretion and retention mediated by variations in local ADH concentrations ensure preservation of the ECF osmotic pressure.
Preservation of ECF osmotic pressure overrides all other considerations in water, electrolyte and pH regulation of body fluids.
Angiotensinase
Angiotensin III - some vasoconstrictor activity is retained (about 40% of the vasoconstrictor activity of Angiotensin II). Angiotensin II and III are equally potent stimulators of aldosterone secretion.
Metabolic degradation of Angiotensins II and III to biologically inactive substances.

tomy does not affect serum ionized Ca^{++} levels as long as the parathyroids are intact. Additionally, alterations in serum ionized Ca^{++} are uncommon in patients with medullary carcinoma of the thyroid, despite frequent coexistence of high levels of circulating calcitonin. Medullary carcinoma of the thyroid is a tumor of calcitonin-producing parafollicular thyroid cells.

Calcitonin can inhibit osteoclast activity. It has been used in postmenopausal women with osteoporosis to reduce the incidence of vertebral fractures. A small effect was seen but there was little reduction in the incidence of peripheral fractures (**Chesnut, C.H. 3rd., Silverman, S., et al.**: A randomized trial of nasal spray salmon calcitonin in postmenopausal women with established osteoporosis: the prevent recurrence of osteoporotic fractures study. Am. J. Med., 109:267, 2000.).

The erythropoietin-red cell complex.

Erythropoietin is a hormone produced in the kidney. The marrow requires erythropoietin for maturation of stem cells and erythrocyte precursors to reticulocytes that then leave the marrow, enter the circulation, and eventually become mature erythrocytes. The locus at which erythropoietin promotes red cell maturation is

Chart 7-2: THE ERYTHROPOIETIN-RED CELL MATURATION COMPLEX

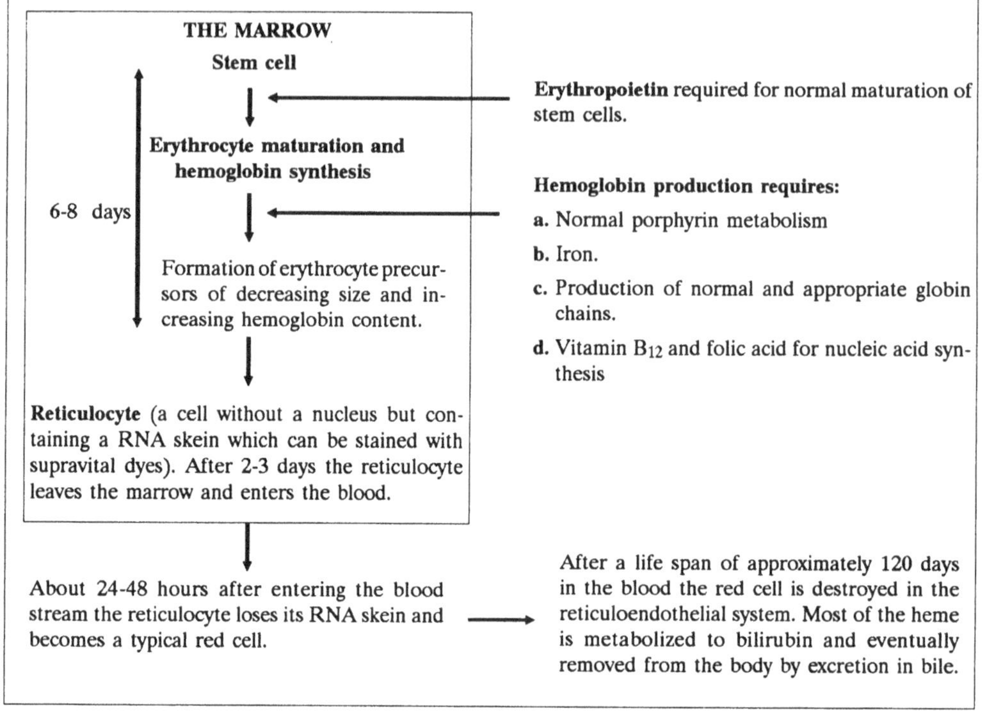
THE MARROW
Stem cell
Erythrocyte maturation and hemoglobin synthesis
6-8 days
Formation of erythrocyte precursors of decreasing size and increasing hemoglobin content.
Reticulocyte (a cell without a nucleus but containing a RNA skein which can be stained with supravital dyes). After 2-3 days the reticulocyte leaves the marrow and enters the blood.
Erythropoietin required for normal maturation of stem cells.
Hemoglobin production requires:
a. Normal porphyrin metabolism
b. Iron.
c. Production of normal and appropriate globin chains.
d. Vitamin B12 and folic acid for nucleic acid synthesis
About 24-48 hours after entering the blood stream the reticulocyte loses its RNA skein and becomes a typical red cell.
After a life span of approximately 120 days in the blood the red cell is destroyed in the reticuloendothelial system. Most of the heme is metabolized to bilirubin and eventually removed from the body by excretion in bile.

indicated in Chart 7-2 on the next page.

Proof of the effects of this hormone is found in individuals with advanced renal failure where erythropoietin production is decreased and there is a concomitant anemia that can be partially reversed by injections of synthetic erythropoietin. An additional component in these patients is the so-called "anemia of chronic disease". This ends a summary of the autonomous peripheral endocrine control systems.

One speculates that these five control systems are autonomous of CNS control because they themselves are designed to preserve CNS function by ensuring that the brain has adequate quantities of glucose, a blood pressure that provides sufficient brain perfusion, serum ionized calcium levels that are within the physiologically permissible levels for accurate transmission of nerve impulses, and a system that, in the long-term, provides an adequacy of hemoglobin-containing erythrocytes. If these systems were dependent on CNS control they would not be able to restore or support deteriorating CNS function.

Diabetes mellitus.

Diabetes is the most common endocrine dysfunction. The diagnosis of diabetes mellitus is made when the fasting (for 8-12 hours) plasma glucose level exceeds 6.6-7mmol/L (SI units) or 60-110mg/dl in conventional units. Typical symptoms include thirst, weight loss, excessive urination and hunger. The cause of diabetes mellitus is a deficit of effective insulin. The main principal causes of this deficit are insufficient circulating insulin or an intracellular deficit of insulin which depends on the the availability and avidity of cell wall receptors for insulin. An important if not main function of insulin is promotion of intracellular glucose ingress. There are two principal types of diabetes mellitus:

Non-insulin dependent diabetes (NIDD).

This is the more common form. Most of the patients are obese, do little exercise and are older than about 45 years. Blood insulin levels are often normal or higher than normal. Patients should be advised to exercise and diet as these increase the numbers and avidities of the insulin receptors. Unfortunately the patient often does not comply with advice. Failure to lose enough weight may require oral hypoglycemics or insulin. Eventual exhaustion of endogenous insulin production will result in an insulin-dependent state.

NIDD is occasionally seen in young people. Most are associated with obesity. At this age symptoms include infections such as vaginitis and acne. One type, "maturity-onset diabetes of the young", is said to be inherited as an autosomal dominant.

Insulin-dependent diabetes (IDD).

About 10% of diabetics have IDD. It is a disease of youth but can develop suddenly at any age. The cause is said to be antibodies directed against the beta cells of the pancreas. Some consider it an autoimmune disease with a complex of virus and beta cell acting as the antigen. Many viruses have been implicated as causative. In addition diabetes is associated with many autoimmune diseases. IDD and an associated ketoacidosis can develop suddenly and rapidly.

The mechanisms of ketoacidosis were depicted in Chart 4-9, page 91. The ketones are strong acids and are excreted as their sodium and potassium salts. Because of the osmotic diuresis there is hypovolemia and a raised blood urea and creatinine.

The clinical features of ketoacidosis are characteristic. Overpowering thirst, air hunger, and often, nausea and vomiting. The breath has a typical sweet and fruity odor and the patient is drowsy and inattentive, responds to questions with confused and inappropriate responses and may, on occasion, drift into a coma. There is hypotension and breathing is by deep gasps through the open mouth.

It is essential to try and determine the cause for the keto-acidosis. Was the patient a diabetic needing insulin? Was the insulin stopped because of financial difficulties or for any one or more other reasons? Is there any intercurrent infection? Microscopic examination of the urine and a chest X-ray are essentials. Treatment is rehydration with fluid and sodium, intravenous insulin as required and potassium as and when needed. Requirements for potassium are best assessed by estimations of serum potassium and regular monitoring by ECGs. The development of hypokalemia or hyperkalemia is difficult to predict by clinical bedside assessments alone.

The complications of diabetes mellitus.

Most complications of diabetes are the result of vascular stenoses and occlusions and microangiopathies of the retina and kidney capillaries and atheromatous lesions in larger vessels.. Atheroma may result in coronary artery stenoses and their related symptomatologies. When the limb vessels are affected common consequences are intermittent claudication, ischemic changes in the feet and toes, infections, and wounds that do not heal and often eventuate in gangrene and finally, amputations.

Diabetic retinopathy is a frequent cause of blindness and visual dysfunctions and a dreaded complication. It results from a selective retinal capillary microangiopathy. The main pathological lesions in the capillaries of the retina and kineys are segmental thickenings of the basement membrane thickenings with focal ruptures and areas of ischemia. In places the capillary wall cells degenerate and in some areas a loss of endothelial cells are demonstrable. Small retinal hemorrhages and microaneurysms are common, presumably because of the weakness of vessel walls. New blood vessels grow from the retina into the vitreous humor and many then rupture. The subsequent fibrosis can detach the retina adding to existing problems. Diabetic retinopathy is a common cause of blindness. The availability of laser coagulation has altered the prognosis and it is said that good metabolic control of diabetes will delay the onset of retinopathy. This is disputed by some.

An angiopathy similar to that of diabetic microangiopathy is said to be responsible for the pathological changes in the Kimmelstiel-Wilson nephropathy.

Other vascular dysfunctions. Diabetes also promotes development of atheromas.

Neuropathies. The neuropathies may be mononeural or multineural in distribution. They result from neural vascular insufficiencies and/or intraneural infarcts. Loss of peripheral sensations often result in wounds that do not heal and chronic ulcers that may be extensive enough or disabling and painful enough to require amputation of an affected limb. Another distressing consequence of a diabetic neuropathy is impotence in males. The neuropathies can affect any one or more nerves and the dysfunctions that result can affect any one or more innervated structures. Diabetic neuropathies are often painful.

Diabetic renal disease. Dysfunctions and renal failure may result from glomerular lesions, from repeated pyelonephritis or from stenoses or occlusions of renal vessels by atheroma. The typical lesions of glomerulosclerosis are a hyaline arteriolar sclerosis involving both afferent and efferent arterioles. It is accompanied by hypertension.

In some patients there is a nodular glomerulosclerosis (Kimmelstiel-Wilson kidney) due to large deposits of basement membrane matrix in the mesangium. Clinically, there are various combinations of proteinuria, hypertension, the nephrotic syndrome and finally, uremia.

Therapy for diabetes mellitus.

There is evidence that good control of diabetes will reduce the incidence of complications though this is disputed by some who maintain that good control does not reduce the incidence of complications.

The current generation of sulfonylureas include glyburide, glimepiride and glipizide. They stimulate insulin release from the pancreas.

An option is a biguanide such as glucophage. The biguanides act by promoting insulin-mediated suppression of hepatic glucose production and by increasing glucose uptake by skeletal muscle. They seldom produce hypoglycemic episodes as they do not increase insulin release from the pancreas. The main site of action is the liver and they should be given with caution if there is any significant hepatic dysfunction.

Finally, if control is unsatisfactory and more medication cannot be given self administration of an appropriate insulin is necessary. The different types of insulin available are well described in standard texts.

Chart 7-3: HYPOTHALAMIC AND PITUITARY CONTROLS

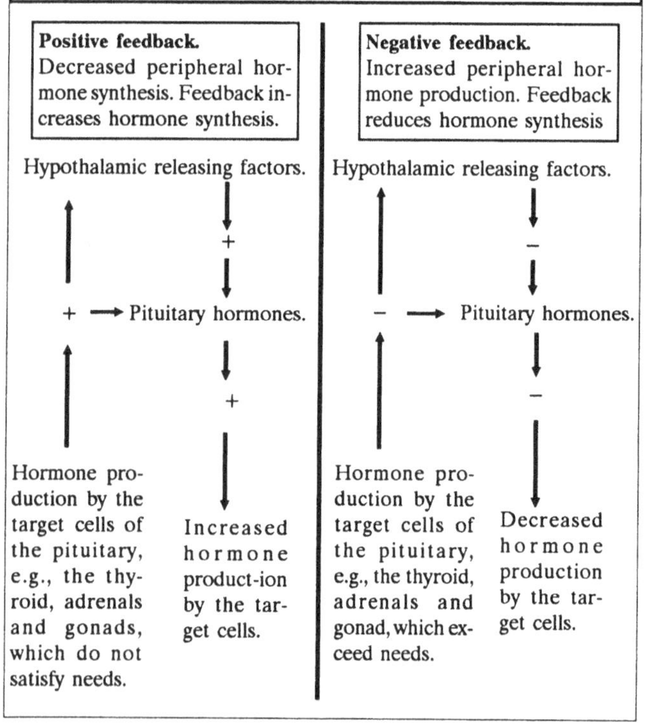
Positive feedback.
Decreased peripheral hormone synthesis. Feedback increases hormone synthesis.
Hypothalamic releasing factors.
+
+
Pituitary hormones.
+
Hormone production by the target cells of the pituitary, e.g., the thyroid, adrenals and gonads, which do not satisfy needs.
Increased hormone product-ion by the target cells.
Negative feedback.
Increased peripheral hormone production. Feedback reduces hormone synthesis
Hypothalamic releasing factors.
–
–
Pituitary hormones.
–
Hormone production by the target cells of the pituitary, e.g., the thyroid, adrenals and gonad, which exceed needs.
Decreased hormone production by the target cells.

Endocrine systems subordinate to the CNS.

Hypothalamic control.

The hypothalamus produces two hormones and many releasing factors. It receives:

- Afferent information about all body systems via the autonomic nervous system.
- Neural commands from cerebral centers and from the medullary cardiac, vasomotor and respiratory centers.
- Feedbacks from the blood levels of pituitary hormones and the products of their targets: thyroid, adrenal, gonadal and other hormones.

Control of hypothalamic production of hormones is by complex positive and negative feedbacks from the products of the pituitary targets.

Chart 7-3 summarizes the mechanisms of pituitary and hypothalamic feedback controls of hormone production by the targets of pituitary hormones; for example, the thyroid, the adrenals, the gonads and other targets.

Chapter 7-4 presents in summary form the complex interactions of hypothalamic hormones and releasing factors, with pituitary hormones and the products of the targets of pituitary hormones. It is a copy of Chart 5-10 on page 109 but is reproduced here for the convenience of the reader. **(Contd. on page 164)**

Chart 7-4: HYPOTHALAMIC HORMONES AND RELEASING FACTORS, PITUITARY HORMONES AND THE PRODUCTS OF THEIR TARGETS - THYROXINE, ADRENAL HORMONES AND GONADAL HORMONES.

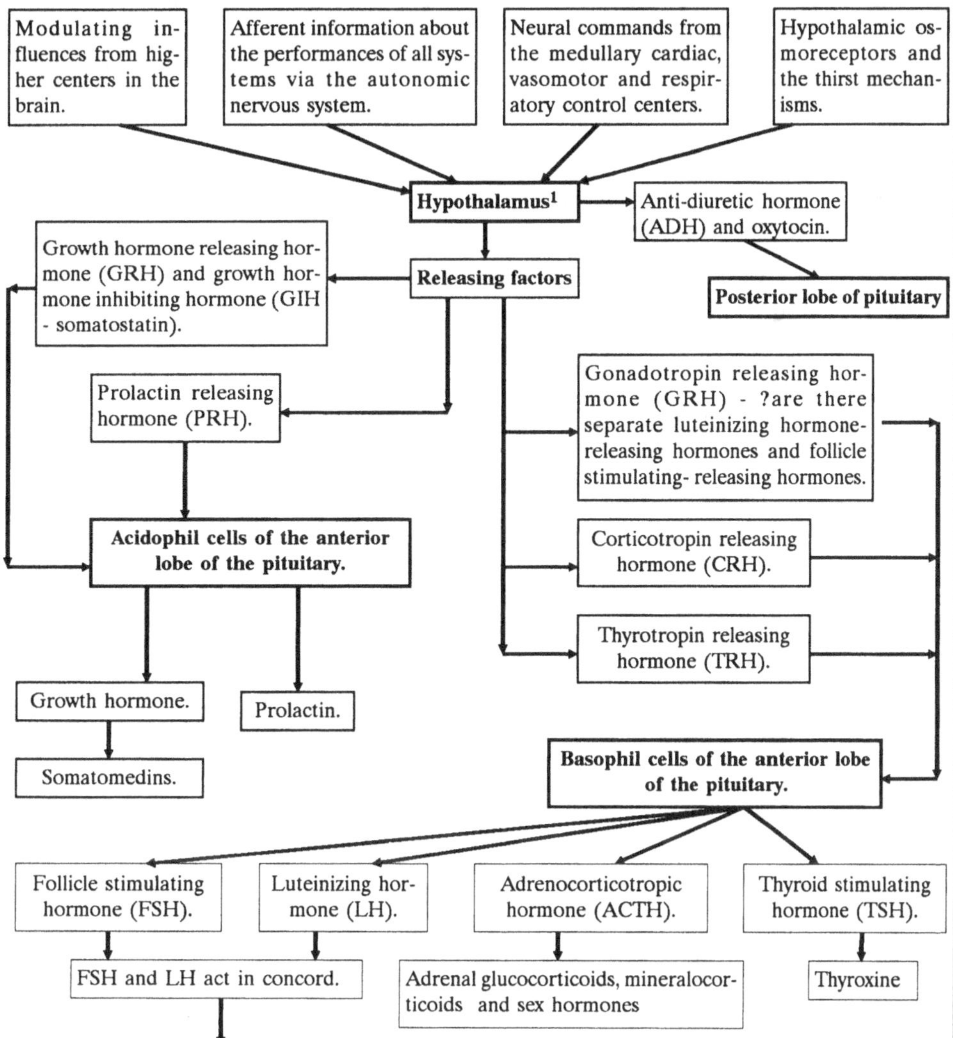
Modulating influences from higher centers in the brain.
Afferent information about the performances of all systems via the autonomic nervous system.
Neural commands from the medullary cardiac, vasomotor and respiratory control centers.
Hypothalamic osmoreceptors and the thirst mechanisms.
Hypothalamus[1]
Anti-diuretic hormone (ADH) and oxytocin.
Posterior lobe of pituitary
Releasing factors
Growth hormone releasing hormone (GRH) and growth hormone inhibiting hormone (GIH - somatostatin).
Prolactin releasing hormone (PRH).
Gonadotropin releasing hormone (GRH) - ?are there separate luteinizing hormone-releasing hormones and follicle stimulating- releasing hormones.
Acidophil cells of the anterior lobe of the pituitary.
Corticotropin releasing hormone (CRH).
Thyrotropin releasing hormone (TRH).
Growth hormone.
Prolactin.
Somatomedins.
Basophil cells of the anterior lobe of the pituitary.
Follicle stimulating hormone (FSH).
Luteinizing hormone (LH).
Adrenocorticotropic hormone (ACTH).
Thyroid stimulating hormone (TSH).
FSH and LH act in concord.
Adrenal glucocorticoids, mineralocorticoids and sex hormones
Thyroxine

1 **In females:** FSH and LH act sequentially on the ovary during the menstrual cycle. FSH promotes estrogen secretion and development of the ovarian follicle. After ovulation estrogen secretion decreases and LH secretion increases with promotion of progesterone production and development of the corpus luteum. If pregnancy results the placenta secretes human chorionic gonadotropin (measured as β-HCG) as well as estrogen and progesterone.

2 **In males:** LH promotes secretion of testosterone by the interstitial Leydig cells of the testis. Testosterone is required for normal spermatogenesis and for maintenance of the secondary sex characteristics of males. FSH maintains the seminiferous tubules and promotes spermatogenesis by converting the primary spermatocytes to secondary spermatocytes. Testosterone is a requisite for the final maturation of sperms and also stimulates seminiferous tubule growth.

1 There is continual feedback control of as-needed hormone production by the final target cell products (thyroxine, corticosteroids, FSH, LH, and ADH) on the one hand and the hypothalamic releasing factors, pituitary hormones, and hypothalamic osmoreceptors on the other.

(Contd. from page 162)

Hypothalamic hormones.

Hormones produced in the hypothalamus.

The **hormones** are **vasopressin (anti-diuretic hormone - commonly called ADH) and oxytocin.** They are packaged as granules that pass to the posterior pituitary via the axons of hypothalamic neurons. When the neurons are stimulated the granules are released from the axon terminals and hormone diffuses into adjacent capillaries and thus reaches the target cell membranes and receptors. ADH acts on the distal nephron and the collecting ducts of the kidney. It is an important regulator of water balance (discussed in detail in a later chapter on water and electrolyte balance - Chart 13-7, page 300). Control of production and release of ADH is by feeback reflexes between cerebral thirst systems and hypothalamic osmoreceptors on the one hand and osmotic pressure of blood which perfuses them on the other.

Hypothalamic "releasing factors".

Releasing factors produced in the hypothalamus are:

— **Thyrotropin releasing hormone (TRH)** which stimulates production of pituitary thyroid stimulating hormone (TSH). TSH stimulates thyroxine production by the thyroid. Control of thyroxine production is determined by feedback reactions between TSH, and TRH on the one hand and thyroxine and triiodothyronine on the other.

— **Corticotropin releasing hormone (CRH)** which stimulates adrenocorticotropic hormone (ACTH) release from the pituitary. ACTH stimulates both corticosteroid and mineralocorticoid production by adrenal cortical cells. Mineralocorticoid production is also increased by excess blood potassium and by angiotensin. In fact, many suggest that angiotensin is the most potent of the stimulators of aldosterone synthesis. Control of corticosteroid production depends on feedback reflexes between blood corticosteroids on the one hand and the hypothalamic releasing factor and pituitary ACTH on the other.

— **Prolactin releasing hormone** stimulates specific pituitary cells to produce prolactin. A prolactin inhibiting factor is also thought to exist because pituitary stalk section increases prolactin section.

— **Gonadotropin releasing hormone** which stimulates FSH and LH production by the pituitary. Both, FSH and LH act on the gonads and genitalia of both sexes.

— **Growth hormone releasing hormone** which stimulates release of growth hormone and growth hormone-inhibiting hormone (somatostatin) which blocks growth hormone release from the pituitary. Growth hormone promotes lipolysis and also stimulates somatomedin production, primarily in the liver. Somatomedin stimulates protein, DNA and RNA synthesis. Growth hormone by itself probably has little direct effect on growth promotion. The main end organs of the pituitary are the thyroid, the adrenals and the gonads and their main products are thyroxine, adrenal steroids and gonadal hormones.

The following hormones are synthesized in the pituitary:

From the acidophil cells.

— Growth hormone and Prolactin.

From the basophil cells.

— Thyroid stimulating hormone (TSH) which stimulates thyroid hormone production by the thyroid.

— Adrenocorticotropic hormone (ACTH) which stimulates steroid synthesis in the adrenals and

— Luteinizing hormone (LH), and follicle stimulating hormone (FSH) which control production of gonadal hormones.

Synthesis of each of the above hormones are regulated by simple feedback systems summarized in Chart 7-3.

The following are hormones produced by the target cells of pituitary hormones.

Thyroxine.

Thyroxine promotes metabolic activity in almost all cells. In the body it comes in two forms: T4 and T3. Control of production is by positive and negative feedbacks with pituitary TSH and hypothalamic TRH. The normal thyroid secretes T4 and only small amounts of T3. Most of the circulating T3 is derived from T4 metabolism outside the thyroid. Most of the thyroid hormones in the circulation are bound to protein, mainly thyroglobulin. It is the unbound fractions that are biologically active.

Hyperthyroid disease.

Symptoms suggestive of **hyperthyroid dysfunction** are fatigue, loss of weight despite an increased appetite and intake, nervousness and excitability, tremors, a characteristic stare, lid lag and sometimes exophthalmos, tachycardia, palpitations and even atrial fibrillation. Physical examination and laboratory studies are diagnostic; an increased T4 and/or T3, a low TSH and a radionuclear study showing generalized or focal increased uptake of iodine. Common causes are autonomous hyperactivity of the whole gland or of a single nodule or tumor, benign or malignant. Treatment is simple and gratifying. Blocking of thyroxine synthesis by an oral thiourylene (propylthiouracil is an example), with ablation by radioactive iodine for those who want this as primary therapy, and for those patients who do not respond to or are intolerant of oral thiourylenes. Surgery is needed for any autonomous benign or malignant lesion causing the hyperthyroidism. If there is a palpable nodule a needle biopsy is advisable before any decision on therapy.

Hypothyroidism.

Hypothyroid disease is a common condition and also one easily missed. Blood TSH is raised but before making a diagnosis of hypothyroid disease it is necessary to be sure that blood free T4 and total T3 are reduced. It has been my experience that many elderly people have high TSH levels but normal blood levels of thyroid hormones. Perhaps with advancing years higher levels of TSH are required to drive thyroid tissue to produce normal hormone levels. Giving thyroxine to an individual who is not hypothyroid can result in the symptoms of hyperthyroidism. This is especially dangerous in the elderly because of possible cardiac dysfunctions, especially atrial fibrillation and hypertension.

The symptoms and signs of hypothyroid disease are rather non-specific. The individual is usually lethargic, somewhat obese, and slow in intellectual and motor activity and responses. There is intolerance of cold and a poor appetite. The response to hormone replacement therapy is usually gratifying.

Hypothyroid disease in children is called **cretinism** and may be the result of a congenital defect of thyroid development or iodine deficiency during pregnancy. A deficiency of iodide in remote areas of the world is a frequent cause of hypothyroid disease and cretinism. Children born to iodine deficient mothers have retarded mental development. Their physical characteristics should arouse suspicion; short stature, a protruding tongue, broad flat nose, widely set eyes and not much hair on the head are fairly typical. If discovered early enough thyroid extract and iodine supplementation throughout life may improve the mental deficit.

Universal salt iodinization was started in 1993 and now some 50 countries have salt iodination programs. Almost 5 billion inhabitants of this planet now have access to iodized salt. Global rates of goiter, mental retardation and cretinism are falling rapidly.

Hashimoto's disease is probably an autoimmune response directed against thyroglobulin in the thyroid. It often results in adult hypothyroid disease. The disease is readily diagnosable by the cytology of needle aspirations but is easily missed because of the rather nonspecific clinical picture. This is unfortunate as it results in a patient with chronic and undiagnosed tiredness from a disease that is easily treated by hormone replacement therapy. Equally important is that any form of hypothyroidism can have unpleasant cardiac accompaniments. They are detailed in the Chapter on Cardiovascular dysfunctions (Chapter 9).

As mentioned previously, hyperthyroid and hypothyroid disease are often symptomless in the initial stages. When untreated or inadequately treated, both can result in major cardiovascular and neurological problems. The corollary is that the wary physician needs to exclude thyroid dysfunction when faced with a difficult clinical problem; the problem could be an accompaniment or an immediate or long-term consequence of the dysfunction.

Adrenal cortex hormones.

The production and control of adrenal hormones is complex. Three groups of hormones are synthesized: the glucocorticoids, mineralocorticoids, and the sex hormones, testosterone and estradiol. Chart 7-5 summarizes the facts. The principal **glucocorticoid** is cortisol. Its production is controlled by variations in ACTH synthesis resulting from positive and negative feedbacks reactions involving the pituitary and hypothalamic releasing factors. The glucocorticoids promote hepatic glycogen synthesis and hepatic gluconeogenesis, mostly from the glycogenic amino acids of protein. They have an anti-insulin effect in peripheral tissues but not in the brain

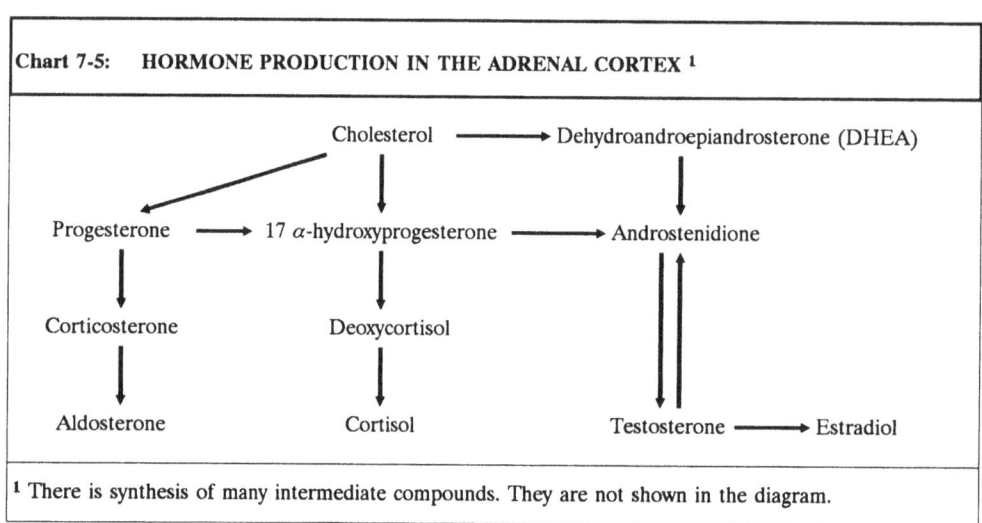

Chart 7-5: HORMONE PRODUCTION IN THE ADRENAL CORTEX [1]

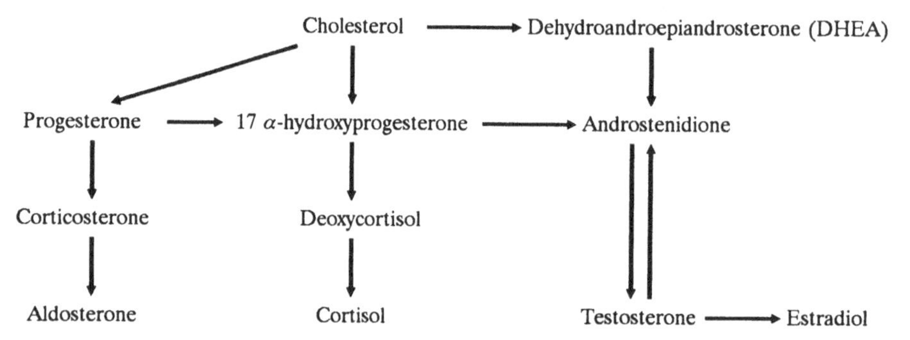
Cholesterol
Dehydroandroepiandrosterone (DHEA)
Progesterone
17 α-hydroxyprogesterone
Androstenidione
Corticosterone
Deoxycortisol
Aldosterone
Cortisol
Testosterone
Estradiol

[1] There is synthesis of many intermediate compounds. They are not shown in the diagram.

or heart so that glucose available to these two organs is not reduced. Corticosteroids also inhibits inflammatory and immunological reactions and promote feelings of "well-being".

Cushing's syndrome and Cushing's disease.

About 70% are due to bilateral adrenal hyperplasia. About 25% have adrenal tumors; both benign as well as malignant tumors. The remainder have autonomous ACTH secreting pituitary tumors. A hyperadrenal syndrome caused by pituitary ACTH-secreting tumors is called Cushing's disease as this was the syndrome of adrenal hormone dysfunction originally described by Harvey Cushing. The other forms of adrenal hypersecretion are usually called Cushing's syndromes. Ultrasounds and CT scans are diagnostic as well as a raised urinary free cortisol. Ectopic ACTH secretion, that is, ACTH over-production for no obvious reasons, is often a paraneoplastic condition that requires a complete physical examination to exclude malignancy, if one is not already present.

Patients with Cushing's disease or syndrome have hypertension because the large amounts of corticosteroids present often have additional aldosterone-like effects which cause sodium and water retentions. Their anti-insulin effects result in diabetes, and patients have an obesity that affects the trunk but not the extremities. There is often muscle wasting and proximal myopathy as well as ecchymoses due to skin fragility. Hypercholesterolemia is common and so is the osteoporosis that results from antagonism of 1,25-dihydroxycholecalciferol. Reduction of 1,25-dihydroxycholecalciferol activity decreases calcium absorption and reduces the activation of bone cells. A secondary hyperparathyroidism and osteopenia can develop and result in vertebral body collapses. Androgen excess is not uncommon and may result in feminine virilism and amenorrhea. Therapy depends on the cause. The patient will often need surgery for tumors and hyperplasias.

Addison's disease.

Addison's disease results from adrenal insufficiency and can result from any one of many causes. Most are idiopathic and these are often attributed to autoimmune reactions. Some are caused by tuberculosis and a variety of other pathogens. Other causes include amyloid disease, hemochromatosis and malignant disease. Addison's disease can also result from pituitary microadenomas that decrease ACTH secretion because of pressure. An uncommon cause is a hypothalamic disorder that interferes with CRH secretion.

The principal adrenal mineralocorticoid is aldosterone. It regulates ECF volume and potassium content by an action at the distal nephron and the renal collecting ducts. It promotes Na^+ reabsorption and K^+excretion. Sodium retention results in water retention in order to preserve ECF osmotic pressure. Control of aldosterone production is by feedback mechanisms involving the juxtaglomerular apparatus and the macula densa.

In Addison's disease there are deficiencies of mineralocorticoids and glucocorticoids. Weight loss, salt deficits and hypoglycemia are common. A prolonged period without food can result in serious hypoglycemia. The blood pressure is low because of the hyponatremia.

It is uncommon for salt deficits caused by an excess of diuretics or abnormal gastrointestinal losses to reduce serum sodium levels. They are assumed from changes in the volume of extracellular fluid as reflected in a raised hematocrit. A decreased serum sodium level suggests significantly greater sodium loss. When there is such a decrease one should always consider Addison's disease or ectopic and often paraneoplastic hypersecretion of ADH which results in dilutional hyponatremia.

In Addison's disease minor infections often result in shock-like symptoms. There may be a diffuse tan all over the body because of MSH over-production and there is increased pigmentation in scars and skin creases, in the ano-genital regions and the areolae. The skin looks dirty at pressure points such as the knees and elbows. The heart is small and postural hypotension and dizziness are common.

Treatment consists of rehydration with water and salt, and hormone replacement therapy. The pigmentations often persist for long periods.

The adrenogenital syndromes.

These syndromes are often congenital and result in children born with anatomical abnormalities that make determination of the gender difficult. Treatment is ACTH suppression by glucocorticoids and this can be difficult in children where a fine balance must be maintained between too little and too much.

In adults the usual causes of adrenogenital syndromes are adrenal adenomas or carcinomas or adrenal hyperplasia, often with associated Cushingoid symptoms and signs. When females are affected there is virilization with hirsutism, acne, deepening voice, decreased breast size, amenorrhea and clitoral hypertrophy. For obvious reasons virilization is difficult to detect in males. However, feminization is not difficult to detect for one feature is a bilateral gynecomastia with testicular atrophy and reduction in penis size.

Growth hormone and acromegaly.

Hypothalamic growth hormone releasing hormone (GHRH) stimulates pituitary production of growth hormone and hypothalamic somatostatin inhibits it. Pituitary growth hormone stimulates hepatic IGF-1 (somatomedin C) mediated growth of bone and other tissues.

Standard texts describe many syndromes of dwarfism due to congenital failure to produce or respond to growth hormone. They are uncommon. Only one clinical condition is described here. It is acromegaly, a condition resulting from excess production of growth hormone.

Acromegaly. In some 90% of those affected acromegaly is the result of GH over-production by a benign GH-secreting pituitary adenoma. Soft tissue swelling of hands and feet are early symptoms. Gradually the bone changes alter the face. The brow and lower jaw protrude and the spacing of teeth increases. The enlarged sinuses and vocal cords result in deepening of the voice. Overgrowth of bone and cartilage result in arthritis and nerve-entrapment syndromes. The skin is thick, coarse and oily and there is weakness and headaches. When increased GH production occurs in children the long bones increase in length and there is an increase in height. In adults the epiphyseal plates have fused so that there is no increase in height.

Serious consequences are diabetes mellitus, hypertension and an increased risk of cardiac dysfunctions. The tumors may produce intrasellar compression syndromes similar to those that sometimes result from pituitary microadenomas or if large they produce extrasellar compression symptoms and signs. Examples are headaches microadenomas or if large they produce extrasellar compression symptoms and signs. Examples are headaches and visual deficits due to pressure on the chiasma and/or optic tracts.

Diagnosis is by measurement of blood IGF-1 levels. Increased levels are almost invariable in patients with acromegaly. CT scans and MRIs are useful for detecting pituitary tumors. If scans do not detect a tumor a lesion elsewhere should be suspected if the clinical features suggest acromegaly and the IGF-1 is raised.

Treatment is by drugs or if necessary by surgery when the tumors are large. Small lesions can be suppressed by bromocriptine (Parlodel - Novartis) or octreotide which is a synthetic form of somatostatin, the inhibitor of GH production.

The menstrual cycle.

In females FSH and LH act sequentially on the ovary during the menstrual cycle. FSH promotes estrogen secretion and development of the ovarian follicle and proliferative changes in the endometrium. After discharge of the ovum at about day 14 the follicle is left as a corpus luteum which produces progesterone as well as estrogen. If pregnancy results the placenta secretes human chorionic gonadotropin (measured as β-HCG) as well as estrogen and progesterone. If it does not corpus luteum secretion gradually decreases. Progesterone withdrawal results in the menstrual flow which contains blood as well as discharged endometrium.

Anovulatory cycles are common, especially as the menopause nears. Progesterone is not produced and menstruation results from bleeding as estrogen levels fall below a threshold. If infertility exists anovulatory cycles are diagnosable by low blood progesterone levels at day 25 or by an endometrial biopsy in the late part of the cycle. It will not show a secretory pattern

Infertility is a common problem. In about ⅓ the problem is a male sperm count which is abnormal. In another ⅓ the cause is a gynecological problem such as blocked fallopian tubes, endometriosis (some dispute that endometriosis causes infertility), other hormonal dysfunctions and pelvic pathology. If the sperm count and morphology is normal investigation of the female partner is desirable; an ultrasound, a blood hormone study, hystero-salpingography and endoscopic lapararoscopy are the investigative tools. Alas, in the remaining ⅓ couples no cause is demonstrable and there is much theorizing about these patients. Insemination with donor sperm, in vitro fertilization and other procedures which might help infertile couples are subjects about which I know very little. They are the final refuges for those desperate to become parents.

The sex hormones in males.

In males LH promotes secretion of testosterone by the interstitial Leydig cells of the testis. Testosterone is required for normal spermatogenesis and for maintenance of the secondary sex characteristics of males. FSH maintains the seminiferous tubules and promotes spermatogenesis by converting the primary spermatocytes to secondary spermatocytes. Testosterone is a requisite for the final maturation of sperms. It is also required for stimulation of seminiferous tubule growth.

Some other miscellaneous endocrine dysfunctions.

Iatrogenic endocrine dysfunctions.

Long-term corticosteroid administration for any one or more of a variety of clinical problems: chronic obstructive lung disease and asthma, the arthropathies, autoimmune diseases, and in transplant immunosuppression have a decreased ability to deal with infections, their wounds heal slowly, some have a Cushingoid appearance, others develop peptic ulcers, and in some there is osteoporosis and ischemic bone necroses. The last can create major problems if the upper femora are involved.

As previously mentioned, endogenous corticosteroid production is decreased when individuals are on long-term steroids for conditions such as chronic obstructive lung disease. They need more corticosteroid if an infection develops, if they are the victims of accidental or deliberate trauma, or if they need surgery.

Microadenomas of the pituitary.

Finally, a not too infrequent endocrine dysfunction is the failure of one or more aspects of pituitary function because of pituitary compression by a local adenoma or microadenoma. It is almost invariably a benign tumor and usually intrasellar. Some tumors are larger and extend to extrasellar tissues with symptoms of increased intracranial pressure and visual disturbances due to pressure on optic tracts and/or chiasma.

Microadenomas are small lesions that rarely require surgical removal. The deficiency syndromes are readily treated by hormone replacements.

Pituitary adenomas and microadenomas are readily diagnosed and treated once clinical suspicion is evoked. Some tumors produce an excess of one or other hormones (e.g., the galactorrhea produced by prolactinomas). Others make their presence known by deficient productions of one or more hormones by compressed pituitary tissue. An example of the latter is cortisol deficiency that can result in circulatory failure in a patient with an infection.

Case history.

Male aged 52 admitted to hospital because of circulatory collapse (unrecordable blood pressure and a thready and rapid pulse) associated with a fairly minor pneumonia. Blood studies showed low levels of thyroid hormones and of cortisol. There was a rapid response to hormone replacement therapy. A CT scan showed a small (0.8cm) pituitary microadenoma. No attempt was made to remove the tumor. Ten years later he remains well and stable on oral thyroxine and a monthly injection of cortisone and testosterone.

Endocrine dysfunctions due to drugs.

Any medication can result in endocrine dysfunctions. Examples are the nephrogenic diabetes insipidus that occasionally results from long-term lithium administration for psychoses. Another example is the toxic effects of chemotherapy affecting the function of one or more endocrine systems.

Other endocrine disorders related to hormone systems controlled directly or indirectly by the CNS are not detailed here. They are well described in standard texts, are many but uncommon. A physician who does not specialize in endocrinology is unlikely to see more than a few, if any, of them during a lifetime of practice. It is only necessary to recognize that the symptoms, signs and ancillary biochemical and radiological studies suggest the existence of some uncommon endocrine disorder. Such patients usually require specialized investigations and therapy from an endocrinologist.

How do hormones effect intracellular change?

This is a complex and evolving subject. It is detailed because many drugs are based on these evolving concepts. At least four different mechanisms are involved.

- The principal mechanism is one mediated by **cyclic AMP**. Chart 7-6 on the next page summarizes the basic processes. Additional text is unnecessary.
- **Thyroxine:** It is one of a group of hormones that bind to nuclear DNA and initiate specific mRNA synthesis. It stimulates the metabolisms of all cells it enters.
- **The steroid hormones:** Many steroid hormones bind to cytoplasmic receptors. The complex of hormone and receptor then binds to nuclear DNA and initiates specific mRNA synthesis. A notable example is estrogen that acts by binding to a cytoplasmic protein receptor. The complex moves into the nucleus and derepresses the part of nuclear DNA that stimulates production of the enzymes needed for synthesis of desired uterine, vaginal and breast proteins.
- **Calcium channels:** The role of intracellular calcium in skeletal muscle contraction was detailed on pages 128-130. Similar effects occur in cardiac muscle and, to a lesser degree in smooth muscle. A notable example of the last is contraction of the muscular component of the walls of arterioles.

  Various calcium channel blockers have been developed to control cardiac dysfunctions. The original ones were nifedipine, diltiazem and verapamil. They each have distinctive qualities. They do not cause bronchial constriction and are useful alternatives to beta-adrenoreceptor blocking agents in patients with chronic

Chart 7-6: CYCLIC AMP: SOME DETAILS ABOUT THE PRODUCTION AND MODE OF ACTION OF THIS IMPORTANT SECOND MESSENGER

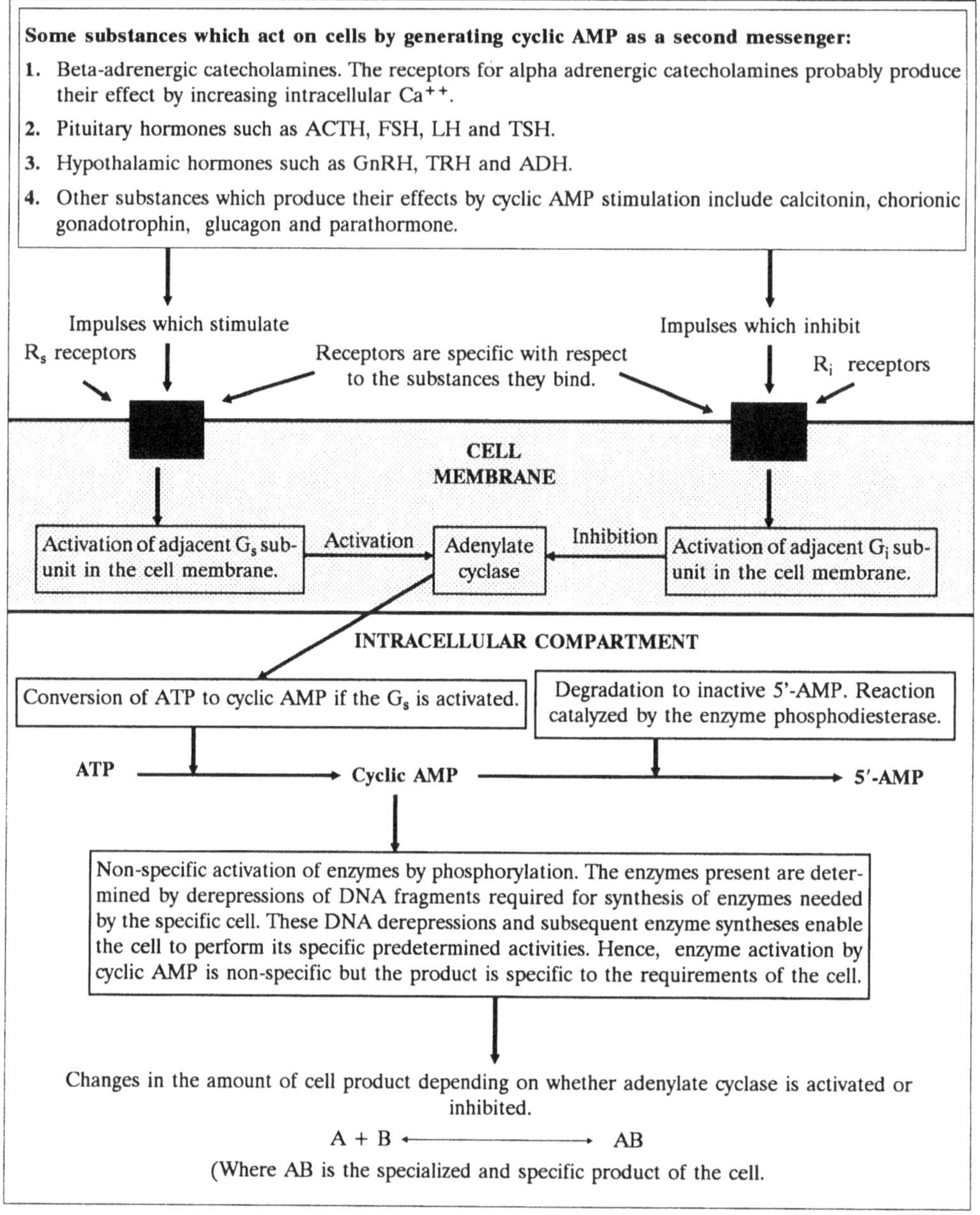
Some substances which act on cells by generating cyclic AMP as a second messenger:
1. Beta-adrenergic catecholamines. The receptors for alpha adrenergic catecholamines probably produce their effect by increasing intracellular Ca^{++}.
2. Pituitary hormones such as ACTH, FSH, LH and TSH.
3. Hypothalamic hormones such as GnRH, TRH and ADH.
4. Other substances which produce their effects by cyclic AMP stimulation include calcitonin, chorionic gonadotrophin, glucagon and parathormone.
Impulses which stimulate
R_s receptors
Receptors are specific with respect to the substances they bind.
Impulses which inhibit
R_i receptors
CELL MEMBRANE
Activation of adjacent G_s sub-unit in the cell membrane.
Activation
Adenylate cyclase
Inhibition
Activation of adjacent G_i sub-unit in the cell membrane.
INTRACELLULAR COMPARTMENT
Conversion of ATP to cyclic AMP if the G_s is activated.
Degradation to inactive 5'-AMP. Reaction catalyzed by the enzyme phosphodiesterase.
ATP
Cyclic AMP
5'-AMP
Non-specific activation of enzymes by phosphorylation. The enzymes present are determined by derepressions of DNA fragments required for synthesis of enzymes needed by the specific cell. These DNA derepressions and subsequent enzyme syntheses enable the cell to perform its specific predetermined activities. Hence, enzyme activation by cyclic AMP is non-specific but the product is specific to the requirements of the cell.
Changes in the amount of cell product depending on whether adenylate cyclase is activated or inhibited.
A + B ↔ AB
(Where AB is the specialized and specific product of the cell.

lung and cardiac dysfunctions.

The microenvironmental control systems

The objectives.

The microenvironmental control mechanisms are autonomous systems that modulate commands from the systems that control. The modulations are designed to optimize responses to commands from the control systems, in concord with local microenvironmental conditions.

The resources.

The microneviromental system has two groups of resources. One is intracellular and the other is extracellular.

The microenvironmental intracellular control systems.

This group of systems include mechanisms for faithful transcription and translation of proteins from nuclear DNA. Enzymes are proteins and are essentials for intracellular reactions. Their functions and modes of action were detailed in Chapter 5. The components of the microenvironmental control systems were also enumerated in that chapter but for the reader's convenience are detailed again.

The system has many components: accurate derepression of DNA fragments required to produce enzymes and other proteins needed by the specific cell; accurate protein synthesis from derepressed DNA operons; mechanisms for repair or deletion of errors of transcription and/or translation; transport systems for moving products of intracellular activity to the exterior; quantitative and qualitative variations in production of cell surface receptors and membrane pumps; the housekeeping systems that use the Golgi apparatus lysosomes and vesicles to prevent intracellular accumulation of undesirable materials; and the mitochondrial enzyme complexes that use oxygen to convert energy substrate from the environment to energy usable for biological activities (i.e., ~P) which is stored in ATP or ADP till needed.

The microenvironmental extracellular control systems.

These systems act in one or both of two ways. Firstly, by changing the diameters and permeabilities of arterioles and metarterioles in the microenvironment, and secondly, by changing the permeabilities and other characteristics of cell wall membranes in capillaries by the contraction of endothelial capillary wall cells. Vascular changes vary the quantity of substrate available to the cell for production of ~P and cell wall changes vary the varieties and quantities of materials that may enter the cells. The principal effectors of changes in vascular calibers and wall permeabilities are local axon reflexes, local changes in pH, pO_2, and CO_2, and a variety of autacoids, a word used by Schäfer (Schäfer, E.A.: The Endocrine Organs: An Introduction to the Study of Internal Secretion. New York: Longmans, Green & Co. 1916.) to describe locally produced hormone-like substances. The autacoids include histamine, angiotensin, the prostaglandins the kinins and locally produced adenosine and are responsible for both vascular changes and cell wall changes.

Therapeutic options for endocrine disease and dysfunctions

The therapeutic options.

The following list is not comprehensive but covers the most common endocrine dysfunctions.

Drugs for treatment of diabetes mellitus. The Diabetes Control and Complications Trial (DCCT) and the United Kingdom Prospective Diabetes Study have shown that good control of diabetes reduces the incidence of retinopathies, neuropathies and nephropathies. The reductions were in the 55-75% ranges.

Weight reduction, exercise and an appropriate diet are essential for both, insulin dependent diabetics (Type 1 diabetics) and non-insulin dependent diabetics (Type 2 diabetics). The American Diabetic Association provide guidelines and diet sheets for Type 1 diabetics.

Type 1 diabetics are usually young people who learn to treat themselves and to recognize symptoms of hypoglycemia and the need to immediately drink a carbohydrate such as plain sugar in water or a fruit juice such as orange juice. Aggressive treatment of children under 12 is not a good idea as their recognition of hypoglycemic symptoms are often unnoticed or disregarded. Type 1 diabetes is thought to be due to a viral infection of the pancreas.

There are a variety of insulins on the market and their durations of action and times to onset of activity are described in standard texts. In the past insulin was derived from bovine and pig pancreases. Immune reactions often resulted in intolerance or resistance, both requiring progressively larger doses of insulin. In 1977 the human insulin gene was cloned and human-type insulin manufactured. It is now in general use.

Usually Type 2 diabetics are treated with oral medications as briefly described in the preceding text. Some stimulate insulin production by the pancreas. They include the sulfonylureas such as glyburide (Diabeta), glimepiride (Amaryl) and glipizide (Glucotrol). They are usually effective in the early stages of Type 2 diabetes. They should not be given to patients with sulfa allergies as these drugs are sulfa compounds.

They can be combined with a biguanide such as glucophage. Alternatively, glucophage can be given as initial therapy and later supplemented with a sulfonylurea if needed. Glucophage does not produce hypoglycemia because it does not stimulate insulin production. Its mode of action depends on promotion of insulin-mediated suppression of hepatic glucose production and the increasing of glucose uptake by skeletal muscle.

Thyrotoxicosis.

Opinions differ as to best treatment for thyrotoxicosis. Some start with drugs and if these do not control the disease it is followed by ablation of the thyroid with radioactive iodine. Others feel that radioactive iodine ablation is the treatment of choice as it almost always succeeds though it may aggravate the eye signs. It has been used for more than 40 years and there is no evidence of a carcinogenic effect. Nevertheless, even the ardent proponents of radioactive iodine feel that it should not be given to patients who are less than 25 years old.

The available drugs are Propylthiouracil and Methimazole. Patients need to take tablets for about a year. Once treatment is stopped there is a 50% chance of a recurrence which is the best treated with radioactive iodine unless the individual is young or prefers surgery (i.e., subtotal thyroidectomy) to radioactive iodine therapy.

Surgery is obviously necessary if the hyperthyroid state results from an autonomous thyroxine-producing benign or malignant lesion. Subtotal thyroidectomy is probably appropriate treatment for a person under 25 who has a recurrence. It used to be primary treatment for the disease but is now reserved for individuals with recurrences or those who refuse radioactive iodine.

Occasionally a patient with thyrotoxicosis presents in an acute state: marked agitation and tremors, a rapid pulse and a high blood pressure, and occasionally, with additional atrial fibrillation. The first step is a beta blocker to slow the pulse and reduce the blood pressure. After control is established treat the thyroid problem.

Myxedema.

The dangers of giving thyroxine to all patients with raised TSH levels was detailed in the preceding text. Always be sure that the blood T4 and T3 levels are lower than normal levels. Giving thyroxine to an individual with normal thyroid function can result in iatrogenic thyrotoxicosis.

Hormone therapy.

Hormone replacements are needed for hypofunctions such as myxedema and the adrenal hypofunctions of Addison's disease. They are also needed as replacement therapies for the compression effects of pituitary microadenomas on cells that control hormone production by the thyroid, adrenals and gonads.

Drugs for suppression of hormone production are needed in conditions such as thyrotoxicosis and acromegaly. Corticosteroid supplements are usually needed for patients on long-term corticosteroids who develop infections, are subjected to trauma or other stresses, and/or need surgery.

Surgery

Surgery will be needed for the autonomous hyperfunctioning hyperplasias or adenomas that sometimes affect the parathyroid glands and the adrenals. Surgery is also required for autonomous hyperfunctioning benign or malignant tumors in the thyroid. Surgery is usually not required for removal of pituitary microadenomas. It is usually reserved for removal of pituitary tumors causing extrasellar compressions of the optic tract and chiasma and/or brain tissue.

This ends the chapter on endocrine and microenvironmental control systems.

8

Diagnosis: The Control Systems

3. Systems for Compensation and Protection

Table of Contents

Notation.

The notation ~P denotes phosphorous with a high energy bond. Depending on the context in which the term is used, ~P may also denote the energy liberated when a high energy phosphate bond detaches from ATP or

ADP.

A general comment on the methodology of clinical assessments.

The comments made **on page 119** about this topic are not repeated. They merit reading before proceeding with this chapter.

The resource systems for protection.

They are three in number:

- **Resource systems for compensation**
- **Resource systems for protective pathology.**
- **Resource systems for protective immunology.**

Systems for compensation.

When systems or organs become dysfunctional related systems attempt to compensate for the dysfunctions. At times they cannot prevent the clinical features of dysfunction from appearing when the individual is stressed. At other times they are ineffective and unable to prevent symptoms appearing at rest.

Neural and hormonal factors.

Afferent information reaches medullary centers and the hypothalamus and reflexes generate responses. The mechanisms were previously detailed on pages 108-110.

Functional reserve.

Normal life continues in the absence of **one kidney** or one lung, provided, of course, that the remaining organ is healthy. Unpaired organs such as the liver have comparable levels of functional reserve.

The heart has similar functional reserve. In a 70Kg man at rest vigorous exercise can increase the cardiac output from a low of 5-6.5L/min to more than 18L/min.

The kidneys have greater functional reserve. Of the 180 liters of water in the daily glomerular filtrate up to 179 liters can be reabsorbed depending on the local levels of antidiuretic hormone (ADH).

Renal handling of sodium shows similar functional reserve. The glomerular filtrate contains approximately 26,000mEq of sodium each day. Aldosterone can reduce sodium excretion to 1mEq/day. When salt intake is high it can allow excretion of as much as 400mEQ/day.

Hypertrophy.

Hypertrophy is the enlargement and increased functional performance of a single biological unit. Hypertrophy usually results in an increase in performance

Hypertrophy can result from pathology (e.g., cardiac muscle hypertrophy consequent on cardiac dysfunctions) or more commonly, because of normal temporary, physiological demands. Examples are the uterine and mammary gland hypertrophies of a normal pregnancy.

Hyperplasia

Hyperplasia is an increase in the numbers of functioning biological units. Typical examples are the hyperplasias seen after renal or liver injury. The ability of liver cells to proliferate is an extreme example of hyperplasia as a compensatory process. It is claimed that after removal of even 75% of a liver, proliferation of liver cells can restore liver mass within two weeks.

There are cells that do not divide. They include the neurons and the cells of cardiac and striated muscle. Cardiac muscle can only respond to increased demands by hypertrophy. When hypertrophy does not satisfy needs cardiac dilation begins for the cardiac muscle cells cannot proliferate.

Hyperplasia and neoplasia are dissimilar. Hyperplasia is cell proliferation in response to demand. Proliferation stops when demands have been met. Neoplasia, both benign and malignant, are uncoordinated proliferations of cells unrelated to needs. Neoplasia is often due to unknown causes, and often continues after the inducing agent or agents have ceased to act. Benign tumors have the capacity for expansile growth and proliferation but they do not infiltrate surrounding tissues. Growth is limited by the pressure of surrounding tissues. Malignant tumors have capacities for expansile as well as infiltrative growth and proliferation not restricted by the pressure of surrounding tissues. They can also form metastatic tumors with similar capabilities. Hyperplastic cells only proliferate in response to demands and proliferations cease when requirements have been met.

Systems for protective pathology and immunology

Systems dysfunctions can result from microorganisms: bacteria, viruses, rickettsiae, fungi, helminths, and parasites; from environmental toxins; from trauma (accidental, self-inflicted, or the result of war, civil conflict, sabotage, or maintenance of law and order); from extremes of temperature or atmospheric pressure; from therapeutic drugs and "recreational" drugs (some such as tobacco and alcohol permitted in most jurisdictions, others not, e.g., the opiate derivatives) and from any of the other causes of disease, as detailed on page 75.

Protection against these injurious agents is necessary, as are mechanisms that compensate for any existing, changeable or immutable dysfunctions caused by them.

Clinical decision-making requires a knowledge of the biological systems for compensation, protection and performance for at least two reasons:

First, when disease exists, to determine which of these mechanisms have not been able to defend adequately. Alternatively, if they are functioning normally, the nature of the overwhelming assault that they were not been able to neutralize.

Second, when organ or systems dysfunction exists, to determine which of the existing mechanisms for protection and compensation require therapeutic amplification.

The inflammatory reaction.

The inflammatory reaction comes in two forms: acute inflammation and chronic inflammation. The pathological features of chronic inflammation are a combination of smoldering acute inflammation combined with the histological features of granulation tissue. Granulation tissue characterizes repair.

Acute inflammation.

Willis described acute inflammation as "the immediate vascular and exudative reaction of living tissue to injury which does not kill the tissue." This is a good and accurate definition. Inflammation is a protective mechanism that originates in the microenvironment but may become systemic. Acute inflammation is designed to protect against injury by animate pathogens and, if possible to eliminate them. It also protects against injury by inert but harmful materials. This is why acute inflammation is usually present in areas adjacent to dead tissue, hematomas, foreign bodies and necrotic malignant tissue.

The initial vascular reaction of acute inflammation is a faster blood flow due to the liberation or activation of vasodilators by damaged tissues. Very soon flow slows because of adherence of blood cells to vascular endothelia that have become sticky. Next, the cells lining the walls of capillaries swell and spaces appear between adjacent cells. The blood vessels become permeable to substances to which they were previously impermeable. Blood cells and plasma traverse the vessel walls.

The exudate dilutes irritants and forms a fibrin clot that retards spread of infection. It also brings soluble and cell-bound antibodies to the area. Important components of the extravascular exudate are the microphages (i.e., polymorphonuclear leukocytes) and the macrophages. Both phagocytose undesirable items such as bacteria and dead tissue. The subsequent course of events depends on any one or more of the following:

- The virulence and numbers of infecting organisms.
- The ability of natural and generated defense mechanisms to destroy or inactivate them, especially the products of generated humoral and cell-bound immunity in the exudate.

- The presence of foreign bodies, undrained pus, hematomas and dead tissue. All retard resolution.
- Coexisting diseases or therapies that decrease the ability of natural and generated immunity to deal with the infecting agent. Examples are HIV\AIDS infections, recent radiotherapy, anti-cancer chemotherapy, prolonged corticosteroid therapy for COPD and/or advanced autoimmune disease, disseminated malignant disease, and chronic cardiac, respiratory, gastrointestinal, hepatic, endocrine and renal dysfunctions.
- Aging is not a disease but a condition where the functional capabilities of most systems are reduced. This reduces the functional reserves often needed to complement the acute inflammatory reaction.
- Vascular insufficiency and sensory deficits affecting the inflamed tissues, especially when these affect limb vasculatures and sensory receptors. Examples are atheromatous stenoses or occlusions of vessels, diabetic and other peripheral neuropathies and the posterior root demyelinations of tabes dorsalis.

Acute inflammation of any severity is usually associated with local and systemic symptoms and signs.

Locally there are pain, swelling, redness, increased temperature, and diminution of function. Examples are the reduction of volitional activity when acute inflammation involves muscles and joints, decreased respiratory activity over an inflamed lung, the reduced gastrointestinal activity of peritonitis, and the neck stiffness of meningitis. Lymphangitis, manifested as red streaks extending from inflamed tissues to enlarged and tender local lymph nodes, is a common additional feature.

Systemic findings depend on the severity of the infection. They include toxemia with fever, myalgia, and a general ill-definable feeling of sickness. A laboratory finding of a polymorphonuclear leucocytosis is characteristic. Severe infections can result in bacteremia, septicemia, metastatic abscesses, shock, extensive destruction of soft tissues (e.g., gas gangrene and the so-called "flesh-eating disease" of some streptococcal infections), hemorrhagic diatheses such as microangiopathic anemia and disseminated intravascular coagulation, and even death. The last is a real possibility when infections are fulminating and rapidly progressive. The features of meningococcal septicemia were detailed in the previous chapter. It is a condition that can result in rapid death.

It is a paradox that the commonest sites for metastatic abscesses are the muscles, spleen and liver. Metastases from malignant disease favor the lungs, the bones, the liver and the brain. Metastatic spread of malignant disease to the spleen or muscles is distinctly uncommon and almost anecdotal.

The possible sequelae of acute inflammation include rapid resolution and restoration to normality. This is usually seen with simple uninfected cuts where inflammation is not protracted by self-replicating organisms or organisms of extreme virulence, or because of rapid and immediate effective therapy. A comparably frequent consequence is suppuration, at times followed by necrosis and gangrene and finally by repair.

The formation of pus.

Pus is fluid containing dead and living cells, dead and living bacteria, the inflammatory exudate and the products of proteolytic digestion of tissue. An abscess is a collection of pus. It presents as a tender, hot swelling that may show fluctuation if its contents are mainly fluid pus. Fluctuation is absent when most of the abscess consists of inflamed tissue surrounding a small collection of pus. The pus may be reabsorbed and the mass gradually decrease in size, especially if antibiotics are given. More common is progression to formation of more pus which requires drainage. The wall of an abscess consists of granulation tissue which, after drainage of pus, collapses and becomes fibrous tissue after organization and repair.

On free surfaces pus results in a purulent discharge - often described as a catarrh. In tissues of loose texture such as subcutaneous tissues it usually presents as a cellulitis or a localized abscess. In pre-existing body cavities a collection of pus is called an empyema (e.g., pleural empyema and gall bladder empyema).

Necrosis and gangrene.

Extensive necrosis is especially prone to occur in anaerobic infections such as gas gangrene or the necrotic tissue lesions occasionally associated with hemolytic streptococcal infections (so-called "flesh-eating" infections). More commonly it results from infections in debilitated individuals or individuals with vascular or neurological deficits involving the inflamed tissues. Alternatively, or additionally, it could result from infection by organisms of powerful virulence, or overwhelming numbers of organisms with usual virulence, or both. A frequent cause of inflammatory lesions that will not heal are ischemia of the lower limbs, especially when the individual is a poorly controlled diabetic. Another less common cause is the osteonecrosis seen when a nutrient artery is occluded in acute osteomyelitis and some traumatic bone lesions.

Repair and organization.

Repair is protective. Its object is to restore the proportions and functions of damaged tissues to normal, or to as near normal as possible. The initial reaction of repair is the simultaneous migration of lymphocytes and macrophages into the damaged tissues and the outgrowth of solid buds from patent capillaries in the area. The macrophages ingest, digest and remove dead tissue and blood clot and concurrently there is canalization of the capillary buds with eventual formation of many arbors of patent capillaries. The appearance is that of a red and delicate velvety surface, hence the name, "granulation tissue". The healing tissue is next invaded by fibroblasts which lay down collagen. As the collagen framework contracts epithelial cells at the periphery of the lesion proliferate and eventually cover any anatomical deficit.

A distinction is made between wounds that heal by "first intention" and those that heal by "second intention". An example of the former is a clean cut, uncontaminated by bacteria and with the skin edges approximated soon after injury. Healing is rapid and a thin linear scar results. An example of the latter is a lesion where tissue is lost and epithelial edges cannot be approximated. Healing requires epithelial proliferation to cover granulation tissue in the base of the tissue deficit. Healing is prolonged and the eventual scar is usually larger and irregular in comparison with the scar of first intention healing. This is seen when significant amounts of tissue have been destroyed. As inflammation subsides there is coexisting repair with granulation tissue and subsequent fibrosis. This can result in contractures and, at times, in functional deficits that result in tissues without functional capability (e.g., a healed myocardial infarct) or stenotic lesions that retard the free flows of body fluids such as blood, urine and gastrointestinal fluids.

Chronic inflammation.

There are many possible causes of chronic inflammation and its manifestations are protean. Common causes include any one or more of the following:

- Infections by especially virulent pathogens and/or numerous pathogens of normal virulence. Chronic inflammation results when the pathogens do not respond or respond poorly to therapy. Alternatively, when therapy is inadequate or incorrect.
- The infectious granulomas. Examples are tuberculosis, syphilis, sarcoidosis, leprosy and yaws.
- Many of the infections caused by fungi, protozoa, helminths and arthropods.
- Intralesional presence of foreign bodies, blood clots, necrotic tissues, and pus that has not been drained.
- The ulceration of malignant disease, often not recognized as such till the lesion is biopsied.
- Persistence of a sinus or fistula (usually with chronic discharge) from a previously inflamed lesion, either because of epithelialization or fibrosis of the track. Fistula in ano is an example.
- The coexistence of chronic disease involving any one or more systems of the body; they all reduce resistance to infections. Examples are chronic infections (e.g., tuberculosis and AIDS), cardiac, neurological, respiratory, endocrine (especially diabetes mellitus), hepatic, and renal disease, subnutrition and malnutrition, obesity and jaundice, chronic alcoholism, and addictions to opiates and other "recreational" drugs.

The pathology of chronic inflammation features a combination of the pathology seen in a smoldering acute inflammation (increased vascularity, macrophages, lymphocytes and neutrophils and at times, small granulomata) and in repair (granulation tissue, fibroblasts and collagen). The clinical features are protean: some examples are a chronic discharging ulcer, sinus or fistula, a symptomless pulmonary shadow, a lesion that has the clinical features of malignancy but which, on biopsy, shows chronic inflammation. Other features suggestive of chronic inflammation are hematomas, collections of undrained pus or serous fluid, intralesional foreign bodies, and foci of dead tissue or bone.

Innate protective mechanisms.

They are many. The following summarizes the main ones:

Epithelial barriers and body fluids.

Intact skin and mucus membranes act as mechanical barriers. In addition, short chain fatty acids on the skin act as metabolic inhibitors of bacteria while the long chain dermal fatty acids[1] inhibit bacteria by a surfactant action.

The body fluids contain many antibacterial agents. An example is lysozyme, a protein found in tears, saliva, leucocytes and macrophages. It hydrolyzes muramic acid in the walls of bacteria, mainly in gram positive organisms. It is maximally effective at ranges near neutral pH.

Other examples are phagocytin and properdin. The former is a protein that can be extracted from white cells by acid. It appears to have a wide range of action against both gram positive and negative organisms. The latter complexes with complement and magnesium ions and thus activates the alternate pathway of complement. This system has been implicated as the inactivator of many viruses and gram negative bacteria.

Phagocytes.

Phagocytes have a protective function which can never be over-emphasized. They ingest, and when possible digest bacteria, dead tissue and small particles of foreign material, some digestible, others not. Much of our knowledge of the role of macrophages derives unchanged from the work of Metchnikoff in the latter part of the last century (Metchnikoff, E. Sur la lutta des cellules de l'organismes centre l'invasion des microbes. Annales Inst. Pasteur 1887; 11:321. - not listed in references as it is usually only available in special scientific collections of rare works). He correctly proposed that there were two types of phagocytes: the microphages and the macrophages. The principal microphage is the polymorphonuclear leukocyte. Eosinophils and basophils can phagocytose but have less phagocytic activity than the neutrophils.

There are two types of macrophages: the sessile and the wandering macrophages **The sessile macrophages:** are present in capillary endothelia and in liver sinuses (the Kupffer cells), and in the blood vessel walls of the spleen, the bone marrow and many other tissues. They phagocytose foreign bodies and bacteria in blood flowing through the structures where they are located.

The wandering macrophages (often called histiocytes) are monocytes that migrate through capillary walls and become macrophages. Other wandering macrophages derive from proliferation and mobilization of the sessile tissue macrophages and the fixed histiocytes present in all tissues. Some may derive from transformation of lymphocytes to monocytes.

Macrophages perform many different functions and are often named accordingly: dust cells and heart failure cells when scavenging dust particles and blood pigment in the air passages; foam cells when filled with lipid; melanophores or chromatophores when filled with melanin; lepra cells in the lesions of leprosy; and Aschoff cells in the lesions of rheumatic fever. Giant foreign body multinucleated cells are characteristic of phagocytes that have ingested material that is not easily digested and eliminated by intracellular enzyme systems.

Immunity.

There are two types of immunity: natural immunity and generated immunity.

Natural immunity.

Natural antibodies are often found in individuals who have not been deliberately immunized or overtly infected previously. They probably result from subclinical infections or as the result of immunization against cross-reacting antigens. They function in the same way as generated antibodies (discussed later in the text).

Some opsonins are not immunologically generated. These natural opsonins do not have specificty. They exist in fresh serum and promote phagocytosis of bacteria by leukocytes, especially gram negative bacteria as well

Chart 8-1: NATURAL KILLER CELLS
1. Natural killer cells are lymphocytes which have surface immunoglobulin recognition receptors and also, receptors for MHC class I molecules. When a natural killer cell is exposed to foreign cells coated with immunoglobulin and without a "self specific" MHC Class I unit it lyses the foreign cell. Lysis is mediated by perforins. It is effected by transcellular passage of toxic granzymes through perforations created by perforins. Destruction of intracellular DNA by granzymes follows.
2. Interaction with a cell which does not have a "self specific" MHC I Class molecule will result in destruction of that cell by natural killer cell perforins which convey granzymes into the cell via perforations. Normal cells are protected because they have MHC Class I molecules which are recognized by natural killer cells as "self specific" molecules.

as inert particles. Like properdin they can activate complement.

Natural killer cells.

Their capabilities and effects are summarized in Chart 8-1. Additional text is not needed.

Generated immunity.

The generated immune response is a defense mechanism induced by any one or more of a variety of antigens: pathogens such as bacteria, viruses, parasites, helminths, and fungi, drugs, and/or by foreign proteins and blood antigens, allogeneic organ transplants and, at times, altered self-antigens.

B and T lymphocytes.

There are many excellent reviews and books on the mechanisms of generated immunity. It could be invidious to cite only one or two and impossible to cite all. Some descriptive differences do occur in many publication and the following summarizes what seems commonly agreed.

The immune response is mediated by B and T lymphocytes. Both B and T cells originate in the marrow. The former continue development in the marrow while the latter migrate to, and further develop in the thymus. Antigen-specific receptors are produced in both types of cells by random splicings and rearrangements of many DNA segments. Arstila and associates[2] have proposed that a large repertoire of specificities exist for both T and B cells - 10^8 T-cell receptor specificities and more for B cells. Clones of new B and T cells continue to appear throughout life, but with decreasing frequency as the individual ages.

B lymphocytes.

Chart 8-2 summarizes the main functional capabilities of B lymphocytes. Additional text is unnecessary.

T lymphocytes and cell-mediated immunity.

Charts 8-3 to 8-5 summarize the developments and capabilities of T lymphocytes. Apart from its participation in cell mediated immunity the CD4 cell has another important function. It can recognize antigen even when the antigen is not coupled to an MHC molecule. This ability to recognize antigen allows it to act as a B cell helper. Most B cell responses require a helper T cell for initiation of humoral antibody production (Chart 8-2), though some do not.

T cell immunity is responsible for immune mechanisms directed against many viruses and fungi, some bacteria (notably the one causing tuberculosis), rickettsiae, and some parasites. A reduction of T cell-mediated immunity is responsible for the many opportunistic infections associated with immunological depression by diseases such as AIDS.

The cytotoxic T cell response also mediates delayed hypersensitivity reactions. An example is the tuberculin reaction. T cell immunity also mediates the Schick test, skin reactions to allergens such as poison ivy (usually an urticarial type rash), perhaps the elimination of tumor cells, and certainly, the rejection of allogeneic transplants. The increasing use and importance of such transplants in clinical medicine has resulted in a whole pharmacopoeia designed to eliminate, or at least reduce T and B cell immunity directed**(Contd. on page 182)**

Chart 8-2: B LYMPHOCYTES, HUMORAL ANTIBODY AND T HELPER CELLS (GENERATED IMMUNITY #1)

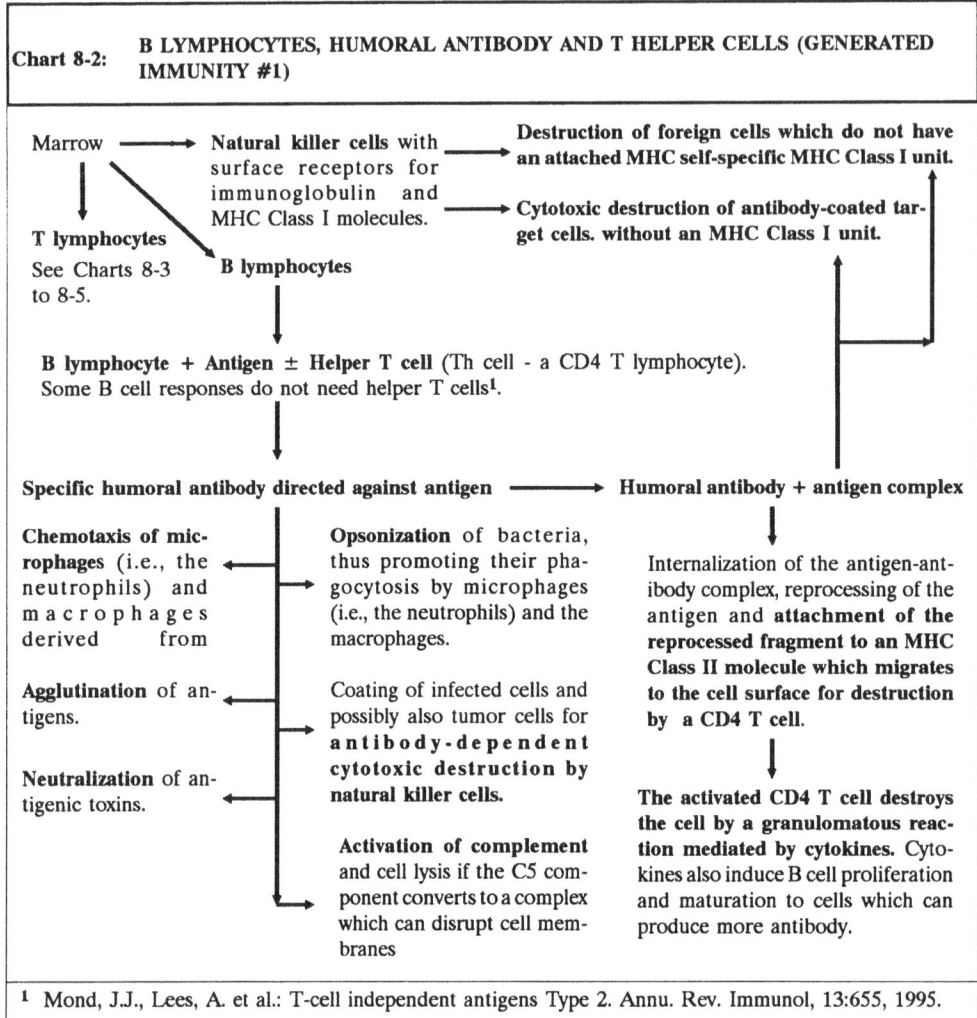

Marrow → **Natural killer cells** with surface receptors for immunoglobulin and MHC Class I molecules.

→ **Destruction of foreign cells which do not have an attached MHC self-specific MHC Class I unit.**

→ **Cytotoxic destruction of antibody-coated target cells. without an MHC Class I unit.**

Marrow → **T lymphocytes** See Charts 8-3 to 8-5.

Marrow → **B lymphocytes**

↓

B lymphocyte + Antigen ± Helper T cell (Th cell - a CD4 T lymphocyte). Some B cell responses do not need helper T cells[1].

↓

Specific humoral antibody directed against antigen → **Humoral antibody + antigen complex**

From specific humoral antibody:

- **Chemotaxis of microphages** (i.e., the neutrophils) and macrophages derived from
- **Agglutination** of antigens.
- **Neutralization** of antigenic toxins.
- **Opsonization** of bacteria, thus promoting their phagocytosis by microphages (i.e., the neutrophils) and the macrophages.
- Coating of infected cells and possibly also tumor cells for **antibody-dependent cytotoxic destruction by natural killer cells.**
- **Activation of complement** and cell lysis if the C5 component converts to a complex which can disrupt cell membranes

From humoral antibody + antigen complex:

↓

Internalization of the antigen-antibody complex, reprocessing of the antigen and **attachment of the reprocessed fragment to an MHC Class II molecule which migrates to the cell surface for destruction by a CD4 T cell.**

↓

The activated CD4 T cell destroys the cell by a granulomatous reaction mediated by cytokines. Cytokines also induce B cell proliferation and maturation to cells which can produce more antibody.

[1] Mond, J.J., Lees, A. et al.: T-cell independent antigens Type 2. Annu. Rev. Immunol, 13:655, 1995.

Chart 8-3: T LYMPHOCYTE DEVELOPMENT (GENERATED IMMUNITY #2.)

T lymphocytes originate in the marrow but develop in the thymus, at first without CD4 or CD8 units

↓

Next, each T lymphocyte acquires both, a CD4 and a CD8 unit

↓

Then, each T lymphocyte loses either a CD4 or CD8 unit and enters the circulation

↓

CD4 (T helper cell - Th cells) and CD8 (T cytotoxic cells - Tc cells) cells only respond to foreign antigens which are bound to an MHC unit. Examples of such antigens are phagocytosed foreign material, intracellular viruses, bacteria and other pathogens, possibly, tumor antigens, and internalized antigen-antibody complexes.

These items are complexed with an MHC Class I or II molecule and presented on cell surfaces for cytotoxic destruction by T lymphocytes. It is only after an initial complexing with an MHC unit that a T cell is able to recognize the complex as foreign material requiring destruction by immune T cell-mediated cytotoxicity.

Self cells do have surface MHC antigens but are not recognized as cells requiring destruction as foreign antigen is not complexed with its MHC antigen.

Chart 8-5: THE CD4 Th T LYMPHOCYTE REACTIONS (GENERATED IMMUNITY #3)

1. **Antigen processing and presentation.**
   a. Intracellular antigens from viruses. pathogens, tumor cells and cell-antigen complexes from tissue transplants.
   b. Antigen bound to specific B cell surface immunoglobulins and internalized by endocytosis.
   In the cell antigen is broken down to peptide fragments which bind to "self" intracellular MHC Class II units. These complexes then appear on the surfaces of the affected cells.
2. **Helper function of CD4 cells.**
   Most B cell antibody production requires initiation by a complex of B cell, antigen and a CD4 T helper cell.

↓

The CD4 cell recognizes and binds to the cell-surface complexes of foreign antigen and MHC Class II unit. T cell surface coreceptors are activated and this eventuates in the final activation of the T cell to express cytotoxicity and produce cytokines.

↓

Cytokine effects (cytokines can also be produced by cells other than CD4 lymphocytes):

When produced by leucocytes in an immune response they are called interleukins **and their effects include:**

1. **Activation of macrophages to kill intracellular pathogens such as mycobacteria, protozoa, and fungi. The final destruction is by a cell-mediated granulomatous inflammatory reaction. This is the type of reaction excited by organisms such as M.Tuberculosis.**
2. An increase in CD8 cytotoxicity.
3. CD4 and CD8 cell proliferation,
4. Stimulation of B cells to proliferate, mature and produce humoral antibody.
5. Cytokines which attract chemicals are called **chemokines.** They include **colony-stimulating factors** which promote proliferation and maturation of stem cells, and **interferons which act by inhibiting viral proliferation.**

Chart 8-4: THE CD8 CYTOTOXIC T LYMPHOCYTE REACTIONS (GENERATED IMMUNITY #4)

Antigen processing and presentation:

The antigens are usually intracellular. They include viruses and some bacteria, phagocytosed foreign protein particles and possibly, also tumor antigens and phagocytosed cell-antigen complexes from tissue transplants.

Peptide fragments derived from this internalized material bind to MHC Class I units. These complexes present on the surfaces of the cells.

All nucleated cells have a Class I MHC unit but are not destroyed because the Class 1 MHC unit is not complexed with foreign antigen. Incidentally, fewer cells have Class II units.

↓

When the CD8 cell recognizes the complex of foreign antigen and MHC Class I unit on the cell surface it attaches to the affected cell and produces perforins.

↓

Perforin effects.

There is transcellular passage of toxic granzymes through perforations created by the perforins. The granzymes fragment and destroy DNA in the cell presenting the antigen-MHC Class I unit complex.

(Contd. from page 179)
against non-self antigens in allogeneic transplants.

Immunological dysfunctions and autoimmune disease

Inherited dysfunctions.

The literature contains descriptions of many syndromes of immunological deficiency resulting from dysfunctions due to inherited genetic abnormalities - B cell deficits (e.g., the Bruton-type X-linked agammaglobulinemia), T cell deficits (e.g., the thymic hypoplasia of the DiGeorge syndrome) and combined B and T cell deficits (e.g., the Swiss type lymphopenic agammaglobulinemia). These conditions are uncommon. The generalist is unlikely to encounter a single case in a lifetime of practice but must be alerted to the possibility of the existence of one when a child presents with recurrent infections, especially opportunistic infections, failure to thrive, bizarre skin rashes, chronic diarrhea and malabsorption syndromes.

Acquired immunological deficiencies.

Decreased immunological competence is a frequent accompaniment of chronic disease, malnutrition, subnutrition, aging, malignant disease, chemotherapy for malignant disease, prolonged corticosteroid administration, and poorly controlled or uncontrolled diabetes mellitus. At present acquired immunological deficiency syndrome (AIDS) due to infection with the HIV virus is the most common cause of demonstrable immunological deficiency.

Acquired immunodeficiency syndrome (AIDS).

HIV is a retrovirus. Retroviruses contain diploid RNA genomes and the enzyme, reverse transcriptase. The enzyme uses its RNA template for production of DNA transcripts. The virus-derived DNA is then integrated into the DNA of the infected cell. When activated the new DNA transcript produces new virus particles that infect other cells, and so the cycle goes on.

The HIV virus has a protein on its surface. This envelope protein is specific for attachment to CD4 receptors and subsequent internalization. Antigenic mutation and variation of this envelope protein are common and this is a major obstacle to development of an effective vaccine. AIDS is probably initiated by attachment of HIV to the CD4 receptors on CD4-T helper cells and CD4 receptors on other CD4 cells. Eventually the virus kills the CD4 cell. AIDS denotes the clinical phase of the disease. It is not diagnosed till the CD4 blood count falls below 200/mm^3 (normal values are 500-1000/mm^3).

Usually AIDS does not kill directly except, possibly, in conditions such as AIDS dementia. Many claim that AIDS dementia results from the direct cytotoxicity of HIV on neurons. Others feel that it results from opportunistic viral infections. Certainly, opportunistic viruses can result in multifocal leukoencephalopathies.

The principal cause of death from AIDS is a decreased ability of the body to deal with infections of any sort. They include bacterial infections such as reactivation of quiescent tuberculosis (many individuals have quiescent M. tuberculosis in their bodies), syphilis and salmonella infections. Opportunistic infections are of particular importance. These are infections caused by normally quiescent pathogens in the body or by infections caused by external pathogens which rarely cause disease. Destruction of CD4 cells makes the patient susceptible to these opportunistic infections. They include infections such as aspergillosis, candidiasis, coccidiomycosis, cryptococcal meningitis, histoplasma infections, and protozoan and helminth infections such as cryptosporidiosis, isosporiasis, microsporidiosis, pneumocystis carinii pneumonia and toxoplasmosis. There is also an increased incidence of Kaposi's sarcoma and lymphoreticular malignancies.

Viral opportunistic infections are also common: cytomegalovirus infections, hepatitis, herpes simplex (shingles) and herpes zoster (genital warts) infections, and human papilloma virus infections resulting in genital warts and even cancer of the cervix. Opportunistic infections can also result from protozoa that rarely cause major infections in individuals with normal immune systems. Neurological complications of HIV infections include the AIDS dementia syndrome mentioned above as well as peripheral neuropathies. Finally, there is the well recognized wasting syndrome of unknown etiology, but probably the result of multiple clinical as well as subclinical opportunistic infections.

The search for therapeutic agents continues and is intense. Usually combinations of inhibitors of proteases and reverse transcriptase in various combinations are temporarily effective in controlling the clinical manifestations of the disease but a fatal outcome usually eventuates, especially when drugs are unavailable or unaffordable. Drug resistance and viral mutants that escape endogenous and exogenous controls are additional causes. Antigenic variants and mutations make the development of effective vaccines difficult.

Types 1-4 adverse immunological reactions.

The effects of interactions between antibody and antigen are not always benign. Four basic types of adverse reactions are described. They were called Types 1-4 reactions by Coombs and Gell[4] and are described in detail on pages 183-187. The first three result from adverse interactions between antigen and humoral antibody. The Type 4 from interactions between immune T cells and antigenic targets. The following is a summary of these reactions:

1. The Type 1 reaction: Systemic and local anaphylaxis.

Chart 8-6 summarizes the principal features of anaphylaxis. Numerous antigens are capable of evoking anaphylactic reactions. Examples are proteins, chemical haptens conjugated to carriers, some carbohydrates, occasional products of food digestion and absorption (unexpected anaphylactic reactions to peanuts are real dangers in children), and fungal antigens (e.g., the antigens of aspergillus).

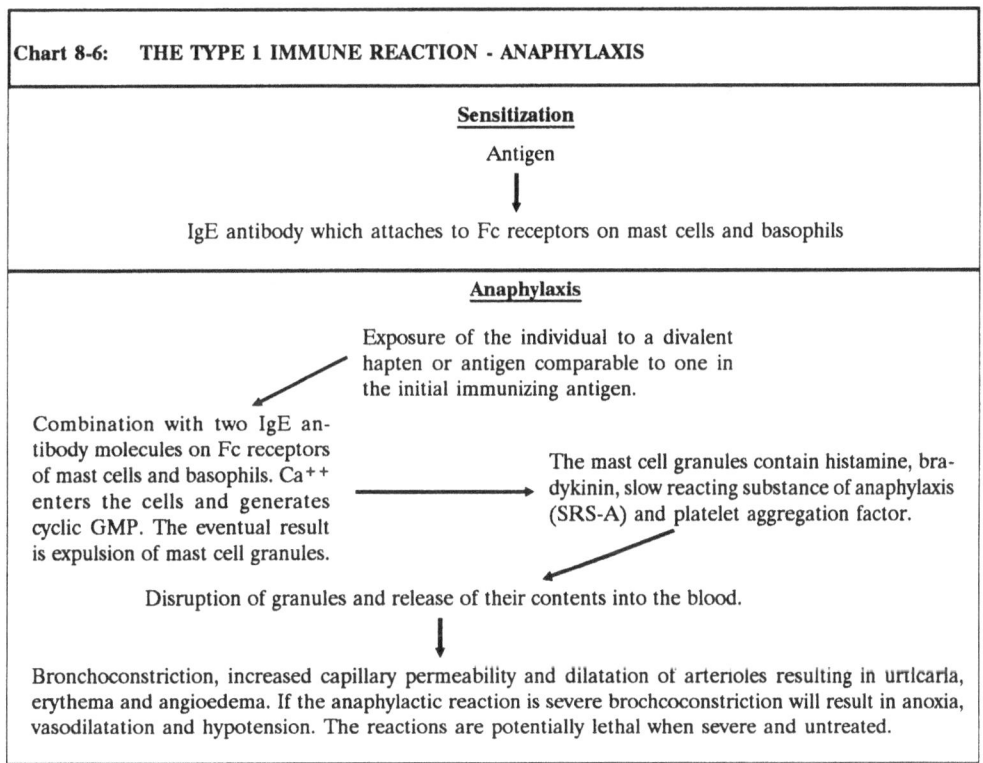

Chart 8-6: THE TYPE 1 IMMUNE REACTION - ANAPHYLAXIS

Sensitization

Antigen

↓

IgE antibody which attaches to Fc receptors on mast cells and basophils

Anaphylaxis

Exposure of the individual to a divalent hapten or antigen comparable to one in the initial immunizing antigen.

↙

Combination with two IgE antibody molecules on Fc receptors of mast cells and basophils. Ca^{++} enters the cells and generates cyclic GMP. The eventual result is expulsion of mast cell granules.

→ The mast cell granules contain histamine, bradykinin, slow reacting substance of anaphylaxis (SRS-A) and platelet aggregation factor.

↙

Disruption of granules and release of their contents into the blood.

↓

Bronchoconstriction, increased capillary permeability and dilatation of arterioles resulting in urticaria, erythema and angioedema. If the anaphylactic reaction is severe brochcoconstriction will result in anoxia, vasodilatation and hypotension. The reactions are potentially lethal when severe and untreated.

The reaction occurs within minutes of giving antigen to an individual who was previously exposed to a comparable hapten or antigen and developed specific antibody directed against it. Chart 8-6 details the sequence which results in anaphylaxis. The consequences of an anaohylacvtic reaction can be severe enough to result in death if uncontrolled

The postulated sequence of events is that the exciting agent should be a divalent antigen that combines with two adjacent IgE molecules attached to the Fc receptors of mast cells or basophils. A channel into the cell opens, calcium enters and proesterase is activated to esterase. This and the increased intracellular calcium generate cyclic GMP results in expulsion of mast cell granules. The result is an extracellular and eventually systemic increase of the products of these granules; among those of special clinical import are histamine, bradykinin, serotonin, slow reacting substance of anaphylaxis (SRS-A) and platelet aggregation factor.

The pathophysiologic consequences are contraction of smooth muscle, especially bronchial smooth muscle and the smooth muscle of the air passages, increased capillary permeability, dilation of peripheral arterioles, urticaria, erythema and angioedema. The anaphylactic reaction may be severe enough to cause a shock-like syndrome with shortness of breath, asthma, urticaria, hypotension and, at times, death if uncontrollable or untreated. Type 1 reactions are often responsible for many less catastrophic diseases; allergic rhinitis, asthma, and occasional rare conditions such as hereditary angioedema.

Localized anaphylaxis usually results from diagnostic skin testing for allergies. The use of too much antigen in skin testing can result in a generalized reaction.

The reaction could be severe enough to cause death from bronchostriction asphyxia. Every physician is well advised to keep injectable epinephrine and oxygen in the office, regardless of the type of medicine practiced.

Case History.

Young man age 16 tottered into my office with difficulty in breathing. Within two minutes respiration stopped. I immediately gave him 0.4ml 1:1000 epinephrine subcutaneously, left the needle in place and started oxygen by mask. When he began to breathe spontaneously I gave another 0.25ml epinephrine. Within five minutes he was back to normal. The history given was that he had just eaten a handful of sunflower seeds. He had done so on many previous occasions without any consequent problem.

2. The Type 2 hypersensitivity reaction.

The mechanics of Type 2 reactions are depicted in Chart 8-7. Type 2 reactions occur when antibody binds to antigen attached to one or more of the different types of blood cells: erythrocytes, platelets, neutrophils and

Chart 8-7: THE TYPE 2 IMMUNE REACTION

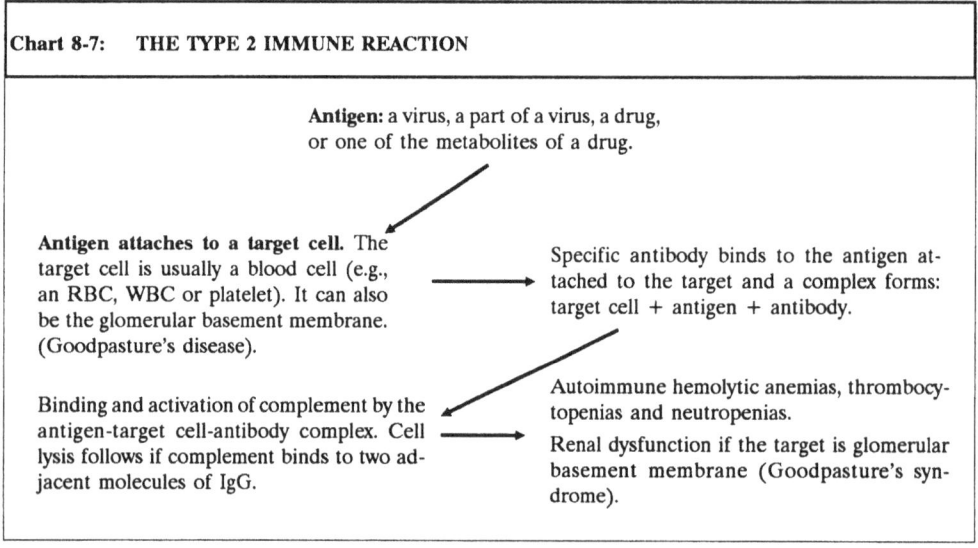

Antigen: a virus, a part of a virus, a drug, or one of the metabolites of a drug.

↓

Antigen attaches to a target cell. The target cell is usually a blood cell (e.g., an RBC, WBC or platelet). It can also be the glomerular basement membrane. (Goodpasture's disease).

→ Specific antibody binds to the antigen attached to the target and a complex forms: target cell + antigen + antibody.

↓

Binding and activation of complement by the antigen-target cell-antibody complex. Cell lysis follows if complement binds to two adjacent molecules of IgG.

→ Autoimmune hemolytic anemias, thrombocytopenias and neutropenias.
Renal dysfunction if the target is glomerular basement membrane (Goodpasture's syndrome).

lymphocytes, or to the glomerular basement membrane in the kidney (Goodpasture's syndrome). Examples of the usual antigens are viruses, parts of viruses, drugs, one of the metabolites of a drug adsorbed on the cell, or altered cell antigens adjacent to any of the above attachments. The usual mechanism of cell injury is the attachment of antibody to antigen to form a complex that binds complement. Activation of complement and subsequent cell lysis results if complement binding is to two adjacent molecules of IGg. Drugs frequently cited as the cause of Type 2 reactions are the antihistamines, the sulfonamides, chlorthiazide and its derivatives, isoniazid, quinidine, quinine, rifampicin, and tetracyclines.

The consequences of autoimmune antibodies directed against any one or more components of blood could be autoimmune hemolytic anemias, drug induced hemolytic anemias, alloantibody-induced hemolytic anemias, autoimmune leucopenias, idiopathic autoimmune thrombocytopenia (ITP - anti-platelet antibody is demonstrable), secondary autoimmune thrombocytopenia, and drug-induced immune thrombocytopenia.

The Coombs test.

The Coombs test is used to detect Type 2 immunological reactions. The test reagent is an antiserum produced in animals injected with human immunoglobulin and complement. Cell clumping when the reagent is added to blood indicates the presence of human immunoglobulin on the surfaces of red cells, or other blood cells. This is the direct Coombs test.

The indirect test is used to detect antibodies in serum. The serum is first incubated with normal red cells in vitro. The red cells are washed and then tested as in the direct test. The test is used by blood banks and by those evaluating possible recipient-donor reactions in transplantation. It determines if there are serum antibodies that can react with and harm the patient's cells.

3. The Type 3 hypersensitivity reaction.

This reaction results from soluble complexes of antibody and antigen, usually formed at a time when excess antigen is present and when the ratio of antigen to antibody is about 3:2 or higher. The complexes lodge on

Chart 8-8: THE TYPE 3 IMMUNE REACTION (IMMUNE COMPLEX DYSFUNCTION)

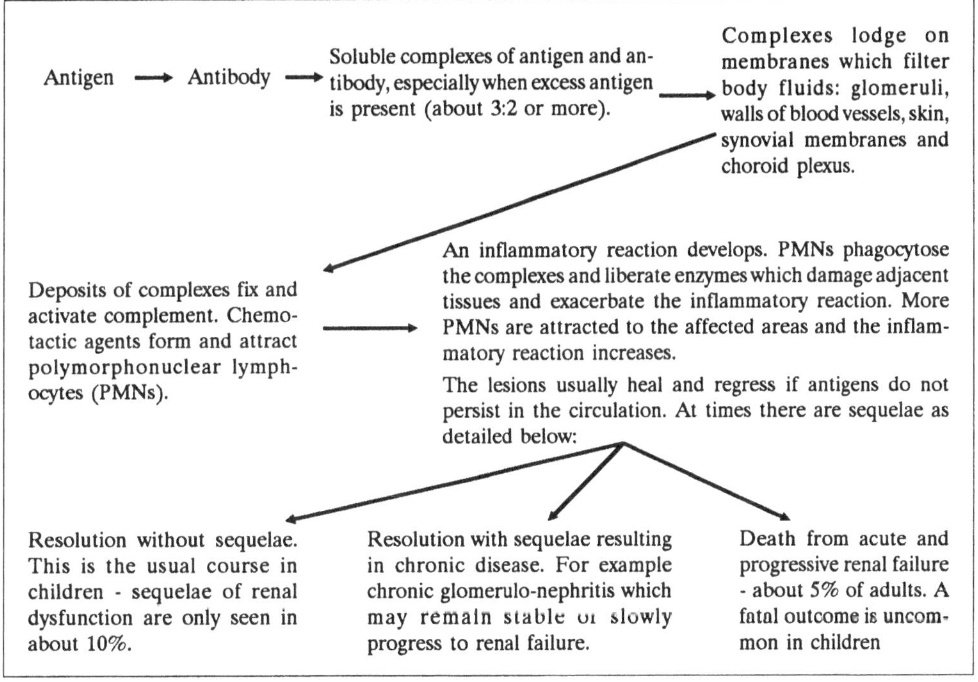
Antigen
Antibody
Soluble complexes of antigen and antibody, especially when excess antigen is present (about 3:2 or more).
Complexes lodge on membranes which filter body fluids: glomeruli, walls of blood vessels, skin, synovial membranes and choroid plexus.
Deposits of complexes fix and activate complement. Chemotactic agents form and attract polymorphonuclear lymphocytes (PMNs).
An inflammatory reaction develops. PMNs phagocytose the complexes and liberate enzymes which damage adjacent tissues and exacerbate the inflammatory reaction. More PMNs are attracted to the affected areas and the inflammatory reaction increases.
The lesions usually heal and regress if antigens do not persist in the circulation. At times there are sequelae as detailed below:
Resolution without sequelae. This is the usual course in children - sequelae of renal dysfunction are only seen in about 10%.
Resolution with sequelae resulting in chronic disease. For example chronic glomerulo-nephritis which may remain stable or slowly progress to renal failure.
Death from acute and progressive renal failure - about 5% of adults. A fatal outcome is uncommon in children

membranes that filter body fluids, especially the glomeruli, the walls of blood vessels, the skin, the synovial membranes and the choroid plexus. The usual antibody is an IgG or IgM molecule. Occasionally IgA may be responsible. The deposited complexes fix and activate complement. Complement activation results in formation of chemotactic factors. Polymorphonuclear leukocytes (PMN) are attracted to the area. An inflammatory reaction begins. The polymorphonuclear granulocytess phagocytose the complexes and there is exocytosis of PMN enzymes such as lysosomal hydrolases, proteases, esterases and glycosidases. The result is damage to adjacent cells and tissues and exacerbation of the inflammatory reaction. More PMNs are attracted to the area with more tissue damage. The lesions usually heal and regress if antigens do not persist in the body.

Immune complex disease.

Immune complex disease can present in many different forms. Three examples are given below: serum sickness, immune complex nephritis, and autoimmune disease. These are the three principal types of immune complex disease.

— **Serum sickness.**

Serum sickness may follow entrance into the body of any one of many agents, usually foreign proteins. The more common examples are heterologous antitetanus, antirabies, and other antisera, and bee venom. It can also result from drugs, especially penicillin, the sulfonamides, dilantin, and arsenicals.

After an incubation period of 5-10 days there is itching, the appearance of different types of skin rashes (usually urticarial), fever, lymphadenopathy, arthralgias and even arthritis, edema of face lips and rarely, the glottis. Neurological deficits and mononeuropathies may develop. Serum sickness is usually a self limiting disease that subsides in about three weeks with little residuum.

— **Immune complex acute glomerulonephritis.**

Causes are many. Examples are streptococcal antigens in the acute glomerulonephritis associated with streptococcal antigens and the acute glomerulonephritis occasionally seen with hepatitis antigen infections, viral gastroenteritis and other viral infections.

Acute glomerulonephritis resulting from streptococcal infection begins about 10 days after a throat infection with group A beta-hemolytic streptococcus. It is thought to be a Type 3 reaction to streptococcal antigens. There is edema of the face, edema of the legs, shortness of breath, hypertension, a raised blood creatinine, and a dark brown urine that results from hemolysed as well as intact red cells, often accompanied by red cell casts, and with oliguria.

Complete recovery is the usual course in children; sequelae are seen in only about 10% of those affected. About 50% of adults do have sequelae. About 2-5% die of progressive acute renal failure. Others develop chronic disease of varying severity. Some develop renal failure in the 3-12 month period following infection. At the other extreme are patients with stable chronic glomerulonephritis who eventually die of some unrelated disease. During life there may be proteinuria and hematuria (often microscopic), a raised but reasonably stable blood creatinine and a similarly decreased but stable creatinine clearance.

— **Autoimmune disease.**

The immune system of an individual does not produce an immune response to self antigens because the binding of self antigens to immature B and T lymphocytes during development results in the programmed destruction of these lymphocytes. Some self antigens are only recognized later. Anergy to the antigen results because there is no tissue damage. Natural killer cells do not destroy cells with these late appearing antigens because they are MHC class I positive. The binding of these molecules to the receptors on the natural killer cells protects them.

However, if one or other self antigen changes there is a real possibility that an immune response against these new antigens will be evoked and produce antibody that could cross-react with self antigens. An immunologically mediated disease directed against self antigens could result. The symptoms and syndromes would vary according to the nature of the antigen and the tissues affected by the perverted immune response.

Changes in self antigens are favored by many factors. The following have been hypothesized:

- **Aging, nonspecific hypergammaglobulinemia, malignancies, immune deficiency diseases, and endocrinopathies.**
- **Viral infections.** The virus and self antigen could combine to form an immunogenic unit that is recognized as a new immunogen.

- **Bacterial infections.** Bacteria such as Bordetella Pertussis liberate substances that can cause nonspecific polyclonal lymphocyte activation and autoimmunity because of their adjuvant effects. Others (e.g., streptococci) have antigenic determinants that cross react with tissue antigens. If these determinants complex with self antigens the complex could become antigenic and excite an immune response against self antigens.
- **Drugs:** The drug, acting as a hapten could combine with host tissues to form immunogenic units. The resulting immune response (if there is one) could cross-react with self antigens and initiate autoimmune disease.

A variety of diseases have been ascribed to presumed autoimmune reactions. Their causations by autoimmune reactions are presumed but difficult to prove except that they often respond to immunosuppression.

The following are the five most commonly accepted into this pathological category:

— **Systemic lupus erythematosus.** LE cells and anti-nuclear and anti-DNA antibodies are often present in significant amounts.

— **Rheumatoid disease.** Rheumatoid factors are present in about 80%, LE cells in 20%. Many patients have positive, but low titers of anti-nuclear antibody.

— **Progressive systemic sclerosis.** There are no specific blood findings. It is presumed that the disease results from immune responses to antigens common to subcutaneous and other tissues.

— **Polymyositis and dermatomyositis** The creatine phosphokinase (CPK) levels are elevated and often, the liver enzyme levels also. The muscle biopsy findings can be diagnostic.

— **Polyarteritis.** It is thought to be an autoimmune disease but the reasons are flimsy. The disease is characterized by a vasculitis and necrotizing arteritis, clearly seen in a biopsy and diagnostic in the right clinical setting.

The findings and symptoms of disease presumed to result from autoimmune reaction are varied. Common findings are any one or more combinations of the following: a rheumatoid-like arthritis; Raynaud's phenomena; muscle weakness; myositis; arteritis; and heartburn due to disturbed esophageal motility. Skin rashes and fever rarely affect progressive systemic sclerosis but may be manifest in any of the others. Renal disease (at times leading to renal failure) is a dreaded complication of systemic lupus erythematosus and polyarteritis but is uncommon in other autoimmune diseases.

4. **The Type 4 immune reaction: Cell-mediated immunity (Delayed hypersensitivity).**

The Type 4 immune reaction is mediated by immune T lymphocytes (Charts 8-4 and 8-5).

As mentioned previously, cell-mediated immunity is the principal mediator of reactions such as the Mantoux tuberculin test and the Schick test. They are also responsible for skin reactions to allergens such as poison ivy (usually an urticarial type rash), and, perhaps most important of all at the present, the rejection of allogeneic transplants.

Because of the increasing frequency of allogeneic transplantation some comment on the agents of destruction of allogeneic transplants is necessary. The precise mechanisms involved are still incompletely delineated. The probable antigens are blood-borne antigen-presenting cells derived from the graft. They express the MHC I and II molecules of the transplant. Most graft destruction probably results from natural killer cells and cytotoxic T cells.

Type 4 reaction protection in tuberculosis.

The WHO[5] estimates that a third of humanity (approximately 2 billion people) are infected with tuberculosis. Only 8 million develop clinical disease each year and of these about 1.6 million die (less than 1% of those infected).

The mortality is so low because the initial infection induces cell-mediated immunity against Mycobacterium tuberculosis var. hominis or Mycobacterium tuberculosis var. bovis or both. Mycobacterium var. bovis is present in the unpasteurized milk of tuberculous cattle and Mycobacterium tuberculosis var. hominis in the cough droplets of infected humans. Droplets 1-5 microns in diameter remain suspended in the air when coughed up by an infected person. They are inhaled by uninfected individuals, phagocytosed by macrophages and deposited in the lung parenchyma. When bacilli are ingested (usually Mycobacterium var. bovis) the primary foci of infection are the tonsils and the intestinal walls. In jurisdictions where there are infected cows up to 20% of tuberculosis results from bacteria ingested in unboiled milk. Cutaneous infection may occur in butchers handling infected meat and transplacental infection (congenital tuberculosis) has been reported.

From the primary focus (called the Ghon focus when the lung is affected) proliferating bacteria and accompanying pathology fairly rapidly spread to the draining lymph nodes; the hilar nodes when primary infection affects the lung, the cervical nodes when the primary focus is in the tonsil and the mesenteric nodes when the primary focus is intestinal. The initial pathology is a granulomatous reaction with frequent central caseation as the disease progresses. What happens next depends on the T cell immunity excited by the primary infection.

The Koch phenomenon.

Resistance to progression of the disease was demonstrated many decades ago by Robert Koch. He found that guinea pigs injected with tubercle bacilli developed the disease and, as a rule, gradually died. At the site of injection there was a persistent ulcer that did not heal. The draining lymph nodes were also infected. If any surviving guinea pig was given a second inoculum of bacteria there was a local inflammatory reaction, often with ulceration, but with eventual healing. The draining lymph nodes were not affected. This resistance was ascribed to hypersensitivity to the bacillus. We now know that it represents cell-mediated immunity directed against Mycobacterium tuberculosis. The tuberculin Mantoux reaction is one of its minor manifestations.

This generated immunity halts progression of the primary infection which then usually subsides with cessation of any systemic or bronchopulmonary spread. Most primary lesions regress and heal with scarring of granulomas and calcification of caseations. At times the generated immunity fails to halt spread of the disease and miliary tuberculosis and multi-organ disease result and progress unless vigorous therapy is started and continued till there is regression and eventual resolution. The only sequelae of generated immunity are two.

The first is a positive Mantoux test which indicates previous infection with M. Tuberculosis. About 24-72 hours after subepithelial injection of tuberculin into an individual with T cell immunity directed against mycobacteria tuberculosis, a raised, warm, red and itchy lesion appears and then disappears in the next few days. It does not mean the patient has active tuberculosis - only that there is immunity. The conversion of a negative Mantoux test to one which is positive suggests recent infection and merits medication directed against M.Tuberculosis.

The second is the frequent persistence of dormant M.Tuberculosis in the body. Reactivation of active disease can result from anything that depresses the individual's immune responses. Example of such items are malnutrition, subnutrition, uncontrolled diabetes mellitus, chronic disease of any sort, malignant disease, chemotherapy, long-term corticosteroids, and decreased immunological competence (e.g., due to HIV/AIDS). Reactivation or an uncontrolled primary infection can result in tuberculous bronchopneumonia, cavitation in the lungs, pleural spread and empyema. Disseminated infection can result in generalized disease (miliary tuberculosis) or to disease localized in one or more tissues such as the meninges, the bones, and the genitourinary complex. Peritoneal dissemination results in tubercles on visceral and parietal peritoneum. Adhesions of tuberculous bowel loops to each other are a common cause of intestinal obstruction in countries where people drink milk, contaminated with bacteria, but not pasteurized or boiled.

References for Chapter 8.

1. Hansen, H.S., Jensen, B. Essential function of linoleic acid esterified in acylglucosylceramide and acylceramide in maintaining the epidermal water barrier. Biochim. Biophys. Acta, 1985; 834:357.

2. Arstila, T.P., Casrouge, A., et al. A direct estimate of the human B and T cell repertoire diversity. Science 1999; 286:297.

3. Mond, J.J., Lees, A. et al.: T-cell independent antigens Type 2. Annu. Rev. Immunol. 1995; 13:655.

4. Coombs, R., Gell, P.: Classification of allergic reactions responsible for clinical hypersensitivity and disease. In: Gell, P., Coombs, R. (Eds.): Clinical aspects of immunology. Oxford. Blackwell Scientific Publications, 1975.

5. WHO Initiative for Vaccine Research. Tuberculosis: Internet: http://www.who.int/vaccine_research/diseases/tb/en/.

9

Diagnosis: The Slave Systems

1. The Gastrointestinal Tract and the Liver

Table of Contents

Notation.

The notation ~P denotes phosphorous with a high energy bond. Depending on the context in which the term is used, ~P may also denote the energy liberated when a high energy phosphate bond detaches from ATP or ADP.

A general comment on the methodology of clinical assessments.

The comments made **on page 119** about this topic are not repeated. They merit reading before proceeding with this chapter.

The gastrointestinal tract - normal physiology

The objectives.

The objectives of the gastrointestinal are the digestion, absorption and transfer to the blood of the products of food digestion and of ingested water, minerals and vitamins.

Bile produced by the liver is essential for absorption of fat. However, the liver has many other functions and for this reason it is considered separately in a subsection at the end of this chapter.

The resource systems of the gastrointestinal tract.

They are four in number:

- **Systems for ingestion.**
- **Systems for digestion.**
- **Systems for absorption and**
- **Systems for intestinal propulsion and evacuation.**

Chart 9-1 is an overview of the system that transfers environmental energy substrate to the intracellular milieu for conversion to energy that is usable for biological reaction. The substrate is the absorbed products of food digestion, absorbed water, minerals and vitamins and inhaled oxygen. The end product is energy stored in high energy phosphate bonds (~P).

Chart 9-1 summarizes the facts. It is a version of Chart 5-5 on page 104, truncated for this chapter.

Ingestion.

The requirements for ingestion of sufficient food include an intact central nervous system for obtaining food, for mastication and for swallowing. Additional requirements are a patent oropharynx, esophagus and gastrointestinal tract. The most important requirement is enough food, safely potable water, and minerals and vitamins. Regrettably, enough food is a frequent deficit for much of mankind. Chapter 15, page 319 et seq., details the

Chart 9-1: ENERGY SUBSTRATE FROM THE ENVIRONMENT TO CELLS FOR PRODUCTION OF ENERGY USABLE FOR BIOLOGICAL ACTIVITIES, i.e. ~P

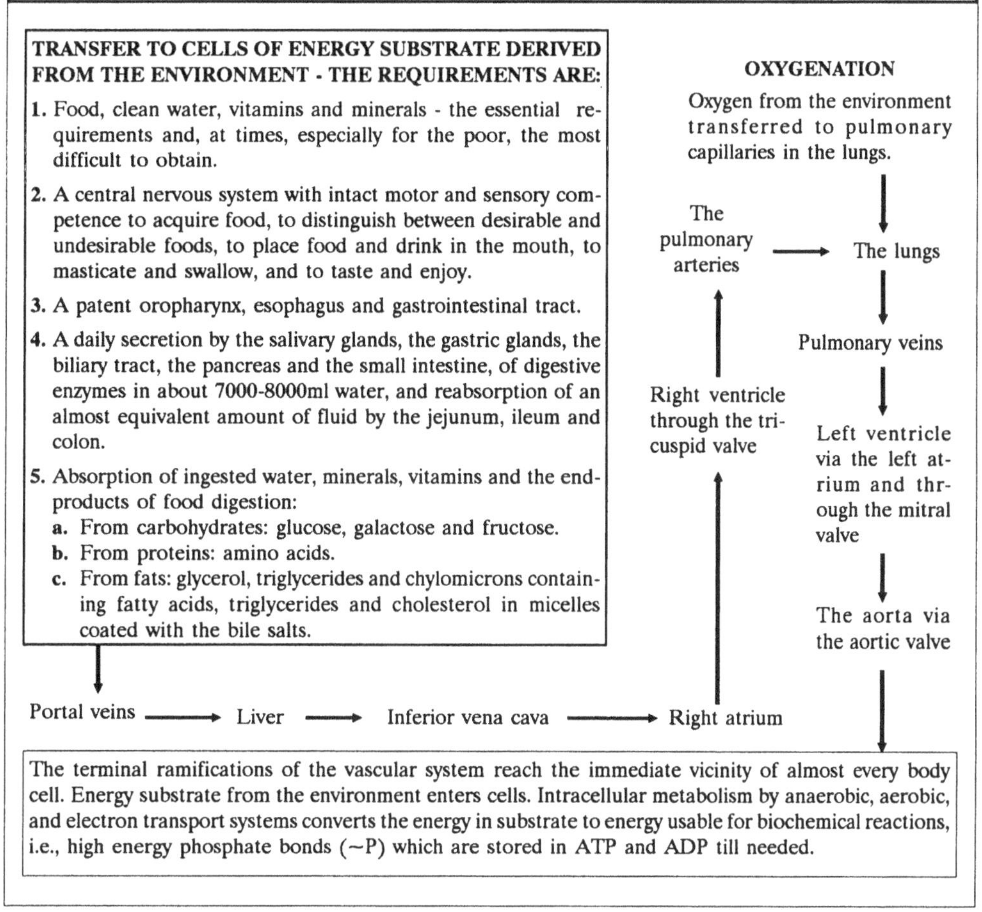
TRANSFER TO CELLS OF ENERGY SUBSTRATE DERIVED FROM THE ENVIRONMENT - THE REQUIREMENTS ARE:
1. Food, clean water, vitamins and minerals - the essential requirements and, at times, especially for the poor, the most difficult to obtain.
2. A central nervous system with intact motor and sensory competence to acquire food, to distinguish between desirable and undesirable foods, to place food and drink in the mouth, to masticate and swallow, and to taste and enjoy.
3. A patent oropharynx, esophagus and gastrointestinal tract.
4. A daily secretion by the salivary glands, the gastric glands, the biliary tract, the pancreas and the small intestine, of digestive enzymes in about 7000-8000ml water, and reabsorption of an almost equivalent amount of fluid by the jejunum, ileum and colon.
5. Absorption of ingested water, minerals, vitamins and the end-products of food digestion:
a. From carbohydrates: glucose, galactose and fructose.
b. From proteins: amino acids.
c. From fats: glycerol, triglycerides and chylomicrons containing fatty acids, triglycerides and cholesterol in micelles coated with the bile salts.
OXYGENATION
Oxygen from the environment transferred to pulmonary capillaries in the lungs.
The pulmonary arteries
The lungs
Pulmonary veins
Right ventricle through the tricuspid valve
Left ventricle via the left atrium and through the mitral valve
The aorta via the aortic valve
Portal veins
Liver
Inferior vena cava
Right atrium
The terminal ramifications of the vascular system reach the immediate vicinity of almost every body cell. Energy substrate from the environment enters cells. Intracellular metabolism by anaerobic, aerobic, and electron transport systems converts the energy in substrate to energy usable for biochemical reactions, i.e., high energy phosphate bonds (~P) which are stored in ATP and ADP till needed.

requirements for an adequate diet and the essential dietary requirements of humans.

Digestion.

Digestion is the catabolism of ingested food by enzymes. The enzymes needed are secreted in water by the salivary glands, the stomach, the small intestine, the pancreas, and the liver, by way of the gall bladder. Chart 9-2 depicts the volumes of water secreted with the enzymes and later reabsorbed in the gastrointestinal tract

The salivary glands and their secretions.

The contribution of saliva to digestion is small. Its main function is the lubrication of the mouth so that a combination of saliva and chewing can convert food to a paste that is easy to swallow and digest in the stomach and intestine.

The stomach.

Gastric secretion is about 2-3 liters per day. Water constitutes 99.5%. The rest is acid, enzymes, and inorganic ions.

There are three types of gastric glands: the parietal cells that produce acid and the chief cells that secrete inactive zymogens such as pepsinogen, prorenin and lipase, and many mucus-producing glands. The acid is HCl with a pH of about 1-2.5. It has many functions:

— It denatures and breaks the intramolecular and intermolecular bonds of proteins thus facilitating subsequent enzyme digestion.

— It activates the inactive enzyme pepsinogen to its active form, i.e., pepsin.

— It provides a pH of 1-2.5 which is optimal for pepsin digestion.

Chart 9-2: INTERNAL TURNOVERS OF WATER [1]

Secreted:		Reabsorbed:	
Saliva	1,000ml	Jejunum	4,500 - 5,500ml
Bile	1,000ml	Ileum	3,000 - 3,500ml
Pancreas	1,500ml	Colon	100 - 1,000ml
Gastric juice	2,500ml	Total reabsorbed	8,000-10,000ml
Small intestine	2,000 - 3,500ml		
Total secreted	8,000 - 10,000ml		

[1] Values are averages of those given by three authors. Many of these values have been derived by extrapolations from animal experiments. For obvious ethical reasons accurate figures for humans are difficult to obtain. The potential magnitudes of losses from disease such as gastroenteritis or sequestrations of fluids in loops of obstructed or adynamic bowel are obvious.

— It kills bacteria and other ingested microbes.

— It solubilizes iron compounds so that they can be easily absorbed and

— It stimulates the production of secretin by the intestines. Secretin promotes the flow of intestinal juices.

Pepsin breaks peptide linkages within protein molecules and hydrolyzes them to proteases and peptones. Few free amino acids are produced so that its contribution to final protein digestion is small.

Other enzymes produced in the stomach include rennin and lipase. In addition, salivary amylase is carried into the stomach by food and continues to catabolize carbohydrates until inactivated by the acidity of gastric juice about 10-20 minutes after ingestion. The result of gastric digestion is an acid chyme that is a liquid mixture delivered to the duodenum by peristalsis.

Intestinal digestion.

About 5-10 liters of secretions are produced each day by glands in the walls of the duodenum, jejunum and ileum. The intestinal secretions contain enzymes as well as hormones. Most of the water secreted is reabsorbed and returns to the circulation.

The following are the principal digestive enzymes produced by the small intestine:

Enzymes that break down protein and nucleic acids:

— **Aminopeptidases** catabolize the peptide bonds of proteins. The final product is a mixture of dipeptides and some amino acids.

— **Dipeptidases** catabolize dipeptides to amino acids. This completes protein digestion.

— **Nucleosidases and phosphatases** that complete the breakdown of nucleic acids started by the nucleases of pancreatic secretions.

Enzymes that catabolize carbohydrates.

- **Disaccharidases.** The principal ones are sucrase which splits sucrose to glucose and fructose, maltase which catabolizes maltose to two molecules of glucose, and lactase which splits lactose to glucose and galactose. The three monosaccharides absorbed are glucose, fructose and galactose.

Other hormones produced by the small intestine:

- **Secretin.** It is produced in and released from mucosal cells consequent on HCl stimulation. Secretin increases pancreatic and intestinal secretions and the production of bile.
- **Enterokinase** that converts inactive pancreatic trypsinogen to its active form which is trypsin.
- **Enterocrinin** that stimulates production of intestinal secretions.
- **Cholecystokinin** that stimulates contraction of the gall bladder, and
- **Pancreozymin** that stimulates the flow of pancreatic juice.

The pancreas.

The volume of daily pancreatic secretion is about 1000-1500ml. Its pH is about 7.5-8.2 and its content is 98% water. The remaining 2% contains enzymes (proteases, amylases, lipases and nucleases):

Trypsinogen. Enterokinase converts it to active trypsin which is an endopeptidase. It hydrolyzes peptide bonds within a protein. The final product is smaller protein fragments and a few amino acids.

Chymotrypsinogen which is secreted in an inactive form and activated by trypsin to chymotrypsin. It is another endopeptidase. Peptidases hydrolyze peptide bonds at the free ends of peptides that have carboxyl groups. Amino acids are produced as these chains shorten.

Amylases. Pancreatic amylase breaks the 1,6 and 1,4 linkages of starch. The result is sequential production of dextrins, erythrodextrins, achroodextrins and finally maltose.

Lipase. Bile salts, calcium ions and other emulsifying compounds significantly increase its activity. It catabolizes fats to a mixture of monoglycerides, diglycerides, free fatty acids and glycerol.

Other pancreatic enzymes include **phospholipases and nucleases.** The latter act on DNA and RNA with formation of the respective nucleotides.

The role of bile in digestion.

Up to 1 liter of bile is produced in the liver each day. In the gall bladder it is concentrated by reabsorption of water. Bile contains pigments, bile salts, cholesterol and various inorganic compounds. It is a secretion and also an excretion. The excretions are compounds such as bile pigments and other toxic substances, including metabolites of drug catabolism. The bile pigments are products of hemoglobin catabolism.

The bile salts.

The bile salts facilitate digestion and are eventually reabsorbed and returned to the liver. The principal **bile acids are cholic and chenodeoxycholic acid. They are synthesized in the liver** from cholesterol and secreted into the bile as conjugated salts of taurine and glycine.

The bile acids have two important functions in fat digestion:

First, they are emulsifying agents that disintegrate fat globules into small particles. This provides a larger surface area for the action of pancreatic lipase. The bile salts also energize pancreatic lipase to maximum activity.

Second is their ability to form micelles. The products of lipolysis are diglycerides, monoglycerides and free fatty acids. These products are maintained in solution by the bile acids which are amphipathic molecules with hydrophobic groups projecting inwards and hydrophilic groups projecting outwards. The core is interdigitating molecules of triglycerides, monoglycerides, diglycerides and cholesterol. These structures are the micelles. They are requisites for absorption of the products of lipolysis as well as the absorption of fat-soluble vitamins (vitamins A, D, E, and the carotenes).

Bile acid recirculation.

After absorption the bile acids separate from the micelle complexes and return to the liver. More than 95% of bile acids are reabsorbed in the intestine. However, the enterohepatic circulation is so frequent (5-15 times a day - the more calories ingested the more cycles) that about a quarter of the bile acid pool escapes into the colon each day. Some is absorbed in the colon and the rest is excreted in the feces (approximately 500 mg/day).

About half the bile acid reabsorption is active and the other half passive. Active absorption occurs in the terminal ileum. If fat digestion and absorption are incomplete the fat digestion products in mixed micelles reaching the terminal ileum interfere with absorption of bile salts and they escape into the colon. Resection or disease of the terminal ileum reduces the absorption of bile salts and diarrhea may result because:

First, if the malabsorption of bile salts is mild, synthesis of bile salts by the liver can maintain the pool and there is little or no effect on fat digestion or absorption. However unabsorbed bile acids escape into the colon and inhibit colonic sodium and water absorption with resultant diarrhea. This type of diarrhea can be decreased by giving cholestyramine which binds and sequesters bile acids.

Second, if bile acid malabsorption is severe, digestion and absorption of long chain fatty acid triglycerides is defective and unabsorbed fatty acids or their derivatives may cause diarrhea.

Intestinal absorption.

The intestinal surface is thrown into folds, each covered with finger-like or ridge-shaped villi. Each villus is 0.5-1.5mm long and they have a density of 10-40/mm^2. The free borders of the villi have hundreds of minute processes termed microvilli. At the bases of the villi are the crypts, simple tubes 0.3-0.5mm deep. There are about three crypts to each villus. It is estimated that these anatomical arrangements provide about 200m^2 of effective small intestinal absorptive surface. Cells are shed from the villi all the time, mostly from their tips. Normally cells are shed at a rate of about 100×10^6 per minute and in this process 30-50g of endogenous protein are delivered to the lumen each day. The entire epithelium is replaced in 3-6 days.

The absorption of the products of carbohydrate digestion.

Carbohydrates are absorbed throughout the small intestine, but mostly in the middle part. The three sugars left after digestion are glucose, galactose and fructose. They are all absorbed by facilitated diffusion; attachment to a cell membrane carrier protein which transfers the sugar into the cell along a concentration gradient. No energy is required. The carrier for fructose is a **uniport transporter**; it needs only one type of molecule, i.e., fructose. The transporter for glucose and galactose are **symport transporters** (SGLT1) because for each transport they require a combination of a molecule of the sugar and two ions of Na^+. Thus, sugar in the intestinal lumen promotes sodium absorption and replacement of diarrheal losses as long as sodium content in the lumen exceeds that in the cells. The excess sodium in the cell is repeatedly extruded by the sodium pump to maintain intracellular osmotic pressure and water follows passively. The process continues repeatedly as long as there is glucose in the lumen and a diffusion gradient for sodium from intestinal lumen into the cell. This is the rationale for giving sodium and glucose for oral rehydration in severe gastroenteritis where sodium loss is often large. It relies on luminal concentrations of sodium which are higher than those in the cells, and the common **symport carrier** for glucose and sodium transport into cells. The glucose promotes intracellular movement of sodium which is important when gastroenteritis is resulting in significant sodium losses in the diarrheal output. The sugar exits the cell by another facilitated diffusion using a different uniport (GLUT2).

The absorption of the products of protein digestion.

The end products are amino acids. Absorption takes place throughout the small intestine. About half the amino acids come from digestion of food protein, about a quarter from digestion of the protein content of the intestinal secretions and the remainder from desquamated epithelial cells. The D-amino acids are absorbed by passive diffusion. Most of the L-amino acids use carrier transport systems.

The absorption of the products of fat digestion.

Absorption takes place throughout the small intestine. The micelles attach to the intestinal brush border and their content of fatty acids and cholesterol enter the mucosal cells by passive diffusion. The bile salt coatings enter the blood and are returned to the liver.

Fatty acids with less than 12 carbon atoms enter the portal blood. The larger fatty acids are converted to triglycerides and some cholesterol is esterified. All then combine with phospholipid, free cholesterol and lipoprotein to form chylomicrons. The chylomicrons leave the intestine in the lymphatic drainage of mucosal cells. Some of the triglyceride is incorporated into very low density lipoprotein (VLDL) which is also transported by lymphatics. Cholesterol metabolism is detailed in a later chapter about cardiac function. Triglyceride metabolism is discussed later in this chapter.

Propulsion in the intestinal tract.

The small intestine. Two types of movement are demonstrable. **Segmental contractions that mix food, water and digestive enzymes** and **peristaltic contractions** that move the intestinal contents onwards to the ileocecal valve. Extrinsic innervation is not required but an intact myenteric nerve plexus is.

The colon. Common gastrointestinal dysfunctions are associated with disturbances of colonic motility. The colon of an adult receives 500-2500ml of chyme each day. It contains undigested and unabsorbed residues of food, water and electrolytes. The usual diet of humans contains some materials, chiefly the cellulose walls of plant cells, which are not easily digested in the small intestine. This residue accumulates and is to some extent digested in the cecum. The contents of the cecum and ascending colon are kneaded by non-propulsive churning movements and they are slowly dried by absorption of water and electrolytes till they have the consistency of mush. Haustral movements, multihaustral contractions, peristalsis and mass movements slowly move the contents of the colon to the rectum. Distention of the rectum arouses the defecation reflex. The nerve centers of this reflex are located in the sacral segments of the cord. It involves coordinated contractions of voluntary and involuntary muscles. If the reflex is not inhibited by higher centers defecation follows.

The gastrocolic reflex and mass peristalsis. These reflexes are evoked by movement of ileal contents into the colon. Humoral and neural factors are involved as it also occurs even when ileal contents cannot enter the colon. Within ten minutes of eating a meal distal colonic activity is at its peak suggesting that the reflex is neurally mediated. An anti-cholinergic drug can inhibit the early response but usually not the later response when hormones released by a meal are reaching peak levels. Fat in the diet stimulates cholestokinin release and this is probably the main stimulus increasing colonic motility after eating. Proteins and amino acids inhibit the response to fat. Carbohydrates do not. The increased activity in the right colon that follows eating initiates mass peristalsis.

The gastrointestinal tract - the dysfunctions

Any one or more of the etiologies detailed on pages 75-77 can affect any one or more of the components of the gastrointestinal tract. The resulting dysfunctions are well described in standard texts. **The comments on methologies of clinical assessments are summarized on page 119 and merit a re-reading before continuing.**

There are some dysfunctions which are unique to the gastrointestinal tract. Examples are potentially lethal infections by pathogens, the malabsorptions syndromes and inflammatory bowel disease, i.e., Crohn's disease and ulcerative colitis. These are described in a little more detail than others. Needless to say the most common gastrointestinal dysfunction does not result from disease but from insufficient food, a frequent affliction of many people in this world of ours.

The symptoms and signs of gastrointestinal dysfunction include any one or more of the following: pain, masses, dysphagia, heartburn, changes of bowel habit, diarrhea and constipation, loss of appetite, weight loss, nausea and vomiting, hematemesis, melena, jaundice, and edema and ascites.

Diagnosis of gastrointestinal dysfunctions are seldom difficult because of the many ancillary procedures available. Examples are blood work, the examinations of stools for blood and pathogens, radiological studies of the upper and lower gastrointestinal tracts, ultrasounds, endoscopies, biopsies, CT scans, and MRIs. Often the clinical suspicion is that the cause of the problem is an irritable bowel syndrome or some other psychosomatic syndrome affecting the intestinal tract. However, all investigations must be done to exclude dangerous pathology before making such diagnoses.

Duodenal ulceration, reflux esophagitis and proton pump inhibitors.

Lykoudis[1] was the first to postulate that a frequent cause of peptic ulceration was bacterial infection. His original postulates were later confirmed by Warren and Marshall[2]. Currently it is felt that most duodenal ulcers are caused by Heliobacter Pylori infections which can be eradicated by therapy which usually results in cure of the ulcer. Nevertheless, there remain some ulcers that are either not caused by H. Pylori or are resistant to treatment by antibiotics. These patients need relief of symptoms and so do many patients with reflux esophagitis.

Conventional antacids are chemical neutralizers of gastric acid or antagonists of H_2 receptors. Often they do not provide adequate relief. A recently introduced group of drugs, the proton pump inhibitors are often effective when antacids do not suffice.

Proton pump inhibitors. These drugs can produce large decreases in gastric acid secretion by binding to the cysteine molecules on gastric H^+/K^+-ATPase. This inactivates the enzyme and stops ejection of H^+ by the parietal cells. The Na^+/K^+-ATPase has been called the proton pump. Given the nature of the enzyme a more probable explanation is that its activation by, perhaps H^+, results in extraction of ~P from intracellular ATP and that this provides the energy for extrusion of H^+ through H^+ channels. Long-term ingestion of proton pump inhibitors increases the risk an increased incidence atrophic gastritis[3].

Subnutrition, malnutrition and obesity.

It is a terrible paradox that many of the people in this world go to bed hungry while minorities of affluence have and eat more than they need, and suffer for this. Sufficient food is essential for good health and for resistance to disease. But overfeeding and obesity results in individuals who are prone to multifactorial dysfunctions such as heart disease, diabetes, arthritis and respiratory disease.

Subnutrition and malnutrition result in weak, apathetic and stunted individuals. Many of their children are mentally retarded. Many syndromes characterize deficiencies of specific dietary components. A diet sufficient in calories and nutrients is an important component of therapy and many factors determine the necessary quantities of food in a diet as well as its essential components. All are detailed and described in Chapter 15 which details therapeutic and other measures for prevention of disease.

Is food scarce? The answer is a qualified no. In wealthy countries farmers are often paid to not farm their lands, or given subsidies to maintain the low prices that prevent the competitive import from, and facilitate profitable exports to disadvantaged communities (this is a major problem and the subsequent text expands on this problem). Subsidized farmers compete monetarily with food and items such as cotton produced locally in disadvantaged states. Well-meaning gifts of food from affluent countries and charitable organizations often have the same effect. They compete with local products and the end-result is a decrease in local productivity. The objectives of the affluent are profits and the gaining of local and international political kudos to the detriment of the impoverished. A consequence is increased suffering for the poor. The need for ending or reducing subsidies and high tariffs is repeatedly stated in one conference after another. Very little seems to get done to effect these reductions. Promises are made about debt reductions but once again little is done. There are other factors responsible for insufficient food. The following are some:

- **The ravages of HIV/AIDS in Africa.** Many are afflicted and are dying or are dead. The decimation of the population and the weakness of those who survive with active AIDS results in decreases of individuals who can work. The fields are not tilled, the seeds are not sown and the little that is produced is not harvested. Many effective drugs are not affordable and the world looks on with sympathy but little else. Horrors await the unfortunates of that continent as the horsemen of the Apocalypse descend on it. They continue to be additionally burdened by the other causes of insufficient food which are itemized below.
- **Poverty.**
- **Drought.**
- **Inadequate irrigation systems and insufficient water.**
- **Corruption.**

- **Inequitable distribution of land.**
- **Lack of skills.**
- **Lack of fertilizers, herbicides and pesticides.**
- **Insufficient seeds.**
- **Genetically modified seeds which give better production but are too expensive for peasant farmers.**
- **Lack of storage facilities.**
- **Lack of an efficient infrastructure for distribution.**
- **Primitive and inefficient farm equipment.**
- **Difficulties in obtaining funds for improvements - banks avoid lending to the poor.**
- **and the all too common global minefields.**

As mentioned above African countries are especially afflicted by insufficient food and its medical consequences. In most Asian countries sufficient food is available to avoid starvation but usually not hunger The main problems are substandard infrastructures. Inadequate road and rail systems for transport create bottlenecks and there are limited facilities for storage and delivery. Often, rodents eat more than humans! Hopefully, with the passage of time these problems will be resolved. At present multitudes in Africa and Asia go to bed hungry and this is immoral and unnecessary, given the potentials of the world's farmlands.

Obesity.

This is a common and numerically increasing affliction in affluent societies. Many criteria have been used to define obesity and papers about the pathophysiology and treatments of obesity are legion. Any excess over desirable weights increases the risks of multifactorial diseases: cardiac disease, diabetes, arthritis and respiratory disease. Thus, obesity is a potential danger to life.

The treatment of obesity is simple. No fad diets or canned liquids are needed. The individual just needs to eat less. To those who say this does not work photographs of concentration camp survivors are mute testimony to their error. The problem is psychological - a desire and often a love of food, as against the knowledge of possible future dysfunctions. A pathetic belief is that possible consequences will bypass the addict. They often do. All who are obese do not develop cardiorespiratory disease, arthritis or diabetes but many others do and a frequent consequence for them is premature death. A relapse from good intentions is common and this is why most of those who lose weight by dieting soon regain their previous weight. They just like eating.

Malabsorption syndromes.

The malabsorption syndromes are disorders that result from absorption deficits of one or more components of ingested food. The possible causes are many:

- **Enzyme deficiencies.** Notable examples are lactase deficiencies and deficits due to pancreatic disease. Many other syndromes due to congenital enzyme deficiencies are described. They are rare but well described in standard texts on genetics. Often they are only recognized when standard investigations of individuals with the symptoms of a malabsorption syndrome fail to demonstrate any of the more common causes.
- **Short bowel syndrome,** the result of extensive bowel resection.
- **Chronic intestinal infections,** bacterial, parasitic or viral.
- **Celiac disease and tropical sprue.**
- **Crohn's disease** affecting the small intestine.
- **Alcoholism** and some drugs.
- **Intestinal lymphoma** is always a possibility when investigations do not identify a cause. The malabsorption results from lymphatic blockages. It is diagnosable by an intestinal biopsy.

The symptoms of a malabsorption syndrome.

The symptoms and signs. Weight loss is common. Any of the malabsorption syndromes can cause deficits of all nutrients or only of specific proteins, sugars, products of fat digestion, vitamins or minerals. The clinical features of many of these deficits are detailed in Chapter 15.

What follows is a description of the salient features of four malabsorption syndromes: lactase deficiency, malabsorption due to pancreatic disease, celiac disease and tropical sprue.

Lactase deficiency.

Lactase is an enzyme that splits lactose to glucose and galactose. A deficiency of the enzyme is inherited as an autosomal recessive and the onset of symptoms is usually between the ages of three and five. Occasional cases first appear in adolescence or early adult life. Secondary lactase deficiencies can result from any of the malabsorption syndromes listed above.

There are ethnic differences in the incidence of lactase deficiency. The incidence is only about 15% in individuals of Northern European origin. Increases begin in the Mediterranean countries. About 65-70% of individuals in South India are affected but the incidence is much lower in the North (20-30%). In people of Sinic origin the incidence rises to almost 100%. In case you have not noticed, Chinese foods rarely contain any milk products, possibly because of the frequency of lactase deficiencies in these populations.

Symptoms result from the presence of undigested lactose in the colon. Water is drawn in and the results are bloating, cramps, flatulence and diarrhea. The diagnosis can be confirmed by a lactose tolerance test. The patient drinks 0.5-1g (laboratories vary in the amounts given) lactose/Kg of body weight. The test is positive if intestinal symptoms appear in an hour or so, concurrent with a rise in blood glucose of less than 1.1mmol/L.

Treatment is avoidance of milk products though some individuals can drink small amounts of milk without the appearance of any symptoms. Milk treated with lactase is available. So are the enzymes that permit home treatment of milk.

Milk is an important source of calcium and individuals with lactose intolerance who avoid all milk products are well advised to supplement their diets with 1-1.5g calcium each day unless they eat foods such as meat and meat products that contain calcium. Also watch for any symptoms of vitamins A, D and riboflavin deficiency. Vitamin supplements are advisable as long as permissible doses are not exceeded.

Malabsorption due to pancreatic failure.

The commonest cause is cystic fibrosis. It is a disease that crosses many physiological borders. It is inherited as an autosomal recessive trait.

The diagnosis is made on the basis of clinical findings, studies of pancreatic exocrine function and the electrolyte concentrations in sweat. There are various ways of inducing sweating. The object is to measure sweat chloride. A value greater than 60mmol/L of chloride in sweat is usually diagnostic of cystic fibrosis. Values less than 40mmol/L are normal while values between 40-60mmol/L are border line, suggestive but not diagnostic. They must be repeated and any borderline values require evaluation in conjunction with the clinical picture and the values of pancreatic exocrine secretions.

The disease is characterized by viscous glandular secretions. The principal symptoms result from blockage of bronchiolar and pancreatic gland ducts by these thickened secretions. In the lungs the results are repeated infections with occasional acute exacerbations and a progressive decrease in pulmonary function. The thickened secretions often cause various atelectases, some large enough to cause lobar occlusions. The mean life expectancy has gradually increased and is now over 30 years. Pneumothorax, hemoptyses, and cor pulmonale may occur. The terminal event is usually an acute on chronic lung infection.

Occlusion of pancreatic ducts by viscous secretions results in replacement of the acini by fibrous tissue and fat. The decrease or absence of pancreatic lipase decreases fat digestion. There is chronic diarrhea and steatorrhea with foul-smelling and bulky stools. Decreases in normal growth are common.

Fortunately there are current preparations of supplemental pancreatic enzymes that can be taken orally (e.g., Pancrease: Janssen-Ortho). They greatly help in reduction of symptoms due to pancreatic insufficiency.

Celiac disease.

The disease is an inherited intolerance of the gliadin fraction of gluten, a protein present in wheat, barley, rye and oats. In afflicted individuals gluten is thought to cause an autoimmune response that damages the intestinal surface so that a biopsy shows a flat mucosa without villi. It is said that the amino acid sequences causing the autoimmune reaction are not present in corn or rice.

Celiac disease is a disease that can be difficult to diagnose because of its protean manifestations. In children symptoms appear when gluten is introduced into the diet. Symptoms vary from mild abdominal discomfort to painful cramps and bloating. Because of decreased fat absorption the stools have an unpleasant smell and are pale and bulky. The children are short and development is slow. They often develop an iron-deficiency anemia. Anemias due to vitamin B_{12} deficiencies can also occur, at times with the concomitant characteristic neurological dysfunctions. Bone growth is abnormal because of calcium deficits.

Adults usually have weight loss, malnutrition, diarrhea with bulky pale stools as well as dysfunctions similar to those seen in children. At times the diagnosis is missed because gastrointestinal dysfunctions are minimal or absent and patients present with isolated consequences of the disease. Examples are presentations with iron deficiency anemias or anemias due to vitamin B_{12} deficits. Other forms of presentation include bone pains and abnormalities of bone growth, menstrual dysfunctions and/or a coagulopathy.

The treatment of celiac disease is simple and recovery is rapid. All foods containing gluten must be excluded. Gluten is present in many commercial products such as ice-creams, hot dogs and sauces. Peruse the label on the article before buying. Women are often diagnosed earlier than men because of menstrual disturbances or a pregnancy anemia that is marked and fails to respond to therapy.

About 10% of celiac disease patients develop **dermatitis herpetiformis** which is an itchy skin rash with small blisters. Some of these individuals have no gastrointestinal symptoms.

Case history.

Young lady who was 19 when seen 15 years ago because of a skin rash. I had never before seen a similar skin rash and did a biopsy of one of the lesions. The pathologist described the histology and commented that the lesion was compatible with a diagnosis of dermatitis herpetiformis. A gastroenterologist did an intestinal biopsy. It showed a flat mucosa without villi. The diagnosis of celiac disease was made. Once a gluten free diet was started her resistant iron deficiency anemia immediately responded to oral iron as did her menstrual dysfunctions. She began to gain weight and is now a healthy mother with two sons aged 10 and 11.

Tropical sprue.

This is an acquired disease. The specific cause or causes have not been identified. Infections with bacteria, parasites or viruses are suggested causes. So are food toxins. The disease occurs predominantly in South India, Southeast Asia and the Caribbean. It can affect individuals native to these areas as well as visitors.

The presentation is one of weight loss, diarrhea and strangely, a sore tongue. Any or all the features of a malabsorption syndrome can appear. For example, anemias due to deficits of iron, folic acid and vitamin B_{12}. Other symptoms include steatorrhea and albumin, calcium and prothrombin deficiencies.

The intestinal biopsy is rarely diagnostic. There may be some villus atrophy but not of the degree seen in celiac disease. Typically there is a mucosal infiltrate of lymphocytes, plasma cells and eosinophils.

There is a good response to a long-term course of a tetracycline.

Childhood diarrhea and oral rehydration therapy.

Some 5-6 million deaths per year result from diseases that cause diarrhea and most of these deaths occur in young children[4]. There are many possible causes but most are impossible to identify with certainty except in research-oriented major hospitals.

The commonest cause is the rotavirus. This organism is said to be responsible for 20% of deaths in children less than five years of age. Another common pathogen is the Enterotoxigenic Escheria Coli (ETEC), accounting for about 10% of all deaths in these children. Other causes include the Shigella bacteria that occasionally result in epidemics, other bacteria such as the Vibrio Cholera and viruses such as the human Calciviruses (HuCV). Recently much interest has centered on HuCV as the cause of infantile diarrhea. It appears to be the second most common cause of diarrhea in children (rotavirus is the first). Confirmation of HuCV infections is the demonstration of HuCV antibodies in children living in countries such as Bangladesh and China (in China the estimate of HuCV antibodies was reported as 99%).

Therapy.

Unfortunately there are no antibiotics that are effective against the viral infections. The use of anti-bacterial antibiotics is limited by the relative infrequency of infantile diarrhea caused by bacteria.

Is there no way to end this holocaust of innocent children. Certainly there is. End poverty, malnutrition and subnutrition, provide clean potable water, and advise on hygiene and good sanitation. Those living in affluent countries must learn to help and share. At present various manipulations, restrictions and subsidies ensure that the rich remain rich and the disadvantaged live out a karma of misery - 4-6 million deaths a year is cause for shame and introspection.

Oral rehydration.

The only therapy available is one that maintains life till the intrinsic defenses of the body arrest the infection and restore normality. Alternatively, till they are unsuccessful and death ensues.

Oral rehydration with a mixture of glucose or sucrose with Na^+ is effective therapy because of the common carrier for glucose and sodium. The physiological basis for this therapy was described on page 194. The first record of the use of this form of therapy that I can find is by Mahalanabis and associates[5]. It is an observation vigorously promoted by the WHO[6], and verified by many others since then[7,8]. Long chain carbohydrates such as rice are as effective as glucose and many reports have confirmed this fact[9].

Incidentally, at one time in the late 1950s I worked for a period in a small missionary hospital in an impoverished part of the world. Children with severe dehydration from gastroenteritis were frequent patients. Most parents and friends in the area and the two nuns who ran the three room hospital knew that the therapy was sugar, salt and water by mouth till the child was strong enough to put down a mush of salted boiled rice. I only learnt about this after arriving. It seems that this protocol had been used by rural populations for centuries. We all thought that the processes were such obvious remedies that no thought was given to publication.

When there was time to spare blood counts could be done using an antiquated microscope in a side room. Intravenous equipment was not available nor a laboratory to do electrolytes. In the late 1950s some young, dedicated and altruistic physicians from a charitable organization in the USA visited our little hospital. They looked horrified at the sight of some of the dehydrated children brought in that morning. A common comment was that mortality would never be reduced without facilities for intravenous rehydration and laboratory services that measured electrolytes. I explained how we extemporized quite satisfactorily. Therapy with subcutaneous saline was very effective. Glucose was never added to the injected saline because of the inflammatory reactions that can result from subcutaneous glucose. The visitors stayed two days and left with astonishments and thanks for the experience. None of the children died. All were up and about in two days.

The saline solution was made each morning with sterilization by boiling. It was given to severely dehydrated infants as two to three subcutaneous injections of 50ml each with the single large antiquated metal syringe available. If necessary up to 100ml per injection was given to children age 7-10. Needles were repeatedly sharpened on a grindstone, sterilized by boiling with the syringe and reused. In the severely dehydrated the large subcutaneous bulges of saline would disappear in a couple of hours. Adequate hydration was evinced by slower disappearance of the bulges and a urine with a gradually decreasing yellow color as hydration improved. Incredibly, despite the absence of any sophisticated laboratory technology this ad hoc therapy resulted in a negligible mortality. As soon as adequate dehydration of the acutely ill child ended, and often simultaneously, the children drank water containing sugar and salt and as soon as possible graduated to a mush of rice with salt. There was no need for packets of oral rehydration minerals. In any case they were not available. Correct the water and salt deficits and potassium and pH will automatically readjust unless there is renal failure.

If there is renal failure as evinced by a negligible urine neither intravenous nor subcutaneou saline will help

Death will eventuate unless the patient can access the sophisticated services available in large hospitals. Remember that the potassium in the packets of ORT is contraindicated in a patient with renal failure.

I describe these anecdotal incidents in a little detail as many physicians will practice in destitute locations such as the one described above. I have heard such physicians commenting on deaths of dehydrated children because of the lack of WHO oral rehydration packages and of equipment for intravenous therapy. Subcutaneous saline is an effective and safe alternative. It is also much less bothersome to the child than an intravenous setup. Also, listen to the mother and the interested villagers. They may appear uneducated but have lots of commonsense and the wisdoms handed down from one generation to the next.

Incidentally, I recently saved the life of a pet cat who was vomiting because of eating some sort of long dead and decayed bird. She refused to allow intravenous rehydration and the veterinarian suggested I take her home and hope for the best, i.e., let her die. Injections of subcutaneous saline in my home saved her life. After two days of therapy, 50ml twice a day, she was up and about, looking for food in the house and creating the domestic turmoil so unique to all cats.

The diarrheas of adults.

Gastroenteritis is a common cause of disease in adults and the following is a short description of their causes and pathologies.

Viral gastroenteritis.

Viral infections are the commonest cause of acute gastrointestinal diarrheas in adults. Many different viruses can cause gastroenteritis. They include rotaviruses, adenoviruses, Norwalk virus, and calciviruses. Transmission is by food handlers who have not washed their hands after defecating or urinating or handling contaminated clothing and diapers or hospital dressings. Many permutations and combinations of fecal-oral contamination are possible. Viral gastroenteritis is also transmitted by the eating of shellfish contaminated by consumption of water in streams, rivers and oceans polluted with sewage. Another cause is contamination by underground seepage of coliforms from human or animal wastes into wells used for drinking water.

The gastroenteritis is usually self curing. While the disease is present some dietary restrictions help. Each physician has different ideas on what these should be. My favorite is clear soup, apple juice or flat ginger ale (not the diet type that has no sugar) and plain crackers, i.e., crackers without salt or cheese, till there is recovery. It is difficult to know what part, if any, this dietary regimen had on recovery. Intravenous or subcutaneous rehydration is only needed in extreme situations, usually in the elderly and in children with profuse and persistent diarrhea.

Therapy. There are no antibiotics that are effective against these viral infections. In both infants and adults the efficacy of antibacterial drugs is limited by the infrequency of gastrointestinal infections by bacteria. Typhoid, cholera and shigella dysentery do occur and immediate ad hoc antibacterials are appropriate when diarrhea is severe and bloody. The results of stool cultures and studies of sensitivities can be obtained in a day or two and determine whether the antibacterial therapy should be stopped or changed. Of course the majorities of jurisdictions where such infections occur do not have the facilities for such tests and entrepreneurs wishing to sell antibacterials are always present.

Hamburger disease.

The disease is so named because it comes from eating undercooked and contaminated ground beef, and/or foods that could have been contaminated by manure. Examples are unpasteurized milk or cheese, or unpasteurized apple juice and cider. Contamination of wells by underground seepage is another danger.

The causative organism is E.Coli 0157:H. The organism is a frequent inhabitant of the intestines of cattle, poultry and other animals. It often contaminates the meat of slaughtered animals. Its presence in manure results in contaminations of unpasteurized milk, cheese, apple juice and cider. Human infections result from contamination of meat by contact with the meat of other slaughtered animals carrying the organism, or by hands inadequately washed after defecation, urination or the handling of bed and personal linens and medical dressings. The organism produces a toxin (verotoxicogenic toxin) that attacks the intestinal mucosa and the kidneys.

Symptoms of infection may be mild or severe diarrhea, often with melena, cramps, vomiting and fever. The disease lasts 2-10 days and begins 2-10 days after eating contaminated food. It is estimated that some 10% of infected individuals will develop a hemolytic-uremia syndrome (HUS). Dialysis and blood transfusions may be needed. Most will recover, but some will die and others will remain with permanent kidney damage.

Prevention includes personal hygiene and the repeated testing of water supplies for contamination. Always cook hamburger, pork or chicken thoroughly up to the center (meat and juices should not be reddish - a taste relished by many but at their own risk) and do not drink unpasteurized milk, apple juice or unpasteurized cider or eat cheese made from unpasteurized milk. Inevitably, personal preferences often override these desiderata.

Campylobacter infections.

Infection results from the species campylobacter jejuni. The organism is resident in many birds and infection results from eating or handling raw or undercooked poultry meats. All poultry products should be cooked thoroughly.

Campylobacteria infections are a common cause of diarrheal disease. Symptoms begin 2-5 days after infection. There are cramps, vomiting and diarrhea, often with blood. Recovery is usual in a week. On rare occasions there are long-term complications. One is an arthritis. Another, strangely enough, is a Guillain-Barré syndrome. It is said that 40% of Guillain-Barré syndromes in the United States are associated with campylobacter infections.

Giardiasis.

The diagnostic difficulties result from the appearance of symptoms some 1-2 weeks after infection. The causative organism is a protozoon, Giardia intestinalis, present in the intestines of man and animals. Infection is via fecally contaminated food or water. Symptoms include cramps, diarrhea, and some weight loss. The disease usually lasts 5-10 days with full recovery. But it can become chronic and result in a malabsorption syndrome. Treatment may not be needed but metronidazole is an effective antimicrobial for this disease.

Inflammatory bowel disease.

All bowel infections result in inflammation of some degree. The appellation "inflammatory bowel disease" disease is reserved for two diseases that cause chronic inflammation of the bowel: Crohn's disease and ulcerative colitis.

Crohn's disease.

Crohn's disease is a chronic inflammation that can affect any part of the digestive tract from mouth to anus. Its etiology is not known but thought by many to be the result of some type of autoimmune response. The inflammation extends deep into the bowel wall. Edema and scarring can result in intestinal obstruction. Extraintestinal tracts can develop with formation of perianal fistulae and fistulae between the intestine and the bladder or vagina.

The symptoms are abdominal pains, cramps and diarrhea, rectal bleeding, weight loss and fever. Children with Crohn's disease are stunted and growth is delayed. Nutritional deficits are common; deficits of protein, vitamins and calories due to malabsorption, inadequate intake of food and intestinal loss of protein. Systemic complications include arthritis, dermatitis, inflammatory conditions of the eyes and mouth, and dysfunctions of the liver and biliary tract.

The prognosis is always guarded. A common picture is one of remissions and recurrences. Others may have a continuum of disease. Therapy is often disappointing. Drug therapy includes 5-ASA agents, corticosteroids and immunosuppressive agents. Antibiotics may be needed for infections caused by strictures or fistulae.

Nutritional supplements are often needed and parenteral alimentation may be required to rest the intestine, or to provide for adequate nutrition by diseased intestine or a "short bowel syndrome" resulting from extensive surgical resection.

Surgery cannot cure Crohn's disease. It is indicated for obstruction, hemorrhage, perforation or large pericolic abscesses that do not respond to antibiotics. Some gastroenterologists recommend resection of affected bowel if control becomes corticosteroid dependent. Unfortunately, recurrence of the disease is usual, often in bowel next to the resected area. The outlook for a patient with Crohn's disease is bleak. At best there will be long periods of remission between recurrences. More common is lifelong episodes of pain, cramps, rectal bleeding, inadequate nutrition and weight loss or an inability to gain weight.

Ulcerative colitis.

Ulcerative colitis is a chronic inflammatory disease of the colon. The characteristic lesions are ulcers of the mucosa with bleeding and production of mucus and pus. It may only affect the rectum and distal colon (ulcerative proctitis) or extend over the whole colon (pancolitis). Theories abound but there are no known and demonstrable causes for Crohn's disease or ulcerative colitis.

The symptoms include bloody diarrhea, abdominal cramps, loss of appetite and weight loss. Anemia is frequent. Systemic complications are similar to those seen in Crohn's disease: skin lesions, arthritis, inflammations of the eye and liver dysfunctions. The maintenance of good nutrition is essential.

Therapy includes 5-aminosalicylic acid (5-ASA) drugs, corticosteroids and immunosuppressive agents. Complications include severe bleeding, perforation and toxic megacolon. The last is a sudden distention of the colon with active colitis and fever. It results from inflammation extending through the full thickness of the colon. The wall of the colon is ballooned and there is a real risk of rupture. If this complication cannot be rapidly controlled surgical resection of the colon will be needed.

Ulcerative colitis and Crohn's disease differ in several ways:

- Crohn's disease can affect any part of the digestive system from mouth to anus. Ulcerative colitis only affects the colon.
- "Skip areas" are frequent in Crohn's disease but uncommon in ulcerative colitis.
- Crohn's disease can affect the whole thickness of the bowel while the ulcers of ulcerative colitis are usually only mucosal. Ulcerative colitis only affects the whole thickness of the bowel when there are major exacerbations, some resulting in "toxic megacolon", as described above.
- Surgery is needed in some 20-30% of individuals with ulcerative colitis. If it involves removal of the whole colon the patient is usually cured of the disease but must put up with the inconveniences of an ileosotomy. Alternatively, with the diarrhea that often follows reconstructive procedures. In Crohn's disease surgery is rarely curative. It is only indicated on an ad hoc basis that depends on the clinical judgments and views of the attending physician.

Maxim:

Always consider the possibility of either one of the two main types of inflammatory bowel disease (Crohn's disease and ulcerative colitis) in any patient who has recurrent diarrhea with or without melena, or with abdominal pains that are not typical of any other gastrointestinal disease. Early diagnosis may or may not help but is always useful for assessments and therapies of any future exacerbations. The day will surely come when the etiologies of these conditions are identified. A previous diagnosis will then expedite cure. X-ray studies of the gastrointestinal tract and endoscopic inspections and biopsies are valuable diagnostic tools.

The irritable bowel syndrome.

The most common of gastrointestinal dysfunctions is probably the so-called "irritable bowel syndrome". The condition is caused by uncoordinated and abnormal motor activities of the intestines. There is abdominal pain and episodes of constipation and diarrhea. As a result of irregular spasms the fecal masses may be retained for a long time while water is absorbed. They are eventually evacuated as hard dry balls. Alternatively evacuation may be as pencil-thin ribbons if there is spasm of the anus, rectum and sigmoid colon.

It is difficult to attribute the symptoms of irritable bowel disease to psychological disturbances. Abnormal myoelectric activity may be present but such abnormalities are often demonstrable in individuals free of bowel symptoms. A patient with irritable bowel has hyperalgesia. A degree of tension in the wall of the colon that would not bother a normal person causes pain in the hypogastrium, the iliac fossae, the perineum and the anorectal region. During the irregular spasms of the sigmoid colon and rectum the internal anal sphincter relaxes. This together with the hyperalgesia, produces a sense of urgency but not the ability to defecate.

The diagnosis of "irritable bowel syndrome" is usually one of last resort, even if the diagnosis is suspected at the initial consultation. A long history of dysfunctions dating back for many years suggests that the diagnosis is correct. The diagnosis should only be made after routine investigations fail to demonstrate organic disease such as malignancies or inflammatory bowel disease. Treatment is usually unrewarding. Many physicians believe that a diet containing lots of fiber are essential for relief of symptoms in this disabling disease that is not a hazard to life. Antispasmodics may help.

Colonic and rectal neoplasms.

The frequency and the potential lethal consequences of these lesions should be known to all physicians. Any patient with a recent history of melena or change in bowel habit must be fully investigated to exclude a colonic or rectal neoplasm; a rectal examination is essential at every annual assessment.. An occult blood study at the annual physical examination is appropriate for all older than 45. The pathology and clinical consequences of colonic neoplasms are so well covered in standard texts that no additional description is includad in this text.

This ends a short summary of the principal features of dysfunctions specific to the gastrointestinal tract. **One important component of the gastrointestinal system is the liver. The liver has important roles in fat absorption and carbohydrate and lipid homeostasis. But it also performs other important functions unrelated to the gastrointestinal tract. For this reason it is considered in a separate section of this chapter. This allows the detailing of all its functions and principal dysfunctions regardless of whether or not they are related to gastrointestinal tract physiology and disease.**

The Liver - normal physiology

An extensive literature on every aspect of liver disease is by the late Sheila Sherlock and easily accessed on the PubMed page of the Internet.

Apart from its other functions an important function of the liver is to metabolize, degrade and eliminate endogenous toxins, drugs and other noxious materials. Renal excretion and pulmonary exhalation assist in these activities.. The topic is long and complex and merits a separate chapter (Chapter 16)..

The objectives.

- **Glucose homeostasis.**
- **Lipid homeostasis.**
- **Protein synthesis.**
- **Detoxification.** The liver metabolizes, degrades and detoxifies many substances; endogenous waste products such as those derived from heme as well as many different drugs. A later chapter (Chapter 16) on drug therapy contains detailed information on these topics.
- **Bile production.**
- **Metabolism of ammonia to urea (the Kreb's-Henseleit cycle)**
- **Vitamin storage and absorption.**

The resource systems of the liver:

The **multifunctional hepatocellular cell** with its many complex separate resource systems is the principal resource system of the liver.

Subsidiary resource systems are:

- A **biliary tract** that transports the products of hepatocellular function to the gall bladder and from there, to the intestine. It is described as a resource because any hindrance to the free flow of bile can result in hepatic dysfunctions.

-- **A patent unobstructed portal and systemic hepatic circulation.** It also is described as a resource because any hindrance to the free flow of portal or systemic bloods can result in hepatic dysfunctions.

Glucose homeostasis.

This topic was detailed on pages 85 et seq. About 5-7% of liver weight is glycogen. Glycogenolysis and gluconeogenesis from protein are the catabolic and anabolic hepatic functions that, in combination and interaction with insulin and glucagon, maintain blood glucose within physiologically desirable and permissible ranges during post-prandial periods or during periods of fasting. Hypoglycemia is one result of advanced liver failure.

The interactions of liver glycogen, insulin and glucagon ensure that the central nervous system is always perfused with enough energy substrate to form ~P, provided that perfusion with blood is sufficient. As repeatedly mentioned before, the central nervous system can only use glucose for production of ~P though, after a period of starvation, some ketones are usable for this purpose.

Lipid homeostasis.

As detailed on page 89, fat[11] is an efficient storage material. One gram of fat can store 9KCal of energy as compared with the 4KCal/gm that is storable as carbohydrate or protein. In addition fat storage does not need much, if any, intracellular water. It is estimated that if humans stored energy as carbohydrate rather than fat the average individual's body mass would increase by a factor of six to eight.

The objectives of lipid homeostasis are the following.

Storage of energy substrate that exceeds immediate needs. The absorbed products of fat digestion and of intracellular catabolism of stored fat accumulate in hepatocytes and fat cells when there are no intracellular energy deficits in any organs and tissues. A frequent result is a fatty liver. When any cell needs energy the stored material is catabolized, and the products are transferred by the blood to cells that have energy deficits. The intracellular enzymes of those cells metabolize the transported fatty acids to the ~P that it needs.

Maintenance of blood triglyceride and cholesterol levels within physiologically permissible and desirable levels. Cholesterol metabolism is detailed in a later chapter on the cardiovascular complex. Triglyceride metabolism is the topic considered here (Charts 9-3 and 9-4 on the next page). Triglycerides are glycerol triesters of fatty acids. They are the basic constituents of fat and the principal sources of energy from lipids. The different fatty acids in animal and plant foods exceed 50 in number. Some are saturated fats, others are unsaturated, some are straight-chain compounds while others are branched-chain structures. Most body fats are complex mixtures of up to 12 different triglycerides

Chylomicrons from intestinal digestion (Chart 9-3) contain about 80-90% triglycerides and about 5-10% cholesterol. Lipoprotein lipase in endothelial cells of adipose tissue and muscle capillaries remove the fatty acids of the chylomicrons. The triglycerides are used locally for energy production or stored as fat in the liver and adipose tissue till there is insufficient substrate for ~P synthesis in the cells or in the cells of other organs

The liver is also the main site for conversion of excess dietary amino acids and sugars to their storage forms which are glycogen, fatty acids and fat. When cells need energy, hepatic triglycerides are packaged with cholesterol into VLDLs. The required triglycerides are removed from the VLDL by endothelial cell lipoprotein lipase and used locally. The VLDLs then become cholesterol remnants.

Protein synthesis.

The liver synthesizes many proteins. They include:

Albumin. The liver produces 150-400mg/Kg body weight each day. Serum albumin cannot egress from capillaries except in small amounts (<0.5%). Exceptions are a few places in the liver and spleen where some capillary walls are discontinuous. Albumin and other proteins retained in the circulation have osmotic pressures (termed oncotic pressure in plasma) that prevents water from moving to the interstitial fluid. **(Contd. on page 207)**

Chart 9-3: COMPOSITIONS OF SOME LIPOPROTEINS

	Chylomicrons	VLDL (hepatic and dietary)	LDL	HDL[2]
Triglycerides	85-95%	50-70%	5-15%	0%
Cholesterol and cholesterol esters	5-10%	15%	40-50%	15-20%
Phospholipids and proteins (including the apoproteins)	~ 5%	20-30%	40-50%	75-85%

[1] Averages of values given by different authors. The significant features are the progressive decrease in triglyceride percentages from VLDL to LDL and then HDL, and the progressive increase of cholesterol percentages from chylomicron to LDL.

[2] HDL contains cholesterol from cells which have extruded unneeded cholesterol and also the cholesterol in chylomicron and VLDL remnants. Some is free and unesterified and the rest is esterified by LCAT. HDL is returned to the liver for endocytosis and utilization of cholesterol for production of bile acids.

Chart 9-4: TRIGLYCERIDE HOMEOSTASIS

The objectives

1. Storage of energy substrate in excess of immediate body needs as fat. The substrate is the absorbed products of fat and carbohydrate digestion.
2. Provision of triglycerides to cells which have deficits of substrate for production of biologically usable energy (i.e., ~P stored in ATP or ADP).
3. Maintenance of blood triglyceride levels within physiologically desirable levels.

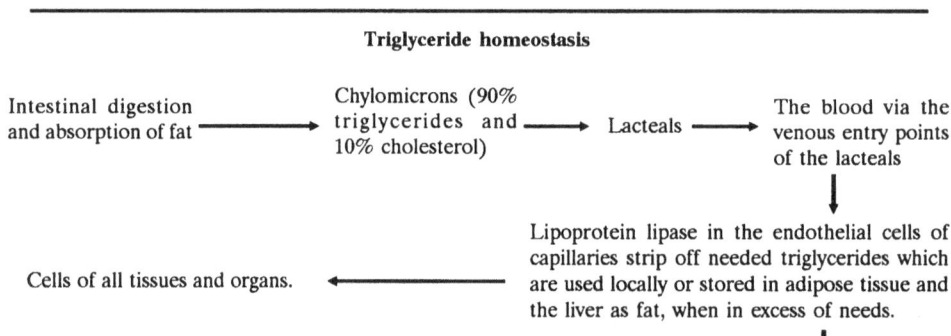

Triglyceride homeostasis

Intestinal digestion and absorption of fat → Chylomicrons (90% triglycerides and 10% cholesterol) → Lacteals → The blood via the venous entry points of the lacteals

↓

Lipoprotein lipase in the endothelial cells of capillaries strip off needed triglycerides which are used locally or stored in adipose tissue and the liver as fat, when in excess of needs. → Cells of all tissues and organs.

↓

If dietary and stored triglycerides do not satisfy body needs the liver synthesizes triglycerides. Hepatic triglycerides are packaged with cholesterol as VLDLs; composition of about 15% cholesterol and 60% triglycerides. They leave the liver in the blood. Endothelial cell and tissue lipoprotein lipase remove needed triglycerides which become available to cells where there are energy deficits. Intracellular enzymes of those cells convert the triglycerides to ~P by beta oxidation and subsequent metabolism in the Kreb's cycle and Electron Transport system.

(Contd. from apge 205)

This maintains intravascular volume.

Many of the clotting factors (e.g., Factors 2, 7, 9 and 10) are produced in the liver.

Prolongation of prothrombin times (the INR), bleeding diatheses and purpura that appear without obvious cause, or after minimal trauma are complications of advanced liver failure.

Other proteins.

The liver produces many other proteins. Examples are transferrin, ceruloplasmin, haptoglobin, various anti-proteases and some of the complement components. As a rule, deficiency syndromes are only seen in advanced liver failure.

Any hepatic decrease of the degradation of plasminogen activator can promote fibrinolysis. Clotted blood from cirrhotic patients will often lyse when allowed to stand due to stimulation of fibrinolysis by increased amounts of plasminogen activator. In patients with advanced liver disease this can result in increased thrombolysis of protective clots.

Bile production.

Bile is the vehicle for removing the products of red cell destruction from the body. Old or damaged red cells account for 80-90% of serum bilirubin. The remainder is derived from enzymes such as catalases and peroxidases. Chart 9-5 on the next page graphically depicts the processes involved in production of bile. Additional explanatory text is not needed. Excess bilirubin in the blood results in jaundice. It is an important physical sign of liver disease. A later section details the differential diagnosis of jaundice.

Conversion of ammonia to urea.

Ammonia is formed in the intestine by the action of bacterial enzymes on the amino acid products of protein digestion and catabolism. The liver converts this ammonia to urea that is subsequently excreted by the kidneys. Increased amounts of ammonia result from gastrointestinal bleeds.

There is an association between hepatic encephalopathy and raised blood ammonia levels but many question whether this is a cause and effect relationship or, at least whether increases in blood ammonia are the only factors responsible for hepatic encephalopathy.

Vitamin storage and absorption.

The fat-soluble vitamins (A, D, and K) are stored in the liver. Bile salts are needed for absorption of these vitamins from the intestine. A vitamin K deficiency syndrome and an accompanying bleeding diathesis can develop when there is an obstructive lesion of the biliary tract. Vitamin D deficiencies in primary biliary cirrhosis can result in bone pains, osteomalacia and fractures.

The Liver - the dysfunctions

The following is a summarized description of the more common liver dysfunctions.

Fatty Liver.

This condition results from fat accumulation in hepatic cells. It is probably the commonest hepatic dysfunction. The risk of developing inflammations, fibrosis or cirrhosis are directly proportional to the amount of fat present.

Nutritional causes predominate. Eating to excess is a common cause. Paradoxically, starvation, protein malnutrition, and bypass surgery for obesity also cause fatty liver. The probable reason is increased lipolysis and mobilization of fat to provide energy when other sources are in short supply. Excessive drinking of alcohol is another common cause as is diabetes mellitus. Less common causes are drugs such as corticosteroids and long-term tetracycline for acne.

The fatty liver of pregnancy is uncommon but of importance. A large amount of fat can be rapidly deposited in the liver resulting in a palpable and tender liver. It usually occurs near term and can result in premature

Chart 9-5: BILIRUBIN METABOLISM AND BILE PRODUCTION

Bilirubin: about 80-90% is from heme in old or damaged red cells.

Bilirubin: about 10-20% is from ineffective erythropoiesis and from catabolism of heme-containing enzymes such as catalases, peroxidases and cytochrome enzymes.

Water-insoluble unconjugated bilirubin (approximately 250 mg per day) enters the blood.

Water-insoluble unconjugated bilirubin in the blood binds to serum albumin.

The water-insoluble bilirubin-albumin complex is transported to the liver. The liver cell membrane separates **unconjugated bilirubin** from albumin and unconjugated bilirubin enters the hepatic cell.

Unconjugated bilirubin binds to Y and Z receptor proteins and is converted to bilirubin monoglucoronide (**conjugated bilirubin**) by the enzyme glucuronyl transferase. It is secreted into bile as a water-soluble diglucoronide[1]. The liver also receives the urobilinogen not excreted in the urine and excretes it in bile.

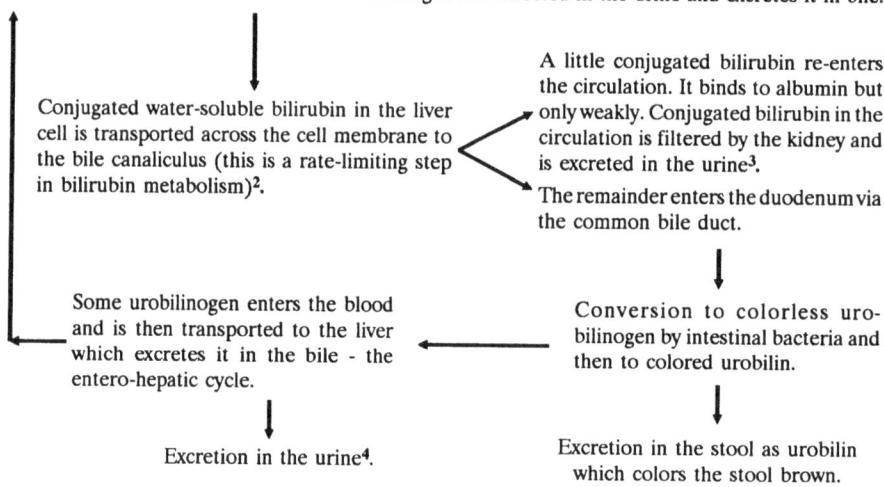

Conjugated water-soluble bilirubin in the liver cell is transported across the cell membrane to the bile canaliculus (this is a rate-limiting step in bilirubin metabolism)[2].

A little conjugated bilirubin re-enters the circulation. It binds to albumin but only weakly. Conjugated bilirubin in the circulation is filtered by the kidney and is excreted in the urine[3].

The remainder enters the duodenum via the common bile duct.

Conversion to colorless urobilinogen by intestinal bacteria and then to colored urobilin.

Some urobilinogen enters the blood and is then transported to the liver which excretes it in the bile - the entero-hepatic cycle.

Excretion in the urine[4].

Excretion in the stool as urobilin which colors the stool brown.

[1] Laboratory tests can separately determine blood levels of conjugated and unconjugated bilirubin. **Water-soluble conjugated bilirubin is called "direct bilirubin"** and **water-insoluble unconjugated bilirubin is called "indirect bilirubin".**

[2] When the capabilities of this rate-limiting step are reduced by cholestasis or liver cell swelling there is a decrease in excretion of bilirubin into the bile and entry of conjugated bilirubin into the blood and excretion in the urine.

[3] Unconjugated bilirubin cannot be excreted in the urine but conjugated bilirubin can. In both, obstructive jaundice and jaundice due to hepatitis conjugated bilirubin accumulates in the blood and its urinary excretion increases. Often conjugation of bilirubin is decreased in patients who have hepatitis. When this occurs the total serum bilirubin is raised but the direct (i.e. conjugated) bilirubin is low.

[4] Usually not more than about 4 mg per day. Significant increases are seen when there is increased production of conjugated bilirubin (e.g., in hemolytic anemias), or when hepatocellular disease damages the excretory systems of the liver cells and conjugated bilirubin is reabsorbed into the blood and excreted in urine.

birth. A similar type of acute fatty liver is occasionally seen in juvenile diabetics.

Non-alcoholic steatohepatitis (NASH).

NASH is described as inflammation associated with fatty liver. Often there are no symptoms and the diagnosis is suspected by raised aminotransferases and an ultrasound showing fatty liver.

Previously it was thought that NASH was a benign condition without significant associated disabilities. However, biopsies have shown fibrotic lesions in some 40% of patients and it is estimated that 5-10% eventually develop typical cirrhosis.

Jaundice.

The physiology of bile production was graphically depicted in Chart 9-5. Normal serum bilirubin levels usually do not exceed 1mg/dL (5-19μmol/L in S.I. units) and of this the direct reacting water-soluble conjugated fraction rarely exceeds 0.4mg/dl (7μmol/L in S.I. units). The remainder is lipid-soluble but water-insoluble unconjugated bilirubin (3-13μmol/L in S.I. units). Clinical jaundice is usually demonstrable when the serum bilirubin exceeds 2 or 3mg/dL (about 30-40μmol/L in SI units). Most hepatic dysfunctions are associated with some degree of jaundice. Therefore, analysis of the causes of jaundice provides a basis for identifying some of the different causes of hepatic dysfunction.

Differential diagnosis of jaundice by examination of blood, urine and stools.

Blood. Total **bilirubin** measures the sum of conjugated and unconjugated bilirubin. The direct reaction measures conjugated bilirubin and the indirect measures the unconjugated fraction. Both are raised in hepatocellular disease; the unconjugated because of its decreased uptake by damaged liver cells and the conjugated because of a combination of hepatocellular injury that reduces egress from hepatocytes into the biliary tract and also, the cholestasis that frequently accompanies hepatocellular injury. When cholestasis is the main cause of jaundice the conjugated fraction predominates. Serum bilirubin levels are usually higher in hepatocellular disease than in obstructive jaundice.

Liver aminotransferase enzymes (SGOT and SGPT levels) are of value in distinguishing jaundice due to hepatocellular disease from that which results from posthepatic biliary obstruction. In acute hepatitis enzyme levels can exceed 1000 units/dL. In posthepatic obstructions elevations of aminotransferase levels are usually modest.

Urine. Bilirubinuria indicates increased serum conjugated bilirubin. An increase is seen when there is heme overload as in hemolytic anemias and absorption of intestinal blood after a hemorrhage or in situations where cholestasis is a prominent feature. Normal urine urobilinogen is less than 4mg/day. It derives from conjugated bilirubin excreted in the bile and first converted to colorless urobilinogen and then to urobilin in the stools.

Stools. Urobilin is responsible for the brown color of stools. Obstructive jaundice is characterized by clay colored stools (the stools are bulky and of grayish color) because conjugated bilirubin does not enter the intestine. Its absence result in deficits of fat digestion and absorption. Bulky gray stools result from the undigested intestinal fat.

Causes of jaundice.

There are three principal causes of jaundice:

- **Prehepatic pathology.**
- **Hepatocellular disease.**
- **Posthepatic obstruction** (so-called "**surgical jaundice**").

1. **Prehepatic jaundice**

The usual cause of prehepatic jaundice is a hemolytic anemia or absorption of blood from a gastrointestinal bleed, or from a large collection of blood (e.g., after rupture of an aortic aneurysm), or from sizable tissue infarcts.

Uncommon causes of prehepatic jaundice with excess unconjugated bilirubin in the blood include hereditary conditions such as **Gilbert's syndrome** which results from deficient uptake of bilirubin by liver cells, and deficient hepatocellular glucuronyl transferase activity.

Neonatal jaundice

Neonatal jaundice merits mention as another prehepatic cause of jaundice. The hepatic cell uptake systems for unconjugated bilirubin (glucuronyl transferase and the Y and Z proteins) are often not mature at birth. An unconjugated bilirubinemia develops but usually subsides in the next two weeks with maturation of the hepatic uptake systems. In premature infants the uptake systems are less mature at birth and take longer to recover. When unconjugated bilirubin levels near 20mg/dL kernicterus is a potential danger. It is a syndrome that results from bilirubin deposits in the basal ganglia with subsequent choreoathetosis and ataxia. Phototherapy is widely used as therapy. The methods used vary and when specialized care is not available standard and accepted pediatric texts should be consulted for details.

2. Hepatocellular jaundice.

Hepatocellular dysfunctions may be global or focal.Focal causes include multiple granulomas, abscesses, cysts and tumors - benign and/or malignant, and if malignant, primary and metastatic lesions. The commonest liver neoplasm is a metastatic malignancy.

Global hepatocellular dysfunctions.

The usual causes are viral hepatitis and dysfunctions caused by drugs and alcoholism. Chronic hepatic disease and hepatic cirrhosis are occasional sequelae. Hepatocellular dysfunctions often decreases the uptake of unconjugated bilirubin, as well as its conjugation and subsequent excretion. Hence, it is often impossible to determine which predominates, hepatic cell dysfunction or intrahepatic cholestasis.

A cholestasis can occur without much, if any hepatocellular dysfunction. Examples are the cholestasis occasionally seen in third trimester pregnancies (possibly due to increased sensitivity to estrogens), cholestasis due to drugs, notably chlorpromazine, and the cholestasis of primary biliary cirrhosis.

Hepatocellular dysfunction due to acute viral hepatitis.

The symptoms and signs of acute hepatitis are usually similar regardless of the cause. Etiology is determined by the clinical setting, the previous history and ancillary laboratory and radiological investigations.

Viral hepatitis has clinical presentations that range from minimal to life-threatening symptomatology. At one extreme the disease can be symptomless and its previous occurrence only recognized by incidental and unexpected findings of antibodies and/or antigens in the blood. The prodrome of clinical disease is 1-2 weeks. Symptoms are often only those of a viral infection - myalgia, fatigue, headaches, and slight fever. If the clinical picture is more advanced there is fever, jaundice, abdominal pain in the right upper quadrant, tender hepatomegaly, and occasional symptoms of immune complex deposits causing polyarthritis, urticaria, and other skin rashes. Serum bilirubin increases, at times to 30-40mg/dl. Bile and urobilinogen are present in the urine, and there is a progressive increase in aminotransferases (SGOT and SGPT) to levels that could exceed 1,000 units. Jaundice increases for 1-2 weeks and then begins to decrease till normality is reached in 4-6 weeks. Progression to acute hepatitis and necrosis are real but uncommon possibilities.

Hepatitis A and B have similar clinical features with a single exception. Recovery from hepatitis A infections is usually complete within three months of the onset. Not so with hepatitis B and C infections. A significant portion (approximately 10-20%) have persistent infections, sometimes subsequent cirrhosis, and occasionally, hepatocellular malignancy.

The hepatitis A virus is a fecal virus usually transmitted by oral-fecal contamination. This is why it frequently affects children and is more common in places where there is overcrowding and poor sanitation.

The hepatitis B virus has a world-wide distribution and, in addition, many asymptomatic carriers exist. The virus can be present in a variety of body fluids: saliva, tears, droplets expelled during a sneeze, menstrual fluid and urine. Transmission can occur by oral or parenteral routes. A particularly important mode of transmission in current society is by intravenous injection of drugs using contaminated needles.

The hepatitis C virus is said to be transmitted mainly by contaminated blood. However, there are almost certainly other factors involved as there are patients with antibodies to Hepatitis C without any previous history of transfusions. Infection can eventuate in cirrhosis and at times, in hepatocellular carcinoma.

Numerous additional hepatitis viruses are being continually discovered. Those interested can find a lot of useful information of the D, E and other viruses on the Internet.

Variations of the usual clinical course of viral hepatitis.

Hepatitis without jaundice. Many patients with viral infections of the liver do not develop jaundice. The ratio of anicteric to icteric cases is about 1:1 in adults. It is estimated that in children the ratio is nearer 1:10. There may be no symptoms. The occurrence of previous disease is subsequently assumed because of the incidental findings in blood of antibodies to a hepatitis virus. Raised aminotransferases are not diagnostic as they can result from any hepatocellular dysfunction. More common than a symptomless dysfunction is a flu like syndrome of fever, myalgia, tiredness and maybe some rhinitis.

Fulminant viral hepatitis. This develops in about 1% of patients with acute viral hepatitis. It is associated with massive liver necrosis. There is increasing jaundice, a decreased prothrombin time, and finally, coma. The mortality is high with only some 20-25% of these patients surviving to subsequently live with the aftermaths of extensive liver damage.

Chronic active hepatitis. The syndrome of chronic active hepatitis includes a number of dissimilar syndromes of hepatic dysfunction. A large percentage are labeled idiopathic as no obvious cause is demonstrable. Approximately 1-5% of patients who have had a B virus hepatitis, and some who have had an anicteric form of the disease, develop recurrent episodes of hepatitis and eventual cirrhosis. Estimates are that the sequelae of hepatitis-B virus infections account for 30-40% of patients with chronic active hepatitis (chronic active hepatitis is an uncommon condition). Non-A and non-B viral infections and adverse reactions to drugs are said to be occasional causes. Usually the cause cannot be identified and these patients are said to have idiopathic disease.

About 70% of the affected patients are adolescent or young women and some 25% are men. At times there is spontaneous restoration to normal or maintenance of a stable cirrhotic state. The disease usually presents with fatigue and a gradual appearance of jaundice. The usual course is one of recurrent jaundice, with eventual development of the stigmata of cirrhosis. Extrahepatic symptoms are common; some examples are arthralgias, skin lesions, and a keratoconjunctivitis sicca syndrome.

Some of those who are not Hepatitis B Ag-positive have anti-nuclear antibodies and the lupus erythematosus factor in the blood. For such reasons the syndrome of chronic active hepatitis has been described by many different names: chronic lupoid hepatitis, autoimmune hepatitis, chronic liver disease in young women and plasma cell hepatitis. It is probable that these are all the same disease: chronic active hepatitis.

The diagnosis is usually based on the clinical history and the histology of liver biopsies. The pathology is one of focal cell necroses, portal and periportal lymphocytes and plasma cells. Bridging areas of necrosis are often seen connecting portal and central areas of lobules and whole lobules may collapse. Cirrhosis is a frequent sequel. Corticosteroids are often of therapeutic value. Otherwise only supportive treatment is possible with the persistent hope that there will be regression or persistence of a stable state.

Hepatocellular dysfunction duc to alcoholism.

The hepatotoxicity of alcohol has been surmised since the recognition by Laennec of cirrhosis. However, its first clear demonstration was probably the study of Rubin and Leiber[12]. Individual variations are a major factor. Some chronic alcoholics do not develop pathology while many others who may consume less do. Presentations vary. The following are some examples:

Acute hepatitis after an episode of binge drinking. There is jaundice, some tender hepatomegaly, occasional purpura, nausea and vomiting. The serum bilirubin is raised (usually the unconjugated fraction but also the conjugated fraction when there are associated cholestatic obstructions. The aminotransferases are also raised but uncommonly to the high levels seen in viral hepatitis. Recovery to the previous level of dysfunction, if any, is usual if the patient stops drinking and there is no underlying liver disease.

Case history.

Patient age 62 who was an enthusiastic maker of wine at home. When the time came to make new wine for the year he found quite a lot left in the old barrel. During the course of the day he drank it all - about a gallon and a half. Two days later he came to the office looking as yellow as a canary. Blood results suggested an acute hepatitis. No treatment was available. I told him to go home and hope for spontaneous recovery. A strict injunction was no alcohol for three months. He recovered completely over the next two weeks. Needless to say my injunction was disregarded. When confronted he assured me that wine consumption was necessary for maintenance of good health. Fortunately there was no recurrence of hepatic dysfunction. He died five years later from a myocardial infarct.

Acute hepatic flare-ups with underlying cirrhosis. This also usually occurs after an episode of binge drinking or a febrile disorder due to any cause (for example, renal and pulmonary infections). Recovery from the acute phase is usual but inevitably there is some progression of the underlying cirrhosis.

Slow progression to liver failure because of associated cirrhosis. This is frequent. With the passage of time the chronic alcoholic develops all the complications and stigmata of advanced cirrhosis and the eventual outcome is usually fatal.

Presentation with a neurological syndrome. Many have been described. Wernicke's encephalopathy is the one most often described. The syndrome is characterized by oculomotor pareses, ataxia of the trunk that affects stance and gait, varying degrees of dementia and disturbed retentive memory.

The mental disturbances are often described as a Korsakoff psychosis. Recovery is possible for about 20% of patients. The remainder gradually deteriorate till supervised existence becomes necessary. Current thinking attributes this syndrome to a thiamine deficiency. Rapid therapy with thiamine does occasionally result in recovery. Unfortunately the usual course is a supervised existence and eventual death from cirrhosis or infections of different sorts.

Some other causes for the acute hepatitis dysfunction syndrome.

Many drugs can cause a hepatitis like syndrome because of toxic or idiosyncratic reactions. Important in the latter group are the anti-convulsant, dilantin (diphenylhydantoin), the anti-tuberculosis drugs, isoniazid and rifampin, and some tranquilizers, notably chlorpromazine and related phenothiazines. Jaundice due to cholestasis from drugs such as oral contraceptives and chlorpromazine was previously described.

Other causes of an acute hepatitis are some poisons, notably mushroom poisoning by amanita phalloides, and poisoning by accidental or deliberate drinking of carbon tetrachloride, a common cleaning agent.

3. Post-hepatic jaundice ("Surgical jaundice").

Common causes are biliary calculi from the gall bladder, carcinoma of the head of the pancreas or of the duodenum in the region of the ampulla of Vater, and infrequently, acute pancreatitis and malignancies of the common bile duct. Other uncommon causes include ampullary stenosis, congenital choledochal cysts and hemobilia from hepatic tumors or rupture of a hepatic artery aneurysm. In poor countries, especially those in Asia, ductal obstruction by Ascaris lumbricoides is a frequent cause of bile duct obstruction.

Jaundice appears early and may be associated with pain and fever if there is associated cholecystitis or liver abscesses. The combination of an enlarged painless gall bladder (presumably because there was no previous inflammation with post-inflammatory fibrosis) and jaundice is said to indicate post-hepatic obstruction by a neoplasm (Courvoisier's law), usually of the head of the pancreas. Pruritus is an extremely bothersome symptom, especially in an individual with common bile duct obstruction due to an inoperable malignancy. The insertion of a drainage stent often relieves the pruritus. If endoscopy cannot manipulate it into the termination of the common bile duct the alternative is external tube drainage of bile via a dilated intrahepatic duct.

"Surgical liver disease" is characterized by jaundice, pale bulky stools and bleeding tendencies due to deficient vitamin K absorption because of the absence of bile salts in the intestine. The bilirubin seldom exceeds 30mg/dL. A significant portion is water-soluble conjugated bilirubin which is absorbed into the blood so that bilirubinuria is also present. The aminotransferases may be normal or raised but not to the levels seen in inflammatory hepatitis. A raised alkaline phosphatase is characteristic of post-hepatocellular obstructions.

Post-hepatic obstruction must be distinguished from hepatic parenchymal disease and intrahepatic cholestasis. Jaundice, raised serum bilirubin and bilirubinuria are present in both. Aminotransferase levels (SGOT and SGPT) are helpful. In post-hepatic obstruction increases are modest. In hepatocellular disease they are more marked and may, at times, exceed 1000 units. Malignant obstructions result in higher serum bilirubin levels (up to 30 mg/dL) than obstructions due to stone (usually less than than 15 mg/dL). Radiological investigations are valuable. CT scans and ultrasounds often readily demonstrate calculi, malignancies and dilated intrahepatic bile ducts. Histological assessments of biopsies can be helpful as can cytological evaluations of fine needle biopsies of the liver. They should not be done unless INRs are normal. Cytological examinations and bacterial cultures of ascitic fluid are helpful adjuncts. Of major diagnostic assistance are endoscopic ERCP and related studies.

Hepatic cirrhosis.

Cirrhosis is the end-stage lesion of various forms of smoldering and unresolved hepatitis. The possible causes are many. They include viral hepatitis, chronic active hepatitis, alcohol related liver dysfunctions, some individuals with fatty livers (NASH), toxic or idiosyncratic reaction to drugs or poisons, long-standing obstruction of the biliary tract (e.g., in primary biliary cirrhosis), chronic hepatic congestion (as in chronic congestive heart failure) and some rare conditions such as hemochromatosis and Wilson's disease (hepatolenticular degeneration).

The following are some of the clinical manifestations of liver cirrhosis:

Jaundice.

This is often precipitated in patients with quiescent cirrhosis by binge drinking, or intercurrent infections of any sort (examples are urinary and pulmonary infections, and viral infections, notably, influenza). Other precipitating factors are any one or more of the following: anemia; trauma in accidents; hypovolemia and hypotension; binge eating and binge consumption of alcohol; adverse reactions to therapeutic drugs; and environmental toxins and the "recreational" drugs.

Inconstant clinical features of hepatic cirrhosis.

They include spider angiomas, palmar erythema, weight loss and a tendency to bleed easily and to develop purpura after minimal or no trauma.

Portal hypertension.

The portal vein delivers blood to the liver from the intestines. At the esophagogastric and anorectal junctions and at the umbilicus, portal and systemic venous systems communicate. At the umbilicus communications are by vessels that follow the ligamentum teres.

Obstruction to portal blood flow in the liver can result from any one or more different causes. The common causes are pressure from regenerated or regenerating nodules, strangulation of intrahepatic vessels by fibrous tissue and anatomical distortions, inflammatory obliteration of intrahepatic veins, and rarely, occlusion of the main hepatic veins (the Budd-Chiari syndrome). Uncommon causes include portal vein occlusions because of adjacent intra-abdominal inflammations, the pressure of tumors or the idiopathic thromboses which are occasionally seen when there is constrictive pericarditis or advanced congestive heart failure.

Obstructions of portal blood flow results in **portal hypertension** with distention of varices at the places where there are portal-systemic communications. An important consequence is dilation of veins at the esophagogastric junction and bleeding, often fatal, from erosion of these dilated varices. An innocuous clinical feature is distended veins radiating radially from the umbilicus - the so-called "Caput Medusae". Collaterals of this type are also seen in obstructions of superior and inferior vena cavae. If the former, drainage is downward to the umbilicus for communication with the systemic circulation via the ligamentum teres. If from the latter, drainage is upward to the subclavian venous system. In the portal hypertension of hepatic cirrhosis blood flow in these subcutaneous varices is in all directions but always away from the umbilicus. Clinical assessments of the directions of flow in periumbilical varices are often informative.

Liver size.

Neither hepatomegaly nor its absence is diagnostic of cirrhosis. The cirrhotic liver may be smoothly enlarged but firm if the cirrhosis is of micronodular variety, or palpably enlarged and nodular if the cirrhosis is macro-nodular (be sure to exclude primary or metastatic malignancy if there is palpable nodularity). No demonstrable hepatomegaly exists in some cirrhotics. In fact liver size may be smaller than normal if fibrosis rather than nodular regeneration predominates.

Ascites.

This is common in advanced chronic liver disease. Contributing factors are portal hypertension combined with a low serum albumin and impaired catabolism of aldosterone with consequent sodium retention and expansion of the extracellular fluid volume.

A serious and not infrequent accompaniment is spontaneous bacterial peritonitis. Characteristic features are pain, fever and a sudden increase in ascites. The diagnosis is easily made by examination of the ascitic fluid which becomes cloudy and has a high neutrophil count.

Progressive renal failure (the hepato-renal syndrome).

This is a frequent terminal event in advanced chronic liver disease. Its cause remains conjectural. Active intrarenal vasoconstriction of indeterminate cause has been suggested as a possibility.

Hepatic encephalopathy.

The encephalopathy is usually precipitated by some extraneous factor or factors. Examples are binge drinking, increased dietary protein, drugs such as opiates like morphine, renal failure and uremia, and a gastrointestinal hemorrhage. The last is probably the most frequent precipitating factor. The bacterial breakdown of blood in the gut results in a significant increase in blood ammonia levels. The sick liver cannot convert this ammonia to excretable urea. It accumulates and a large body of opinion ascribes development of hepatic encephalopathies after gastrointestinal hemorrhages from esophageal varices to the effects of ammonia on the brain. The subject is controversial and other precipitating factors have their champions.

The symptoms and signs have no special characteristics. An initial irritability and inability to sleep progresses to bizarre behavior, nonsensical speech, abnormal emotional reactions and finally delirium, coma and often, death. A rhythmic flapping of hands (asterixis) is often said to be characteristic but this is frequently seen in other preterminal situations.

Development of hepatocellular carcinoma.

The development of a hepatocellular carcinoma must always be suspected when there is clinical deterioration in any individual with stable chronic liver dysfunction. Hepatocellular carcinoma is said to develop in 15-20% of patients who have cirrhosis following unresolved injury from viruses, hepatotoxins, or any one of the more uncommon causes detailed above. Blood α-fetoprotein levels are often raised and this, together with an abdominal ultrasound and liver biopsy are diagnostic aids for identifying malignant change.

Malignant change can often be identified by a palpable nodule though a definite diagnosis always requires a biopsy, usually by final needle aspiration. It is always important to remember that the commonest hepatic neoplasm is a metastatic tumor; common sites for the primary are the lungs, the breasts and colon and the prostate. An occasional α-fetoprotein estimation is appropriate for those at risk from cirrhosis or previous hepatitis B or C infections, though admittedly, the therapeutic outlook for primary hepatic tumors is bleak.

Intrahepatic cholestasis.

Cholestasis is always present in post-hepatic obstructions for obvious reasons. It is also a common accompaniment of many hepatic dysfunctions that result from viral hepatitis, alcoholic liver disease, drug-induced and various other forms of liver disease. In these dysfunctions the cholestasis is usually attributed to compression of the biliary ductules by swollen liver cells. As previously mentioned, cholestasis can also result from oral contraceptives. The cholestatic jaundice of pregnancy is a third trimester complication of women with increased sensitivity to estrogens. The laboratory features often mimic the features of "surgical post-hepatic obstruction" but the clinical setting, the history and the results of an abdominal ultrasound and a CT scan that excludes calculi, malignancies and dilated intrahepatic ducts usually suffice to distinguish this syndrome from "surgical jaundice".

Primary biliary cirrhosis.

The disease is uncommon and typically affects women aged 30-55. The cause is unknown though associations with autoimmune diseases and autoimmune reactions have been suggested as possible culprits. Characteristic lesions are portal inflammation, destruction of bile ducts, periportal cholestasis, and areas of duct proliferation. Fibrotic changes develop later and finally, the characteristic changes of cirrhosis are demonstrable. There is little initial evidence of damage to hepatocytes.

Pruritus and jaundice are the usual early clinical features. Later, xanthomata appear and there is hyperpigmentation. Bone pains, fractures and osteomalacia are the result of vitamin D deficiency and bleeding disorders are consequent on deficits of vitamin K. The laboratory findings have three distinguishing characteristics - marked increases in alkaline phosphatase levels, high levels of blood cholesterol and anti-mitochondrial antibodies. There is fibrosis between the portal areas, and a consequent cirrhosis with few regenerating nodules. The average survival after onset is about 5-10 years. Death is due to cirrhotic liver failure caused by fibrosis.

Therapeutic options for gastrointestinal and hepatic diseases

Prevention and therapy.

- Therapy for duodenal ulceration, the malabsorption syndromes and lactase deficiencies have been detailed and do not need reiteration.
- The avoidance of gastrointestinal infections by fecal-oral contamination is important. So is the routine testing of water supplies which might be contaminated by underground seepage. Cook food well to avoid "Hamburger disease" from undercooked beef and Campylobacter infections from undercooked poultry.
- Therapy for gastrointestinal infections have been detailed and especially oral rehydration therapy.
- There does not seem to be a current consensus on appropriate non-surgical treatment of Crohn's disease or ulcerative colitis.
- Therapy for liver disease are mainly preventive measures that avoid viral and alcohol disease. Pre-hepatic jaundice due to autoimmune hemolytic disease has its own therapy. Post-hepatic jaundice due to non-malignant bile duct obstructions by calculi or other comparable causes are some of the few gastrointestinal conditions that are amenable to surgical cure. Malignant lesions causing post-hepatic obstructions are rarely curable by excision. These obstructions often result in intense pruritus that is severe enough to need endoscopic stenting of the common bile duct obstruction or, if this is not possible, external tube drainage of the bile by a tube inserted in a dilated bile duct. by transhepatic needling.

Therapeutic options for acute abdominal pain:

The "acute abdomen".

Abdominal pain of recent onset has many causes. It is a complex commonly called the "acute abdomen". Speedy assessment and analysis are essential because some types of acute abdomen are potentially fatal without surgery in the immediate or near future. Others do not need surgery and may even worsen if operated on. These are some of the reasons for considering the "acute abdomen" in detail. **The important question when assessing**

a patient with abdominal pain of recent onset is whether surgery is needed - at times, life saving surgery.

Some of the signs and symptoms that assist in diagnosis are the responses to the following questions:

- What is the type and location of the pain: superficial type pain, deep pain or deep pain that is referred to specific locales?
- Was the pain maximum at onset or did it gradually increase in intensity?
- Did the pain move from its original location to another locale?
- Does the intensity of pain fluctuate from time to time and is there any time when it completely disappears? Are there any palpable masses and if there are any are they tender?
- Is there any previous history of abdominal surgery and if there is what was the reason for the surgery?
- Is there any fever, leukocytosis or vomiting?
- Are there any recent alterations in bowel habit?
- Is there any history or current or previous hematemesis or melena?
- Is the patient taking any drugs that can adversely affect the gastrointestinal tract? Examples are acetylsalicylic acid, non-steroidal anti-inflammatory drugs, and anticoagulants. All three can cause bleeding and the first two can result in gastric perforations.
- Is the patient taking oral contraceptives or getting hormone replacement therapy? Both can precipitate vascular thromboses in mesenteric vessels.
- Finally, are there any associated medical conditions that could result in embolic occlusion of mesenteric vessels (e.g., atrial fibrillation). Intracardiac emboli can disseminate even if these patients are adequately anticoagulated. About 1% do even with effective anticoagulation. There is an annual cumulative incidence of about 5% in patients not taking anticoagulants

The "acute abdomen":

The more frequent causes of acute abdominal pain are detailed below:

1. Inflammation without luminal obstruction.

This is the most common cause of acute abdominal pain. It is usually called gastroenteritis, gastritis or enteritis, depending on whether the whole intestinal tract is affected or only the upper or lower tracts. The usual causes are viral or bacterial infections from ingestion of contaminated food and/or water, either directly or after fecal-oral contact.

Gastroenteritis. Typical symptoms are vomiting, with or without diarrhea, and colicky abdominal pains, usually referred to the midline. **Typically, tenderness on palpation is absent or minimal** and the condition is limited and self-curing. However, on occasion, the disease can take a much more serious course with melena, dehydration, hyponatremia and hypotension, and a hemolytic uremia syndrome, especially in children. Characteristic of this syndrome is acute and progressive renal failure, a hemolytic anemia, fragmented red cells, and thrombocytopenia. In extreme cases acute gastroenteritis can result in death, especially in the elderly and in the very young, or when adequate water and electrolyte replacement is not provided or is unavailable. A fatal outcome is also possible if infections result from virulent bacteria such as the typhoid bacillus, shigella, vibrio cholera and infections with certain strains of E.Coli.

2. Inflammation with luminal obstruction.

Common and typical examples are acute appendicitis (luminal obstruction by fecoliths, enlarged lymphoid tissue, etc.), acute cholecystitis (luminal obstruction of the cystic or common bile duct by one or more calculi) and acute diverticulitis (obstruction of the neck of one or more diverticula by fecal material). The symptoms are typical and similar to those previously described as the symptomatology of acute appendicitis (page 68). They begin with central abdominal referred type colicky pain (epigastric, periumbilical or hypogastric depending on whether disease involves the gall bladder, the appendix, or diverticula in the sigmoid colon), with fever, leucocytosis and vomiting. **When inflammation spreads to the surface the overlying pain-sensitive parietal peritoneum also becomes inflamed. Palpation of the area results in pain and guarding, i.e., tensing of the overlying muscle.** The pain now becomes sharp and localized to the peritoneum overlying the inflamed organ. Rectal examination of a patient with acute abdominal pain is needed to exclude inflammation of parietal peritoneum adjacent to an inflamed appendix lying in the pelvis.

Rebound tenderness reflects the irritation of an inflamed parietal peritoneum as it is first made to adhere to a sticky and inflamed visceral peritoneum and then rapidly stripped away from this adhesion. The overlying muscle is rigid, probably as a protection against this type of pain. The subsequent course is variable. Occasionally, there is spontaneous resolution, with or without the aid of antibiotics. Alternative courses are resolution after surgical excision of an inflamed appendix or gall bladder, progression to abscess formation, and then to resolution with antibiotic therapy or perforation to the exterior or into the rectum or into the abdominal cavity with localized or generalized peritonitis. If adequate treatment is not available or provided these conditions have significant mortality rates.

3. Perforation, torsion, rupture and vascular occlusions.

Typically the onset is sudden with pain maximum at the time of the incident. For diagnosis the following are all helpful: a history of previous peptic ulcer; of an ovarian cyst; of a pregnancy where an ultrasound has not been done to exclude an extra-uterine gestation; of medication with drugs that could produce vascular occlusions. Examples are oral contraceptives or estrogens taken for relief of menopausal symptoms. They can cause thromboses of mesenteric vessels. Patients with atrial fibrillation can discharge arterial emboli even when adequately anticoagulated.

Typically pain is localized to the parietal peritoneum overlying the affected tissue. If the perforation discharges a significant amount of liquid (e.g., a perforated duodenal ulcer) pain is generalized and the abdomen has a board-like rigidity. Typically, there is a later temporary amelioration of this pain as uninfected peritoneal fluid is secreted to dilute the discharge. Inevitably, if untreated, the pain subsequently increases with generalized peritonitis and eventual death. An erect X-ray of the abdomen usually shows gas under the diaphragm

The discharge of blood (e.g., from a ruptured tubal gestation) does not usually result in generalized rigidity. Hypogastric pain and rigidity do exist, often with significant hypotension and exquisite pain on pelvic examination. A ruptured tubal gestation is usually accompanied by vaginal bleeding. Immediate surgery is often lifesaving. If there is time, a pregnancy test and an ultrasound examination can be invaluable for confirmation of the clinical diagnosis. Other cause of acute gynecological emergencies include the torsion or rupture of ovarian cysts, conditions that also need surgery.

Torsions and vascular occlusions (venous or arterial) of the intestine have pain and muscular guarding localized to the affected tissue. In both conditions it is usually possible to demonstrate palpable and tender masses.

Acute pancreatitis must always be considered when there is acute upper abdominal pain with rigidity and rebound tenderness. It helps if a gall stone is demonstrable on ultrasound or the serum amylase is raised. The peritoneum covering the pancreas is parietal peritoneum and spread of inflammation to this structure is the reason for the pain, rigidity and rebound tenderness. Surgery is definitely not required, at least in the early stages. Antibiotics are frequently given to prevent secondary infections. If the serum amylase is not significantly raised acute pancreatitis is often distinguishable from a perforated peptic ulcer by the absence of radiologically demonstrablc gas under the diaphragm.

4. Intestinal obstruction:

The four features that typify intestinal obstruction are central abdominal colicky pain of the referred type, vomiting, abdominal distention, and absolute constipation. Often, depending on the site of obstruction, one or more of these clinical manifestations may be absent or delayed in appearance. Thus, vomiting is not an early feature in obstruction due to neoplasms of the distal colon (commonly, the sigmoid colon) and absolute constipation is not an early feature of obstructions affecting the small intestine. The pain of intestinal obstruction is usually of a stepladder type with progressive increase of pain. In some instances such as intestinal obstruction due to **volvulus, or a strangulated hernia** it is sudden and often maximum at the onset and a mass may or may not be palpable. A common cause of intestinal obstruction are adhesions from previous surgery for an intraabdominal problem such as inflammation, strangulated or obstructed hernias and neoplasms, especially in the elderly. Alternatively, it could result from an **obstruction associated with and caused by perforation of an inflamed colonic diverticulum or neoplasm with localization by omentum and coils of intestine** This is why a good and accurate history about previous illnesses and symptoms is essential, especially symptoms suggestive of neoplasm; for example, melena or change of bowel habit. Incidentally, **all hernia orifices must be examined when assessing an acute abdomen.**

Case history.

A 93 year old patient of mine was seen in the emergency room because of generalized abdominal pain. She was sent home with a diagnosis of constipation and a bottle of lactulose! The daughter phoned me the next morning to ask if I could come to the house to see her mother as her pain was much worse. Clinical examination immediately showed a large strangulated inguinal hernia. She was surgically treated within the hour. Despite needing resection of a small segment of small bowel recovery was uneventful. The cause of her abdominal pain was missed because the young male resident felt too embarrassed to examine the pubic area of a 93 year old woman. She died four years later from the disseminated metastases of a colonic neoplasm removed 10 years previously.

A tender palpable mass with pain and rebound tenderness of the overlying parietal peritoneum usually indicates strangulation, infarction or an acute inflammatory process that is also causing obstruction. For example, acute diverticulitis or appendicitis associated with a localizing surround of omentum, bowel loops and perhaps early abscess formation. Alternatively or additionally it could denote an obstruction accompanying perforation of an inflamed diverticulum or colonic neoplasm. It is important to identify patients with such lesions because surgery is usually necessary and often lifesaving.

Intestinal obstruction is distinguishable from the silent abdomen of **adynamic ileus** by an increase in bowel sounds; they often acquire a characteristic tinkling quality.

In underdeveloped or emerging countries (use whichever terminology suits you) a common causes of intestinal obstruction is **tuberculous peritonitis** with adherence of intestinal loops to each other. There are scattered tuberculomas on the surfaces of the omentum and intestinal walls. Surgery is only indicated for life-threatening situations or when conservative measures (gastrointestinal suction and intravenous fluids) do not relieve symptoms. Usually no more than entero-enteric bypasses are possible. Aanastomotic breaks are frequent. Vigorous treatment of tuberculosis is essential as soon as the diagnosis is made and this often reduces the incidences of anastomotic leaks.

Children in these countries often develop **intestinal obstruction from roundworm infestations,** especially ascaris infections. When misdiagnosed, unnecessary surgery, or worse may result.

5. Gynecological conditions causing acute abdominal pains:

Gynecological conditions can cause acute abdominal pains. **Ruptured tubal pregnancy** was mentioned previously. More common causes are **acute salpingitis** and **intraperitoneal bleeding from a ruptured corpus luteum at the time of ovulation (termed "mittelschmerz").**

Acute salpingitis presents as bilateral lower abdominal pain of gradual onset. Often it progressively increases and is accompanied by fever that is usually higher than the typical 100°F or so found when the pathology is acute appendicitis. Other features include leucocytosis, lower abdominal tenderness, guarding and rebound tenderness that is frequently bilateral, and often an associated purulent cervical discharge. Bimanual examination may demonstrate tenderness in the fornices, and thickened and tender tubes. It is important to distinguish salpingitis from appendicitis; surgery is not needed for the former but is for the latter. Important clues are bilateral pain from the onset, the results of a pelvic examination, fever exceeding 100^0F and the absence of referred type central abdominal pain preceding its onset.

Another common gynecological cause for abdominal pain are the small bleeds that often occur from the developing follicle at the time of ovulation - the so-called **"mittelschmerz"** (middle pain). Onset is sudden and acute, usually some two weeks or so after the previous menstruation. There is lower abdominal tenderness and guarding but these are rarely marked and there is no fever or leucocytosis. Spontaneous resolution can be expected in the next 48 hours.

Much more serious is the hemorrhage from a ruptured tubal gestation. The patient may know she is pregnant or that there has been a missed menstrual cycle. A beta-HCG pregnancy test can rapidly confirm or refute the diagnosis. Abdominal pain is of sudden onset, maximum at the beginning, and accompanied by lower abdominal tenderness and guarding as well as vaginal bleeding. Hypotension from intraperitoneal bleeding is common. The patient is pallid and air hunger is a frequent symptom. The condition is one of extreme gravity and immediate surgery is required. A pelvic ultrasound can be diagnostic if time, the equipment and the operator of the equipment are all immediately available.

Ruptures and torsions of ovarian cysts and uterine fibroids. Hemorrhages into cysts and acute degenerations of fibroids with hemorrhages into their substances do not usually need surgery. Spontaneous resolution with reduction in size and organization by granulation tissue usually eventuates. Differential diagnosis may be difficult but clinical examination and judgment and an ultrasound help. Hemorrhagic or other forms of degenerations of large fibroids rarely need surgery unless there is rupture into the abdominal cavity. Most will gradually decrease in size and fibrose if left alone. Torsions of peduculated fibroids do occur and usually require surgical excision.

In sum, surgery is needed if there is hypotension and evidence of intraabdominal bleeding, especially if a rapid beta-HCG for pregnancy is positive. If there is no evidence of bleeding there is time for ultrasound and other investigations to determine whether or not surgery is needed for any torsion, rupture or degenerative change.

6. Water and electrolyte balance in the acute abdomen.

Major water and electrolyte deficits often coexist with conditions causing an "acute abdomen". They result from vomiting, diarrhea and sequestration of water and electrolytes in loops of distended and obstructed or adynamic bowel. Chapter13 details the pathophysiological mechanisms that control water and salt balance and the pH of body fluids and the solutions available for intravenous replacements of lost water and electrolytes.

Concluding comments.

This ends a summarized description of normal and dysfunctional gastrointestinal and hepatic function. This chapter omits descriptions of the benign and malignant tumors of the intestinal tract and liver. They are well detailed in standard texts and all physicians know, or should know that their existence always needs exclusion.

References for Chapter 9.

1. Lykoudis, J. The truth about gastric and duodenal ulcer. Athens, Greece. 1966.
2. Marshall, B.J., & Warren, J.R. Unidentified curved bacilli in the stomach of patients with gastritis and peptic ulceration. Lancet 1984; 1:1311.
3. Kuipers, E.J., Lindell, R.L. et al. Atrophic gastritis and Heliobacter pylori infection in patients with reflux esophagitis treated with omperazole or fundoplication. N. Engl. J. Med. 1996; 334:822.
4. Diarrheal diseases. WHO fact sheet. http:/www.who.int/vaccine and access "diarrheal diseases".
5. Mahalanabis, D. et al. Use of oral glucose electrolyte solution in the treatment of paediatric cholera. Journ. of Trop. Paediatrics and Environmental Child Health 1974; 20:82.
6. World Health Organization. 25 years of ORS - Joint WHO/ICDDR,B Consultative meeting on ORS formulation, 1994. Internet: WHO/CDR/CDD/95.2.
7. Avery, M.E. Oral therapy in acute diarrhea. The underused simple solution. N. Engl. J. Med. 1990; 323:891.
8. Victoria, C.G., Bryce, J. et al. Reducing deaths from diarrhea through oral rehydration therapy. Bull, of the WHO, 2000; 78:1246.
9. Gore, S.M., Fontaine, O. et al. Impact of rice based oral rehydration solution on stool output and duration of diarrhea: meta-analysis of 13 clinical trials. Brit. Med. J. 1992; 304:287.
10. Gore, S.M., Fontaine, O. et al. Efficacy of rice based oral rehydration. Lancet 1996; 348:193.
11. Metabolism and Nutrition. In Smith, L.H., Thier, S.O. (Ed.): Pathophysiology. The Biological Principles of Disease. Philadelphia. W.B. Saunders Company, 1981, p. 501.
12. Rubin, and E. Lieber, C.S. Alcohol-induced hepatic injury in nonalcoholic volunteers. N, Engl, J, Med. 1968; 278:869.

10

Diagnosis: The Slave Systems
2. The Respiratory Complex

Table of Contents

Notation.

The notation ~P denotes phosphorous with a high energy bond. Depending on the context in which the term is used, ~P may also denote the energy liberated when a high energy phosphate bond detaches from ATP or ADP.

A general comment on the methodology of clinical assessments.

The comments made **on page 119** about this topic are not repeated. They merit reading before proceeding with this chapter.

Respiration - normal physiology

The objectives.

The system complex has three objectives:

The first is the transport of environmental oxygen into cells in amounts that satisfy energy needs. Oxygen is needed for oxidative catabolism of energy substrate from the environment in the Kreb's cycle and the Electron Transport systems. Anaerobic metabolism of 1mole of glucose yields 8moles ATP. This is not enough for biological needs. The combination of anaerobic and aerobic metabolism of 1mole of glucose yields 38moles ATP and this suffices for most current energy needs.

The second is removal of carbon dioxide from cells. This is needed for regulation of intracellular pH (details on page 303, Chapter 13.

The third is minor compared to the first two. It is protection of the lungs from toxins and pathogens.

Oxygenation.

The CNS receives about 20% of the total resting oxygen consumption of the body. Glucose is the obligatory substrate for production of usable energy in the CNS though, as previously mentioned, after four or five days of fasting ketones can provide for some of the energy needs of the brain. CNS needs for oxygen are continuous for the body does not have oxygen reserves. If oxygen is in short supply the requirements of the brain have priority over all other systems.

Abrupt cessation of the cerebral circulation results in loss of consciousness in 20-40 seconds and brain death will follow after about four minutes of total anoxia. Restoration of the circulation in the interim could result in recovery but with residual deficits of mentation and other CNS functions. Abrupt stoppages of cerebral blood flow usually result from asphyxiation (accidental, criminal or judicial), or from cardiac arrest (e.g., the cardiogenic shock of a large infarct or because of an arrhythmia such as ventricular fibrillation).

More often the decrease of cerebral perfusion is gradual, and usually a feature of preterminal states. Initially there are poor judgments and inappropriate responses to questions. Later there is confusion that gradually progresses to stupor, coma and finally, death if oxygen deficits continue.

There are many other causes of confusion and coma, all detailed in the chapter on the nervous system. Before concluding that cerebral dysfunction results from preterminal anoxia, hypoglycemia as a cause needs exclusion as well as head injuries that are not recognized because of the absence of external signs of trauma.

Maxim

Always check the blood sugar of every patient unconscious for no obvious reason. Severe hypoglycemia has effects similar to those of acute anoxia.

The resources systems for delivery of oxygenated blood to cells:

The respiratory complex has three principal resource systems for transferring inhaled oxygen to cells. Figure 10-1 itemizes the needed resources. In summary they are:

- **Respiration**, a process that brings environmental oxygen in contact with alveolar walls.

(Contd. on page 223)

Chart 10-1: THE REQUIREMENTS FOR OXYGENATION OF CELLS

1. An atmosphere with sufficient oxygen and a pO_2 which permits normal oxygenation of blood without supplemental oxygen. At high altitudes pO_2 decreases till, at some point, adequate oxygenation of blood needs supplemental oxygen.
2. A functioning brain stem. Neurons in the brain stem control respiration. They:
   - **a)** Automatically sends rhythmic discharges to the respiratory muscles at about 15-20 per minute. Active contraction of respiratory muscles results. The muscles relax between discharges.
   - **b)** Receive afferent information via chemoreceptors and baroreceptors in the carotid and aortic bodies, from medullary receptors which respond to pH changes in the cerebrospinal fluid and by transmission along autonomic and somatic (e.g., from the respiratory muscles) afferents without interruption by receptors. The control centers compute and decide if functional changes are needed. If they are, commands are transmitted by efferent nerve impulses and/or quantitative changes in circulating hormones. These commands modify the rates and depths of respiration. At all times there are functional integrations with the neuron effectors of the vasomotor, cardiac and hypothalamic centers. **This coordinates respiratory changes with alterations of cardiac output and peripheral vasomotor tone.**
3. Airways which are patent enough to let sufficient inspired air reach the alveoli.
4. At least ⅔ of a normal lung - preferably two normal lungs.
5. **The principal requirements for normal ventilation:**
   - **a)** A rigid chest wall.
   - **b)** The elastic recoil of the lungs.
   - **c)** A negative intrapleural pressure which ensures continual apposition of parietal and visceral pleura.
   - **d)** Production of surfactant.
   - **e)** No hindrance to the normal diffusion of oxygen through the alveolar walls, the lung interstitium and capillary walls, into the blood. Common causes include consolidations, alveolar wall thickenings, interstitial fibrosis, asthma and chronic obstructive lung disease (chronic bronchitis and emphysema).
   - **f)** A normal pulmonary venous and arterial blood flow. Perfusion of lung segments which are not aerated (**i.e., ventilation-perfusion imbalances**) reduce oxygenation of pulmonary blood.
   - **g)** Hemoglobin in adequate amounts and with normal oxygen binding capacities. No significant anemia or genetic, or fortuitous hemoglobin mutants which might hinder and/or decrease oxygen binding to or release from hemoglobin.
   - **h)** A normal mitral valve and a left ventricular output of adequate volume and pressure.
6. Healthy cells or, at least, cells which are sufficiently viable to have active and functioning enzymes for oxidative catabolism of the absorbed products of food substrate digestion, and of water, minerals and vitamins. First, anaerobically, then by oxidative metabolism in the Kreb's cycle and finally, by metabolism in the Electron Transport System to energy usable for biological needs, i.e., high energy phosphate bonds (~P) stored in ATP and ADP till needed.
7. The following are some factors which could adversely affect well controlled chronic lung disease and precipitate an exacerbation and/or respiratory failure:
   - Infections affecting the lungs and/or any other system, especially if accompanied by systemic components (fever, toxemia, septicemia, bacteremia, or metastatic spread). Also, any new disease affecting the lungs or other systems, or reactivation of a previously well controlled medical problem.
   - Malignant disease, either from a lung primary, metastases from a lung primary, or metastases from malignancy in other sites such as the breast, colon or prostate.
   - A myocardial infarct, valvular dysfunction and/or arrhythmia.
   - A pulmonary embolus.
   - Subnutrition and malnutrition.
   - Trauma resulting in brain injuries and cerebral failure or in a flail chest or in blood from facial and oropharyngeal injuries blocking the air passages.
   - Adverse reactions to drugs and excessive sedation.
   - Supplemental oxygen not available, or not affordable, or not acceptable to patient because of discomfort from nasal cannulae and/or masks.
8. Exclude poisoning of cells by cyanide and comparable cytotoxic agents.

This is a checklist of items which should be sequentially considered as etiology or as a precipitating factor when dealing with a recent pulmonary dysfunction or an exacerbation of a pre-existing dysfunction (e.g., increased dyspnea not yet diagnosed). Examples are an acute pneumonia, a pulmonary embolus or an exacerbation of chronic obstructive pulmonary disease (COPD).

(Contd. from page 221)

- **Oxygenation of blood (Chart 10-3 on page 227) and**
- **Delivery of oxygenated blood to the interiors of cells.** This last resource depends on a normal cardiovascular complex and circulating blood, two topics which get detailed attention in Chapters 11 and 12.

The anatomy and dynamics of respiration

The respiratory cage.

It consists of the ribs, the intercostal muscles, the accessory muscles of respiration and the diaphragm. The bones of the respiratory cage are 12 pairs of ribs, 12 thoracic vertebrae, the sternum, and the joints and ligaments connecting these bones. The muscles of respiration are the external and internal intercostal muscles.
The accessory muscles are the diaphragm, the sterno-mastoids and the abdominal muscles (rectus abdominis, transversus abdominis, and the external and internal obliques). During inhalation the ribs rotate at the costovertebral joints. The displacement is both upwards and outwards - the so-called "bucket-handle" movement. The result is an increase in both the antero-posterior and transverse diameters of the thorax. The diaphragm is an important and probably principal muscle of respiration at rest. Contraction results in its descent and consequent inhalation, relaxation in exhalation due to its ascent. Its vertebral fibers attach to the second and third lumbar vertebrae and the medial and lateral arcuate ligaments. The sternal fibers to the lower xiphoid process and the costal fibers to the lower six ribs, interdigitating with the transversus abdominis. The efferent motor innervation is from the phrenic nerve and the afferents return along the same nerve.

The bones of the respiratory cage are essential for normal ventilation. Without their rigidity and the negative intrapleural pressure the cage would not be able to pull out the lungs during inhalation. The negative intrapleural pressure ensures that the visceral pleura adheres to the parietal pleura that lines the respiratory cage.

Consequences of losses of this rigidity are seen in the ineffective respirations of individuals with a flail chest following severe trauma. Decreases of rib cage rigidity can be therapeutically created by thoracoplasties that remove ribs to permit collapse and subsequent healing of lung segments containing tuberculous tension cavities.

The lungs.

These are complex structures with multiple branching airways ending in alveoli. They also contain many blood vessels as well as fibers of collagen and elastin. Each bronchus divides approximately 23 times and becomes terminal bronchioles, each about 0.6mm in diameter. Subsequent divisions result in respiratory bronchioles that are about 0.4mm in diameter, and finally, alveolar ducts, atria, alveolar sacs, and alveoli.

Cartilage disappears from the walls of these air ducts at about the 11th. division and from then on radial traction maintains the patency of the air ducts. The spontaneous retractions of the lungs at the end of inhalation results from the elasticity of their collagen components, and the surface tensions of the liquids lining the alveoli.

The average diameter of an alveolus is about 250 microns. There are some 300 million alveoli so that total alveolar surface area is some 70m^2, many times the body surface area. However, at any one instant the capillaries are only partially filled with blood so that the effective alveolar surface area is probably about 35-40m^2. During exercise the blood in the capillaries increases so that the effective alveolar surface area could increase to 60m^2. At rest, only about 100ml of blood is in the lung capillaries at any one time. The amount increases proportional to activity. At rest, a red cell passing through the pulmonary vessels is exposed to alveolar air for only about 0.75 seconds. The time decreases with exercise. During this period adequate gas exchanges take place.

Respiratory system receptors and control systems.

The vagus nerve transmits afferent information from lung receptors to the respiratory center. Information about the peripheral effects of respiration (pO_2, pCO_2, pH and blood pressure) is transmitted directly by the blood, or by autonomic nerves without interruption, or after initial recording in peripheral receptor complexes such as the carotid and aortic bodies and subsequent transmission by vagus and glossopharyngeal nerves.

The lung receptors.

They include the following:

Stretch receptors located in bronchi and bronchioles. They discharge during inhalation and the discharges stop when inhalation ends. Their stimulation results in bronchodilation, an increase in heart rate and decreased peripheral vascular resistance.

Irritant receptors are responsible for the cough reflex. They are located subepithelially, mainly in the posterior wall of the trachea and at the bronchial bifurcations as far as the respiratory bronchioles. There are many at the carina. Any one or more of many factors stimulate these receptors. Some examples are irritants, mechanical stimulation, anaphylaxis, pulmonary congestion, pneumothorax, hyperpnea, and microemboli. Stimulation results in coughing.

Type J lung receptors locate in the interstitium surrounding the alveoli. They are stimulated by interstitial fluid collections caused by high pulmonary capillary pressures. Stimulation of the J receptors results in the rapid and shallow breathing, hypotension and bradycardia.

The receptors of the carotid and aortic bodies. These are chemoreceptors located at the bifurcations of the carotid and in the aortic arch. A low pO_2, high pCO_2 and/or low pH stimulates these receptors. In man hypoxic stimulation of receptors does not occur till high pCO_2 levels fail to stimulate as in the late stages of pulmonary failure. At this stage a low pO_2 is the only stimulus of these centers. Administration of supplemental oxygen to these patients can further reduce the respiratory stimulation.

The respiratory center.

It is located in the medulla, close to the cardiac and vasomotor centers. All three centers integrate and interact to produce coordinated respiratory, cardiac and vasomotor changes, as and when needed. The neurons of the respiratory center have intrinsic automaticity and rhythmicity. They discharge during inhalation and cease discharging when the subject exhales. Somatic nerve discharges pass down the spinal cord to motor neurons which activate the appropriate muscles. A raised pCO_2 stimulates the respiratory center as does a decreased arterial pH. A low pCO_2 depresses the center as do analgesics, sedatives and anesthesia.

Higher cerebral centers can modify the activity of the respiratory center. Stress and anxiety can result in hysterical hyperventilation with lowering of pCO_2, often with paresthesiae, tetany, and even convulsions. Other examples are inhibition of the respiratory center during swallowing, speaking, laughing and crying. Fever stimulates the center via the hypothalamic temperature regulating center. When a person sleeps there is spontaneous depression of the respiratory center and a decrease in the rates of its rhythmic discharges. Sedatives and analgesics at bed time magnify this decrease.

The neural response to exercise is probably responsible for the immediate increase in ventilation as exercise begins. There are two causes. First, a conditioned response to exercise and a feedback stimulation by proprioceptors in the muscles of respiration. Second, the neural response that results from stimulation of peripheral and central chemoreceptors by the raised pCO_2 of exercise and lactic acidemia if exercise is vigorous.

A system that maintains the constancy of CSF pH also provides for the long-term alterations needed by those living at high altitudes. It is a pumping mechanism, probably located in the choroid plexus and ependyma, which pushes H^+ions into the CSF. H^+combines with local HCO_{3-} to form H_2CO_3 which then dissociates to H_2O and CO_2. CO_2 diffuses out and is removed.

The pleural membranes and negative intrapleural pressure.

The pleura is a mesothelial membrane that covers the lungs. At the hilum it reflects onto the lateral surface of the mediastinum, the inner surface of the rib cage, and the superior aspect of the diaphragm. In man the two pleural cavities are completely separate.

The visceral pleura is insensitive to pain; pneumonia is painless until inflammation spreads to the parietal pleura. The latter is sensitive to pain. The pain is a typical sharp and localized superficial type pain. It is felt when the patient breathes deeply or coughs - the cause of pain is inflamed parietal pleura rubbing against the underlying inflamed but painless visceral pleura.

There is a potential space between parietal and visceral pleura surfaces. Normally the space is essentially non-existent because of a negative intrapleural pressure. Only a film of liquid remains to lubricate the two pleural surfaces so that they can easily glide over each other. The negative intrapleural pressure is essential for normal respiration. During inhalation it maintains the apposition of parietal and visceral pleural surfaces. This allows the lungs to expand as the respiratory cage enlarges. During exhalation the same apposition resists the complete alveolar collapse that would otherwise occur because of the intrinsic elasticity of the lung and the surface tension of the fluid that lines alveoli. When the intrapleural negative pressure is zero, as it is in a pneumothorax, the lung collapses against the mediastinum and does not expand on inhalation. There is dyspnea, pain, absent breath sounds and a ventilation-perfusion imbalance.

The pleural space is kept free of gas because the total gas pressure of venous blood is less than the total alveolar gas pressure of 760mm Hg (Chart 10-2). Venous blood has a total gas tension of about 706mm Hg (a pO_2 of 40mm Hg + pCO_2 of 46mm Hg + pH_2O of 47mm Hg + pN_2 of 573mm Hg = 706mm Hg). This difference of 54mm Hg (760 - 706 = 54mm Hg) is sufficient to exceed by a small amount the forces driving fluid into the pleural space. During quiet breathing the negative intrapleural pressure is about -6 cm water on inhalation and about -2.5 cm. on exhalation.

Surfactant and hyaline membrane disease.

Surfactant is a phospholipid produced by alveolar Type 2 cells. It reduces the surface tension on alveolar walls by reducing the attraction to each other of molecules in the fluids lining the alveoli. The alveoli remain patent at low transpulmonary pressures and expand with the usual inspiratory forces.

A thin film of liquid lines the alveoli. The molecules of this liquid are close to each other and adjacent molecules attract each other resulting in surface tension. Most physiologists use the Laplace Law to explain why surfactant prevents surface tension from collapsing alveoli when they are small. However, the law only applies to hollow, distensible structures, presumably without deficits in their circumferences. All alveoli have an opening for an air duct at some point in their circumferences.

One wonders if a better explanation for surfactant action could be based on Newton's general law of gravitation. This law states that there is always a gravitational force between two bodies, the attraction being proportional to the product of their masses and inversely proportional to the square of their distance apart (the inverse-square law of gravitation). Surfactants are amphipathic molecules with hydrophilic and hydrophobic ends. Attachments of their hydrophobic ends to alveolar walls and their hydrophilic ends to fluid lining alveolar walls could result in separation of the molecules of alveolar fluid. This would increase the distances between the latter. If this does occur, an application of Newton's law of gravitation would show a considerable decrease in attraction of alveolar fluid molecules to each other because the attraction is inversely proportional to the squares of their distances apart.

Clements discovered surfactant in the 1950s. He subsequently determined that its function was to prevent lung collapse at low pressures. His studies were honored by a special publication of Biochim. Biophys. Acta[1]. In 1959 Avery and Mead[2] showed that lung extracts from babies with hyaline membrane disease were deficient in surfactant. Hyaline membrane disease is a frequent concomitant of premature births. If birth cannot or should not be delayed till enough surfactant is present, steroids given to the mother for 24-48 hours before birth can often stimulate maturation of the fetal lung to produce surfactant. Replacement therapy with exogenous surfactant and various new techniques of ventilation have also increased the survival rates of premature infants with hyaline membrane disease. About 7% of babies are born prematurely. Many have respiratory difficulties because of surfactant deficits. Many are now saved by artificial ventilations till their lungs mature and start producing their own surfactant.

Resistance to breathing.

Nose breathing contributes at least 50% of the total resistance encountered on inhalation. With mouth breathing the resistance is less - about ⅓ of total resistance. The pharynx, glottis, larynx and extrathoracic trachea contribute small additional amounts of resistance. The remainder is due to airways resistance from variations in their calibers and tone, in the thickness of their mucosal linings, and in the amounts of bronchial secretions. These factors are of special importance in many lung dysfunctions, especially the various types of chronic obstructive pulmonary disease (COPD). Resistance is best measured by the forced vital capacity, especially the forced expiratory volume in the first second of exhalation (FEV1) as a percentage of the total forced expiratory volume (FEV). The normal is about 80%.

The pulmonary circulation.

The pulmonary circulation is a low pressure system. The mean pulmonary arterial pressure is 14mm Hg and the mean left atrial pressure is 9 mm Hg so that the driving force across the pulmonary vascular bed is small; about (14 - 9) = 5mm Hg. About 10-20% of the circulating blood volume is in the lungs at any one time depending on variations in posture and other factors. About 10% of this blood is in the capillaries and 60% in the pulmonary veins.

The pulmonary arterial bed pressure is much lower than the oncotic pressure of the plasma proteins. Normally, this prevents transudation of fluid into the alveoli and also results in rapid reabsorption of alveolar fluids. The ability of the pulmonary vascular bed to dilate is considerable. It results from the opening of closed capillary channels and passive dilation of these vessels. When the limit of distensibility is reached the transmural pressure increases and eventually exceeds the oncotic pressure of plasma proteins. The result is pulmonary edema.

Systemic venous return varies as intrathoracic pressure and as a result right ventricular output varies with the rate and/or depth of respiration. The pulmonary venous reservoir is substantial and variations in right ventricular output ensure maintenance of left ventricular output within small limits.

There are usually three bronchial arteries. They originate from the thoracic aorta or upper intercostal arteries and supply oxygenated blood to the lower trachea and the bronchi as far as the respiratory bronchioles. They also vascularize the vasa vasorum of the large pulmonary vessels. Venous drainage is by the azygos veins going to the right atrium, and by anastomoses with pulmonary veins.

Oxygenation of cells.

Chart 10-2: INHALED AIR AND ALVEOLAR AIR AT SEA LEVEL

Atmospheric air composition	
Nitrogen	78%
Oxygen	21%
Argon	0.9%
Carbon dioxide, xenon, etc.	0.1% or less
Total	100%

Partial pressures of inhaled air	
Water vapor	47mm Hg
Nitrogen	563mm Hg
Oxygen[2]	150mm Hg
Carbon dioxide, xenon, etc.	0mm Hg
Total	760mm Hg

Partial pressures of alveolar air	
Water vapor	47mm Hg
Nitrogen	568mm Hg
Oxygen[3]	105mm Hg
Carbon dioxide	40mm Hg
Total	760mm Hg

[1] Figures for partial pressure of water vapor varies from author to author as it depends on atmospheric humidity. The amount of water vapor in the atmosphere is variable - usually around 1%.

[2] Calculated on the basis of 47mm Hg for water vapor pressure: (760-47) x (20.93/100) = 149.23mm Hg.

[3] Lower than inhaled air because of mixing with CO_2 remaining in the alveoli.

Partial pressure of a gas defined.

Dalton's law of partial pressure states that the total pressure exerted by a mixture of gases is the sum of the pressures each would exert if it alone occupied the entire volume. Atmospheric air has a pressure of 760mm Hg, and this figure is the sum of the partial pressures of nitrogen, oxygen, carbon dioxide, water vapor, and other gases such as neon, argon and xenon. If water vapor is present it must be subtracted from the total pressure before the partial pressures of the gases are estimated. The water vapor in alveolar air exerts a pressure of about 47mm Hg. Hence, the sum of all gas partial pressures in alveolar air is 760-47=713mm Hg. Chart 10-2 summarizes the compositions and partial pressures of gases in the atmosphere and in alveolar air.

Oxygenation of blood.

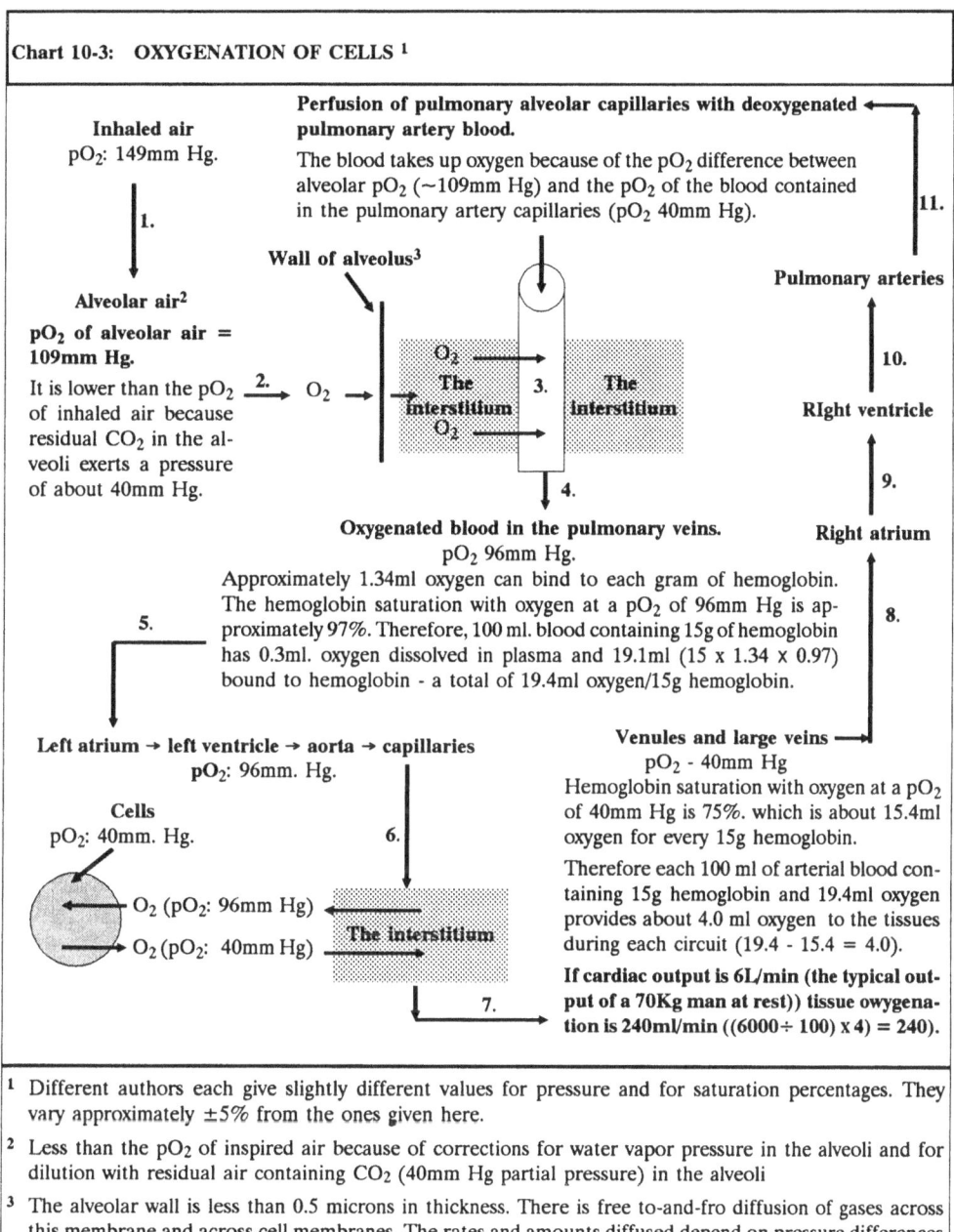

Chart 10-3: OXYGENATION OF CELLS [1]

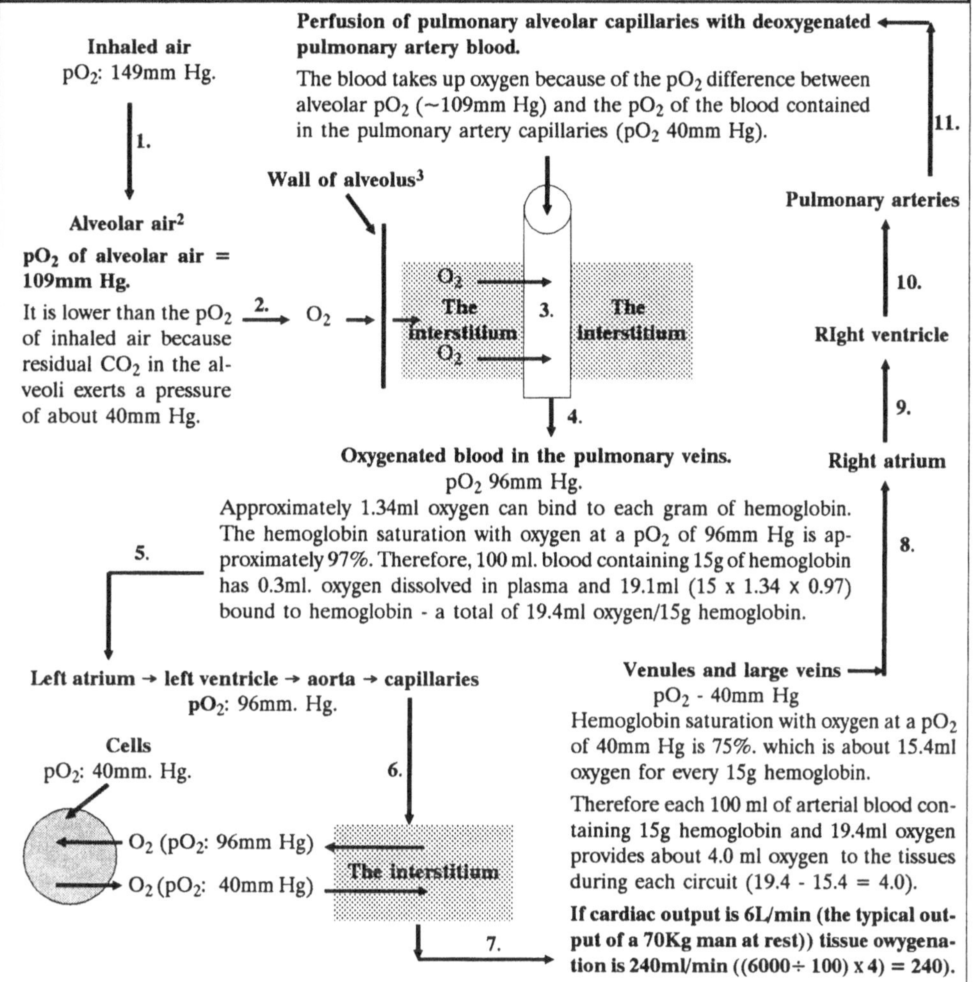
Inhaled air
pO_2: 149mm Hg.
1.
Alveolar air[2]
pO_2 of alveolar air = 109mm Hg.
It is lower than the pO_2 of inhaled air because residual CO_2 in the alveoli exerts a pressure of about 40mm Hg.
2.
O_2
Perfusion of pulmonary alveolar capillaries with deoxygenated pulmonary artery blood.
The blood takes up oxygen because of the pO_2 difference between alveolar pO_2 (~109mm Hg) and the pO_2 of the blood contained in the pulmonary artery capillaries (pO_2 40mm Hg).
11.
Wall of alveolus[3]
O_2
The interstitium
O_2
3.
The interstitium
4.
Pulmonary arteries
10.
Right ventricle
9.
Right atrium
Oxygenated blood in the pulmonary veins.
pO_2 96mm Hg.
Approximately 1.34ml oxygen can bind to each gram of hemoglobin. The hemoglobin saturation with oxygen at a pO_2 of 96mm Hg is approximately 97%. Therefore, 100 ml. blood containing 15g of hemoglobin has 0.3ml. oxygen dissolved in plasma and 19.1ml (15 x 1.34 x 0.97) bound to hemoglobin - a total of 19.4ml oxygen/15g hemoglobin.
5.
8.
Left atrium → left ventricle → aorta → capillaries
pO_2: 96mm. Hg.
Cells
pO_2: 40mm. Hg.
6.
O_2 (pO_2: 96mm Hg)
O_2 (pO_2: 40mm Hg)
The interstitium
7.
Venules and large veins
pO_2 - 40mm Hg
Hemoglobin saturation with oxygen at a pO_2 of 40mm Hg is 75%. which is about 15.4ml oxygen for every 15g hemoglobin.
Therefore each 100 ml of arterial blood containing 15g hemoglobin and 19.4ml oxygen provides about 4.0 ml oxygen to the tissues during each circuit (19.4 - 15.4 = 4.0).
If cardiac output is 6L/min (the typical output of a 70Kg man at rest)) tissue owygenation is 240ml/min ((6000÷ 100) x 4) = 240).

[1] Different authors each give slightly different values for pressure and for saturation percentages. They vary approximately ±5% from the ones given here.

[2] Less than the pO_2 of inspired air because of corrections for water vapor pressure in the alveoli and for dilution with residual air containing CO_2 (40mm Hg partial pressure) in the alveoli

[3] The alveolar wall is less than 0.5 microns in thickness. There is free to-and-fro diffusion of gases across this membrane and across cell membranes. The rates and amounts diffused depend on pressure differences between the two sides of the membranes.

Chart 10-3 summarizes how blood is oxygenated. Chart 10-1 has already summarized the requirements for transport of oxygenated blood into cells.

The average male uses 250 ml of oxygen per minute in the basal state. Women about 5-10% less. The CO_2

production of the average male is 200 ml/minute at rest and the lungs eliminate about 300 liters each day at rest. Atmospheric air is composed of 79.03% nitrogen and 20.93% oxygen. The rest (0.04%) consists of carbon dioxide and rare gases. Atmospheric water vapor exerts a pressure of about 47mm Hg which varies according to locations (47mm Hg is the pressure at sea level). Hence, the other components of the water vapor saturated gas reaching the alveoli exert a pressure at sea level of 760 - 47 = 713mm Hg. In consequence the pressure of oxygen has been reduced to (760-47) × (20.93÷ 100) = 149.23mm Hg. At the end of exhalation residual air containing C02 (pCO_2 of ~ 40mm Hg) remains in the alveoli. This as well as the saturation of alveolar air by water vapor (partial pressure of 47mm Hg) results in an alveolar oxygen tension of about 105-115mm Hg at sea level (Chart 10-2). This is the gas that equilibrates with and oxygenates pulmonary capillary blood (pO_2 ~40mm Hg).

Most of the oxygen is transported to the tissues in chemical combination with hemoglobin. Approximately 1.34ml oxygen can combine with each gram of hemoglobin that carries it to the tissues as oxyhemoglobin - 15 gm of hemoglobin can transport about 15×1.34 = 20.10ml oxygen per 100ml blood when blood is fully saturated with oxygen. The actual amount of oxygen carried is less because at the arterial pO_2 of 96mm Hg the saturation of hemoglobin with oxygen is 97%. Hence, arterial hemoglobin carries 19.1 ml oxygen (15 x 1.34 x 0.97). About 0.3 ml oxygen dissolves in plasma so that the total oxygen content of arterial blood is 19.4ml (19.1+0.3) per 100 ml blood when hemoglobin is 15g/dL. Chart 10-3 on the previous page shows how blood oxygenates cells. Additional descriptive text is not needed.

The oxygen dissociation curve.

The amount of oxygen carried by blood is related in a nonlinear fashion to the partial pressure of oxygen in blood and is defined by a sigmoid shaped oxyhemoglobin dissociation curve (Chart 10-4). The upper portion of the curve is flat so big changes in oxygen tension at those levels only result in small changes in oxygen

Chart 10-4: OXYGEN SATURATIONS OF HEMOGLOBIN AT DIFFERENT PARTIAL PRESSURES

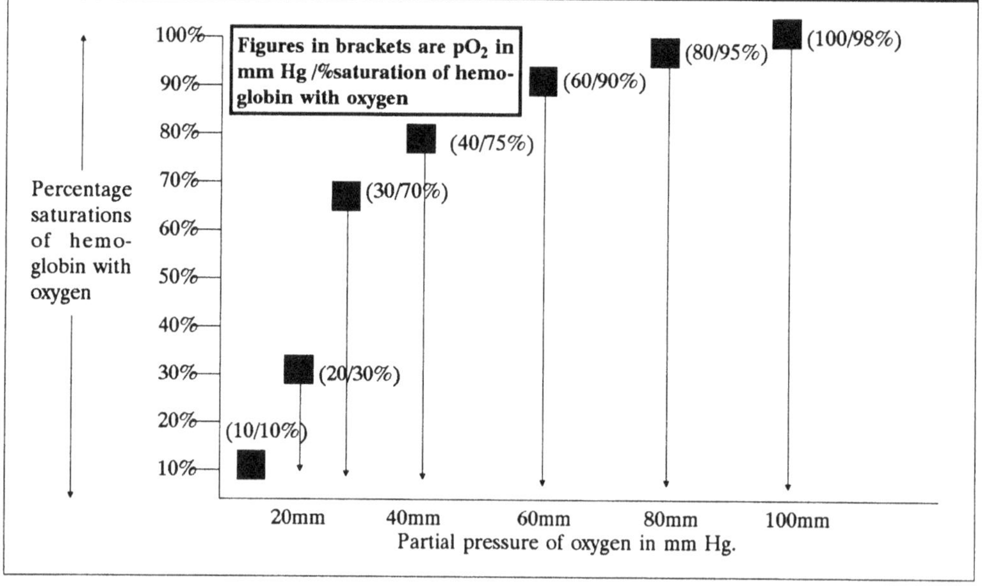
Figures in brackets are pO₂ in mm Hg /%saturation of hemoglobin with oxygen
Percentage saturations of hemoglobin with oxygen
100%
90%
80%
70%
60%
50%
40%
30%
20%
10%
(10/10%)
(20/30%)
(30/70%)
(40/75%)
(60/90%)
(80/95%)
(100/98%)
20mm
40mm
60mm
80mm
100mm
Partial pressure of oxygen in mm Hg.

content or saturation.

At oxygen tensions normally found in alveolar air hemoglobin becomes oxygenated at a rapid rate quickly becoming almost fully saturated. At high altitudes where pO_2 can be as low as 60 mm Hg (normally 105 mm Hg at sea level) blood leaving the pulmonary capillaries will still be 85-90% saturated. The subsequent release of oxygen in the tissues is augmented by the steep portion of the curve where small changes in oxygen tension are associated with large decreases in the percentage saturations of hemoglobin with oxygen. In the lungs a fall in CO_2 shifts the curve to the left so hemoglobin can take up more oxygen at a given oxygen tension.

The amount of DPG (2,3-diphosphoglycerate) affects the curve. It decreases the affinity of hemoglobin for oxygen. DPG levels increase in anemia and hypoxia. The curve shifts to right and more oxygen is given up to the tissues. At high altitudes this mechanism provides some compensation for the respiratory alkalosis that exists.

Reductions of oxygenation by pathology affecting the alveolar membranes and the cell wall.

Gases diffuse freely across cell walls. An important consideration in the oxygenation of cells is free diffusion of gases across alveolar membranes. Hindrances to this free diffusion of oxygen and CO_2 across alveolar membranes are important causes of pulmonary dysfunctions. The usual causes are exudates, fluids and pathology that has resulted in thickening and fibrosis of the alveolar walls (all discussed in detail later).

Carbon dioxide transport.

This topic is considered on page 303 in Chapter 13. Carbon dioxide is a product of intracellular metabolism and must be removed to maintain acid-base balance.

Pulmonary mechanisms for protection.

The lungs are directly connected to the exterior. Mechanisms must and do exist to protect it against toxins. and pathogens. The principal protective agents are macrophages, mucus and ciliary movements and the cough reflex.

Macrophages are plentiful in the lung. They act as non-specific scavengers of particulate material.

The mucus glands. Bronchi have two types of glands that secrete mucus; mucosal goblet cells and submucosal glands that secrete serous fluid as well as mucus. Mucus contains 95% water, 3% carbohydrates and fats, and 2% glycoproteins which are polypeptides with saccharide side chains. The glycoproteins lubricate and protect the mucosa and make mucus viscous.

Ciliated cells. Each ciliated cell has about 275 cilia and each cilium has nine peripheral and two central fibers anchored to basal corpuscles. They show spontaneous unidirectional and coordinated movement. Cilia are in the watery phase and mucus lies on top of this subphase. Ciliary action moves the overlying mucus sheet to the mouth at about 2 cm. per minute. Ciliary clearance is decreased by any one or more of the following: environmental pollutants, cigarette smoking, hypoxia, increased local oxygen and drying.

This ends a short description of the normal and abnormal physiology of the lung.

Dysfunctions of the respiratory complex.

This subsection provides an overview of lung dysfunctions. It certainly does not intend to contend with the many comprehensive and well written standard texts that exist. The object is to provide illustrative examples of how the qualitatives of pulmonary dysfunctions are identifiable by comparisons with the desired and permissible limits of normal function.

Symptoms and signs of pulmonary dysfunctions.

Any of the etiologies detailed on pages 75-77 in Chapter 3 can affect the lungs. Usually, diagnosis and decision are not difficult as many ancillary methods of investigation are available: bacteriological, cytological and microscopic examination of sputum, chest X-rays, CT scans and MRIs, respiratory function tests and determinations of blood gas levels. Occasionally immunological studies can be of some use as well as sleep analyses. All these topics are well described in standard texts and the rest of this chapter merely summarizes the more important and frequently encountered pathologies.

The most common symptoms of pulmonary dysfunctions are cough and shortness of breath. The latter is commonly called dyspnea. Breathing is usually shallow and rapid but the degree of discomfort experienced varies from one individual to another. In general a respiratory rate that exceeds 22 per minute merits evaluation. It is easy to mistake hysterical over-breathing for dyspnea due to lung pathology. The latter must be excluded before making a diagnosis of psychogenic dyspnea.

Pain occurs when the parietal pleura is inflamed. A retrosternal soreness on coughing is charcteristic of tracheitis with or without associated acute bronchitis.

Chart 10-1 summarizes the causes of respiratory dysfunction and is a useful checklist for localizing the cause of the dysfunction.

Hypoxia.

The metabolic needs of tissues require both a satisfactory pO_2 and an adequate blood flow. **Hypoxia** exists when these needs are not met. There are many possible causes. The following are some:

- Congenital cardiac malformations such as reverse flow through a patent ductus arteriosus and congenital pulmonary AV fistulae.
- Decrease in tension of inhaled oxygen. This is found at high altitudes. Also when an individual rebreathes exhaled air.
- Increased oxygen requirements as in vigorous muscular exercise.
- Reduction of the oxygen carrying capacity of blood because of anemia or congenital or acquired genetic defects in the oxygen-carrying or releasing capacities of hemoglobin.
- Failure of the respiratory system to adequately oxygenate blood because of its depression by neurological dysfunction, by alcohol and/or by drugs.
- **Lung disease.**

  The clinical features of most result from combinations of any one or more of the following:

  - The immediate effects of acute parenchymal disease due to infections by bacteria, viruses, parasites, and environmental toxins. When infections extend to the parietal pleura there is pain on inspiration as the pain sensitive parietal pleura rubs against the pain insensitive visceral pleura. A "rub" is audible on auscultation as the two layers of pleura rub against each other.
  - Malignant tumors and benign tumors that are large. Multiple malignant tumors are frequently present Most are metastatic from other sites: e.g., the breast, the colon and the prostate, or a lung primary.
  - An acute increase in bronchial resistance because of a bronchitis.
  - **Ventilation-perfusion imbalance.** This is a frequent cause of hypoxia and an important consideration in any lung disease. Shortness of breath is a common symptom when lung tissue is perfused with blood but not aerated. A typical example is the pneumonic lung. It can be seen with almost any lung disease. Extreme examples are the collapsed lung of a spontaneous or induced pneumothorax, and large areas of atelectasis. The respiratory rate and excursions are increased to maintain oxygenation of blood and these responses are perceived as shortness of breath.
  - Restrictive and obstructive lung disease in single or mixed patterns.
  - Allergic reactions producing obstructive symptoms (expiratory rhonchi). They include asthma and various uncommon pathologies mentioned below. It is possible that most of these conditions are due to or aggravated by bronchial trees that are easily irritated.
  - Atelectasis.
  - Pulmonary emboli.
  - Pleural disease, usually secondary to underlying parenchymal disease but occasionally of primary origin.
  - Breaches of the negative intrapleural pressures resulting in pneumothorax and, at times, in a dangerous tension pneumothorax.

- Breaches of chest wall rigidity, usually because of severe trauma but occasionally surgically induced for underlying parenchymal disease such as tuberculosis. The pattern of disease is often of mixed type.
- Histotoxic hypoxia results from inactivation of mitochondrial enzymes by poisons or disease.

Shortness of breath (dyspnea) is a common symptom which accompanies all lung dysfunctions. Exceptions are the occasional lung dysfunctions only discovered on routine X-rays. It helps determination of the qualitatives of the dysfunction, and a return to normal respiratory rates indicates a good response to therapy and also the extent of recovery. A failure to return to normal respiratory rates indicates therapeutic failure for any one of the many reasons detailed in Chart 16-1 on page 340.

Parenchymal lung diseases.

Acute parenchymal disease.

The **commonest causes are infections** resulting in acute bronchitis and the acute and chronic pneumonias. The usual pathogens for acute infections are viruses, mycoplasma infections and bacteria: the pneumococcus, streptococcus, staphylococcus, hemophilus, mycoplasma and legionella in acute infections. M. Tuberculosis and fungi such as histoplasma in chronic infections. Pneumonia due to opportunistic infections are increasingly common as infections with HIV become pandemic. Another frequent cause of parenchymal disease is **malignant disease, primary, but more often metastatic.** This also is readily recognized by the history, X-ray findings and biopsies, when necessary.

Acute pneumonias are not difficult to diagnose: fever, shortness of breath, occasionally the pain on breathing that occurs when inflammation involves and extends to the parietal pleura, the characteristic auscultation sounds of bronchial breathing, rales and rhonchi, decreased air entry, dullness to percussion and radiological findings. Equally easy is diagnosis of **parenchymal disease due to malignancy.** In all acute pneumonic processes there are frequent **ventilation-perfusion imbalances** contributing to the shortness of breath that accompanies the disease.

Chronic parenchymal diseases.

Chronic parenchymal diseases are often more difficult to diagnose. The patient frequently presents with weight loss, night sweats, occasional fever and increasing shortness of breath or the diagnosis may be consequent on a routine chest X-ray of an otherwise symptomless individual. The history often helps in making the diagnosis.

Lung function tests, sputum cultures, cytological examinations of sputum, bronchoscopies and when necessary, biopsies are useful for diagnosis and assessment. The usual spirometric pattern shows decreased diffusing capacity and hypoxia. Most of the reduction in diffusing capacity is probably due to an alveolo-capillary block caused by accumulation of fluid on the alveolar membrane or, in chronic disease, the result of thickening of the alveolar membrane by disease and associated interstitial fibrosis.

Any chronic parenchymal disease can result in emphysema. The topic is discussed in the section on emphysema.

The causes of chronic parenchymal disease of the lung.

There are three principal groups: parenchymal disease of allergic etiology, parenchymal disease due to inhalation of toxic substances, and finally, parenchymal diseases of unknown etiology.

The following are some examples:

— **Unresolved infections.** The causes are numerous. The following are some:

- **Tuberculosis.** Primary infections, reactivation infections and reactive infections due to decreased immunity resulting from AIDS infections.
- **Fungal, mycotic and parasitic disease.**
- **Opportunistic infections** in patients with AIDS.
- **Bronchiectasis.** Most brochiectasis results from unresolved severe respiratory infections, especially the pneumonias complicating measles, pertussis and adenovirus infections in children. Prophylaxis is im-

munization against measles and pertussis in children, annual influenza vaccination and a one time inoculation with pneumococcal vaccine in older people. Antibiotics must not be withheld when indicated.

The pathological lesion is dilation and peribronchial fibrosis due to inflammatory effects in bronchial walls. The normal expansile forces of respiration pull on the bronchial walls and there is dilatation of these structures and stagnation of secretions. The reduction of bronchial wall elasticity by inflammation results in decreased spontaneous contraction during exhalation. The result is pooling of secretions during exhalation and recurrent infections.

Patients cough up purulent sputum and associated hemoptyses are common as are finger clubbing and exertional dyspnea. Chronic inflammation persists with recurrent exacerbations of infection. The bacterial flora is usually mixed and treatment of infections is arbitrary. Antibiotics are chosen ad hoc until one finds the best choice for the individual patient. Lobar resections are often possible in individuals with localized areas of bronchiectasis. Otherwise therapy is merely supportive; a combination of antibiotics, bronchodilators and physical therapy to promote drainage. As mentioned later, bronchiectasis is one of the causes of chronic obstructive lung disease (COPD)

— **Allergic alveolitis.**

These include conditions such as farmer's lung, pigeon breeder's lung and other comparable conditions.

— **Toxic agents.**

Toxic agents causing chronic parenchymal disease include pneumoconioses due to dust and fibers. Examples are coal dust, asbestos, silica, beryllium and a variety of other agents. Other causes are the inhalation of toxic gases such as nitrogen dioxide (silo-filler's disease), radiation and some drugs.

— **Parenchymal disease of unknown etiology.**

These include lung disease as part of the syndrome of a collagen disease such as rheumatoid arthritis, scleroderma, lupus, polymyositis and dermatomyositis. Another group is caused by granulomatous disease such as sarcoidosis, and a final group is idiopathic disease. The last has many different names according to the radiological and biopsy findings: idiopathic alveolitis, fibrosing alveolitis, desquamative alveolitis, etc.

Restrictive lung disease.

The cause may be pulmonary or extrapulmonary.

The former (i.e., pulmonary causes) include a post-pneumonectomy syndrome as well as occasional sequelae of most of the conditions detailed in the preceding section on parenchymal lung disease.

The latter (non-pulmonary causes) include chest wall disease (e.g., extreme scoliosis), pleural disease such as the fibrothorax which occasionally follows surgery or untreated intrapleural hemorrhage, and diseases of respiratory muscles (e.g., the result of prolonged starvation or end-stage amyotrophic lateral sclerosis).

A restrictive pattern is characterized by decreased vital capacities, decreased lung volumes and decreases in total lung capacity. It is important to show that the last (i.e., decreased total lung capacity) exists, and that there is no obstruction to the passage of air to the alveoli, before deciding that a lung problem results from restrictive lung disease alone.

In restrictive lung disease without an obstructive element the FVC is reduced but if there is no obstruction the FEV/FVC ratio will be about 80%. Emphysema often has a restrictive component because of reduction in the effective alveolar membrane.

Chronic obstructive lung disease (COPD)

The usual causes are chronic bronchitis and emphysema. Some cases of bronchial asthma develop COPD and so do many cases of chronic bronchiectasis. COPD is characterized by dyspnea, first on exertion, then at rest and finally, by persistent dyspnea even when supplemental oxygen is provided.

It is diagnosable by spirometry. Patients with COPD have decreased FEV1/FVC ratios (forced expiratory volume in the first second of exhalation/forced expiratory vital capacity). This is because the initial part of forced exhalation depends on the force of contraction of the expiratory muscles, the elastic recoil of expanded lungs, and the absence of any tracheal or bronchial obstruction. The latter part of exhalation is essentially passive, depending on the elastic recoil of the lungs and the absence of more than normal resistance between the alveoli and the main, lobar, or segmental bronchi. Normal individuals can exhale 80-85% of their VC in the first second. An obstructive problem is probably present when this falls below 70%. The following are a few observations on each clinical condition that can result in COPD.

Chronic bronchitis.

Chronic bronchitis is a reaction of the bronchi to repeated exposure to irritants and/or repeated infections. The commonest cause is cigarette smoking. As many as 50% of patients who smoke two packs of cigarettes a day will eventually have enough productive cough to be diagnosed as chronic bronchitics.

There is mucus gland hyperplasia as well as other signs of inflammation in the bronchial wall. The condition is characterized by a persistent cough, excess mucus production and expectoration (not socially acceptable so the patient often swallows the product). Symptoms range from the morning cough of a smoker to a condition that is disabling because of hypoxia, hypercapnia and cor pulmonale.

Emphysema.

Emphysema is an anatomic change of the lung characterized by dilated terminal air spaces and destruction of their walls. The changes may predominate in the center of the lobules (centrilobular emphysema). Alternatively, the distribution is even throughout the lobule (panacinar emphysema). Some patients may have both emphysema and chronic bronchitis as well as COPD but COPD is not an invariable concomitant of emphysema.

The obstructive element of emphysema may result from one or both of the following:

- Decreased lung recoil resulting in excessive in situ collapse of airways during exhalation. Collapse of airways results in air trapping with an increase in residual volume (RV) because of decreased lung recoil. The total lung capacity (TLC) is also decreased but not in proportion to the RV and the RV/TLC ratio rises.
- Mechanical obstruction due to inflammation, mucus gland hypertrophy and accumulated secretions.

Whatever the cause, the obstructive element is diagnosable by spirometry; the FEV1 and FEV1/VC ratio is decreased.

The main theories on the cause of emphysema hypothesize that cigarette smoke and polluted air reduce the ability of the pulmonary macrophage system to clear inhaled microorganisms. Recurrent low grade infections develop with leucocytic infiltrates that release proteolytic enzymes which damage tissue. The severity of the resulting emphysema would depend on the ability of the individual to inhibit proteolysis, a function of alpha1-antitrypsin. This has not been proven but emphysema does occur in individuals with decreased anti-proteolytic mechanisms.

In homozygotes for alpha1-antitrypsin deficiency an emphysematous type of chronic airways obstruction can develop with onset in early middle age. They account for less than 2% of COPD patients. The diagnosis should be suspected in emphysematous patients under 50, in patients with a family history of COPD and in non-smokers with chronic airway obstruction.

Exacerbations of COPD.

The following are some causes:

- **Infections.** Often unrecognized except for increased shortness of breath at rest. The usual cause is a mixed bacterial infection of diseased lung. Precipitating factors include viral upper respiratory tract infections, inadequately treated right ventricular failure, exposure to toxic fumes of industrial and automobile pollution, and the development of some additional disease affecting the lung. Often, only blunderbuss single or multiple broad spectrum antibiotic therapy is possible. The topic of therapy is controversial and detailed later in this chapter. Additional causes of exacerbations include:

- **Pulmonary emboli.** Typically there is a sudden onset of acute dyspnea. This could also mean a sudden myocardial infarct or an acut internal pneumothorax
- **Mucus impaction** with atelectasis.
- **Bronchospasm** secondary to exposure to allergens or irritants.

Other causes of COPD.

Any of the parenchymal diseases detailed in a previous section can result in COPD if chronic and prolonged.

Type A and Type B patients with COPD.

COPD patients with emphysema but little bronchitis are designated Type A patients while those with little emphysema but severe bronchial disease are designated Type B patients.

Type A patients are deep breathers and maintain blood gases close to normal. They are therefore called pink puffers. The principal symptom is effort intolerance because of shortness of breath. The chest is typically barrel-shaped and breath sounds are heard poorly. Chronic cor pulmonale is uncommon in these patients.

Type B patients are apt to be cyanotic and are designated "blue bloaters." Wheezes and basal rales are heard on auscultation. Arterial blood gases show a decreased pO_2 and when the disease is advanced the pCO_2 is raised. The development of cor pulmonale is common as the disease progresses.

Respiratory and biochemical changes in COPD.

The hypoventilation of COPD results in an increased pCO_2 and a decreased pH. Bicarbonate is reabsorbed in the kidneys resulting in additions to pCO_2. A pCO_2 over 70mm Hg depresses the respiratory center and then ventilation depends on hypoxic stimuli. This is why in advanced COPD supplementary oxygen can, at times, reduce the hypoxic drive.

Bronchial asthma.

Asthma is best defined as episodic and reversible airways obstructions in response to one or more stimuli that in normal individuals would not induce such a response. As a rule the individual has a reactive bronchial tree that has marked sensitivity to a variety of stimuli that can provoke episodes of bronchospasm. Examples of such stimuli are allergens, infections, irritants, bronchoconstrictors, cold weather and exertion or emotional factors.

It is hypothesized that on exposure to environmental allergens IgE develops in these individuals and attaches to mast cells. When allergens are inhaled and the bronchial tree is reactive there is an immune reaction with release of mast cell mediators and consequent bronchospasm. Sputum and eosinophilia in the blood are often present.

Many asthmatics may not have an allergic basis for their reactions especially if the first attacks begin after the age of 30. Recurrent infections and inhalation of bronchial irritants appear to be major causes of bronchospasm in such patients. There are also aspirin sensitive asthmatics.

Diagnosis is not difficult. The history is one of recurrent attacks of non-exertional dyspnea with wheezing and rhonchi. Spirometry shows marked slowing of exhalation during attacks and improvement with bronchodilators.

A severe attack, called status asthmaticus, may be life threatening. Childhood disease often abates during teen-age or early adult life. Late onset asthma sometimes progresses to chronic airway obstruction, especially in patients whose attacks are accompanied by or related to infections and who have concurrent chronic bronchitis. Frank anatomic emphysema does not appear to result from bronchial asthma. The hyperinflated chest of some asthmatic individuals should not lead to this diagnosis.

Respiratory failure defined.

Campbell has defined respiratory failure as blood gas levels of pO_2 below 60mm Hg or a pCO_2 above 49mm

Hg. Normal arterial blood has a pO_2 greater than 80mm Hg (96mm Hg in young healthy adults).

Cor pulmonale.

Cor pulmonale is a frequent consequence of progressive lung disease, especially COPD. It has been defined[3] as an:

> "alteration in structure or function of the right ventricle resulting from disease affecting the structure or function of the lung or its vasculature, except where the alteration results from disease of the left side of the heart or congenital heart disease."

When hypoxemia is absent or slight and pulmonary artery pressure is normal a low output type of cor pulmonale is a common result. There are few signs of congestive heart failure.

When pulmonary hypertension is significant the changes are those of right ventriclular dysfunction. First there are ECG changes, then right ventricular hypertrophy and an increase in right ventricular pressure which results in fluid exudates into the alveoli. Basal rales are audible and finally, congestive failure develops with peripheral edema and a raised jugular venous pressure. Congestive heart failure may develop insidiously or suddenly during an acute exacerbation of the underlying lung disease.

The following are some reasons for development of congestive heart failure:

- Increased hypoxemia with increased pulmonary artery pressure and increased right ventricular strain.
- Associated myocardial dysfunction resulting from any one or more of many causes - usually arrhythmias and/or coronary artery occlusions or stenoses.
- Increased demand for oxygen and hence, of an increased cardiac ouput because of infections, thyrotoxicosis, anemia, or new unrelated disease of other organs and systems.

Dependent edema is common in these patients even in the absence of overt congestive heart failure and tachycardia may be marked, even in the absence of heart disease. A common ECG change is a dominant R wave in the right precordial leads. Another reliable sign is increasing heart size. Occasionally, oxygen therapy can result in decreased pulmonary hypertension and reduction of right ventricular hypertrophy. ACE inhibitors and diuretics are the usual medications prescribed. Beta blockers should not be given for associated heart disease because of the frequent overlap of putative cardio-selective β_1 blockers with pulmonary β_2 blockers.

Pulmonary neoplasms.

The commonest lung tumor is a metastatic tumor. They are often multiple. Common sites of origin are the breast, the colon, the prostate and the lung itself. Benign neoplasms of the lung do occur but the dreaded lesion is a primary lung cancer. Smoking is a definite risk factor. Any persistent cough of recent origin or a hemoptysis merits exclusion of a lung tumor as the cause. Many methods of investigation are available; X-rays, CT scans, sputum cytology and fine needle biopsy are options. The possibility of lung malignancy in any patient with persistent respiratory symptoms of recent origin is well known to all physicians. These topics are well described in standard texts and additional text is not necessary in this monograph.

One uncommon pulmonary tumor merits mention. It is the pleural mesothelioma and exposure to asbestos is a definite risk factor for developing such a lesion.

Miscellaneous causes for other lung dysfunctions

Atelectasis.

This is a common accompaniment of any type of lung disease. Atelectasis is a decrease in the volume or number of functional lung units, decreases due to occlusions or collapse. Common causes are blockage by inflammatory exudates, pressure from space occupying lesions and localized bronchiolar occlusion by fibrous tissue contraction.

The oxygen tension in pulmonary arterial blood is lower than in isolated atelectatic tissue so that oxygen is rapidly absorbed. Nitrogen is more slowly absorbed. With complete obstruction all gas in an obstructed unit could be absorbed in a few hours. As air is absorbed some edema develops and contributes to the radiographic density seen. Later the edema fluid is absorbed. Shortness of breath is common and rapid shallow breathing is usual when there is atelectasis of significant degree. Blood flow to the affected area continues and the shunt effect of this ventilation-perfusion imbalance results in hypoxia and an additional increase in the rate of breathing.

Pneumothorax.

When the space between visceral and parietal pleura is breached air enters the pleural space, the negative intrapleural pressure is lost, the parietal and visceral pleura part company and the lung collapses because of its intrinsic elasticity. There are three principal types of pneumothorax: internal, external and tension pneumothorax.

Internal pneumothorax results from puncture of the visceral pleura. In younger age groups the usual cause is rupture of congenital pleural blebs present because of fortuitous deficits in the elastica of alveolar walls. In older individuals rupture of pleural blebs are usually an accompaniment of COPD.

Other causes include rupture of congenital cysts, of the cysts of staphylococcal pneumonia, of cavities and of perforation of the esophagus, during instrumentation or from progression of esophageal cancer. Trauma in motor vehicle and other accidents can tear the visceral pleura or even cause rupture of a bronchus

External pneumothorax is the result of a tear in the parietal pleura. Causes include penetrating injuries and compound fractures of the ribs. An iatrogenic external pnemothorax does occasionally follow an aspiration or biopsy. It used to be employed as therapy for collapsing tuberculous tension cavities before surgery after a course of drug therapy became the option of choice.

Tension pneumothorax. Occasionally a ball-valve mechanism in the breached visceral pleura prevents free communication between the pleural space and the atmosphere. It allows increasing amounts of air to be pumped into the pleural space. Increasing intrapleural pressure results. This occurs especially during coughing. The mediastinum shifts to the opposite side. The function of the other lung is adversely affected resulting in much respiratory distress. In addition venous return is impeded leading to circulatory collapse. This can be a life-threatening emergency. Treatment is immediate decompression by insertion of a needle into the pleural cavity. It should be left in place till a drainage tube can be inserted.

Pleural effusions.

Effusions of 100-500ml are detectable on X-rays. Clinical detection usually requires an effusion of greater volume. **There are two types of effusions: exudates and transudates.**

Exudates have a specific gravity greater than 1015 and a protein content greater than 3g/100ml. They are usually caused by infections or tumors. The fluid is cloudy and dark yellow in color. Its principal cellular contents may be neutrophils, lymphocytes or malignant cells.

Transudates have a specific gravity less than 1015 and a protein content that is less than 3g/100ml. The usual cause is congestive heart failure.

The pleural effusion of a primary tuberculous infection.

It is often termed idiopathic. It usually begins with acute pleural pain and a febrile illness with high ESR. The effusion may or may not be evidence of a primary tuberculous infection. The demonstration of enlarged hilar glands and/or a primary Ghon focus will clinch the diagnosis. Resolution is the rule - often with some fibrosis and calcification.

Culture of the pleural fluid shows TB bacilli in many cases. Many tuberculosis specialists feel that these individuals should be treated as patients with tuberculosis, even if the bacilli are not demonstrable, as 20-30% of adolescents with such an effusion will eventually develop clinical disease.

Therapeutic options for diseases and dysfunctions of the respiratory complex

Therapy for infections are various antibiotics for bacterial, mycoplasma and legionella infections. A major problem is the development of increasing numbers of patients with drug resistant tuberculosis. Therapies for pneumothorax and atelectases have been described. Therapies for most chronic lung diseases include the avoidance of smoking, of occupational hazards and of allergens if they are identifiable.

Therapy for stable chronic obstructive lung disease (COPD).

The rest of this section provides the therapeutic options for treating COPD.

Bronchial irritants.

Smoking tobacco remains the main cause of COPD. Anyone hoping for control of COPD must stop smoking. COPD is a serious problem with significant mortality. The WHO[4] claims that by 2000 COPD had become the fourth leading cause of global mortality. Before dying these patients endure long periods of restrictions in daily activities, progressively less effective therapy and significant disabilities.

The FEV_1:FEV ratio

A diagnosis of COPD requires spirometric demonstration of a FEV_1:FEV ratio of less than 0.7 and failure of lung function to return to normal after administration of bronchodilators, though, of course, there is frequent amelioration. It has been shown[5,6] that mortality and disability are directly related to decreases in the FEV_1:FEV ratio and not to symptoms such as the increased secretion of mucus. The causes of a decreased FEV_1:FEV ratio were previously detailed.

$Alpha_1$-antitrypsin deficiency.

This is an uncommon cause of COPD. Its existence was mentioned in the previous text. It should be considered when any non-smoker develops emphysema before the age of 50. To date, replacement therapy programs have not been demonstrably useful though some CT reductions in density are seen at times[7].

Therapy for stable disease.

Between exacerbations therapy is aimed at retarding or stopping progression of disease.

Smoking. The studies of Anthonisen and associates[8] have clearly demonstrated that cessation of smoking decreases future mortality from COPD. It is essential that the patient stop smoking and every attempt should be made to facilitate this; counseling on the dangers of continuing to smoke, descriptions of the miserable life when COPD progresses to a long premortem period of limited activity and continual oxygen therapy, and prescription of nicotine patches and other aids such as bupropion (Zyban; GlaxoSmithKline) which claim to help individuals to stop smoking.

Other irritants. The air of most industrialized cities have high concentrations of lung irritants: examples are fumes from gasoline combustion, from factory smokestacks and from power generating plants. The only way to avoid these irritants is to move to a more pastoral or less industrialized and populated environment. An ideal that is often not possible for any one or more of many reasons.

Bronchodilators. The aim should be maintenance of bronchial dilation. There are three types of bronchodilators: the agonists, typified by salbutamol (Ventolin; GlaxoSmithKline), the anti-cholinergic agents, typified by ipatropium (Atrovent; Boehringer Ingelheim) and the phosphodiesterase type-4 inhibitors such as theophylline. An important precaution when prescribing an anticholinergic is to be sure there is no glaucoma; these agents can worsen existing glaucoma.

Recently these agonists and anti-cholinergic have been marketed as long-acting agents; salbutamol as salmetrol (Serevent; GlaxoSmithKline)[9] and the anticolinergics as tiotripium (Spiriva; Boehringer Ingelheim)[10]. They have the advantage of keeping the bronchioles almost continuously dilated and there seem to be fewer exacerbations and improved well-being.

The phosphodiesterase inhibitor, theophylline, has been used for many years to produce bronchodilation. The β_2 agonists and the anticholinergics seem to be more effective. However, a 2001 paper by ZuWallack and associates[11] claim that a combination of salmeterol and theophylline gives an improvement over treatment with either one alone.

Corticosteroids. The role and effectiveness of corticosteroids in quiescent disease are controversial. They do seem to reduce the incidence of exacerbations but a survey of the literature suggests that they do not change the rate at which lung function declines. However, a study by Calverly and associates[12] suggest that a combination of salmeterol and a steroid (fluticasone) results in improved lung function and fewer exacerbations. The combination is marketed as Advair (GlaxoSmithKline).

Oxygen.

The following are some indications for oxygen therapy:

— A pO_2 of less than 60mm Hg. The ideal is said to be provision of continuous oxygen for 19 hours each day.

— A pO_2 less than 55-60mm Hg during exercise or during sleep, even if the resting pO_2 exceeds 60mm Hg. Oxygen desaturation occurs in up to 40% of patients who have pO_2s greater than 60mm Hg at rest. They should receive oxygen during the sleep period.

— Nocturnal oxygen is required for most patients with cor pulmonale.

Immunizations. A report by Nichol and associates[17] contends that vaccinations against influenza can result in a 50% reduction of serious illness and death in COPD. Comparable figures feature in subsequent reports. Reports on the value of immunization against pneumococci are not as persuasive.

Therapy for COPD during exacerbations.

The typical features of a respiratory infection are usually absent unless there is pleural infection or actual consolidation. Exacerbations of COPD are usually characterized by any one or more of the following: increased dyspnea, wheezing or increased wheezing, cough and increased sputum production. Physical examination usually reveals increased expiratory rhonchi but little else and unless there is pneumonic consolidation the chest X-ray shows little change from previous ones.

The organisms responsible for exacerbations and their treatment. Viral infections account for 30-40% of exacerbations with concomitant or subsequent bacterial infections in some 50%. The role of bacteria in precipitating infections is difficult to prove as some 25-50% of individuals with COPD have bacteria in their airways. The major organisms implicated include Hemophilus Influenza, streptococcus pneumonia, and Moraxella catarrhalis. Mycoplasma pneumonia and chlamydia pneumonia are probable additional causative organisms and this is an important consideration when deciding on an antibiotic.

Several clinical trials have shown the value of antibiotics in acute exacerbations[14,15]. Erythromycin, clarithromycin and tetracycline. are effective against Mycoplasma P., H. Influenza. Many feel that they are the drugs of first choice when treating exacerbations. Mycoplasma pneumonia causes 15-50% of all pneumonias in adults and an even higher percentage in school children[16].

Eryhthromycin and clairithromycin are also effective against streptococci, staphylococci and most gram positive and many gram negative organisms, including H. Influenza. They are also effective against M. Legionella. Some feel that neutrophils should be demonstrable in the sputum before antibiotics are given. Others give them whenever there are exacerbations. The latter practice has been shown to increase the rate of resolution by a small but significant margin. For small exacerbations the ideal antibiotic would be erythromycin or clairithromycin or doxycycline. For more serious exacerbations blind ad hoc combination therapy is usually needed; amoxicillin and doxycycline or a combination of erythromycin or clarithromycin and ciprofloxacin. More potent antibiotics are available if the initial ones fail. They are best reserved for second line therapy to reduce the chances of resistance developing. Antibiotic selection is an ad hoc process because the bacteriological data about causation usually states that the pattern is one of mixed bacterial populations in patients with COPD.

When a patient is known to respond to an antibiotic or antibiotic combination in an acute exacerbation it is a good idea to give a prescription for the antibiotic so that therapy can start immediately an exacerbation begins. Needless to say, early examination and assessment by the treating physician is essential.

Bronchodilators. Rapid relief from brochoconstriction is essential. An effective combination is a nebulizer solution of a 2ml nebule of an anti-cholinergic such as ipatropium (Atrovent; Boehringer Ingelheim) with a 2.5mg nebule of the β_2 agonist, salbutamol (Ventolin; GlaxoSmithKline). A nebulizer is small and relatively inexpensive so that patients with frequent exacerbations of COPD are well advised to buy one and start nebulizer therapy at the first sign of an exacerbation. The effects are not always immediately dramatic as some causes of acute exacerbations are structural; for example, bronchial wall thickening from inflammation.

Oxygen. Almost all patients with exacerbations of COPD will need supplemental oxygen. It may be given by nasal cannula (2-3L/min) or by a venturi-type mask (28%). Careful monitoring is needed as in some patients hypoxia is the only drive for ventilation when there is associated severe hypercapnia.

Corticosteroids. The objective of corticosteroid therapy is reduction of inflammation. There is much evidence that corticosteroids hasten resolution and reduce treatment failures. For patients sick enough to be hospitalized intravenous therapy is the initial step with later graduation to oral corticosteroids. Those who are on long-term corticosteroids do seem to have fewer exacerbations. Corticosteroids reduce the endogenous protective response to an infection. If given they are best given with antibiotics in any acute exacerbation.

Clearing of secretions and physiotherapy. Once the acute phase has passed patients should be advised to clear secretions by vigorous coughing. Physiotherapy may help dislodge mucus plugs.

Chapter 10 References.

1. Pulmonary surfactants. Special issue in honor of Professor John A. Clements: Biochim. Biophys. Acta, 77:1408, 1998.
2. Avery, M.E. & Mead, J. Surface properties in relation to atelectasis and hyaline membrane disease. AMA J Dis. Child. 1959; 97:517.
3. Inter-Society Commission, Pulmonary Heart Study Group: Circulation 1970; 41:A12.
4. Murray, C.J. Lopez, A.D. et al. The Global Burden of Disease 2000 Project: global program on evidence for health policy discussion, paper number 36. Geneva: WHO, 2001.
5. Fletcher, C. & Peto, R. The natural history of chronic airflow obstruction. B.M.J. 1977; 1:1645.
6. Peto, R., Speizer, F.E., et al. The relevance in adults of airflow obstruction but not of mucus hypersecretion, to mortality from chronic lung disease: results from 20 years of prospective observation. Am. Rev. Resp. Dis. 1983; 128:491.
7, Dirksen, A., Dijkman, J.H. A randomized clinical trial of alpha(1)-antitrypsin augmentation therapy. Am. J. Respir. Crit. Care Med 1999; 160:1468.
8. Anthonisen, N.R., Connett, J.E., et al. Smoking and lung function of Lung Health Study participants after 11 years. Am. J, Respir. Crit. Care Med. 2002; 166:675.
9. Rennard, S.I., Anderson, W., et al. Use of a long-acting inhaled β_2 adrenergic agonist, salmetrol xinafoate, in patients with chronic obstructive lung disease. Am. J. Respir, Crit. Care Med., 2001; 163:1087.
10. Vincken, W., van Noord, J.A. et al. Dutch/Belgian Tiotropium Study Group. Improved health outcomes in patients with COPD during 1 year's treatment with tiotropium. Eur. Respir. J., 2002; 19:209.
11. Zu Wallach, R.L. Mahler, D.A. et al. Salmeterolol and theophylline combination therapy in the treatment of COPD. Chest 2001; 119:1661.
12.Calverly, P.M.A., Pauwels, R. et al. Combined salmeterol and fluticasone in the treatment of chronic obstructive pulmonary disease: a randomized controlled trial. Lancet, 2003; 361:449.
13. Armstrong, H.G. Principles and practice of aviation medicine. Baltimore: Williams & Wilkins, 1939. (obtained from Online quote by Weg. J. & Haas, C.F. in Online Postgraduate Medicine, April 1998).
14. Anthonisen, N.R., Manfreda, J. et al. Antibiotic therapy in exacerbations of chronic obstructive pulmonary disease. Ann. Int. Med. 1987; 106:196.
15. Murphy, T. &Sethi, S. Bacterial infection in chronic obstructive pulmonary disease. Am. Rev. Resp. Dis. 1992; 146:1067.
16. Mycoplasma pneumonia: http://health.allref.com/mycoplasma-pneumonia-info.html.
17. Nichol, K.L., Margolis, K,L, et al. The efficacy and cost effectiveness of vaccination against influenza among elderly patients living in the community. N. Engl. J. Med. 1994; 331:778.

11

Diagnosis: The Slave Systems
3. The Cardiovascular Complex

Table of Contents

Notation.

The notation ~P denotes phosphorous with a high energy bond. Depending on the context in which the term is used ~P may denote the energy liberated from a high energy phosphate bond.

A general comment on the methodology of clinical assessments.

The comments made **on page 119** about this topic are not repeated. They merit reading before proceeding with this chapter.

The objective

The cardiovascular system has three components: the heart, the vasculature and the blood. The function of the heart is to pump blood and the function of the vasculature is to provide conduits which deliver blood to all cells. The blood is a complex component of the system and merits a chapter of its own (Chapter 12).

The resource systems of the cardiovascular complex:

- **Heart muscle** which contracts and pumps.
- **A coronary circulation** which provides the heart with environmental energy substrate for conversion to ~P.
- **A cardiac electrical conduction system** to ensure rhythmic and coordinated contractions of its chambers.
- **Cardiac valvular anatomy** to ensure orderly progression of blood into and out of the heart.
- **A patent and extensive vascular complex** of conduits.
- **The blood.**

Signs and symptoms that suggest cardiovascular dysfunction.

They include any one or more of the following:

- Dyspnea (i.e., shortness of breath).
- Chest pain.
- Swollen legs.
- Cough and hemoptysis.
- Alterations in rhythm and rate of the pulse.
- Hepatomegaly and splenomegaly.
- Pericardial pain when infections involve the parietal pericardium.
- Murmurs that suggest existing valvular disease and headaches and other symptoms of uncontrolled hypertension.
- Emboli and cardiac dysfunctions form infections of the heart and/or its valves.
- Syncopal episodes.
- Tiredness.
- Stroke and transient ischemic attacks.
- Intermittent claudication and the other features of vascular insufficiency of the limbs, the kidneys and/or intestines.

The cardiovascular complex - normal anatomy and physiology

The heart.

The heart provides propulsive force. It has four chambers, two atria and two ventricles. The main pump elements are the ventricles. The right ventricle perfuses the lungs and the left ventricle perfuses the rest of the body.

Each ventricle has inflow and outflow valves and on each occasion the former close before the latter open so that there is no backflow.

The left ventricle develops pressures that usually exceed 120mm Hg during contraction. This pressure declines to almost zero during its filling phase (diastole). Pressures for the right ventricle are about 20mm Hg during systole and 0 during diastole. The differences in pressure equate with differences in wall thicknesses - 8-15mm for the left and 3-5mm for the right ventricle.

Pressure drops from over 120mm Hg at the aortic origin to about 35mm Hg at the origin of the capillaries. There is an additional fall of pressure of about 15mm Hg in the capillaries. The venules have a pressure of about 10mm Hg at their origins and zero when the vena cavae enter the heart.

The objectives.

The objective of the cardiovascular complex is propulsion of enough blood to cells to satisfy prevailing needs.

The heart is the pump and the cardiovascular system provides the conduits that reach every cell in the body (the cornea and cartilage are the few exception). All materials needed by the cells and required to be removed from cells are transported in the blood. The blood is contained in the cardiovascular conduits and its functions and objectives are detailed in the next chapter.

The resource systems.

They are:

— **Heart muscle contraction.**

— **A coronary circulation which provides substrate for production of energy (~P) usable by the heart.**

— **The anatomy of the heart with valves that ensure unidirectional flow.**

— **An intrinsic electrical system which ensures appropriate rates and rhythms.**

— **Extrinsic medullary control systems which can modify rates and contractile forces.**

Each resource has many minor systems which repeatedly, automatically and autonomously interact with each other to attain the objective or objectives of the resource. The interactions cease when the set-points of all the allosteric enzymes are reached. Alternatively till there is no more ~P and/or substrate left for biochemical reactions. Subsequent reflexes from the CNS medullary centers assist by changing heart and respiratory rates and the tonic contractions of arterioles in the peripheral vasculature.

Chart 11-1 is an overview of the intrinsic and extrinsic mechanisms that attempt to maintain maximum cardiac output. The chart is similar to Chart 5-6 on page 106 but is replicated here for the convenience of the reader.

Heart muscle.

The stroke volume is the left ventricular output per contraction. It is about 70-90/ventricular contractions in a 70Kg man at rest. Obvious physiological causes for an increase include activity of any sort. The stroke volume depends on factors intrinsic to the heart and to others that are extrinsic. Two principal intrinsic factors determine the force of cardiac contraction.

The first of these is cardiac contractility which is the intrinsic ability of cardiac muscle to vary its contractile force and velocity independent of muscle fiber length.

The second is the Starling principle of heterometric regulation.

In 1914 a publication by Starling and associates[1] showed that the force generated by contracting cardiac muscle was proportional to the degree of its previous stretching. They also found that when the ventricle was over-stretched the systolic pressure decreased.

The Starling effect is called **heterometric regulation.** It has been suggested that heterometric autoregulation occurs because more cross-bridges between actin and myosin form when muscle is stretched. Failure occurs when sarcomeres are stretched beyond their normal lengths with a corresponding decrease between cross-bridges. The Starling effect is important for matching the outputs of the two ventricles when pulmonary and

Chart 11-1: **THE INTERACTIONS OF THE MINOR SYSTEM COMPONENTS OF A RESOURCE SYSTEM OF THE CARDIOVASCULAR COMPLEX. I.E. THE HEART**

The heart is a system of the cardiovascular complex. It pumps blood into the conduits of the vascular complex.

The objective:

Propulsion of blood sufficient to satisfy tissue needs in the prevailing circumstances (i.e. at rest or during moderate or severe exercise). The objective requires optimization of the heart rate and the contractile force of the left ventricular muscle because **output per minute = Beats per min x Stroke volume (i.e., output in ml/left ventricular contraction).**

The heart rate at rest is about 70 beats per minute and the stroke volume is about 70-90ml/ventricular contraction in a 70Kg man at rest. Hence, the output at rest of such an individual is about 5-6.5L/min

The main resources.

1. **The contractile force of the left ventricle.**
2 **An intrinsic electrical system for normal rhythm or well compensated rate and rhythm of an arrhythmia.**
3. **A valve system which ensures unidirectional flow.**
4. **A coronary circulation which provides substrate for production of energy (~P) for heart muscle.**

Each resource system has many minor systems components which rapidly interact by automatic and autonomous to-and-fro interactions and repeated iterations till all the allosteric set-points of the enzymes involved in the reactions are reached or substrate is finished or not responsive and/or more ~P is not available. At all times **the microenvironmental control mechanisms** are intimately involved in interacting with any one or more of the resources to obtain an optimal result in concord with conditions in the microenvironment.

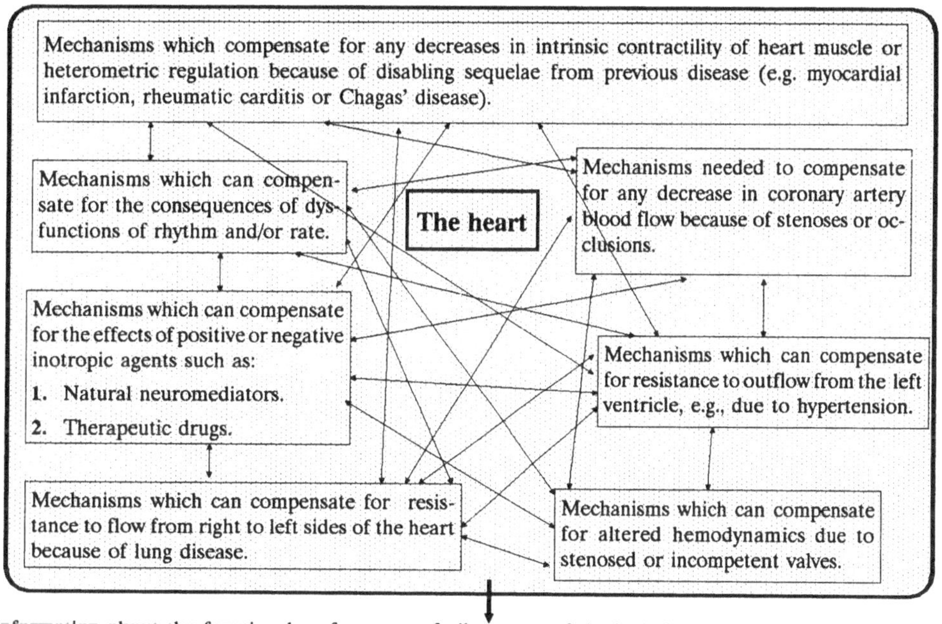
Mechanisms which compensate for any decreases in intrinsic contractility of heart muscle or heterometric regulation because of disabling sequelae from previous disease (e.g. myocardial infarction, rheumatic carditis or Chagas' disease).
Mechanisms which can compensate for the consequences of dysfunctions of rhythm and/or rate.
The heart
Mechanisms needed to compensate for any decrease in coronary artery blood flow because of stenoses or occlusions.
Mechanisms which can compensate for the effects of positive or negative inotropic agents such as:
1. Natural neuromediators.
2. Therapeutic drugs.
Mechanisms which can compensate for resistance to outflow from the left ventricle, e.g., due to hypertension.
Mechanisms which can compensate for resistance to flow from right to left sides of the heart because of lung disease.
Mechanisms which can compensate for altered hemodynamics due to stenosed or incompetent valves.

Information about the functional performance of all systems of the body is transmitted continuously to the hypothalamus and to the medullary cardiac, vasomotor and respiratory centers. If function is deemed inadequate the CNS sends appropriate commands to the resource system or systems of one or more principal systems. For example, when cardiac performance is suboptimal, medullary centers send coordinated and integrated commands to the cardiac beta receptors, the peripheral vasculature and the respiratory apparatus. Transmission is by autonomic and somatic (to the respiratory muscles) efferents and by quantitative changes in hormones produced in the hypothalamus (e.g., ADH) or hormones controlled by hypothalamic releasing factors via the pituitary.

In addition, hypotension is sensed by the JG apparatus, renin production is stimulated with eventual production of angiotensin II and III. Both are potent vasoconstrictors.

systemic venous returns are momentarily dissimilar.

The coronary circulation.

The majority of cardiac dysfunctions result from coronary artery stenoses or occlusions so that comment on the coronary circulation is a priority. The heart weighs about 250-300g and it is supplied with blood by two coronary arteries: the right and left coronaries. The right coronary supplies the right ventricle and part of posterior wall of the left ventricle. The left coronary supplies the left ventricle through the anterior descending and circumflex vessels.

The term, dominance, is used to indicate the vessel that gives off the posterior descending artery. In man 90% come off the right artery. It supplies blood to the AV node and the inferior wall of the left ventricle. Dominance is not synonymous with predominant. The left coronary artery is the predominant vessel of the myocardium. Branches come off the main artery and its principal branches. The left anterior descending artery is the most important branch of the left coronary artery. It supplies most of the left ventricle. Branches penetrate the myocardium and have precapillary sphincters followed by a capillary network. Collateral vessels exist between the branches of adjacent vessels. They are usually small pre-existing arterial channels without intervening capillaries. In man they are mainly in the subendocardial area and when blood flow is gradually decreased these collaterals open up.

The normal coronary circulation is about 5% of cardiac output or about 250ml/min. Coronary blood flow and myocardial oxygen needs are related. Control of the volume of coronary blood flow is effected, in the main, by local vasodilator metabolites. Additionally, decreased pO_2 stimulates coronary blood flow and so does an increased pCO_2 and a reduced pH. The vessels have α and β receptors but the correlations of coronary flows with myocardial needs for $\sim$P substrate is also seen in the denervated hearts of cardiac transplants.

Coronary filling occurs mainly in diastole. In systole flow is less than the mean and at peak of systole the left coronary flow can fall to zero. In the left coronary about 1/5 of flow takes place in systole and 4/5 in diastole. In the right ventricle the difference is not so great because of the lower intraventricular pressures and smaller muscle mass. The decreased flow in systole is due to compression of the vessels by the contracting ventricles. The subendocardial vessels tend to be compressed the most so that subendocardial flow is mainly diastolic. When there is tachycardia systole occupies an increasing part of the cycle and the compression effect is more marked. This could be one reason why angina can be precipitated by exercise in individuals with occlusive coronary artery disease.

It is difficult to evaluate the effects of neurogenic factors on the coronary circulation because they not only affect coronary flow but also the heart and the changes in the heart in turn affect the coronaries.

Normal cardiac electrophysiology.

The object is preservation of normal rate and rhythm and to modify them according to needs.

The intrinsic cardiac electrical control system.

The atria have an intrinsic rhythmicity of about 55 contractions per minute and the ventricles of about 15-30/min. The refractory period of heart muscle is about 0.25 seconds. It is essential that the pacemaker of the heart (the sino-atrial node (SA)) generate contraction impulses at rates that are too fast to permit atrial and ventricular muscle to recover and contract at their own rates before stimulation by another impulse from the SA node.

The cardiac impulse begins in the SA node which is located in the posterior wall of the right atrium just below the opening of the superior vena cava. It has an intrinsic natural rhythmic electrical discharge of about 72 impulses per minute. The contractions of the specialized muscle fibers of the sino-atrial node generate action potentials in the atrial and ventricular musculature. The contraction wave generated in the SA node spreads in a concentric manner through both atria and results in the atrial contractions seen in late diastole. The P wave of the electrocardiogram results from atrial depolarization and subsequent repolarization. Its normal duration is about 0.08 seconds.

About 2/3 of ventricular filling is passive and begins as soon as the mitral and tricuspid valves open. The remainder occurs in late diastole when passive flow is augmented by atrial contraction. The third heart sound, when heard, is associated with this rapid filling phase. After the age of 40 it is often pathological in origin though it may also occur in fever and is usually physiological when heard in young individuals.

The impulse generated at the SA node is not only transmitted to atrial muscle but also to the Purkinje fibers which are specialized muscle fibers capable of transmitting impulses much faster than cardiac muscle; the rate of the former is about 2m/sec while the rate for cardiac muscle is about 0.4m/sec. The Purkinje fibers arise in the SA node and converge by many internodal paths on the AV node.

The atrioventricular (AV) node is located in the posterior wall of the right atrium near the tricuspid valve. Purkinje fibers (the bundle of His) originate in the AV node, pass into the ventricular septum and then divide into right and left branches that spread through the ventricles and terminate on their endocardial surfaces. The atria and ventricles are separated by fibrous tissue except where they are connected by the bundle of His.

Electrical activity of the Purkinje fibers depolarize ventricular muscle cells and the QRS complex of the electrocardiogram represents this wave of depolarization. The Q wave is the first downward deflection. It is followed by an upward R wave and finally a downward S wave. The time from the end of the P wave to the beginning of the QRS complex is 0.08-0.1 seconds . The duration of the QRS complex is also 0.08-0.10 seconds. Following the QRS complex there is a pause, the ST segment located at the baseline of the electrocardiogram. This is followed by a T wave that represents ventricular repolarization.

The right ventricle receives blood at almost zero pressure and pumps it into the pulmonary artery at a peak systolic pressure of 25 mm Hg. The left ventricle also receives blood at about zero pressure but pumps it into the aorta at a peak pressure that usually exceeds 120mm Hg. The two ventricles each eject similar volumes so that the left ventricle has to perform about 5-7 times the work of the right ventricle.

Ventricular contraction has two phases. The **first is the isometric phase** during which there is contraction without volume change. As soon as intraventricular rises above intraatrial pressure the tricuspid and mitral valves close. The contraction of the papillary muscles prevents their eversion into the atria. The QRS complex begins immediately before and terminates soon after the beginning of this phase of ventricular contraction. The first heart sound is a consequence of mitral and tricuspid valve closures.

The second phase of ventricular contraction is the ejection phase. When ventricular pressures exceed aortic and pulmonary artery pressures the valves open and blood enters the arteries. About ⅔ of the blood is ejected in the first ⅓ of systole. Towards the end of this period the aorta begins to distend and then recoil from the impact of the ejected blood. Flow slows till aortic pressure exceeds ventricular pressure and then the valves close. The second heart sound results from closure of pulmonary and aortic valves. As a rule the ventricles do not empty completely. The normal end-systolic volume of the left ventricle is about 40 ml. As the normal end-diastolic volume is about 130ml the average stroke volume is about 80 ml. Hence, the usual ejection fraction is about 70% $((80/120) \times 100 = 67\%)$. When the myocardium is weak there is a decrease in ejection fraction so that this is a figure which is useful for assessing left ventricular fraction.

The cardiac valve system.

Efficient pumping is ensured by the presence of two unidirectional valves in each ventricle. One is located at the junction with the atria and opens into the ventricles. The other is located at the junction of ventricles and great vessels and opens into the pulmonary arteries and the aorta. These latter valves open and close passively depending on pressure gradients.

The atrial valves have their lower surfaces and edges tethered to the papillary muscles of the ventricular walls by means of thin strands called chordae tendineae. The papillary muscles contract at the same time as the ventricles and so prevent eversion of the valves into the atrial cavities during ventricular contraction. Necrosis of a papillary muscle or rupture of one or more chordae tendineae results in an incompetent valve with regurgitation of blood into the atria during ventricular contraction. So will myxomatous degeneration of a valve, a condition usually associated with aging. The mitral and/or aortic valves are the valves most frequently affected by myxomatous degeneration.

Murmurs.

Blood flow in the blood vessels is usually laminar. The outermost layer of blood in the vessel is almost stationary. The speed of each concentric layer of blood increases the nearer it is to the center of the vessel where the rate of flow is highest. Normal laminar blood flow is silent but as velocity increases the flow becomes turbulent. Turbulence also results when blood flows through an obstruction.

Turbulent flow results in murmurs. Turbulence can also result from increased velocity of blood flow. **Murmurs due to increased velocity of blood flow** are often audible over the vascular goiters of Grave's disease and over arterio-venous aneurysms and fistulae. **Murmurs due to narrowing of blood vessels** are more common. The carotid bruit heard as blood passes through a carotid artery or limb vessel narrowed by atheroma are examples. Turbulent flow is also responsible for most **heart murmurs.** The normal flow of intracardiac blood does not result in turbulence. But when a **valve is stenosed** blood flowing through it accelerates and becomes turbulent. If the **valve is incompetent** blood flows back through it with increased velocity because of the pumping action of the next chamber or because of aortic recoil. When murmurs are heard, knowledge of the dynamics of blood flow through the heart helps to diagnose anatomical stenosis or incompetence of a valve. Modern technology has reduced this art to a study of echocardiograms.

Mitral stenosis and aortic regurgitation result in diastolic murmurs, **mitral regurgitation and aortic stenosis** in systolic murmurs. Mitral murmurs are best heard at the apex and aortic murmurs at the base of the heart. Many different murmurs characterize **congenital heart disease.** The point in the cardiac cycle where the murmur is best heard depends on the direction of abnormal blood flow. For example, the blood flow through a septal defect is usually from left to right so that the murmur of an interventricular defect is systolic.

Decreased blood viscosity can also be a cause of turbulent flow. This may be why systolic murmurs are frequently heard **in anemic patients.**

The Korotkoff sounds.

The Korotkoff sounds are the sounds used to measure systolic and diastolic pressures. When the brachial artery is constricted by a pressure higher than the systolic pressure no blood passes through and no sounds are heard. As the cuff pressure decreases to less than the systolic pressure blood squirts through. Because of the arterial narrowing by the cuff, flow is turbulent and staccato sounds are heard. Flow remains turbulent till the diastolic pressure is reached. At this point flow becomes laminar once again and the sounds cease. Near the diastolic pressure the sounds are often audible but muffled. This is the period when flow is continuous but still turbulent. The correct diastolic pressure is probably the pressure noted when the sounds disappear.

The extrinsic control systems of the cardiovascular system

The medullary centers.

There is a collection of neurons in the medulla that control heart rate, the peripheral vasculature and respiration. Their artificial division into cardiac, vasomotor and respiratory centers is probably not justifiable as the neurons are closely integrated with each other and the hypothalamus. They have a common path for effecting changes which is neural discharges to the autonomic nervous system and neural impulses to the hypothalamus. The latter result in quantitative and/or qualitative changes in hormones controlled by the CNS. The hypothalamus also discharges nerve impulses. They accompany those from the medullary centers to the reticular system of the upper spinal cord and then to its intermedio-lateral column. Autonomic nerves emerge from the intermedio-lateral column at different levels. They synapse once before their final synapse. The autonomic nervous system was described in detail on pages 130-134. Somatic nerves transmit commands to the striated muscles of respiration.

The neurons of the medullary centers are tonically active, discharging impulses even at rest. Neurons from the cardiac center discharge impulses that descend in the vagus and slow heart rates. This cardioinhibitory effect can be eliminated by atropine which increases the heart rate. The impulses from the vasoconstrictor center synapse with cells in the intermedio-lateral column and are then widely distributed to arterioles. The result is continuous peripheral vasoconstriction. The automatic rhythmicity of the respiratory center was detailed in the preceding chapter. All three centers are continuously active which makes functional changes easier as there is no zero baseline.

Increased activity of the medullary centers and hypothalamus result in integrated changes of cardiac, and respiratory rates and peripheral vasoconstriction. An example is the usual response to hypovolemia and shock. The blood pressure increases, and there is acceleration of the heart rate and faster respiration. The increase in heart rate is effected by autonomic beta adrenergic sympathetic fibers that liberate norepinephrine at their terminals. Increased autonomic peripheral arteriolar vasoconstrictions cause the initial blood pressure changes.

The receptors and their afferents.

Impulses from the receptors of most systems reach and affect the activities of the medullary centers. The interactions and integrations of these centers ensure that, after receiving information from the receptors, they make appropriate adjustments in heart rates, stroke volumes and the calibers of the arterioles. The microenvironmental pericellular and intracellular control mechanisms optimize peripheral responses in concord with conditions in the cellular microenvironment. **The following are some of the more important receptors:**

The pressure receptors of the aortic arch and carotid sinus. Their principal function is the recording of changes in blood pressure. Reflexes evoked by impulses from these receptors are the principal reflexes involved in immediate short-term cardiovascular regulation. Pressure sensitive nerve endings exist in the walls of the aortic arch and in the walls of the internal carotid arteries at their origins. Stretching of the nerve endings generate action potentials that travel to the cardiovascular centers via the glossopharyngeal nerve from the carotid sinus, and the vagus nerve from the aortic body. They are the afferent limbs of a negative feedback reflex centered on the medullary centers and mediated by autonomic nerves

The responses are greatest in the physiological range and are of special importance in maintaining flow adjustments to changes such as those resulting from alterations in posture. When the blood pressure rises there is an increased neural discharge from the receptors. These travel to the medullary centers where integrated responses result in increased parasympathetic and decreased sympathetic activity with slowing of the heart rate, a decrease in myocardial contractility, reduction in vasoconstrictor and venoconstrictor tone, and finally, restoration of blood pressure to physiologically acceptable levels. The converse occurs when blood pressure falls. The discharges from the receptors decrease. There is increased sympathetic and decreased parasympathetic activity and the heart rate, myocardial contractility, respiratory rates and peripheral vasomotor tone increase. This converse reaction is an important component of the responses to hypovolemic hypotension caused by hemorrhage, losses of plasma in extensive burns, or of extracellular fluid as in extreme gastroenteritis or vomiting, or sequestration of fluids in distended and immobile loops of bowel.

The chemoreceptors of the aortic and carotid bodies. The carotid and aortic bodies have chemoreceptors as well as receptors that sense changes in blood pressure. The chemoreceptors are stimulated by increased pCO_2 or H^+ concentrations as well as decreased pO_2 concentrations. The principal effects are on respiration. A low pO_2 increases discharges from these receptors and results in increases in ventilation with associated peripheral vasoconstriction and bradycardia. The pO_2 effect is usually only seen when the pCO_2 is very high.

Brain stem receptors. They respond to hypoxia and ischemia but are only activated when pressure falls to less than about 70mm Hg. A widespread generalized vasoconstriction is induced in an attempt to maintain blood pressure. This reflex is probably responsible for the Cushing reflex. This is a high blood pressure occurring as the CSF pressure rises. Presumably the raised blood pressure decreases blood flow in the brain stem and the CNS ischemic response is activated in order to maintain adequate blood flow to the brain despite the ischemia resulting from increasing CSF pressure.

Ventricular receptors. These receptors are located in the walls of the left ventricle and are stimulated by stretches resulting from increases in ventricular pressure. Afferent impulses travel along the vagi to the cardiovascular centers and any increase in discharge results in a reflex bradycardia and peripheral vasodilation.

Atrial receptors. Both atria have stretch receptors. Some discharge during atrial systole and others in late diastole when atrial filling is maximum. The Bainbridge reflex is a tachycardia consequent on stimulation of atrial stretch receptors; its physiological effect is probably small.

Atrial distentions also results in production of **atrial naturiuretic peptide (ANP).** This hormone is produced in response to atrial distention and also, by raised angiotensin levels. It inhibits release and actions of aldosterone, angiotensin II and renin. It increases water and salt excretion and may play an important role in regulation of water and salt balance. Its diuretic effect could be one factor in reducing a raised venous pressure.

Modifications of cardiovascular responses by cerebral and hypothalamic influences.

Examples are the effects resulting from pain, emotional stress, impulses from thermal control centers, from overstimulation of the labyrinth, and from the need to coordinate circulatory and metabolic needs during exercise. The nature of modulation because of pain or emotional stress are somewhat similar. When the stimuli are not extreme the usual response is a tachycardia and raised arterial blood pressure. Extreme pain or emotional stress results in bradycardia, hypotension, fainting, and in occasional instances, circulatory collapse. Stimulation of thermal receptors by excess heat or cold results in hypothalamic reflexes that travel to the medullary centers and induce vasodilation or vasoconstriction, as needed, for maintenance of body temperature within physiologically desirable limits. Excessive heat (as from saunas and steam baths) can result in marked peripheral vasodilation. This diversion of blood can precipitate coronary spasm and angina, or even myocardial infarction in individuals with coronary artery disease.

The hypothalamus.

The hypothalamus is a control center as well as a gateway for cerebral modulations. As a control center it maintains body temperature by varying autonomic discharges to vascular smooth muscle, sweat glands and arteriovenous shunts. It coordinates circulatory and metabolic needs during exercise by vasodilation of muscular beds, constriction of non-muscle beds and release of catecholamines into the blood. Two important coordinated hypothalamic reflexes are the "defense reaction" and the "playing dead" reaction. The former is often called the "fight or flight" reaction. It is evoked by danger and results in sympathetic cholinergic vasodilation of skeletal muscle vessels, generalized sympathetic vasoconstriction of other blood vessels, an elevation of blood pressure, and increases in plasma catecholamines, heart rate and cardiac contractility.

The "playing dead" reaction is used by some animals as their defense mechanism and is probably similar to what happens in psychogenic fainting.

Chemical effectors.

Most extrinsic effectors are chemicals liberated at the terminals of autonomic nerves, or by angiotensin and aldosterone formed consequent on renin production by the kidneys. ANP may act as a modulator.

Acetylcholine is released at the post-ganglionic terminals of the vagus nerves. It decreases heart rate, at times to the point of vagal arrest. In the atria it decreases contractility and often increases conduction velocity. However, at the AV node there is decreased speed of conduction, at times leading to AV block. The general effect is that of a negative cardiac inotrope.

Norepinephrine is liberated at the post-ganglionic endings of the cardiac sympathetic innervation. Additional effects can result from circulating catecholamines (e.g., by **epinephrine** released by the adrenal medulla and circulating **norepinephrine** which has escaped uptake at the nerve terminals). The catecholamines act on the β_1 receptors of the SA node. Heart rate and contractility increase as does conduction velocity in the atria and AV node. The general effect is that of a positive inotrope that can be inhibited by drugs that block β_1 receptors - drugs of common use in individuals with cardiac dysfunctions.

The vasculature

The anatomy of blood vessels.

The arterioles are muscular vessels. Metarterioles diverge from them. These vessels have thinner musculatures.

They may act as through channels to the venules. More often a capillary network diverges from a metarteriole. At the point where the capillaries branch off the metarterioles there is a thin band of muscles around the vessel and this controls the amount of blood that can enter the capillary.**The capillaries** have diameters of 4-8μ. They have no smooth muscle in their walls which consist of only a layer of endothelial cells lying on basement membrane. The wall thicknesses of capillaries average 1μ. Anatomical variations described by Majno[2] recognized three types of capillaries:

- **Continuous capillaries** which have no recognizable intercellular openings between cells. They are seen in muscle, nerve and adipose tissue. Tight junctions exist that only allow the passage of small molecules. There is no barrier to diffusion of gases, wateror lipid soluble substances across cell walls.
- **Fenestrated capillaries** which have spaces of 800-1000Å between cells (15-20 times that of continuous capillaries). Gaps may be open as in the renal glomeruli or closed as in endocrine glands and intestinal villi. Large molecules such as proteins can pass through these vessels.
- **Discontinuous capillaries.** Large intercellular gaps are present in the cell walls of these sinusoid capillaries. They are seen in liver, bone marrow and spleen. Cells can pass through the walls of these vessels. Presumably, in these organs (the spleen and liver) extravasated cells and other materials are returned to the circulation by tissue turgor or via the lymphatics.

The capillaries and the Starling forces.

The description by Starling of the forces acting between capillaries and interstitial fluid is a somewhat simplistic but generally useful way of showing how interchanges take place between capillaries and surrounding interstitial fluid. Exceptions to the generalization are the sinusoids where intercellular spaces are large enough to let cells escape into the interstitium. The anatomical structures of most capillaries do not permit egress of any protein molecules in the blood. The smallest is albumin with a molecular weight of 69,000 and a radius of about 7.5nμ.

The Starling model proposed that pressure at the arteriolar end of a capillary was about 35mm Hg and about 15mm at the venular end. The oncotic pressure of proteins in the interstitial fluid is about 25mm Hg. At the arteriolar beginning of the capillary, fluid and gases (e.g., oxygen) traverse the capillary walls and enter the interstitium because of the pressure gradient (35mm Hg - 25mm Hg = 10mm Hg). At the venular end of the capillary interstitial pressure exceeds intracapillary pressure by 10mm Hg and materials that need removal from the tissues (e.g., CO_2, waste products, metabolites and toxins) enter the capillaries.

Control of blood vessel caliber and permeability.

Vascular tone.

All vascular smooth muscle shows basal tonic contraction even when completely denervated. This is due to an intrinsic property of smooth muscle. There are continuous vasoconstrictor discharges from the medullary vasomotor centers. Sympathetic constrictor fibers vary basal tone by altering the effects of medullary discharges.

Vascular tone is important for maintenance of blood pressure. In spinal cord injuries there is a fall of blood pressure due to loss of vascular tone below the point of transection due to the absence of medullary vasoconstrictor impulses, decreased venoconstriction and reduced venous return. Several days later vascular tone begins to return perhaps because of increased myogenic tone or potentiated spinal reflexes. The vessels also become much more sensitive to circulating catecholamines, probably due to degeneration of local mechanisms which normally inactivate catecholamines.

Extrinsic mechanisms for control of vascular tone.

The aorta and large arteries have abundant elastin in their walls. During systole they stretch and during diastole the recoil from stretch ensures flow to the periphery. The smaller arteries and arterioles have less elastin but are well supplied with circular muscle fibers that lets them contract when necessary. The veins have little of either elastin or muscle and are readily distended. In summary, the large and medium sized arteries store pressure, the small arteries and the arterioles regulate flow and vary peripheral resistance, the capillaries allow egress and ingress of cell requirements, while the veins store blood. At any one time only about 5% of the blood is in capillaries but this suffices for the requisite interchanges between cells and the blood The venous system contains 50% of blood volume, about 30% is in the pulmonary circulation and the heart and the remaining 10-15% is located in the large arteries and the arterioles.

Flow through the arterioles and metarterioles are principally regulated by autonomic influences and by angiotensin. Vasoconstrictor nerves to the arterioles also innervate the metarterioles and their terminal sphincters and in this way play a role in determining the area of the capillary bed perfused with blood.

Angiotensins II and III are probably the most potent of all vasoconstrictors in the body. Their origins and mechanisms of synthesis and action were extensively detailed on pages 158 and 159.

Flow through capillaries is controlled by local axon reflexes and by local metabolites such as the kinins and prostaglandins, adenosine and histamine affecting the precapillary sphincters. Additional items that vary the diameters of capillaries are local pCO_2, pO_2 and pH levels. The capillary bed has a large area - over $6000m^2$. As previously mentioned, at any one time the capillaries only contain about 5% of total blood volume but this 5% suffices for the critical exchanges and interchanges needed for normal physiology.

Cardiac dysfunctions.

The symptoms and signs of cardiovascular dysfunctions.

Important symptoms are chest pain, dyspnea, tiredness, alterations in the rhythms and rates of the pulse, palpitations, and syncopal episodes. Additional symptoms include the transient (TIAs) or prolonged syndromes of vascular insufficiency affecting the heart, the cerebrovascular circulation and/or the limb and renal vessels. Pain is a frequent presenting symptom. These were all detailed at the beginning of this chapter.

The pain of esophageal spasm or reflux esophagitis can resemble anginal pain and always enters the differential diagnosis of angina. Palpation and auscultation help to identify cardiac hypertrophy, valvular disease of the heart, hypertension and peripheral vascular occlusions. The electrocardiogram (ECG) is a valuable tool for assessing cardiac dysfunction and so are more sophisticated investigations such as echocardiograms and myoviews of the heart, ultrasound studies of peripheral blood vessels, and angiograms of any one or more parts of the cardiovascular complex.

The scope of the problem of cardiovascular disease.

Cardiovascular disease is the principal killer of humans. The data is well documented and summarized in WHO publications about its MONICA (MONItoring CArdiovascular disease) Project. They group all cardiovascular diseases into a single category. This is appropriate because geographic incidences of cardiac disease differ. The WHO group includes all cases of:

— Congenital heart disease.

— Hypertension.

— Coronary heart disease.

— Cerebrovascular disease.

— Peripheral vascular disease.

— Heart failure.

— Rheumatic heart disease and

— Cardiomyopathies

According to the Monica project, in 1999 a third of all global deaths (a total of 16.5 million deaths of whom 8.6 million were women) resulted from cardiovascular disease; more than the total global deaths from cancer, tuberculosis, HIV/AIDS and malaria. Most of these deaths occurred in countries with medium or low incomes which is understandable as these populations constitute some ⅔ of humanity and also because most of them cannot afford or avail themselves of appropriate therapies.

Chart 11-2: THE ANALYSIS OF SEVERE CHEST PAIN OF RECENT ORIGIN: ? UNSTABLE ANGINA OR MYOCARDIAL INFARCTION

THE PROBLEM

Patient with recent onset of severe chest pain resembling angina. Unless the pain is obviously anginal and/or associated with hypotension, first exclude any possibility that it is pain of chest wall origin by palpation (e.g., costochondritis) or of esophageal origin. Drinking 50ml of a 2:1 mixture of an antacid such as Maalox mixed with viscous xylocaine. often relieves pain due to esophageal reflux. If it does not the pain could be cardiac pain due to unstable angina or myocardial infarction.

Relieve pain as soon as possible and give oxygen when necessary and appropriate.

Then, check for any additional dysfunctions. Treat any identified dysfunctions and then reassess the clinical situation. Non-invasive and invasive procedures for assessing myocardial function and investigating the coronary circulation should only start after a full cardiovascular assessment.

Q. Is the heart muscle healthy, i.e., no cardiomyopathy or disabling sequelae from previous disease (e.g., myocardial infarction, rheumatic carditis, Chagas' disease, and/or any form of endocarditis, cardomyopathy or valvular stenoses or regurgitations due to previous infections?)

Q. Is there any previous history suggestive of coronary insufficiency, e.g., angina? Is there any previous history of myocardial infarction?

Q. Is there any significant resistance to outflow from the left ventricle, e.g., due to uncontrolled or inadequately controlled hypertension?

Q. Is there chronic (e.g., COPD) or acute (e.g., pneumonia or a pulmonary embolus) lung disease severe enough to provide significant resistance to blood flow from right to left sides of the heart? If there is, provide therapy which could reduce the resistance (e.g., steroids and/or antibiotics for an acute exacerbation of pre-existing COPD).

Q. Are there any symptoms or signs suggesting vascular occlusive disease of the limb vessels (claudication pains impalpable pulses, cyanosis, ulcers which do not heal, or gangrene), the carotids (e.g., murmurs, TIAs and cerebrovascular emboli), the renal vessels (decreased renal function) and/or the mesenteric blood supply (e.g., postprandial angina)?

Q. Are there any arrhythmias causing deleterious abnormalities of rate and/or rhythm? Does the electrocardiogram show abnormalities of rhythm or rate or features which suggest myocardial ischemia?

Q. Are there any biochemical abnormalities suggestive of myocardial ischemia or infarction? Is the troponin T or CPK raised?

Q. Are the CNS control centers compromised by disease or drugs (e.g., opiates or barbiturates)?

Q. Are there inappropriate amounts of cardiac negative inotropic agents present (normal neuromediators and\or therapeutic drugs)?

Q. Is there adequate compensation for any incompetent or stenosed valves with restrictions or regurgitations of intracardiac flow and ventricular outflow?

Q. Are there any factors which could precipitate ischemic symptoms in a previously well-controlled situation. Examples are fever; infections; trauma; pulmonary embolism; pregnancy; anemia; thyrotoxicosis; overdosage with thyroxine given for control of myxedema; a sudden increase in weight through overeating or drinking of fluids in excess of needs; the development of hypertension; exacerbation of controlled hypertension by discontinuation of medication; arrhythmias; uncontrolled or inadequately controlled diabetes; physical over exertion; stress; domestic crises; excessive heat and humidity; thiamine deficiency; and binge drinking of alcohol or taking of "recreational" drugs?

If possible treat or ameliorate any identified dysfunction or dysfunctions. Then return to the patient.

Non-invasive and invasive investigations of the coronary circulation are only appropriate. after making these initial assessments.

The MONICA project estimates that by 2010 cardiovascular disease will become the main cause of death in developing countries. This is also understandable. As the standards of living in developing countries rise deaths from diseases associated with socioeconomic inadequacies (e.g., subnutrition, malnutrition, gastroenteritis, tuberculosis, HIV/AIDS and malaria) will decrease, and individuals will live longer and die from diseases currently more common in the affluent. Also as national capital rises there will be more access to drugs, invasive investigations, invasive therapies and surgery - most measures currently unavailable to the disadvantaged. The WHO anticipates decreases in mortality because of changes in lifestyle. One wonders. It is not easy to get large groups to stop smoking, eat so-called "healthy" foods, and exercise. One wonders if physicians who attempt, usually with little success, to change the lifestyles of individuals should not instead target their enthusiasms to vigorous campaigning for better socioeconomic conditions for the disadvantaged. Many artificial barriers of subsidies ensure retention of existing living standards in the developed world, at the expense of the impoverished. For example, in many impoverished African countries farmers cannot sell the food or cotton and natural resources available at prices that are competitive with the imports of the subsidized products of farmers in affluent countries, or the altruistic donations of free foods and other materials. The principal reasons are the subsidies given to food producers in North America and Europe and well-meaning but misguided charity. Another example is failure of drug manufacturers to address the problems of the third world (the 10/90 gap is detailed and discussed in the final chapter of this book). Copy-cat drugs are in vogue but not drugs that cure the diseases caused by parasites, helminths and fungi in poor countries.

The analysis of a cardiac dysfunction.

Assessments of cardiovascular dysfunctions always require systematic functional assessment of the minor systems of each resource used by the system. All deviations from physiologically permissible limits must be identified. Chart 11-2 on the previous page summarizes the factors that need consideration and correction, if possible.

Dysfunctions resulting from cardiac ischemia.

The normal physiology of the coronary circulation was described earlier in this chapter. Insufficient perfusion of the myocardium with blood is a common cause of cardiac dysfunction. The usual cause is atheromatous disease of the coronary vasculature.

Atheromatous disease.

Atheromas are the commonest cause of disease caused by vascular pathology. They can cause disease that is serious and occasionally fatal, and are often widespread in distribution within the body.

The atheromatous plaque is a collection of lipid (fatty acids, triglycerides, cholesterol and phospholipids) deposited in the intima of blood vessels. The plaque is usually in an eccentric location and it increases in size by a combination of peripheral fibrosis and an increase in the amount of contained lipid. Progressive increase in the size of the plaque results in degenerative changes in the adjacent elastica and media with resulting weakness of the affected vessel. Symptoms consequent on atherosclerosis differ according to whether the artery is a small or large vessel. Before proceeding a short digression is needed to detail the facts of cholesterol metabolism.

The normal physiology of triglyceride and cholesterol production, transport and metabolism.

The details of lipid metabolism are complex and there are variations in the descriptions provided by different authors, though the basics are usually described in similar ways. Chart 11-3 on the next page summarizes the basics of cholesterol metabolism and Charts 9-3 and 9-4 on pages 205-206 summarize the compositions of the different lipoproteins and the facts of triglyceride homeostasis. The unmasking of the mechanisms of lipid metabolism would not have been possible without the identification of LDL receptors by Brown and Goldstein in 1975[3]. For this and subsequent observations they received Nobel prizes in 1985.

The lipoproteins.

Lipids are insoluble in water and blood. They are absorbed as micelles which are hydrophilic because of coating with bile salts. The bile salts are removed in the intestinal mucosa and replaced by a hydrophilic coating of intestinal phospholipid and apolipoprotein. This enables the water insoluble lipid components to be transported

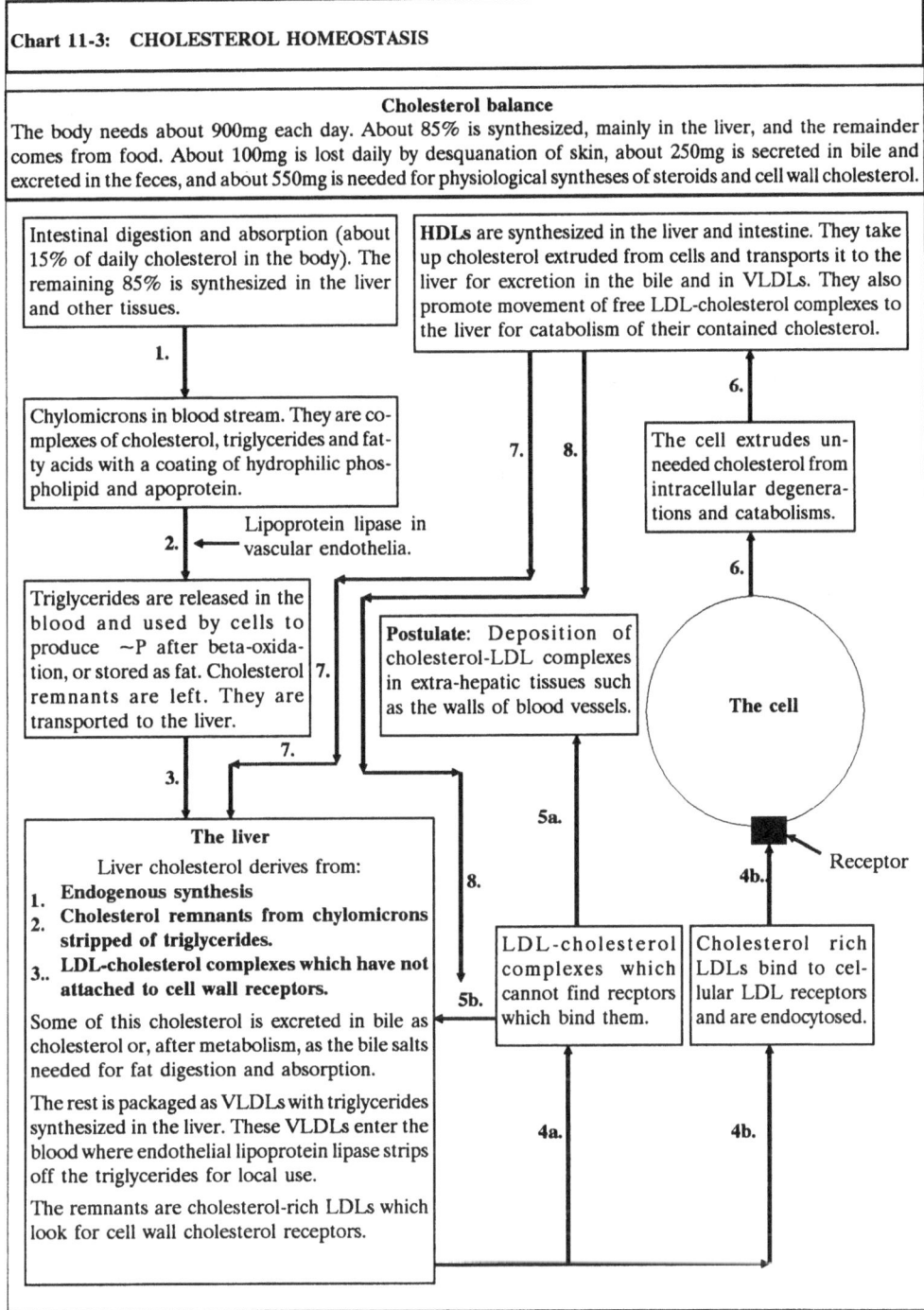

Chart 11-3: CHOLESTEROL HOMEOSTASIS

Cholesterol balance

The body needs about 900mg each day. About 85% is synthesized, mainly in the liver, and the remainder comes from food. About 100mg is lost daily by desquanation of skin, about 250mg is secreted in bile and excreted in the feces, and about 550mg is needed for physiological syntheses of steroids and cell wall cholesterol.

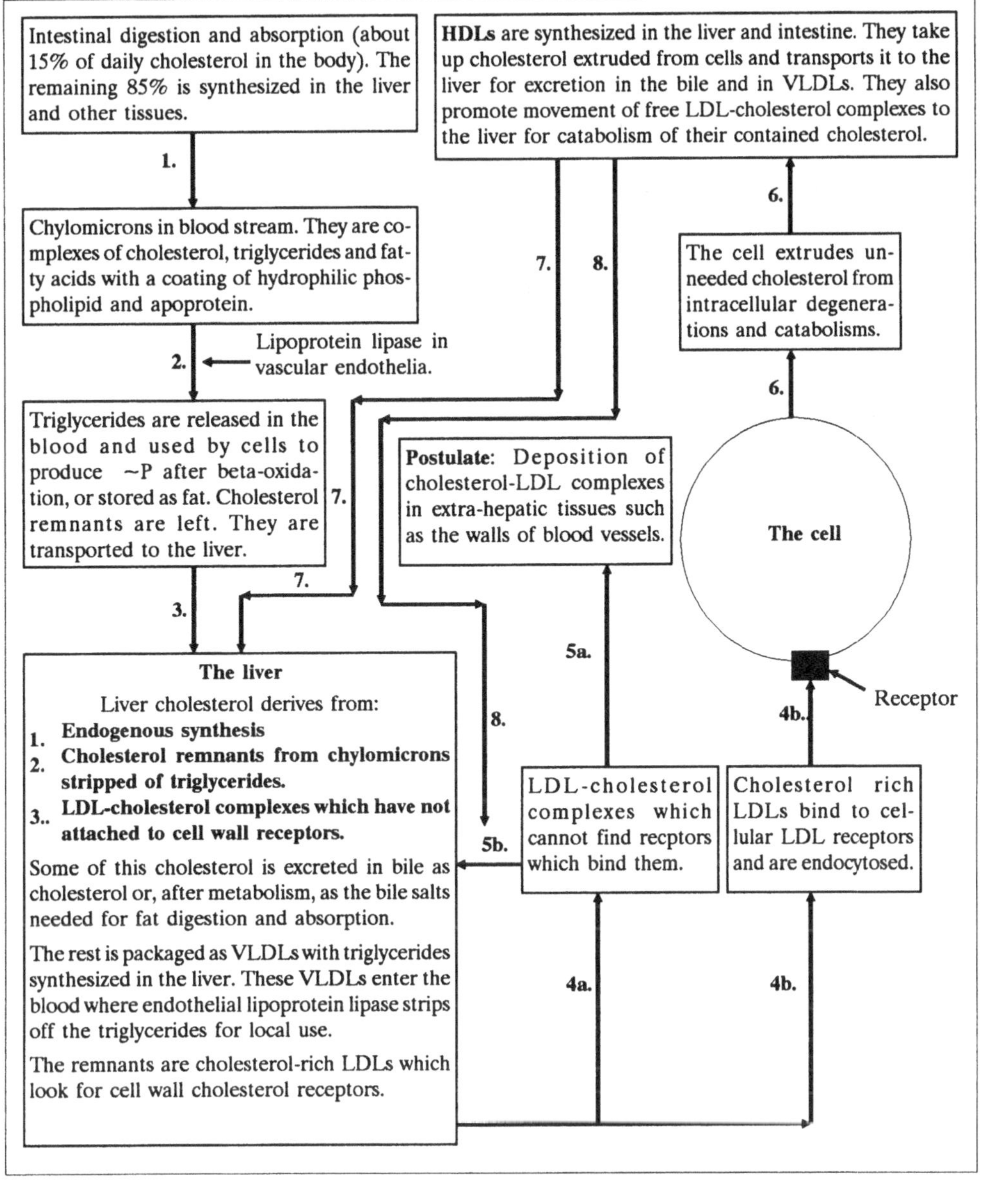
Intestinal digestion and absorption (about 15% of daily cholesterol in the body). The remaining 85% is synthesized in the liver and other tissues.
HDLs are synthesized in the liver and intestine. They take up cholesterol extruded from cells and transports it to the liver for excretion in the bile and in VLDLs. They also promote movement of free LDL-cholesterol complexes to the liver for catabolism of their contained cholesterol.
1.
6.
Chylomicrons in blood stream. They are complexes of cholesterol, triglycerides and fatty acids with a coating of hydrophilic phospholipid and apoprotein.
7.
8.
The cell extrudes unneeded cholesterol from intracellular degenerations and catabolisms.
2.
Lipoprotein lipase in vascular endothelia.
6.
Triglycerides are released in the blood and used by cells to produce ~P after beta-oxidation, or stored as fat. Cholesterol remnants are left. They are transported to the liver.
7.
Postulate: Deposition of cholesterol-LDL complexes in extra-hepatic tissues such as the walls of blood vessels.
The cell
7.
3.
5a.
The liver
Liver cholesterol derives from:
1. Endogenous synthesis
2. Cholesterol remnants from chylomicrons stripped of triglycerides.
3.. LDL-cholesterol complexes which have not attached to cell wall receptors.
Some of this cholesterol is excreted in bile as cholesterol or, after metabolism, as the bile salts needed for fat digestion and absorption.
The rest is packaged as VLDLs with triglycerides synthesized in the liver. These VLDLs enter the blood where endothelial lipoprotein lipase strips off the triglycerides for local use.
The remnants are cholesterol-rich LDLs which look for cell wall cholesterol receptors.
8.
Receptor
4b.
LDL-cholesterol complexes which cannot find recptors which bind them.
Cholesterol rich LDLs bind to cellular LDL receptors and are endocytosed.
5b.
4a.
4b.

in the blood as a uniform suspension. The complex of cholesterol, triglycerides, free fatty acids and hydrophilic phospholipid and protein (apoproteins) enters the intestinal lacteals, and eventually, the blood stream as milky particles termed **chylomicrons**. This is one type of triglyceride-rich lipoprotein. The other type of triglyceride-rich lipoproteins are the very low density lipoproteins (VLDL) - see Charts 9-3 and 9-4 on page 206 for details. The compositions of the lipoproteins and the facts of triglyceride homeostasis were summarized on page 206. A description of cholesterol metabolism and homeostasis follows.

Cholesterol.

Cholesterol homeostasis is summarized in Chart 11-3 on the next page and little additional text is needed.

The liver produces about 80-85% of the cholesterol needed by the body and the rest derives from the absorbed products of digested food. In fact almost all cells can synthesize cholesterol. Cholesterol is essential for survival. It is used for:

— The formation and maintenance of all cell membranes.

— Production of steroid hormones: notably, the corticosteroids, the mineralocorticoids, and the sex hormones - estradiol, progesterone and testosterone.

— Production of hepatic bile acids. Their salts are essentials for intestinal fat digestion and absorption.

— Production of dermal vitamin D precursors when skin is exposed to sunlight.

Receptors for LDL-cholesterol complexes decrease in number when the cell has sufficient cholesterol. It is postulated that the complexes that have not bound to receptors are deposited in extrahepatic tissues such as the walls of arteries. This is the basic hypothesis used by those who feel that raised blood cholesterol and LDL levels predispose to formation of coronary artery atheromas. They also claim that raised HDL levels have a protective effect by returning cholesterol to the liver for metabolism there. Also by promoting the movement of LDL-cholesterol complexes to the liver for catabolism of their contained cholesterol. Receptor production decreases when the cell has enough cholesterol. No comments are made about the use of statins for lowering blood cholesterol levels and their effects on the courses of coronary artery diseases. These topics were extensively discussed in the first chapter of this book (pages 17-22).

Factors affecting blood cholesterol levels.

Numerous factors affect blood cholesterol levels. Eating foods that contain high levels of saturated fats (e.g., hydrogenated vegetable oils, especially palm and coconut oils) and foods with high levels of cholesterol are said to raise blood cholesterol levels. Most foods of animal origin contain cholesterol (meat and poultry, fish, shellfish, dairy products, cheese and eggs are some examples). The importance of diet in raising blood cholesterol is probably marginal as about 85% of body cholesterol derives from endogenous synthesis.

Other factors that result in raised cholesterol levels include age (cholesterol levels tend to increase with age), genetics, diabetes, and smoking. Vigorous exercise can reduce LDL levels and increase levels of HDL. Moderate alcohol consumption can also raise HDL levels.

Cardiac dysfunctions resulting from raised blood cholesterol.

There is certainly an association between blood cholesterol levels which are higher than normal and atheromatous disease. For obvious ethical reasons human studies to prove a cause and effect relationship are difficult. The syndrome of inherited hypercholesterolemia does result in increased coronary atheromatous disease and fatalities. However, this is not necessarily comparable to the much smaller raises of blood cholesterol seen in the usual patient with coronary artery disease though the relationship is suggestive.

The ideal level of blood cholesterol that should not be exceeded varies from one author to another. The average recommended is about 150-250mg/dl (SI: 4-6.5mmol/L). If this or the LDL level is raised attempts should be made to reduce these values. Theoretically, the first choice should be dietary; the appropriate dietary restrictions were detailed above. In practice, diet is rarely enough. It is unpleasant, non-compliance is the rule rather than the exception, the reductions in serum cholesterol levels are usually only modest and the diets must be continued for years to have maximum effects.

Drugs are commonly prescribed if dietary restrictions fail to reduce blood levels of cholesterol, LDL-cholesterol and triglycerides to desirable levels. The statins are the current vogue, while drugs that reduce absorption of dietary cholesterol and fat (e.g., gemfibrozil) seem to be out of favor at present.

Alcohol and the French paradox.

The WHO MONICA[6] study showed that mortality rates from CHD in France approximated those in China and Japan and were much lower than those in comparable industrialized countries. This does not mean that the French are immortal. They do die of CHD and other diseases such as hepatic cirrhosis but the percentages of CHD deaths in the population are much lower than in the USA.

The incidence of risk factors are similar in the USA and France; smoking, consumption of saturated fats, blood cholesterol levels, and lack of exercise. In fact, the French probably eat more saturated fats as meats and milk products such as butter and cream. The only significant difference is the consumption of alcohol. The protection by wine extends to other neighboring countries: Spain, Italy, Portugal and Yugoslavia.

It is suggested that the undesirable effects of a diet containing a lot of saturated fat are counteracted by alcohol consumption. The protective effect of alcohol extends to both genders, to the elderly and to smokers and non-smokers. Consumption of 25-50g/day is ideal. A steady consumption of 25-50g/day can reduce the risk of CHD by as much as 40%. Excessive drinking or binge drinking has the opposite effect - it increases the risk of coronary heart disease (CHD).

There is a lot of evidence that alcohol inhibits platelet aggregation and that this is why it decreases CHD. Some have conjectured that the protective effects of alcohol result from raised HDL levels. Alternatively, from oxidants in red wine: resveratrol, epicatechin and quercetin. All remains unproved except for the fact that alcohol in moderation does provide some protection from CHD.

The pathological features and the syndromes of clinical dysfunction that result from atheroma.

Atherosclerosis of small and medium-sized vessels can result in stenosis and, at times, total occlusion. The stenosis or occlusion results from any one or more of the following:

- **Gradual and progressive increase** in the size of the plaque.
- **Acute occlusion** due to any one or more of the following:
  - **Thrombosis** on its roughened surface or on the surface of a plaque that has softened, ruptured and produced an ulcerated surface.
  - **Hemorrhage into the plaque.** This last possibility may not only result in an ulcerated surface but also release thromboplastic substances that promote surface coagulation[7].

Emboli from plaques.

The emboli are probably fragments of atheroma broken off the surface of a plaque. The consequences result from ischemia in the area of distribution, e.g., myocardial infarction, transient ischemic attacks or, if the embolus is large, a stroke.

The clinical consequences of decreased flow along affected vessels depend on which vessels are narrowed or occluded by atheromatous plaques.

The coronary arteries.

A number of dysfunctional syndromes can result from atheromatous disease of the coronary arteries. The following is a list of some:

- Angina of effort, unstable angina, or microvascular angina.
- Myocardial infarction.
- Sudden death - usually thought to result from ventricular fibrillation or a major and extensive infarct.
- Death in the convalescent period (i.e., in the two weeks or so following infarction). The usual causes are lethal arrhythmias, rupture of infarcted and softened cardiac muscle or chordae tendineae, and progressive and uncontrollable cardiac failure due to a large infarct.
- If, in the recovery phase reperfusion is inadequate there will be persistent angina of effort, or unstable angina, with or without accompanying congestive heart failure.
- De novo congestive heart failure, at times the result of a silent infarct and at others, the result of slowly progressive ischemic sclerosis of the myocardium. The latter is not uncommon in the elderly.

Anginal pain is often the first indication that there is coronary artery disease. Often it is the first herald of serious cardiac dysfunction. Alternative presentations that I have seen are sudden onset of dyspnea, confusional states, profuse sweating, sudden arrhythmias, and even loss of consciousness due to a low blood pressure. It is appropriate to emphasize that ischemic heart disease due to coronary artery disease does not always result in symptoms. A significant number of myocardial infarctions are free of pain; quoted figures vary from 15%-25%. This is not uncommon in the elderly. The diagnosis may be made on a cardiogram done as part of an annual physical examination - one year a normal ECG and the next year an ECG that shows a previous infarct.

Anginal pain typifies myocardial ischemia. It is deep pain of referred type; a pain that is dull, aching, often severe, sometimes catastrophic and devastating and, at times, a herald of death. As is normal with referred visceral pain, cardiac angina is usually localized to areas which are not where the heart is anatomically located but to dermatomes from which the heart developed: T1-T5. Typically, the pain is felt in the substernum and is often accompanied by a sensation that the patient describes as a squeezing or constriction of the chest. Because the heart develops from dermatomes T1-T5 the pain may be felt anywhere from the first rib to the xiphoid process and along the ulnar aspect of the upper limb (T1). The pain can spread or, at times, be referred to other locales; the shoulder and outer aspect of the upper limbs (C5-6), the neck (C3), or the epigastrium (T6). This localization of pain in the C3-6 and T6 areas may represent abnormalities in dermatome differentiation or fringe summation effects in the neuron pools.

There are **four basic types of anginal pain:**

— **Angina of effort** occurs when there is a temporary discrepancy between myocardial oxygen needs and available oxygen. It usually results from excessive exertion by an individual with coronary artery insufficiency, typically, the result of atheromatous stenoses of the vessels. Usually the pain is readily relieved by rest and by vasodilators such as nitrates.

— **The pain of unstable angina** characteristically occurs at rest or when no significant physical or emotional stress exists. It is not relieved by rest and ECG and biochemical studies do not indicate that there has been any myocardial infarction. Often, the pain comes and goes. The syndrome is often followed by a subsequent infarct and vigorous and immediate investigations and treatment are needed. Esophageal pain can be similar at times and must be excluded before major invasive investigations start. Relief of pain by an orally administered mixture of a liquid antacid and viscous xylocaine is fairly diagnostic of an esophageal etiology.

— **The pain of myocardial infarction** is similar but usually much more severe and unremitting and usually associated with characteristic ECG and biochemical changes. **Variants are non-Q wave infarctions and subendocardial infarcts.** The typical ECG changes of myocardial infarcts are absent but the biochemical changes suggestive of myocardial infarction are present; raised Troponin-T and CK-MB (see pages 66-67).

— **Microvascular angina** (described as Cardiac Syndrome X by some cardiologists)[8] is a controversial entity; its existence is denied by many and its actuality can rarely be proved. It is a syndrome where typical anginal symptoms exist without angiographic evidence of coronary artery disease. The symptoms have been ascribed to spasm in the cardiac microvasculature induced by any one of many factors: e.g., stress.

Atheromatous disease affecting other arteries.

The carotid arteries. Symptoms usually result from dislodged emboli that occlude a cerebral vessel. They may present as transient ischemic attacks, strokes of varying severity, and even death if occlusion is sudden and devasularizes large amounts of brain tissue, or lodge in vital areas of the brain. Particularly dangerous are ulcerated plaques for it is not uncommon for loosely bound and potentially embolic platelet plaques to attach to their surfaces. The carotid bifurcation is the usual location of the atheromatous plaque.

The peripheral blood vessels, especially of the legs. Again, symptoms may be absent even when the dorsalis pedis and posterior tibial vessels are not palpable. Alternatively the presentations may vary from claudication pain (calf pain appearing on exercise and disappearing with rest), traumatic and inflammatory ulcerations (usually on the legs) that refuse to heal, pallor, coldness and cyanosis of the toes and finally, gangrene. The coexistence of diabetic neuropathies and vascular disease will exacerbate the clinical problems. They certainly increase pain when it is present.

Occlusions of subclavian vessels are not uncommon. Suspicion is aroused by palpably unequal radial pulses and different blood pressures in the two arms. Confirmation is readily made by a doppler ultrasound. No therapy is needed unless there is unbearable effort angina of the affected arm, weakness of the affected limb or marked and repeated vertebro-basilar dysfunctions due to steal syndromes.

The mesenteric arteries. Unusual syndromes may occur. An example is abdominal angina which is intestinal pain occurring after a meal if the vascular supply of the intestine is impaired. Acute mesenteric vascular occlusion is a real entity presenting as an abdominal emergency. There is a sudden onset of severe abdominal pain with overlying guarding and rebound tenderness. A vague mass is usually palpable. In extensive infarctions where the superior mesenteric artery is occluded extensive surgical excision may be needed. Some of these patients need subsequent lifelong intravenous alimentation to preserve nutritional status. The infarction is usually due to an embolus, often from a clot in an atrium that is fibrillating. Thrombotic occlusions are uncommon. I have only seen it once. The patient was a young woman who had no demonstrable risk factors except for a two month history of taking oral contraceptives.

Atherosclerosis of large vessels. In large vessels such as the aorta and the innominate and subclavian trunks occlusions are uncommon. Exceptions are the leg vessels. Femoral, popliteal and multiple small vessel occlusions are common. Surgery can help when there are femoral occlusions with reasonable vascular run-offs. More commonly, in large vessels there is fragmentation of the adjacent elastica and atrophy of the surrounding media as the atheromatous plaque increases in size . The vessel wall weakens and dilates and aneurysms often develop. The weakened wall of the aneurysm can rupture with life-threatening loss of blood.

Cardiovascular dysfunction caused by inflammatory disease of the heart and blood vessels.

Myocarditis.

There are many causes of myocarditis - infectious agents, collagen diseases, trauma, poisons, irradiation, drugs, and finally, when no obvious cause is demonstrable, the label is idiopathic or viral myocarditis.

Two types of myocarditis are of special importance in certain populations. One is rheumatic heart disease and its complications, conditions that are not uncommon in populations where antibiotics for treatment of streptococcal sore throats are either unavailable, unaffordable, or both. The second is the myocarditis of Chagas' disease. It is caused by Trypanosoma Cruzi, may appear in an acute or a chronic form, and is one of the most common causes of heart disease in Central and South America. Incidentally, it has been suggested that Charles Darwin was infected with T.Cruzi during his travels in South America and that his death resulted from Chagas' disease.

Rheumatic fever and rheumatic heart disease.

The cause is probably some sort of hypersensitivity or autoimmunity to products of Group A beta hemolytic streptococci. The infection begins 2-3 weeks after a streptococcal infection, usually of the throat. The cardiac lesions are foci of fibrinoid degeneration with infiltrates of chronic inflammatory cells and giant multinucleated cells - the Aschoff bodies. The consequences are a myocarditis, often with subsequent fibrosis, and an endocarditis with involvement of valves and later stenosis or incompetence of these structures. Various extracardiac lesions can develop. Examples are acute migratory arthritis affecting the large joints, immune complex disease (the subject, including immune complex nephritis, was detailed on pages 184-186), polyarthritis, chorea, subcutaneous nodules and erythema marginatum (for more details see the modified Jones criteria[9]).

The diagnosis of rheumatic carditis can be difficult in the absence of associated clinical features such as arthritis and the neurological manifestations mentioned above. Fever and fatigue are common and the ESR is high. Suspicious clinical features are shortness of breath appearing 2-3 weeks after a streptococcal throat infection, especially if the condition was not treated with penicillin. Occasionally fleeting heart murmurs are heard in the initial stages and there are occasional arrhythmias. Later clinical cardiac decompensation develops, clinching the diagnosis Penicillin is effective therapy.

There does not seem to be any consensus about the duration of therapy except that the patient should receive penicillin for a "long time". Late sequelae include valvular stenoses and regurgitations. The Mayo Clinic recommendation is that antibiotics be continued for several years as recurrences are common in the first 3-5 years after the first infection (Ref: http://mayoclinic.com/invoke.cfm?id=DS00250&dissection=7).

Chagas' disease.

The disease results from Trypanosoma Cruzi infection and is a frequent cause of heart disease in Central and South America. Estimates are that 50,000 individuals die of the disease each year and that 16-18 millions have the chronic form of the disease.

The acute phase is only seen in a small minority of those infected. There is fever, lymphadenopathy, a characteristic swelling of the eyelids (the Romana sign) and often an acute myocarditis. Benznidazole is effective therapy in the acute phase. There is little therapy available for chronic disease apart from ad hoc treatment of the complications listed below.

The chronic form has cardiac manifestations (arrhythmias, myocardial fibrosis, thromboembolism and eventually, congestive heart failure) and gastrointestinal manifestations (megacolon and megaesophagus).

The diagnosis is made by showing IgG antibodies to T.Cruzi in serum[10]. The IDRI issued an Internet statement in 2002 (ww.idri,org etc.) claiming that 100,000 immigrants from South and Central America are infected with T.Cruzi and may be contaminating blood for transfusion in the US. They claimed that no test was available to screen blood for T.Cruzi. A1966 publication described a test that was able to detect IgG antibodies to T.Cruzi in serum[10]. A subsequent publication in 2002 (Umezawa, e.s., Luquetti, A.O. et al. Serodiagnosis of chronic and acute Chagas' diseases with Trypanosoma Cruzi recombinant proteins : results of a collaborative study in six Latin American countries. J. Clin. Microbiol. 2004; 42:449.) describe testing which they claim had 99.4% specificty for T.Cruzi.

Immigration from South and Central America is increasingly common. When any patient from these areas complains of symptoms suggestive of cardiac disease a diagnosis of Chagas' disease is always a possibility

Endocarditis.

This is a bacterial infection, transmitted in the blood to the endocardium and valves. Two types are described: acute and subacute bacterial endocarditis. Predisposing factors are valvular disease from previous rheumatic heart disease, congenital lesions of the heart and prosthetic heart valves. Uncommon predisposing factors are hypertrophic cardiac cardiomyopathy and mitral valve prolapse. At present the most common cause is probably the injection of prohibited opiates, cocaine and other drugs by intravenous injection. Commonly, the injected materials and the needles are infected. Often they are repeatedly used by different individuals without any attempts at sterilization of equipment between infections.

Acute bacterial endocarditis can result from any one of many potent pathogens: staphylococci, group A streptococci (usually from a skin or puerperal infection), pneumococci and monilia. One cause is embolism from an infection elsewhere. A more common current cause is intravenously injected so-called recreational drugs. The incidence is progressively increasing. Often there is no pre-existing cardiac pathology in patients afflicted with acute bacterial endocarditis.

Subacute bacterial endocarditis. The usual infecting agent is Strep. Viridans. The usual target is a congenital lesion such as a septal defect or an acquired valvular lesion, especially valves damaged by previous rheumatic fever. The infection can be precipitated by recent dental work, by urethral instrumentation or by a variety of other seemingly trivial procedures or infections. Transient bacteremia is frequent after dental extractions.

Another often unrecognized cause of subacute bacterial endocarditis is enterococcal infection in elderly men; usually consequent on a current occult or symptomatic prostatic or genitourinary infection.

Symptoms and signs.

Acute and subacute endocarditis have essentially similar symptoms and signs. They only differ in evolution, intensity and consequences.

Fever, weight loss, anorexia, and, for some reason, arthralgias are common. Usually, with acute bacterial endocarditis the symptoms are acute and fulminant. In the subacute form they tend to be less acute, more insidious and evolve gradually. In the latter there is usually a history of a cardiac dysfunction and the murmurs of stenosed or incompetent valves are often heard on auscultation. Often the symptoms can be predated to a previous dental procedure or instrumentation. Blood cultures are usually positive and help to identify the appropriate antibiotic needed. Anemia is common.

Infection results in **valvular vegetations**. The vegetations of subacute bacterial endocarditis are usually small and located on the valve edges. They may result in embolic manifestations but metastatic suppurations are uncommon as the usual infecting organism is of low virulence. Typical features of embolization in this disease are tender subcutaneous purplish nodules on the hands and soles and mucocutaneous petechiae and splinter hemorrhages under the nails. In contrast, the emboli of acute bacterial endocarditis usually contain many virulent bacteria and metastatic embolic suppurations are common. At times vascular occlusions result in gangrene, especially in acute bacterial endocarditis.

Cardiac murmurs frequently exist when there is acute bacterial endocarditis and valvular disease but none are typical. An exception is the murmur of regurgitation which develops when the chordae tendineae are destroyed by infection. The vegetations of the acute form are usually large, friable and filled with bacteria. The infection can destroy the valve and extend to the adjacent myocardium. Infection and rupture of the chordae tendineae will result in regurgitation, typical murmurs and cardiac failure. Septic emboli and metastatic abscesses are common in acute bacterial endocarditis. Bacteremia is continuous with clearance by the spleen and liver. Splenomegaly is common but surprisingly, hepatomegaly is not.

Therapy is long-term antibiotics to which the bacteria in the blood culture are sensitive. The usual antibiotic for the strep. viridans infection of subacute bacterial endocarditis is penicillin.

Maxim.

Patients with rheumatic, arteriosclerotic, congenital or syphilitic valvular heart disease, congenital cardiac defects such as septal defects, prosthetic valves and probably, any other form of heart disease must always receive prophylactic antibiotics before dental work, before any type of instrumentation or surgery, and if there is an on-going or recent abortion. Bacteremia capable of causing endocarditis are frequently present in these clinical situations.

Cardiovascular dysfunction caused by endocrine and nutritional disease.

Heart disease caused by, or worsened by concurrent thyrotoxicosis, is easily overlooked. The disease causes a rapid heart rate, often recognized by the patient as palpitations, an increased systolic blood pressure and occasionally atrial fibrillation.

Thiamine deficiency (beri-beri - initially shown to be the result of removing thiamine from rice husks during their polishing) presents as dry and wet forms. Wernicke's encephalopathy is characteristic of the dry form. In addition to the ataxia, ophthalmoplegia and confusion there is stiffness, weakness, anorexia and weight loss.

Heart disease is typical of the wet form of thiamine deficiency. In affluent countries a common cause of beri-beri is alcoholism combined with an inadequate diet, probably because the vitamin is water soluble and readily washed out of the body. The contribution of thiamine deficiency to a cardiac problem is easily missed and this is unfortunate as the results of treatment are successful and rapid. Peripheral edema unresponsive to therapy is a suggestive symptom.

Case history.

The patient was a 60 year old male with angina, massive peripheral edema and a history of previous coronary artery disease for which bypass surgery had been done. He was on large, but ineffective doses of diuretics. On questioning the patient told me that he drank twelve bottles of beer a day and ate little. The attending cardiologist was skeptical about my suggestion but within 48 hours of taking large doses of thiamine almost all the edema had gone. I had the advantage of having seen and treated many cases of wet beri-beri in previous years in India. For the rest of his life (approximately three years) he only required a small dose of a beta blocker and 10 mg of lisinopril (an ACE inhibitor) daily together with a large dose of thiamine to remain symptomless. Congestive heart failure was controlled but he continued to smoke and his drinking habits remained unchanged; not surprisingly, death occurred three years later.

Cardiac dysfunction caused by increased afterload.

Hypertension.

Hypertension is the commonest cause of increased afterload. Congestive heart failure due to uncontrolled hypertension is common; especially in affluent societies where congestive heart failure due to the consequences of rheumatic carditis are increasingly uncommon because of vigorous and rapid diagnosis and treatment of streptococcal infections. Indeed, in the Framingham cohort study[11] most of the population attributable risk (male and female) for congestive heart failure was credited to hypertension, with myocardial infarction running second, albeit, a close second. The population attributable risk was calculated by a complex statistic that estimated prevalence with hazard ratio; the figures for population attributable risk were 39% for males and 59% for females with respect to hypertension. For myocardial infarction they were 34% for males and 13% for females.

Most patients with hypertension have essential or primary hypertension with no demonstrable cause. Only a minority (less than 10%) have hypertension resulting from other pathology (secondary hypertension). Some causes of secondary hypertension are renovascular disease (e.g., stenosis of renal arteries, usually by atheroma or disease of the renal parenchyma) and adrenal disease (primary aldosteronism, Cushing's disease and syndrome, and pheochromocytoma). Other causes include oral contraceptives, coarctation of the aorta, toxemia of pregnancy, hyperthyroid disease and aging. Aging replaces the elastin of large vessels with connective tissue and thus decreases their ability to distend when subjected to pressure. The result is an increase in cardiac afterload.

Primary essential hypertension.

Many years ago the diagnosis of hypertension was based on a resting blood pressure of 100 + age for systolic and less than 90mm Hg for diastolic. Later this was reduced to repeated resting levels of 140/90 or more in adults from 18-49 and 160/95 in adults over 50. Current recommendations are more stringent. Thus the sixth report of the Joint National Committee on the Detection, Evaluation and Treatment of High Blood Pressure[12] recommends that systolic pressure be less than 130mm Hg with an optimum of less than 120. These stringent recommendations could result in a lot of possibly unnecessary medication[13] as at least 50% of the over 55 years population have systolic pressures in excess of 130mm Hg.

There may be no symptoms attributable to hypertension discovered during routine examinations. When symptoms are present common complaints are headache that is typically occipital in location, present when the individual awakes in the morning, and gradually disappearing after a few hours. Other complaints include fatigue, dyspnea, and angina of effort if there is any associated cardiac or coronary disease.

In addition to being a risk factor for coronary artery disease and congestive heart failure, untreated or uncontrolled hypertension is a major risk factor for stroke. It can also result in kidney failure, and in blindness. If untreated and progressive, benign essential hypertension can evolve to malignant essential hypertension. Papilledema develops together with severe headaches, vomiting and visual disturbances. Within two years death ensues from renal or cardiac failure or a cerebrovascular bleed. The pathological lesions of malignant hypertension are necrotizing arteriolitis with fibrinoid necrosis of vessel walls. This is a syndrome that was not uncommon in days before anti-hypertensive medication was available, and it is still seen in countries where people do not have access or the finances to obtain these drugs.

The etiology of essential hypertension.

The following are some of the proposed postulates:

Genetic and racial susceptibility. The postulate is that these factors are responsible for the initial increase in peripheral resistance and that the subsequent pathological changes in the vessels are secondary to peripheral vascular spasm.

Vascular pathology is the primary cause. This theory was proposed some years ago by Folkow. He hypothesized that continuing psychogenic stress stimulated sympathetic activity via its effects on the hypothalamus. He proposed that individuals likely to develop hypertension had increased sensitivity of arterial smooth muscle to this stimulation (probably a genetically determined sensitivity). The consequence was gradual hypertrophy of arteriolar walls with increased thickness of their media, a decrease in the ability of these muscles to dilate, progressive increase in blood pressure and eventually hypertension that became permanent.

The urinary output theory of Guyton. This theory postulates that the primary problem is renovascular insufficiency with respect to sodium excretion. The consequence is retention of water and sodium and development of the hypertensive state.

There is no incontrovertible proof of the exclusive validity of any one of these theories. The cause of hypertension is probably a combination of one or more of these theories in varying degrees, each determined by the affected person.

Cardiac dysfunction caused by increased preload.

The commonest cause is chronic obstructive lung disease COPD. The clinical features and causes of COPD and cor pulmonale were detailed on pages 233-235. It is an important cause of increased preload and of right-sided congestive heart failure.

The cardiomyopathies.

The cardiomyopathies are myocardial diseases that usually eventuate in cardiac failure. Three principal types are described: dilated cardiomyopathy, hypertrophic cardiomyopathy and restrictive cardiomyopathy. All result in ventricular dysfunction. They are more easily divided into two groups: ischemic and non-ischemic cardiomyopathies.

Ischemic cardiomyopathy is much more common than the non-ischemic type. The usual cause is coronary artery stenoses and occlusions. Some of these cardiomyopathies result from slow and progressive myocardial fibrosis consequent on ischemia. Others could result from the cumulative effects of repeated small subclinical ischemic episodes.

Non-ischemic cardiomyopathies occur more frequently in younger people. Known causes include viral infections, genetic factors, amyloidosis, hemochromatosis and alcoholism. Often no cause is identifiable and the dysfunction is called an "idiopathic cardiomyopathy". Three subtypes are described. Dilated cardiomyopathy, hypertrophic cardiomyopathy due to abnormal growth and hypertrophy of heart muscle, and restrictive cardiomyopathy when ventricular filling is reduced because of increased and unexplained rigidity of the myocardium. The dilated variety is the most common and represents some 80% of non-ischemic cardiomyopathies.

Clinical features. The associated cardiac muscle dysfunctions of the cardiomyopathies result in the slow development of congestive heart failure and an echocardiogram that shows a decreased ventricular ejection fraction. Arrhythmias are common and are occasionally severe enough to result in syncope or sudden death from ventricular fibrillation. Thromboembolism is an occasional concomitant.

Arrhythmias.

These are common problems that a physician is often required to assess and treat. They are changes in the rates and/or rhythms of the heart beat. There are three basic types: the tachycardias, the premature beats and the bradycardias. Many different types of arrhythmias are recognized and described in standard texts dedicated to electrocardiography. Given the limitations of space, and the objectives of this monograph one only provides an overall view of arrhythmias. The emphasis is on those most frequently encountered and those that have imminent lethal potential.

Normal values:

Each of the small boxes in an ECG tracing represents 40msec (0.04sec). A rough estimate of the heart rate can be obtained by dividing 1500 by the numbers of these small boxes between two consecutive and similar waves (P waves, R waves, etc.) Of course this is only valid when there are no irregularities of rhythm.

The PR interval is the distance between the beginning of the P wave and the beginning of the QRS complex. It should not exceed 0.2sec.

The duration of the QRS complex should not exceed 0.1sec.

The QT interval is the time from the beginning of the Q wave and the end of the T wave complex. It should not exceed 0.45sec. Prolongation may result from inherited defects. It is possible that some sudden deaths in otherwise healthy young adults are due to genetic inheritance of long QT intervals (the Romano Ward syndrome - inherited as an autosomal dominant). More commonly, it is due to drugs such as sotalol and amiodarone, myocardial infarction, myocarditis or any diffuse myocardial disease and electrolyte disturbances.

The general assessment of an arrhythmia.

The following questions are pertinent when there is an arrhythmia:

- What drugs are the patient taking? Are there any clinical causes and/or biochemical findings suggesting that an electrolyte abnormality exists? Common causes of arrhythmias are digitalis, beta blockers, other negative inotropes and abnormalities of potassium balance.
- Is there any evidence of clinical, ECG, biochemical or echocardiogram abnormalities suggesting myocardial infarction, valvular disease, cardiomyopathies, inflammatory cardiac disease or any other cardiac dysfunction?
- Is the patient confused or comatose? Heart blocks and ventricular arrhythmias frequently result in disturbances of mentation and even death.
- Is there any clinical evidence of myocardial pain? How much discomfort is resulting from the arrhythmia? Any tachycardia can cause anginal-type discomfort or pain if the patient has unsuspected or known coronary artery or myocardial disease. The sudden onset of atrial fibrillation is a frequent cause of anginal-type pain when the ventricular rate is fast. Even myocardial infarction can result if the ventricular rate is rapid. Most coronary filling occurs during diastole. When there is tachycardia systole occupies an increasing part of the cycle and coronary perfusion is reduced. In addition rapid and repeated compression of myocardial vessels by rapidly contracting ventricles will reduce the perfusion of myocardial vessels in the subendocardium.
- **Ventricular fibrillation** results from sudden coronary occlusions or as gradual progressions from ventricular premature beats to ventricular tachycardias and finally fibrillation. Another precursor of ventricular fibrillation are **torsade des pointes. Sudden death** is a constant danger with these arrhythmias. **If the pulse is not palpable immediate CPR is essential and then, whether or not a pulse is palpable, electrical defibrillation as soon as the necessary equipment is available.**
- Can the dysfunction be reversed or is reversal needed? When ventricular fibrillation exists (sudden unexplained collapse and unconsciousness) rapid action is essential as detailed above.

  Less urgent are cardioversions for atrial fibrillations of recent onset. An attempt to reverse fibrillation by electrical defibrillation is appropriate if the arrhythmia is of recent onset and the patient is seen within a few hours of onset. If seen later than this, effective anticoagulation prior to defibrillation is desirable.

  Some cardiologists feel that conversion to normal rhythm by cardioversion is not needed. Perfectly satisfactory physical activities can continue as long as those with fibrillation are given medication (beta blockers or calcium channel blockers) to control heart rates. Personal experience requires that I concur. In any case all individuals with established atrial fibrillation and most with paroxysmal fibrillation should receive anticoagulants.
- Does the patient have an extracardiac condition that has caused the arrhythmias? Thyrotoxicosis may present with atrial fibrillation and tachycardia as the only clinical features.

The bradycardias.

Bradycardia is normal in trained athletes and those who do manual labor. The causes and forms of pathological bradycardias are many. Common causes include overdosage with digitalis (especially if the patient is elderly or any renal failure is present), beta adrenergic blockers and acidosis or hyperkalemia. Of course, bradycardias also often reflect underlying cardiac disease or degenerations.

Heart blocks.

The usual causes are delays at the AV node or in one or more branches of the bundle of His.

Complete heart block usually results from degenerative changes in the conducting systems of elderly people or from cardiac disease. The ventricles beat at their own rhythms of 40-50 per minute and there is AV dissociation as the atria continue to beat at their own rates. The low cardiac output may result in congestive heart failure and deficits of neurological and renal function.

Stokes-Adams attacks. The syndrome results from ventricular asystole or tachycardia (tachycardia, flutter or fibrillation) occurring in patients with complete heart block. It is often accompanied by cerebral insufficiencies: seizures, neurological deficits, confusion, coma and finally, death.

Partial heart blocks are more common. **First degree block** is usually symptomless. The ECG abnormality is a prolonged PR interval. All the impulses reach the ventricles. In **second degree blocks** some impulses may not reach the ventricles. Many different types are described (2:1 block, 3:1 block and the Wenckebach phenomenon are examples).

Bundle branch blocks. Blocks can affect one or other of the branches of the bundle of His. **Left bundle branch block** is often the result of cardiac disease. The ECG of bundle branch blocks shows a QRS complex which exceeds 0.12sec and are usually deformed. In left bundle branch block there are positive ECG deflections in leads I and V6 and negative deflections in leads III and V1. The ECG pattern of right bundle block is the reverse. The ECG pattern of LBBB usually merits investigation to exclude coronary artery insufficiency and so does RBBB first appearing after middle age. The ST segment is often raised in LBBB.

Premature beats.

Most supraventricular tachycardias are harmless responses to physical or emotional stress or are inherent biological variations.

Ectopic foci of irritability are frequent. They are atrial or ventricular in location. When a focus of this type discharges an electrical impulse there is an **atrial or ventricular premature beat (an extrasystole)** which interrupts the normal cardiac rhythm. Atrial premature beats rarely indicate underlying cardiac disease. The usual causes are physical or mental stress, or excessive consumption of tea, coffee, or alcohol. The P wave differs from other P waves in the ECG but is followed by a normal QRS complex.

Ventricular premature beats are seen in the ECG as bizarre and wide QRS complexes with each following a normal conduction pattern. In patients without organic heart disease they are not dangerous, but the presence of many VPBs usually merits assessment for occult heart disease. When significant cardiac disease exists, or when there is sudden ischemia VPBs can presage ventricular tachycardia or even a fatal ventricular fibrillation.

The tachycardias.

Sinus tachycardia. Most atrial tachycardias result from harmless increases in the rates of SA discharges. The usual causes are physical or mental stress, or excessive consumption of tea, coffee, alcohol or recreational drugs.

Paroxysmal atrial tachycardia. The cause is rapid discharges from one or more ectopic foci or a re-entry circuit. If the normal impulse from the sino-atrial node reaches the ectopic focus when it is in a refractory state the concentric movement of the SA impulse is blocked and retraces its track. The second time it reaches the ectopic focus the latter is excitable and takes over. Often a new and faster atrial rhythm develops. Usually normal rhythm is eventually re-established, at times with the help of drugs. Re-entry circuits are a frequent cause of recurrent and of rapid paroxysms of atrial tachycardia. If uncontrollable by drugs ablation of the aberrant foci by electrocoagulation may become necessary.

Atrial flutter is an extreme form of re-entry tachycardia. The atrial rate often exceeds 250/min. As the AV node cannot conduct impulses at rates that exceed 230/min many P waves often precede each QRS complex.

Atrial fibrillation results in a rapid pulse, usually in the 100-170 range, and it is irregularly irregular. It is occasionally seen in individuals without heart disease but associated heart disease is more common. The arrhythmia may be paroxysmal or continuous. An ever present danger is stroke from cardiac emboli and anticoagulation is usually required, regardless of whether the fibrillation is paroxysmal or continuous. One must always bear in mind that thyrotoxicosis or digitalis excess can cause this arrhythmia. The cause of atrial fibrillation is probably multiple dissimilar and separate re-entry circuits affecting the atria.

Ventricular tachycardia is usually associated with organic heart disease, digitalis or trauma, especially trauma due to an electric shock; on rare occasions there is no associated cardiac dysfunction. Its principal danger is that it can readily progress to ventricular fibrillation and death. The ECG shows sequential broad and bizarre QRS complexes. The P waves are usually fused in these complexes but are occasionally demonstrable. A variant is the **torsade des pointes** which differs from ventricular tachycardia by variations in the QRS patterns. In ventricular tachycardia they are usually similar; often they look like soldiers on the march.

Ventricular flutter and fibrillation. The causes are the same as those that cause ventricular tachycardia. The ECG pattern is one of complete disorganization of wave amplitude and rhythm. The effective pumping of blood ceases, the pulse disappears, the patient loses consciousness and death will ensue if some cerebral perfusion with oxygenated blood is not re-established in about four minutes.

Ventricular fibrillation is a common cause of death in patients with acute myocardial infarcts. Rapid cardiopulmonary resuscitation (CPR) is essential as well as defibrillation as soon as the necessary equipment is available. Occasionally if the individual is lucky CPR started immediately will suffice.

The ECG of ventricular fibrillation may be difficult to distinguish from torsade des pointes; the latter has a somewhat more regular ventricular rhythm. The distinction is not too important as both need attempts at rapid resuscitation and defibrillation.

Valvular disease.

The mitral and aortic valves are the ones commonly affected.

Mitral valve stenosis. Most stenoses are consequent on previous rheumatic carditis or previous bacterial endocarditis. Entry of blood into the left ventricle is reduced, the left atrium dilates and heart failure develops with hypertrophy and dilation of the right ventricle because of pulmonary hypertension. Complications include atrial fibrillation, thrombus formation in the left atrial appendage and embolic phenomena from the thrombus.

Mitral valve regurgitation. Most mitral valve incompetence has causes similar to those of mitral valve stenosis. Additional possible causes are rupture of the chordae tendineae by endocarditis or myocardial infarction. Another cause is myxomatous degeneration of the valve, usually its posterior cusp; contrary to what is sometimes said, only a small minority of these patients suffer from Marfan's syndrome. Any valve may have myxomatous degeneration and its consequences but the mitral is the one usually affected. Cardiac failure is a frequent consequence.

Aortic stenosis. Aortic valve and mitral valve disease frequently coexist. The causes of the "non-calcific type aortic stenosis" are similar to those of mitral valve disease and it often coexists with aortic regurgitation. "The calcific" type usually occurs in males in their sixties or seventies. Aortic stenosis results in left ventricular hypertrophy and dilation and eventually heart failure develops. The blood pressure may be low and aortic stenosis is frequently associated with angina due to the myocardial ischemia caused by insufficient coronary artery perfusion. Aortic stenosis, especially calcific aortic stenosis, always carries the risk of sudden death.

Aortic insufficiency. The usual causes are either previous rheumatic heart disease or syphilis. Other causes include bacterial endocarditis and other miscellaneous but uncommon causes. Left-sided failure develops with hypertrophy and dilation of the left ventricle. Angina may occur due to inadequate coronary perfusion. Usually, if syphilis is the cause there is associated narrowing of the coronary orifices and this is an important cause of the angina experienced by these patients. In aortic insufficiency the diastolic pressure is low and this results in the characteristic Corrigan waterhammer pulse that results from increased pulse pressure.

The murmurs and their variations are not detailed here. They rarely provide an accurate and definitive diagnosis but were invaluable when echocardiograms were not available to make the precise diagnoses required for modern cardiac surgery. They remain invaluable diagnostic tools in the many areas where neither echocardiograms nor cardiac surgery are available.

Failure of compensation.

Chronic congestive heart failure begins when the heart is unable to pump enough blood to satisfy the metabolic requirements of cells and physiological systems. Symptoms are first discernible on severe exertion, then on moderate or mild exertion, and finally, at rest. Alternatively, it can be acute at inception.

Acute cardiogenic failure and shock.

When a myocardial infarct results in ischemic death of 20-25% of the left ventricle the ventricular contraction can rarely supply enough biological fuel and oxygen to satisfy metabolic needs. Acute left ventricular failure results with hypotension, cerebral dysfunction and often, despite immediate and vigorous therapy, death ensues. Cardiogenic shock is almost always fatal when approximately 40% of the left ventricle stops contracting because of acute ischemia or progressive myocarditis. Of course, any sudden myocardial insult, however small, can result in sudden death from a lethal arrhythmia such as ventricular fibrillation.

The distinction between acute and chronic failure is often blurred as many individuals developing acute failure have suffered from previous chronic congestive failure for a long time.

Chronic congestive heart failure.

There are four categories of chronic congestive heart failure: left-sided and right-sided failure and high output and low output failures. The distinction between these categories is somewhat artificial and overlapping and combinations are the rule rather than the exception.

Low-output and high-output failure.

Low output failure is characteristic of myocardial contractile failure due to ischemic heart disease, myocarditis or cardiomyopathy. It can also result from disease that prevents proper filling and emptying of the heart: e.g., valvular disease, cardiac arrhythmias such as atrial flutter and fibrillation, pericardial disease and the obstructive effects of chronic lung disease. Another important cause is the high pressure afterload of untreated or inadequately treated hypertension.

High output failure is usually the result of extra-cardiac causes: anemia, thyrotoxicosis, beri-beri, arterio-venous fistulae, and Paget's disease are examples. The physiology is complicated by a direct negative inotropic effect on cardiac metabolism by thyrotoxicosis and beri-beri, and the myocardial anoxia and hypofunction associated with anemia. In all such cases the basic cause of heart failure is the failure of coronary blood flow to satisfy myocardial demands for biological fuel.

Left-sided and right-sided heart failure.

Typically, **left-sided failure** is associated with decreased emptying of the left ventricle and renal hypoperfusion. The latter is probably an early cause for the fluid retention seen and due to an aldosterone effect mediated via renin and angiotensin. The latter stimulates aldosterone secretion and its consequent sodium and water retention.

Common causes of left-sided failure are hypertension, coronary artery disease, valvular dysfunctions and various other uncommon conditions. Fluid accumulates behind the ventricle and dyspnea and orthopnea are early symptoms. However, as the causative disease or diseases progress fluid accumulation extends to the right side of the heart with increased pedal edema, systemic venous distention and congestive hepatomegaly.

Right-sided failure result from tricuspid or pulmonary valve dysfunction but a much more common cause is lung disease, especially COPD and environmental toxins or recreational pollutants (e.g., tobacco smoke). Many other lung diseases can cause such failure. A common one is the fibrosis associated with long-standing asthma and its concomitant recurrent infections. A characteristic of right-sided failure is the early onset of exertional dyspnea, often severe.

The symptoms of congestive heart failure.

Initially, overall circulatory compensation is maintained by cardiac muscle hypertrophy in conjunction with intrinsic contractility of heart muscle, the Starling effect, and sympathetic stimulation of β_1 receptors by effectors such as norepinephrine. Subsequently, if pathology progresses there is decompensation with cardiac dilation and the appearance of the following clinical features.

- **Dyspnea.** This is the most common symptom of congestive heart failure. The dyspnea is usually associated with chronic fatigue and weakness. As the disease progresses so does dyspnea; at first, exertional dyspnea and finally, dyspnea at rest. In between are characteristic variations. Examples are orthopnea which is dyspnea when the individual lies down. It results from intrathoracic pooling of extremity blood. Another example is cardiac asthma. The patient wakes up at night with severe dyspnea because of augmentation of intravascular fluid as the result of reabsorption of peripheral edema when the individual reclines. There are moist rales at the lung bases, a raised jugular venous pressure and cough, at times with some sputum tinged with blood.

- **Edema.** Fluid retention results in pitting edema of the legs, basal bilateral rales are heard on auscultation of the lungs, there is demonstrable distention of jugular veins because of raised venous pressure and fluid accumulations may develop in serous spaces such as the pleural, peritoneal and pericardial spaces.

  The principal cause of the edema is reduced renal perfusion and consequent renin production. Angiotensin and aldosterone levels increase with retention of water and sodium. The aldosterone effect is accentuated if, in addition, the hepatic dysfunction from congestion decreases the catabolism of aldosterone.

- **Congestive organomegaly.** Because of venous congestion hepatomegaly and splenomegaly are frequently seen in uncontrolled congestive heart failure.
- **Weight loss.** Patients with congestive heart failure usually lose weight. Regular daily weighing to assess therapeutic responses to diuretics is a good idea. However, many individuals with heart failure regularly lose weight because of inadequate oxygenation A better way of assessing the response to diuretics is determination of the hematocrit. A low hematocrit suggests retention of fluid.
- **Myocardial function:** there is a deficit in ventricular contractility. The defect in contractility may arise from a primary myocardial lesion such as a myocardial infarct or from secondary ischemia due to coronary insufficiency. The ejection fraction is readily measured by an echocardiogram. In myocardial failure it decreases from its normal value of 60-70% and in severe failure may be as low as 20%.
- Therapy for congestive heart failure is discussed in the next section.

A note on interstitial edema.

The volume of the interstitial fluid is about 12 liters. The interstitium consists of a matrix of collagen fibers enclosing a fluid gel, mainly composed of hyaluronic acid. The normal capacity of the gel is about 3.5 liters of fluid. When interstitial fluid pressure reaches zero the gel has expanded to its limit and free fluid accumulates. An accumulation of more fluid results in the typical pitting of dependent edema because the fluid accumulation does not have the mobility of the gel.

The gel is an important feature of the interstitium because approximately 20% of the body is interstitial water. Without the restraining effects of the gel on water movements humans would be musculoskeletal structures standing in a large bag of water moved downwards by gravity.

Therapeutic options for cardiovascular diseases and dysfunctions

Options for coronary artery disease and other miscellaneous dysfunctions.

The latter part of this section details the therapeutic options for treatment of congestive heart failure. The following are some of the therapeutic options for treatment of other cardiac dysfunctions:

Atheromatous disease. Recognition and treatment of coronary artery disease is essential. The ability of the statins to reduce the size and incidence of atheromas is questionable, at least in my opinion (see meta-analyses of the results of statin therapy as detailed on pages 17-22 of the first chapter). There is no doubt about the deleterious effects of tobacco smoking.

Atheromatous disease is a systemic dysfunction that can affect the limb, renal, cerebral and mesenteric vessels. A systematic search of the vasculature is needed to identify and treat the effects of extra-cardiac atheromatous vascular disease.

Relief of pain. Usually angina on effort is easily relieved by cessation of the effort and a few puffs of sublingual nitrate. Angina at rest (unstable angina) may be a harbinger of myocardial infarction. It is usually relieved by sublingual nitrates. The pain of myocardial infarction may be reduced by sublingual nitrates but is often so devastatingly painful that pain can only be relieved by an opiate such as morphine given intravenously.

Therapy for angina. A beta blocker often suffices to reduce the incidence and intensity of angina. The addition of an ACE inhibitor often helps if a beta blocker does not control angina. An alternative is a combination of lisinopril with or without a diuretic. This is especially valuable in patients with pulmonary disease because beta blockers can block lung β_2 receptors; even the ones that claim to be β_2 selective. The mode of action of beta blockers was detailed in the section on the autonomic nervous system (pages 130-134). Reduction of weight to normal proportions if the subject is obese, and regular exercise are valuable adjuncts to medications.

Invasive investigations and therapies. Cardiologists seem to differ in their approach to invasive investigations and therapies. Some feel that none are needed if the patient is well controlled by medications. Others feel that they are always needed. Most are somewhere in the middle, using judgment and experience to determine appropriate procedures. An angiogram has little risk and provides definitive information on stenoses and occlusions. A subsequent or concurrent angioplasty does have some risk but it is small. If angioplasty is not technically possible the only options are vigorous medical treatment and/or bypass surgery. Often even the latter is not possible and in any case, angioplasties and bypass surgeries have significant incidences of restenoses.

A colleague once said to me: "if your patient can walk up a flight of stairs without angina or dyspnea you are treating him correctly and he does not need any additional invasive investigations and therapies". I think there was much wisdom in that advice.

Control of hypertension. This is important. Hypertension is a risk factor for coronary insufficiency due to increased back pressure on the left ventricle outflow. Untreated or inadequately controlled hypertension is probably the primary risk factor for stroke. Diuretics are described in detail on page 308, Chapter 13. Their combination with ACE inhibitors are ideal for control of blood pressure.

Endocarditis and valvular disease. Subacute endocarditis is usually due to a strep. viridans infection of a previous valvular dysfunction, congenital defects, prosthetic heart valves and a few other conditions that are uncommon. Long-term antibiotics are needed, usually as penicillin but with guidance based on bacteriological sensitivity studies of the blood.

De novo acute bacterial endocarditis results from metastatic bacteremia and/or injections of "recreational drugs" - either the drugs are contaminated and/or the needles and syringes. Blood cultures identify the causative organisms and sensitivity tests determine the appropriate antibiotic.

Valvular disease. As with atheromatous disease therapy depends on the views of the attending physician. Some feel that the only therapy for mitral and/or aortic valve disease is surgical valve replacement. Others reserve surgery for situations when cardiac decompensation cannot be controlled by drugs. Finally, there is the question of patient agreement to recommended therapy. After enough information has been provided to let the patient give informed consent many will refuse if they are not greatly disabled. A lifetime of expensive anticoagulants (none are inexpensive) and the dangers of unpredictable infections and emboli are often sufficiently daunting to result in a negative decision. Can medication alone prevent premature death. It often can. An example follows:

Case history.

Female age 72 with mitral stenosis and regurgitation, atrial fibrillation and congestive heart failure when first seen 24 years ago. She was terrified of surgery and refused mitral valve replacement. Since I first saw her the only treatment was digoxin and anticoagulation with warfarin. Congestive failure was readily controlled till she developed hypertension and angina 4 years ago. She was intolerant of any diuretic and also of most ACE inhibitors. Eventually she was able to take one ACE inhibitor, lisinopril (Zestril; Zeneca). She remains well controlled - no angina, hypertension or any congestive heart failure. A beta blocker was not tried as she was well controlled with digoxin. The combination of digoxin and a beta blocker has the potential for reducing the heart rate to unacceptable levels.

Arrhythmias. The therapeutic possibilities were detailed in the text No additional text is needed.

Congestive heart failure - therapeutic options

The Framingham study showed mortality rates for congestive heart failure as 17% for one year, 30% at two years and 56% at five years (Ho, K.K., Anderson, K.M., et al. Survival after the onset of congestive heart failure in Framingham Heart Study subjects. Circulation 1993; 88:107.) .

Control and, if possible, removal of any factors that could have exacerbated failure in a previously stable patient. Examples of precipitating factors include any one or more of the following: fever; infections; trauma; pulmonary embolism; acute exacerbations of previously well-controlled COPD; pregnancy; anemia; thyrotoxicosis; a sudden increase in weight through overeating; excessive fluid intake; binge drinking and eating; the development of hypertension; exacerbation of controlled hypertension by discontinuing medication; arrhythmias; uncontrolled or inadequately controlled diabetes; physical over-exertion; and excessive heat and humidity. If any one or more of these factors exist they should receive vigorous attention and, if possible, control or correction.

Treat any treatable underlying cause for the failure. For example, patients with rheumatic myocarditis and bacterial endocarditis need antibiotics. Those with coronary artery disease will usually benefit from judicious medication, or unblocking or bypass procedures when indicated.

Try to prevent progression of underlying disease. Individuals with failure due to endocarditis must receive appropriate antibiotics. Vigorous control of diabetes and hypertension is essential. Tobacco smoking is an absolute no-no. In addition, individuals with atheromatous coronary artery disease should be advised on control of cholesterol and the benefits of exercise.

Medications: Numerous drugs are available for treating congestive heart failure. The two principal groups are those that do not have a direct effect on the heart and those that do.

The principal members of the first group are diuretics, angiotensin-converting enzyme (ACE) inhibitors, angiotensin receptor blockers and spironolactone.

There are hundreds of references about the value of **ACE inhibitors** as peripheral vasodilators and reducers of afterload and preload. Almost all unequivocally support the use of ACE inhibitors in the treatment of hypertension and congestive heart failure. Only one comprehensive reference[14] is included in this chapter. **The diuretics** get detailed consideration in Chapter 13, page 308. Patients with heart failure often have raised aldosterone levels despite administration of ACE inhibitors; **spironolactone** is an antagonist of aldosterone and in small doses (e.g., 25mg per day) is unlikely to cause uncontrollable hyperkalemia but regular ECG and blood estimations of potassium and sodium are necessary.

The second group are drugs that directly affect heart function: **the beta blockers and calcium channel blockers.**

In general calcium channel blockers should not be given as therapy for congestive heart failure. It is a negative cardiac inotrope and and a clinical trial that ended in 1988[17] showed that calcium channel blockers had no beneficial effect on patients being treated for congestive

The beta blockers are also negative cardiac inotropes. They conduction times of the contraction impulse., reduce cardiac contractility and, in these ways, compensate for the decreased oxygen available as the result of reduction in coronary blood flow. Until recently they were not given to patients with heart failure because of reported adverse effects in advanced heart failure. Recently small doses of beta blockers have been shown to significantly reduce mortality in congestive heart failure[15]. The merits of beta blockers as adjuncts to congestive heart failure therapy was confirmed in the MERIT-HF study[16]. The investigators concluded as follows:

> "... treatment with once daily metoprolol Cr/XL added to standard therapy improved survival and lowered the risk of sudden death and death from worsening heart failure in patients with with mild to severe chronic heart failure secondary to left ventricular systolic dysfunction of ischemic or non-ischemic causes."

However, in the study they state that: "Study drug was permanently stopped early in 13.9% of the metoprolol CR/XL group and in 15% (presumably the placebo was stopped) of the placebo group". The reasons for stopping beta blocker therapy are not stated. The 13.9% in the study group who stopped taking metoprolol presumably did so because of adverse effects. A beta blocker is a negative cardiac inotrope and occasional negative effects must be expected in patients with advanced congestive heart failure given beta blockers. It is

negative effects must be expected in patients with advanced congestive heart failure given beta blockers. It is noteworthy that 63% of the patients in each group were taking digitalis which would add to the cardiac slowing of a beta blocker. The point is that beta blockers can produce adverse reactions and worsening failure in some patients. Regular monitorings are essential when beta blockers are given for congestive heart failure.

Case history.

Patient age 62 of with a previous history of three myocardial infarcts. Cardiac status was well controlled on a diuretic and an ACE inhibitor. An angiogram five years previously had shown that his heart was not suitable for any surgical bypass procedure. On one occasion he went to a local Emergency department with chest pain which was diagnosed as a costochodritis. The physician who saw him was shocked that he was not taking a beta blocker and insisted that he start doing so immediately despite his showing the physician a note that I had asked the patient to always keep in his wallet. The note stated that beta blockers had an adverse effect on his congestive heart failure.

I saw him two days later with severe unstable angina. The unstable angina ended 24 hours after gradually stopping the metoprolol over a period of three days. Beta blockers should be given to patients with severe failure with care, and perhaps preferably, not at all. Any apparently deleterious effect mandates cessation of the drug.

Digitalis. A positive inotrope such as digitalis increases cardiac contractility but also, cardiac oxygen requirements; if available oxygen does not suffice angina or even infarction could result. Digoxin is usually only given to patients with heart dysfunction associated with fibrillation. There are many studies on the effects of digoxin in cardiac dysfunction not associated with fibrillation. A large body of evidence now suggests that digoxin can reduce the symptoms and signs of heart failure (dyspnea, and pulmonary and peripheral edema) in patients with sinus rhythm who are already receiving diuretics[18]. In addition[19], contrary to accepted dogma, digoxin seldom resulted in undesirable side effects. Unfortunately (in my opinion) many currently view digoxin as a drug of last resort in the treatment of congestive heart failure.

Digitalis slows the heart rate and it is paradoxical that it acts as a positive cardiac inotrope. The explanation is as follows. Digitalis inhibits cell membrane Na^+K^+-activated ATPase. Less ~P is available and intracellular sodium increases as there is not enough energy available to keep Na^+ out against its concentration gradient. The sarcotubular system of heart muscle takes up calcium to maintain the osmotic balance between intracellular and extracellular environments. The amount of calcium that can be released to the myofilaments during excitation is increased and the result is a positive cardiac inotropic effect. Other effects of digitalis are slowing of the heart rate.

Digitalis is an effective cardiac drug but not in favor with cardiologists at the moment. Probably because the use of beta blockers is now widespread as an adjunct to the standard treatment of cardiac failure. They slow heart rates and so does digitalis. If combined much caution must be exercised. Digoxin is very useful when a beta blocker is contraindicated because of pulmonary disease such as COPD.

The heart rate can be reduced to potentially hazardous levels by a combination of digitalis and a β **blocker. Additionally, the margin separating digitalis toxicity from therapeutic effectiveness is small. Hence, the need for regular monitoring of the clinical status and serum digoxin levels of patients receiving digitalis.**

Spironolactone. The medication given to a patient with congestive heart failure often varies according to the treating physician's biases and experience. In general, current treatment is a beta blocker, an ACE inhibitor, and a loop diuretic. The addition of spironolactone to this combination can often improve survival rates[20] and a recent paper by McMurray and O'Meara[21] comments on the complexities resulting from spironolactone added to existing therapy. Treatment of congestive heart failure requires assessments at least once a month. Clinical conditions frequently change and so does the need for changes in medication.

The need for repeated assessments when treating patients with congestive heart failure.

Some eight years ago I met a previous patient of mine on the street. After the usual greetings he told me that he had been seeing another physician for the preceding two years because he thought I had been seeing him at unnecessarily frequent intervals. The physician had told him that the medications he was receiving (40mg

furosemide and 20mg lisinopril daily) were fine. He had previously responded negatively to a beta blocker and told the physician this. The man had had two previous infarcts. He told the other doctor he did not think he needed to be seen more often than at six month intervals. The doctor agreed. He renewed his prescriptions for a year and gave an appointment to see him in six months.

The patient asked if I would see him again as his legs were swollen and he was breathless. For various complex reasons he did not wish to see the other physician. I agreed and asked him to phone my office and make an appointment. When examined he had marked peripheral edema, a raised jugular venous pressure and bilateral pleural effusions, clinically and radiologically demonstrable. Rather than increase his furosemide I asked him to take some metalozone which acts at a different point of the renal tubule and has a synergistic, or at least additive effect when combined with furosemide. I also started him on 0.125mg digoxin daily rather than a beta-blocker as there was a previous history of intolerance to this group of drugs. Within a week his increased peripheral edema had almost disappeared and in two weeks a repeat chest X-ray showed that the pleural effusions had gone. He remains alive and well controlled more than eight years later.

The object of detailing this clinical problem is not self-aggrandizement. It is that when treating any patient with congestive heart failure repeated assessments are necessary. The syndrome has a high mortality and changes are frequent and potentially lethal. Frequent adjustments of medications are needed.

This ends the chapter on the cardiovascular system and its dysfunctions.

Chapter 11 References.

1. R.Patterson, S.W., Pipers, H., Starling E.H. J.Physiol. 1914; 48:465.
2. R:G.Majno. In: Handbook of Physiology, Section 2: Circulation, vol.III ed. by W.F.Hamilton and P.Dow. Washington, D.C. American Physiological Society, 1965.
3. Brown, M.S., Goldstein, J.L. Regulation of the activity of the low density lipoprotein receptors in human fibroblasts. Cell 1975; 6(3):307.
4. Grundy, S.M., Pasternak, M., et al. Assessment of cardiovascular risk by use of multiple-risk factor assessment equations. A statement for health-care professionals from the American Heart Association and the American College of cardiology. Circulation 1999; 100:1481.
5. Grundy, S. Hypertriglyceridemia, atherogenic dyslipidemia and metabolic syndrome. Am. J. Cardiol. 1998; 81:18B.
6. Renaud, S. & deLorgeril. Wine, alcohol, platelets and the French paradox for coronary heart disease. Lancet 1992; 339:1523.
7. Paterson, J.C. In: Symposium on atherosclerosis. National Academy of Sciences. Washington D.C. National Research Council, 1954.
8. Hutchison, S.J., Poole-Wilson, P.A., et al. Angina with normal coronary arteries: a review. QJM. 1968; 268:677.
9. Special Committee Report of the American Heart Association. Circulation 13:617, 1956.
10. Umezawa, E.S., Nascimento, M.L., et al. Immunoblot assay using excreted-secreted antigens of Trypanosoma Cruzi in serodiagnosis of congenital, acute and chronic Chagas' disease. J. Clin. Microbiol. 1996; 34:2143.
11. Levy, D., Larson, M.G., et al. The progression from hypertension to congestive failure. JAMA 1996; 275:1557.
12. Sixth report of the Joint National Committee on the Detection, Evaluation and Treatment of Hypertension. Arch. Int. Med. 1997; 157:2413.
13. Port, S., Demer, L., et al. Systolic blood pressure and mortality. Lancet 2000; 355:175.
14. Fletcher, M.D., Yusuf, S. et al. Long-term ACE inhibitor therapy in patients with heart failure or left-ventricular dysfunction: a systematic overview of data from individuals. Lancet 2000; 355:1575.
15. Lechat, P., Packer, M., et al. Clinical effects of beta-adrenergic blockade in chronic heart failure. Circulation 1998; 98:1184.
16. MERIT-HF Study Group. Effect of metroprolol CR/XL in chronic heart failure: Metoprolol CR/XL Randomized Intervention Trial in Congestive Heart Failure. Lancet 1999; 353:2001.
17. The Multicenter Diltiazem Post Infarction Trial Research Group: The effect of diltiazem on mortality and reinfarction after myocardial infarction. N. Engl. J. Med. 1998; 319:385.
18. Digoxin: New Answers; New Questions. Lancet editorial review article, Jul. 8, 1989.
19. Guyatt, G.H., Sullivan, M.J.J., et al. A controlled trial of digoxin in congestive heart failure. Am. J. Cardiol. 1988; 61:371.
20. Pitt, B,, Zannad, F. et al. The effect of spironolactone on morbidity and mortality in patients with severe heart failure. Randomized Aldactone Evaluation Study Investigators. NEJM 1999; 341:709.
21. McMurray, J,J, & O'Meara, E. Treatment of heart failure with spironolactone trials and tribulations. NEJM 2004; 351:526.

12

Diagnosis: The Slave Systems
4. The Blood

Table of Contents

Notation.

The notation ~P denotes phosphorous with a high energy bond. Depending on the context in which the term is used, ~P may also denote the energy liberated when a high energy phosphate bond detaches from ATP or ADP.

A comment on the methodology of clinical assessments.

The comments made **on page 119** about this topic are not repeated. They merit reading before proceeding with this chapter.

The blood is an important resource system of the cardiovascular complex. It fills the cardiovascular complex and the heart repeatedly pumps it around the body so that it can reach every vascularized cell via the conduits of the vascular system.

The functions of the blood.

1. Preservation of intravascular volume.

The most important function of the blood is maintenance of intravascular volume and hence, of cerebral perfusion. The blood maintains intravascular volume because of its content of plasma protein, especially the smallest protein which is albumin (MW:69,00 Radius:7.6nm). Intravascular protein exerts an osmotic pressure (termed oncotic pressure when applied to intravasular proteins) that pulls in fluid from the interstitial compartment of the ECF and thus preserves the volume of the intravascular fluid. The capillaries do have pores but they are not large enough to allow albumin molecules to egress. Exceptions are the discontinuous capillaries in organs such as the spleen where spaces between endothelial cells are big enough to allow escape of protein and cells. They return to the circulation because of tissue turgor pressure and lymphatic drainage.

Blood and extracellular fluid have the same osmotic pressures but slightly different compositions because of the oncotic pressure contribution of intravascular protein to the osmotic pressure of plasma. Blood: Protein 15mEq/L and Cl^- 105mEq/L - Interstitial fluid: Protein 5mEq/L and Cl^- 115mEq/L.

Most movements of water between the interstitial and the intravascular compartments are rapid to and fro movements between the contents of capillaries and the surrounding interstitial fluids. Water passes freely between the interstitial compartment of the ECF and the capillaries so that the osmotic pressures of both are identical. This and the retention of plasma proteins which exert oncotic pressures preserve the volume of the intravascular fluid and hence, of the blood and cerebral perfusion with oxygen and glucose. If intravascular volume is not preserved the result would be hypoperfusion of tissues with eventual cerebral failure and death. This is why preservation of the isotonicity of the ECF must take priority over all other considerations in the physiology of the water and electrolyte balance - volumes and electrolyte contents in the different compartments of the body fluids and regulation of pH and body temperature.

2. Other functions of the blood.

- Delivery of energy substrate to cells (the absorbed products of food digestion, and absorbed water, minerals and vitamins).
- Delivery of oxygen to cells.
- Carbon dioxide removal from cells and its transport to the lungs for exhalation.
- Transport of the catabolic products of stored glycogen, fat and protein in cells where there is enough ~P to cells that have energy deficits.
- Delivery of waste products and other toxic substances to organs where they can be processed, made harmless and excreted mainly by the liver and the kidneys and to a lesser extent, by the lungs.
- Transport of hormones. Most are important messengers for biological control mechanisms.
- Maintenance of body temperature within physiologically permissible levels.
- Initiation of immune responses and the transport of humoral antibodies and immune cytotoxic cells.
- Participation in acute and chronic inflammations and in repair.
- Blood contains clotting factors. They and the platelets provide the hemostasis needed to plug deficits in

the walls of its vascular conduits.

The constituents of blood.

The blood contains red cells, white cells and platelets. All cells are suspended in plasma (35-45ml blood cells/100ml blood).

The red cells provide oxygen to tissues and remove carbon dioxide. Men have 4-5-6 x 10^6 red cells/μL (SI units: 4.5-6 x 10^{12}/L) of blood. The numbers are slightly lower for women. The white cells are the principal components of systems for natural and generated immunity. Blood contains 4,500-11,000/μL (SI units: 4.5-11 x 10^9/L) white cells and 140-400 x 10^3/μL platelets (SI units: 140-400 x 10^9/L). The red cell to white cell ratio is about 10^3 so that the hematocrit is essentially the percentage of red cells to plasma in blood. **The platelets** are required for hemostasis and control of clot formation. The role of **white cells** in generated immunity and phagocytosis were detailed on pages 179-181 in Chapter 8.

The Plasma maintains of intravascular volume because of its content of plasma proteins that cannot traverse the walls of most blood vessels. It also transports essential substances to and from cells as detailed previously.

The origin and life cycle of red cells.

Red cells are produced in the marrow from pluripotential stem cells. Maturation in the marrow to anuclear cells with contained hemoglobin takes 4-5 days. The released cells - the reticulocytes - contain a skein of RNA that can be stained with methylene blue. Within 1-2 days of entering the circulation the reticulocytes lose their internal skeins and become mature red cells Chart 7-2 on page 160 graphically depicts the processes of maturation and development.

Red cells remain in the circulation for about 120 days. Subsequent destruction is in the reticuloendothelial system. The metabolism and excretion of heme in the bile was detailed in Chart 9-5 on page 208. Approximately 1% of the circulating red cells are destroyed each day and are replaced by an equal number of reticulocytes. The reticulocytes remain demonstrable for 1-2 days and the count is a useful index of red cell production. It is raised when most anemias are responding to treatment, but remains unchanged if treatment is not succeeding. The normal reticulocyte count is 25-125 x 10^3/μL (SI units: 25-125 x 10^9/L). Some red cells are destroyed in the circulation. Most of the released hemoglobin is bound to haptoglobin. Free plasma hemoglobin rarely exceeds the hemoglobin binding capacity of haptoglobin except in some hemolytic anemias (see later). Incidentally, the ranges of normal values for all hematology seem to vary from one laboratory to another.

Erythropoietin stimulates erythrocyte unipotential stem cells to differentiate to immature primitive erythrocytes. It is a hormone produced in the kidney in response to decreased renal tissue pO_2. A deficiency contributes to the anemia of chronic renal disease and failure. Parenteral erythropoietin is available for correction, or, at least partial correction of this type of anemia.

The anemias.

Anemia is any reduction in the ability of hemoglobin to convey a sufficiency of oxygen to the tissues. When defined thus there are three principal causes for anemia:

— **Not enough hemoglobin.**

— **Defective hemoglobin** - hemoglobin which cannot bind sufficient oxygen.

— **Excessive loss** of hemoglobin due to causes intrinsic or extrinsic to the red cells.

Hemoglobin synthesis.

The synthesis of hemoglobin is summarized in Chart 12-1.

Normal heme synthesis requires the initial combination of glycine and succinyl CoA by the enzyme ALA synthetase. Subsequently a number of different porphyrins is produced. The last is protoporphyrin 9. It combines with iron to form heme that then binds to the appropriate globin to form hemoglobin. Hemoglobin synthesis needs:

— **Functionally viable and active pluripotential and unipotential marrow stem cells** and accurate derepression, transcription and translation of the fragments of genetic DNA needed for production of blood cells.

— **Vitamin B_{12} and folic acid** are obtained from food but when deficient the result is delayed erythrocyte maturation and hemoglobin synthesis. Other causes of impaired DNA synthesis and consequent anemia

Chart 12-1: HEMOGLOBIN SYNTHESIS

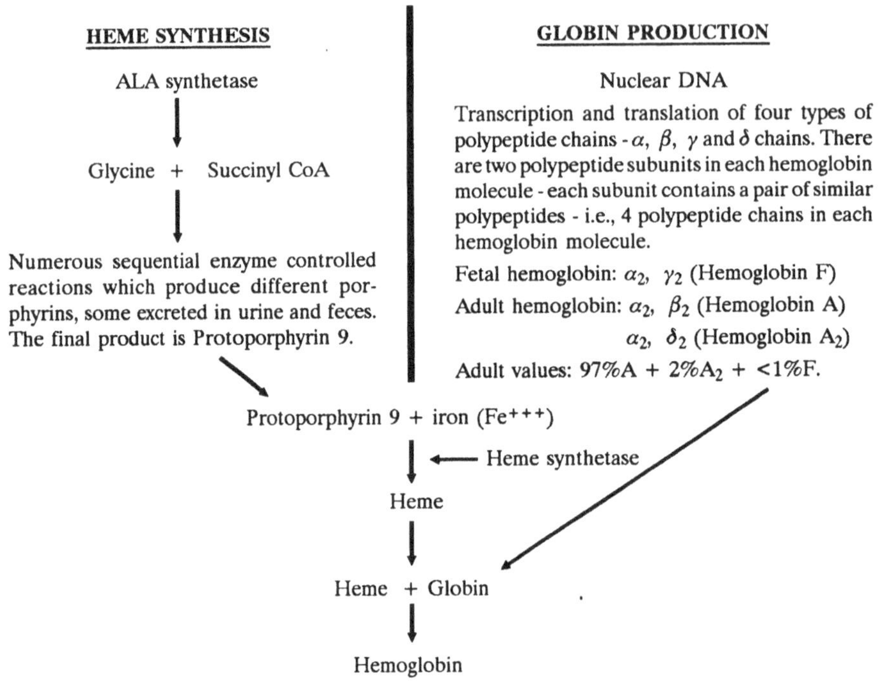
HEME SYNTHESIS
ALA synthetase
Glycine + Succinyl CoA
Numerous sequential enzyme controlled reactions which produce different porphyrins, some excreted in urine and feces. The final product is Protoporphyrin 9.
GLOBIN PRODUCTION
Nuclear DNA
Transcription and translation of four types of polypeptide chains - α, β, γ and δ chains. There are two polypeptide subunits in each hemoglobin molecule - each subunit contains a pair of similar polypeptides - i.e., 4 polypeptide chains in each hemoglobin molecule.
Fetal hemoglobin: α2, γ2 (Hemoglobin F)
Adult hemoglobin: α2, β2 (Hemoglobin A)
α2, δ2 (Hemoglobin A2)
Adult values: 97%A + 2%A2 + <1%F.
Protoporphyrin 9 + iron (Fe+++)
Heme synthetase
Heme
Heme + Globin
Hemoglobin

Abnormalities resulting from defective heme synthesis:

The commonest cause is iron deficiency. With the possible exception of the anemias of "chronic disease" (or so-called refractory anemias), iron deficiency anemia is the most common anemia seen in clinical practice. Various porphyrias due to mutant genes do occur but are rare - examples are acute intermittent porphyria and porphyria cutanea tarda.

Abnormalities resulting from abnormal globin synthesis:

Numerous globin mutants have been identified. Some increase hemoglobin affinity for oxygen while others decrease it. Others result in unstable hemoglobins and associated hemolytic anemias. Others are so-called "exterior mutants" because they distort cell structure; an important member of this last group is Hemoglobin S - the cause of sickle cell anemia. Mutants are also responsible for the thalassemia syndromes. Sickle cell anemia and the thalassemia syndromes are not uncommon in clinical practice and their causes and principal manifestations are detailed in the text.

A note on HbA_{Ic}

HbA_{Ic} is a variant of hemoglobin A. It has a glucose molecule attached to the valine at the end of each β chain. Control of diabetes correlates well with blood levels of HbA_{Ic} - good control is associated with low blood levels of HbA_{Ic}.

include chemotherapy, radiation, vigorous immunosuppression and the aplastic anemias.

— **Iron.** One of the commonest anemias is due to iron deficiency. It binds to protoporphyrin 9 to form heme.

— **Normal globin chain synthesis.** Each globin has two dissimilar polypeptide chains and each of these chains consists of two similar polypeptides; i.e., four polypeptide chains for each type of globin synthesized. The adult patterns are:

97% Hemoglobin A - hemoglobin $\alpha_2 \beta_2$ (2α and 2β chains).

About 2% Hemoglobin A_2 - hemoglobin $\alpha_2 \delta_2$ (2α and 2δ chains).

Less than 1% hemoglobin F - hemoglobin $\alpha_2 \gamma_2$ (2α and 2γ chains).

Hemoglobin electrophoresis can determine the type and quantity of blood globin constituents and is used to identify dysfunctions such as the different thalassemia syndromes.

The Aplastic Anemias.

About half the cases are of unknown etiology. A few are inherited, e.g., the Fanconi syndrome. In this syndrome there are frequent additional abnormalities such as mental retardation, brown pigmentation of the skin and skeletal deformities. The usual causes of an aplastic anemia are radiation or chemotherapy. Other causes include occasional idiosyncratic reactions to drugs such as chloramphenicol (the incidence varies from one publication to another. The ranges are 1:30,000 to 1:100,000 exposures).

Marrow aplasia can also result from extensive bone metastases as well as occasional infections - hepatitis and miliary tuberculosis are the ones most often cited in the literature. There is usually a pancytopenia and because of this, the dysfunction is thought to result from functional deficits of pluripotential stem cells.

The symptoms of the aplastic anemias and of marrow aplasia are similar. In addition to the symptoms which result from all anemias (tiredness, shortness of breath and pallor) there are recurrent infections and fever due to the granulocytopenia. The associated thrombocytopenia results in purpura and petechiae, easy bruising, hematomas and, at times, hemorrhages. The red cells are usually normochromic and normocytic.

The macrocytic anemias.

The mean corpuscular volume of red cells is 82-92μ^3 (SI units: 82-92fl). Macrocytes are larger than 92μ^3 and microcytes are smaller than 82μ^3.

The principal causes of a macrocytic anemia (i.e., red cells with higher than normal mean corpuscular volumes - MCVs) are Vitamin B_{12} or folic acid deficits or both, in combination. Vitamin B_{12} and folic acid are requisites for normal nucleic acid synthesis. Deficits result in abnormal megaloblastic precursors of red cells, anemia, and neurological deficits when the anemia results from a Vitamin B_{12} deficiency (Chart 12-2).

Vitamin B_{12} deficiency anemias.This vitamin is found in meats, eggs, and to a lesser degree in milk and milk products. It is virtually absent in plant foods. The daily requirement is 1-5μg and total body stores vary from 2000-5000μg. Only about 0.1% of the body stores of vitamin B_{12} are used each day so that even if absorption stops completely (e.g., after total gastrectomy) it takes years for deficiency syndromes to appear. Only about 0.1% is lost each day.

Vitamin B_{12} is also synthesized by intestinal bacteria but this Vitamin B_{12} is poorly absorbed because it must first bind to "intrinsic factor" in gastric secretions. The stomach produces intrinsic factor in an acid medium and proximal to B_{12} synthesis by intestinal bacteria, thus reducing the chances of B_{12} absorption in the terminal ileum.

Bacterial destruction or consumption of B_{12} in intestinal diverticula is another cause of B_{12} deficiencies. The anemia is megaloblastic and B_{12} levels are low but the Schilling test is normal. The condition often requires a B_{12} injection each month for maintenance of blood levels of the vitamin.

Pernicious anemia. This disease usually begins in individuals older than forty. It is due to lack of gastric intrinsic factor and is usually associated with achlorhydria. A low serum Vitamin B_{12} level and a positive radioactive Schilling test are diagnostic. The red cells are macrocytic and normochromic. Occasional nucleated megaloblasts are seen in the peripheral blood smear and there is often a leucopenia with hypersegmented polymorphonuclear

Chart 12-2: THE MEGALOBLASTIC MACROCYTIC ANEMIAS DUE TO VITAMIN B_{12} OR FOLIC ACID DEFICIENCY - A SUMMARY

	Vitamin B_{12}	**Folate**
Dietary sources	Meat, eggs, milk and milk products.	Vegetables with leaves, nuts, fruit and liver.
Requirements	~5μg/day in deficiency states. Normally only about 0.1% of body stores are used each day Total body stores are 2000-5000μg so that any deficiency may take many years to present with the typical clinical picture.	Approximately 1mg/day
Sites and mechanisms of absorption	Initial combination with gastric intrinsic factor and subsequent absorption of the complex in the terminal ileum.	Proximal small bowel.
Principal causes of deficiency	1. **Absence of intrinsic factor** because of pernicious anemia or past history of total gastrectomy. 2. **Intestinal causes:** Bacterial growth and utilization of B_{12} in diverticula or blind loops, extensive resection of the terminal ileum, fish tapeworm (Diphyllobothrium latum) infestation - common in Finland.	1. Nutritional deficiencies, usually the result of alcoholism. 2. Increased needs in pregnancy and lactation. 3. Therapeutic drugs: e.g., dilantin, metformin, sulfasalazine and methotrexate. 4. Malabsorption syndromes: e.g., tropical sprue, celiac disease, and extensive small bowel resections.
Dysfunctions	1. **Hematological:** Macrocytic anemia - increased MCV, megaloblastic marrow, low serum Vitamin B_{12}, normal serum and red cell folate, and a Schilling test which is positive if the cause is pernicious anemia. 2. **Neurological**: Peripheral neuropathies and dorsal and lateral column demyelinations in the spinal cord (subacute combined degeneration). Clinical features include bilateral paresthesiae and inabilities to perform fine movements, progressing to incoordination and unsteady gait. 3. **Psychiatric:** Confusional states and psychoses, sometimes progressing to dementia ("megaloblastic madness").	1. **Hematological:** Macrocytic anemia - increased MCV, normal serum Vitamin B_{12}, decreased serum and red cell folate, Schilling test negative for pernicious anemia (usually not done if serum Vitamin B_{12} is normal), megaloblastic marrow. 2. **Deficits in pregnancy:** Possibility of spina bifida or anencephaly resulting from neural tube defects. Needs are also increased during lactation. **Note:** The macrocytic anemia of vitamin B_{12} deficiency may resolve with oral folic acid. The neurological manifestations will not so that, if given folate for a macrocytic anemia due to vitamin B_{12} deficits, a patient with pernicious anemia may present without a macrocytic anemia but with seemingly primary neurological disease.
Therapy	Parenteral B_{12} results in a good and rapid response of hematological abnormalities (an increased reticulocyte count is a good index of response), and of the low grade fever and sore tongue which are often present. The neurological deficits respond slowly and some dysfunction may persist.	Good response and resolution of hematological abnormalities when given oral folate or just a normal nutritious diet.

cells.

The usual symptoms of anemia are present, and occasionally, neurological deficits. A sore tongue is not diagnostic as it also occurs in folate and iron deficiencies. Peripheral neuropathies and subacute combined degeneration of the spinal cord may appear. The latter is a posterior and lateral column demyelination in the spinal cord. Often the earliest manifestations are inability to perform fine movements such as typing and knitting. Subsequent features are general weakness and paresthesiae involving the limbs. Eventually a spastic and uncoordinated gait develops. The abnormalities are typically bilateral. Mental changes are not uncommon in vitamin B_{12} deficiencies and can range from trivial irritability to dementia (termed "megaloblastic madness").

Few conditions respond as dramatically and rapidly to treatment as pernicious anemia. After parenteral Vitamin B_{12} is injected the reticulocyte count starts to rise. Within 48 hours a significant response is seen and anemia soon disappears with its concomitant symptoms. Unfortunately, neurological deficits do not respond as rapidly and some residual disability is common.

Folic acid deficiencies. Folic acid is abundant in leafy vegetables, in nuts, and in the liver. The daily requirements are about 50mg. When insufficient folic acid is absorbed body stores suffice for only a few weeks. The daily requirements are easily satisfied by a diet containing 1mg folic acid.

The anemia is similar to the megaloblastic anemia of Vitamin B_{12} deficiency and the diagnosis depends on estimation of serum and red cell folate.

Causes: The commonest cause is dietary insufficiency due to malnutrition. Often there are associated deficiencies of other vitamins.

- Alcoholics readily develop folic acid deficiency syndromes because of inappropriate diets. Also, alcohol seems to suppress the metabolic effects of folate.
- The dietary requirements are increased in pregnancy because the fetus requires substantial amounts of folate. There is some evidence that increased intake of folic acid during pregnancy reduces the incidence of neural tube defects. Most multivitamins recommended for pregnant women usually contain 1mg folic acid (e.g., Materna: Wyeth-Ayerst).
- Drugs that can interfere with folate utilization include dilantin, metformin, sulfasalazine (a drug used for treatment of inflammatory bowel disease) and the diuretic, triamterene. Methotrexate can cause a folate deficiency because it inhibits the conversion of folic acid to tetrahydrofolic acid by the enzyme, dihydrofolate reductase. These patients need additional folate or folinic acid (citrovorum factor) to avoid a deficiency syndrome.
- Folate is absorbed in the proximal small intestine. Hence, absorption is decreased after extensive small bowel resection and when malabsorption syndromes such as celiac disease and tropical sprue are present. Also, absorption can decrease when there is bacterial utilization of folate in blind loops or diverticula.

  Treatment of macrocytic anemias due to folic acid deficits is simple. The response to oral folic acid is usually rapid. A good balanced diet will often suffice.

  Folic acid supplementation is especially important in pregnant women. Requirements are increased because of fetal use of folic acid. There is also evidence that deficits can result in various fetal malformations, especially neural tube defects with occasional spina bifida and/or anencephaly.

Megaloblastic macrocytic anemias not due to B_{12} or folic acid deficiency. Many agents used in cancer chemotherapy interfere with nucleic acid synthesis. All can cause megaloblastic anemias.

The erythropoietin deficiency anemias.

The anemia of chronic renal disease. Erythropoietin is a requirement for normal maturation of stem cells in the marrow. A deficiency is the cause of the anemia of renal disease and possibly also, of some of the anemias of chronic disease and the so-called "refractory anemias". The anemia of renal disease results from decreased erythropoietin production by the kidney because of decreased O_2 tension in perfusing blood. It is also probable that there is a decreased bone marrow response to the hormone. The anemia is typically normochromic and normocytic. Serum ferritin is usually within the normal range but serum iron is low. The current availability of erythropoietin that can be administered parenterally has been of great help in the management of these patients.

Other causes of anemia in patients with renal failure include decreased red cell survival and a bleeding tendency of uncertain cause; purpura is a common concomitant of chronic renal failure.

The anemias of chronic disease - often designated as the refractory anemias. This is probably the most common anemia that a practitioner will encounter. The anemia is usually normochromic and normocytic. A characteristic feature is a normal or elevated serum ferritin with reduced serum iron.

These anemias are often associated with many infectious and non-infectious diseases such as rheumatoid arthritis and disseminated malignancies. At other times the patient is an elderly individual with no obvious abnormality. Many studies have shown that these anemias probably result from failure of stem cell maturation secondary to reduced erythropoietin production. Others feel that the principal cause is failure of macrophages to release iron.

Hematinics are of no value in treatment of the anemias of chronic disease and the so-called refractory anemias.

The microcytic anemias.

Most microcytic anemias result from quantitative and/or qualitative dysfunctions of hemoglobin production. Chart 12-1 summarized the process of hemoglobin synthesis. It shows that iron is an essential requirement for hemoglobin synthesis. Iron deficiency is the most common cause of a microcytic anemia. Most of the other causes result from inheritance of mutant genes (e.g., the thalassemias and sickle cell anemia).

Iron deficiency anemia.

Iron is essential for formation of of heme. A standard diet contains some 10-15mg iron but most is complexed to organic foods so that only 1-1.5mg is available for absorption. Absorption takes place throughout the intestine but especially in the duodenum. After absorption iron binds to serum transferrin which is a plasma globulin; as a rule only 30-40% of the binding sites are saturated. Most of the iron that exceeds needs is stored in cells as ferritin. Serum ferritin levels are a good measure of iron stores (1ng/ml serum ferritin represents about 10 mg stored iron). Normal values for serum ferririn are 20-200ng/ml (SI units: μg/L).

Iron requirements.

Iron in the blood is used by stem cells and red cell precursors in the marrow to produce hemoglobin. About 21mg iron are needed each day and most of this comes from hemoglobin catabolism recycling. About 1-1.5mg

Chart 12-3: LABORATORY DIAGNOSIS OF THE PRINCIPAL MICROCYTIC ANEMIAS

	Iron deficiency anemia	Anemia of chronic disease	Thalassemias
Serum iron	Decreased	Decreased but usually less than the decrease seen with iron deficiency anemia	Normal
Iron binding capacity	Increased	Decreased	Normal
Serum ferritin	Decreased	Normal or increased	Increased

are lost each day in urine, feces, sweat and lost cells and this is the daily dietary requirement. In females approximately 30mg are lost at each menstrual period - an additional requirement of 1mg per day. Pregnancy increases iron requirements; 400mg for the fetus and an average of 125mg for blood lost during the delivery (about 250ml blood) for a total of an additional 525mg iron or about 2mg per day.

The diagnosis of an iron deficiency anemia.

The red cells are hypochromic and microcytic and the hematocrit is decreased (usually the hematocrit is normal in the thalassemias). Serum iron is decreased, the iron binding capacity of serum increases and the serum ferritin is low. When a microcytic hypochromic anemia does not show the characteristics of an iron deficiency anemia, a thalassemia, one of the so-called "refractory anemias" (anemia of chronic disease) or an anemia due to renal disease (serum creatinine raised), it is worth doing an erythrocyte protoporphyrin assay - protoporphyrin is the precursor of heme. Hemoglobin is a complex of heme, iron and globin. It will not form if heme is absent.

The symptoms of iron deficiency anemias.

As a rule the symptoms are nonspecific; weakness, shortness of breath, a patient who is easily fatigued, is pale and has a sore tongue. Characteristic but uncommon features are brittle nails and nails that are spoon-shaped (called koilonychia). Blood loss from menorrhagia is a common cause.

The causes of iron deficiency anemias.

Blood loss: The most frequent cause of iron deficiency anemia is blood loss. Commonest is excessively heavy menstrual periods. The patient must be specifically asked about the blood loss at each menstrual period as measured by amounts of protection used.

Case history.

Patient age 47 came to see me for tiredness. Routine questioning, examination and blood tests showed a hemoglobin of 8g/100ml due to an iron deficiency anemia. Upper and lower gastrointestinal barium studies were normal. This was in the days before colonscopy was readily available. Treatment with oral iron did not result in any significant improvement. After explaining the potential dangers of intramuscular iron injections she agreed to have a course of these injections. A course was given but with no effect on her anemia, serum iron or ferritin. On repeated questioning about her menstruation she told me she had to use diapers at night to control soiling of bedsheets. She thought this was quite normal for perimenopausal women. Provera and oral contraceptives were of little help in reducing the bleeding. Eventually she had a hysterectomy. The postoperative response to oral iron was gratifying. Within two weeks of surgery she had a normal hemoglobin.

Aspirin ingestion is another common cause, especially as so many individuals, with or without cardiac disease, ingest aspirin daily. Non-steroidal anti-inflammatory drugs can also cause gastric bleeding. A daily loss of 50-75ml blood may not discolor the stools but testing for fecal occult blood will demonstrate blood loss.

An investigation of iron deficiency is rarely adequate without fecal occult blood studies, a sigmoidoscopy and, when appropriate, upper and/or lower GI series, and even a colonoscopy if the cause remains unidentified, and especially if the stools are positive for occult blood. Even if the occult blood is negative and there is no history of ingesting medications that can cause gastric bleeding, an iron deficiency anemia merits radiological examination of the gastrointestinal tract and/or a colonoscopy. Frequent causes of iron deficiency anemia are hemorrhoids, inflammatory bowel disease and most important of all, malignant colorectal lesions.

Diet. An inadequate diet is an uncommon cause of an iron deficiency anemia except in the elderly who live alone, have little money and live on some sort of subsistence diet. Women with severe menorrhagia require iron supplements and so do women during a pregnancy and also postpartum.

Treatment of iron deficiency anemia.

Treatment is simple. Stop taking aspirin or non-steroidal anti-inflammatory drugs. Subsequent daily oral ferrous gluconate, fumarate or sulfate will usually suffice to restore hemoglobin to normal levels. Progress is easily monitored by blood red cell and hemoglobin levels and by the reticulocyte count. Parenteral iron is not without risk.

Iron deficiency due to menorrhagia requires a gynecological assessment which includes a pelvic ultrasound and an endometrial biopsy. If no abnormality is identified the menorrhagia is called dysfunctional uterine bleeding. Various combinations of estrogen and provera or provera alone, in different dosages, are administered by physicians. At times they control bleeding but if it continues and results in persistent significant anemia a hysterectomy is the only available remedy, especially in perimenopausal women with discomfiting menorrhagia with low hemoglobin levels.

An initial intravenous transfusion of stored blood is indicated if the hemoglobin is low (about 6.5g/100ml or less) and accompanied by dyspnea and hypotension. The patient might require gastrointestinal or gynecological medication or surgery. Ideally, any surgery which is not urgent should wait till the anemia has returned to normal values. An exception is a situation where there is bleeding that cannot be controlled without surgery. Examples are uncontrollable dysfunctional uterine bleeding, traumatic injuries of abdominal organs and ruptured tubal pregnancies.

Microcytic anemias resulting from inheritance of mutant genes.

Transmission may be heterozygous or homozygous. Normal adult hemoglobin is:

95-98% Hemoglobin A (2 x α and 2 x β polypeptide chains)
2% Hemoglobin A_2 ((2 x α and 2 x δ polypeptide chains) and
<1% Hemoglobin F (2 x α and 2 x γ polypeptide chains).

The two principal types of gene mutations are:

- Mutations that alter the rates of production of one or more of otherwise normal polypeptide chains. Common examples are the thalassemia syndromes. Hemoglobin electrophoresis is of value for determining quantitative and diagnostic differences in the different hemoglobins.
- Mutations that result in production of abnormal hemoglobins. Many such mutants have been described. Some decrease affinity for oxygen, others increase it, others are unstable hemoglobins with readily induced hemolytic anemia and some are mutants that affect cell membrane structure. An important example of the last group is Hemoglobin S, the cause of sickle cell anemia.

The thalassemias.

Alpha chain thalassemia. The severity of homozygous α chain thalassemia depends on how many of the four alpha gene loci are deleted. The deletion of all four is incompatible with life (hydrops and erythroblastosis fetalis) as all three normal human hemoglobins must contain α polypeptide chains. At the other extreme is a single gene deletion where the individual is a carrier but with little hematologic change apart from a small microcytic anemia of thalassemia type. Intermediate deficit syndromes result from deletions of two or three of the alpha genes. The heterozygous state is difficult to identify because an associated increase of A_2 or F cannot occur. The subject of the alpha chain thalassemias is complex and the clinical findings variable. For those who want more details a text on hematology is recommended.

Beta chain thalassemia: Beta thalassemia has a genetic predilection for people of Mediterranean and Asian Indian ancestry. **The homozygous form is a serious disease** (Cooley's anemia). Both alleles for beta chain synthesis are affected and HbA cannot be produced. Hemoglobin F comprises 30-90% of the circulating hemoglobin. The red cells are hypochromic, hepatosplenomegaly is common and so is retardation of growth and iron overload. The anemia is severe and patients are transfusion dependent. Iron overload results in severe diabetes mellitus and eventual death from cardiac or hepatic failure. Death is common before the individual reaches adulthood and few live beyond 30 years.

Chelating agents to remove iron include desferoxamine and deferiprone. The pros and cons of each are discussed at the end of this chapter.

The heterozygous form of beta chain thalassemia is a fairly benign condition though anemia can be significant. The cells are hypochromic and very microcytic, a feature that helps to distinguish this condition from an iron deficiency anemia. Variant hemoglobin patterns are common. In some A_2 is greater than normal (normal is less than 3%), in others hemoglobin F is higher than the upper limit of normal which is 2%. In others, both A_2 and F are increased. Serum iron and ferritin are usually high normal or increased and the iron binding capacity is normal.

Sickle cell anemia.

The responsible structural mutant is hemoglobin S. **Heterozygous progeny** are said to have a "sickle cell trait". Severe symptoms are uncommon in heterozygotes unless hypoxia is severe. Such episodes are probably responsible in heterozygotes for the **occasional episodes of hematuria and renal infarction resulting from occlusive lesions in the regions of the renal papillae.**

Homozygotes have red cells with HbS. At a decreased oxygen tension the hemoglobin is distorted into rigid strands of abnormal shape. The red cell shape distorts into sickle shaped structures. Red cell fragility increases and hemolysis occurs. The distorted red cells increase blood viscosity. The slower blood flow additionally decreases local oxygen tension, and increases sickling. Eventually blood vessels are occluded by stacks of sickled red cells.

Clinical symptoms begin in childhood. There is a marked racial susceptibility. The sickle-cell gene is said to have originated in Africa where the trait is present in some 40% of the population. About 10% of their American descendants are heterozygotes for the gene but only a small proportion (less than 1%) develop the full-blown homozygotic syndrome. Characteristic features of the homozygotic disease are an anemia, some jaundice, recurrent abdominal and limb pains, chronic and recurrent ulcerations of the legs, recurrent infections, and in older patients, cardiac and hepatic disease. Vaso-occlusive lesions can affect any tissue or organ and result in cumulative dysfunctions of different systems. Acute occlusions result in so-called "crises" which are bouts of acute pain, sometimes excruciating. Death may result from acute infarction of a vital structure or from gradual failure of cardiac, hepatic or renal function. Particularly distressing are vascular changes in the eye; occlusive lesions, aneurysms, vitreous hemorrhages and eventual blindness.

Anemias resulting from increased destruction of red cells.

The causes of increased red cell destruction are intracellular and/or extracellular.

Intracellular cause of intravascular hemolysis.

These include any one or more of the following.

— **Membrane defects** resulting in spherocytosis, elliptocytosis, stomatocytosis and other more uncommon abnormalities, enzyme abnormalities of various sorts and abnormalities of porphyrin metabolism. The last are uncommon but when present result in abnormal heme production. In addition to initiating microcytic anemias, abnormal heme can also result in a hemolytic anemia. A clinically important cause of intravascular hemolysis due to an enzyme deficiency is glucose-6-phosphate dehydrogenase (G6PD) deficiency.

— **Glucose-6-phosphate dehydrogenase (G-6-PD) deficiency.** In G-6-PD deficient individuals there is hemolysis from external stresses. The red cell is unable to regenerate reduced glutathione and cannot defend itself. The stresses include drugs such as the antimalaria drugs primaquine and quinine and the sulfonamides and analgesics. The hemoglobin dissociates into Heinz bodies which attach to the red cell membrane.

  Inheritance is sex-linked and major hemolytic events are rarely seen in females. The hemolytic event may be trivial or life threatening with flank and abdominal pains, shock and dark urine from a major intravascular hemolysis.

Extracellular causes of intravascular hemolysis.

Common extracellular causes of intravascular hemolysis include **mismatched blood transfusions** and **Type 2 immune responses to a complex of red cell, white cell or platelet and any one or more of a variety of antigens. Examples of such antigens are drugs, viruses, parts of viruses and metabolites of drugs. Antibody to the foreign material binds to this complex. The complex of antigen, blood cell and antibody attracts complement. Cell lysis occurs when complement binding is to two adjacent IGg molecules. A variety of syndromes of intravascular hemolysis can result. The Types 1-4 abnormal immune responses and the Coomb's test were detailed on pages 183-187 in Chapter 8. Other extravascular causes include infections.** On a world-wide basis malaria is probably the commonest cause of intravascular hemolysis. **Other causes include lead poisoning, snake venom,** microangiopathic anemia **and** disseminated intravascular coagulation.

Some laboratory findings in abnormal intravascular hemolysis.

- **Increased marrow activity.** The bone marrow can increase red cell production by about 6-8 times the usual levels. This is why chronic hemolytic states are not always associated with anemia - compensated hemolysis. When new red cell production cannot keep up with the rate of destruction anemia and reticulocytosis are seen. Of course, the situation is different if hemolysis is acute because it takes a few days before marrow red cell production can increase.
- **Hemoglobinuria.** When hemoglobin enters the blood following red cell hemolysis it binds to haptoglobin. The complex is then catabolized in the liver. The binding capacity of haptoglobin is about 100mg hemoglobin per 100ml plasma. When this capacity is exceeded hemoglobin is excreted in the urine. Hence, free hemoglobin in blood and urine suggests fairly severe intravascular hemolysis.
- **Other laboratory findings.** Most of the laboratory findings in hemolytic anemias will vary according to the cause. Among these are the Coomb's test, tests for cold agglutinins, for osmotic fragility, for autohemolysis, hemoglobin electrophoresis, special stains for Heinz bodies and globin inclusions, and various enzyme assays. Common findings are reticulocytosis, polychromatophilia, large "shift" erythrocytes and occasional nucleated red cells when hemolysis is severe.

Microangiopathic anemia and disseminated intravascular coagulation.

These two conditions are probably linked by a common etiology; intravascular coagulation and consequent depletion of fibrinogen. Normal mechanisms exists for dissolution of intravascular clots (Chart 12-4) with an eventual increase in blood levels of fibrinogen-fibrin split products.

Microangiopathic anemia.

Chart 12-4: CLOT LYSIS

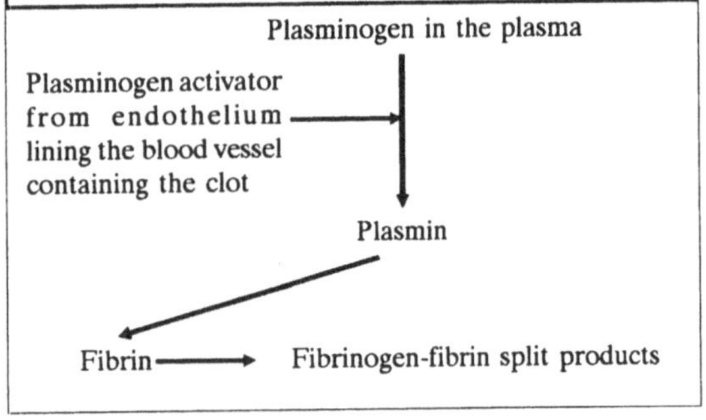
Plasminogen in the plasma
Plasminogen activator from endothelium lining the blood vessel containing the clot
Plasmin
Fibrin
Fibrinogen-fibrin split products

This is probably just a less dangerous variant of disseminated intravascular coagulation.

Both conditions may be associated with the hemolytic uremia syndrome of children and with obstetric emergencies such as severe eclampsia, a retained dead fetus and abruptio placenta. Other causes include major sepsis (bacterial, viral or protozoal - especially, severe malaria) and disseminated malignant disease. Microangiopathic anemia and disseminated intravascular coagulation are also seen at times after transfusion reactions, and in patients who are or who have been in shock.

The hemolytic anemia of microangiopathic anemia is thought to result from red cells that are damaged as they squeeze through fibrin networks or plugs.

Disseminated intravascular coagulation.

It is claimed by many that disseminated intravascular coagulation is only a more serious variant of microangiopathic anemia. Not only does hemolysis result from damage to red cells as they squeeze through fibrin networks and plugs but a hemorrhagic diathesis also develops because of intravascular consumption of clotting factors as the result of disseminated intravascular coagulations. As a consequence there are associated petechiae, ecchymoses, subcutaneous hemorrhages and bleeding from mucus membranes.

The diagnosis is suggested by a thrombocytopenia, by reduced blood levels of fibrinogen and by the presence of fibrinogen-fibrin split products in the plasma. Split products result from the fibrinolysis of fibrin by plasmin

(Chart 12-4).

The blood groups and blood transfusion.

The ABO blood group system.

Many blood group systems have been identified. The principal ones are shown in Chart 12-5. The ABO group is always present and the Rh group is common (the anti-Rh D, but not the E and C). Most of the others are uncommon but may be present and may cause transfusion reactions.

Chart 12-5: THE ABO BLOOD GROUP SYSTEM

The H gene codes for the H antigen which is the substrate for the A and B antigens. O blood has unchanged H antigen and as H isoagglutinins are not present in the other blood groups individuals with O blood are universal donors.

At the H gene locus there are two alleles, H and h. Heterozygotes (HH) code for the H gene which is the precursor of the A and B antigen. Homozygotes do not. Their red cells have no H antigen but the plasma has a full complement of isoantibody; Anti A, Anti A1 and Anti B. This blood group phenotype is very uncommon. It is named Bombay type blood and individuals with this blood type can only receive blood from other individuals with Bombay type blood.

Blood group	Red cell antigens	Serum agglutinins
O[1]	H	Anti A + Anti A_1[2] + Anti B
A	A	Anti B
B	B	Anti A + Anti A_1 in a few individuals.
AB[3]	A AND B	None[3]

1 Universal donor as the other blood groups do not have anti-H agglutinins.

2 Two alleles, A and A_1, exist at the A locus. Two dissimilar blood groups result, A_1 and A_2. A_1 has both A and A_1 while group A_2 only has the A antigen. The result is six dissimilar blood groups: O, A_1, A_2, B, A_1B and A_2B. The A and A_1 antigens are quantitatively and qualitatively dissimilar. One consequence is that some 25% of individuals with this blood type have anti-A_1 serum agglutinins.

3 Universal recipient as no red cell agglutinins are present in the plasma.

The object of blood group typing and cross matching is to ensure that transfused red cells do not meet their corresponding agglutinins in the recipient.

Numerous other minor blood groups exist in addition to the ABO blood group. Examples are the Kell, Duffy, Lewis and many other blood groups. It is said that there are thousands of blood group phenotypes. Hence, except in emergencies of great urgency, blood should never be transfused without cross matching. The object is to ensure that the recipient does not have agglutinins that can agglutinate donor red cells. Such agglutinins could be variants of the ABO group or agglutinins in another uncommon group or groups. If the transfused red cells meet an agglutinin to one of their components a transfusion reaction will result.

The red cells of the ABO group have antigens on their surfaces and antibodies to other red cell antigens in their plasma. It is said that the latter so-called natural antibodies probably result from immunization by A and B type antigens which are present in plants eaten as food. The red cell antigens are widely distributed and are demonstrable in saliva, semen, and many internal organs.

Maternofetal incompatibility.

ABO blood group incompatibility is responsible for about 5% of fetal deaths - for example a type O mother could have natural antibodies against A and B antigens. If the father is not type O the fetal red cells and tissues and the placenta (the placenta is mainly of fetal genotype) would have A, B or both antigens and could be destroyed by antibodies from the mother.

The Rh blood group.

The Rh blood group system is of major clinical importance. The system has many antigens but D is the most antigenic and of principal clinical importance. It is said that about 15% of Caucasians (presumably white skinned individuals of European origin) are Rh negative. Unlike the ABO system, Rh negative individuals do not have natural anti-Rh antibodies in their plasma. However, an Rh negative individual will generate anti-Rh antibodies from a previous transfusion of Rh positive blood or from the blood of an Rh positive fetus.

Hemolytic disease of the newborn.

Fetal blood leaks into the maternal circulation at the time of delivery and also during the pregnancy. Maternal anti-Rh agglutinins develop if the fetus has Rh-positive blood and the mother is Rh-negative. The agglutinins can cross the placenta and enter the fetal circulation causing hemolysis (hemolytic disease of the newborn). Sensitization usually results from fetal blood entering the maternal circulation at the time of parturition so that the first child is usually normal. With each subsequent pregnancy the chance of hemolytic disease developing increases if Rhogam has not been given.

If hemolysis is severe the fetus will die in utero or be born with severe anemia, edema and jaundice. Another serious complication can be kernicterus with early death due to deposition of bile pigment in the basal ganglia. In the fetus and newborn the blood brain barrier is not well developed and bile can traverse this barrier.

Causes of previous maternal sensitization are a previous pregnancy with an Rh positive fetus during or after which she did not get Rhogam. Alternatively, a previous blood transfusion with Rh positive blood.

Rhogam.

Rhogam is anti-Rho(D) antibody. It stops the mother from reacting with antibodies to fetal Rh-positive blood. It should be given to all Rh-negative mothers if the fetus could be Rh-positive because the father is, or if she received any Rh positive blood in a previous pregnancy or a previous blood transfusion. Rhogam is usually given at 28 weeks and again after the baby is born, It prevents sensitization to Rh factor and it is claimed that it also prevents release of existing antibodies in subsequent pregnancies. This passive immunization has greatly reduced and almost eliminated hemolytic disease of Rh-positive newborns who have Rh-negative mothers.

Transfusion reactions.

Blood or plasma transfusions are invaluable adjuncts to clinical therapeutics. However, they are not without dangers. The following lists some of these dangers:

Transfusion of mismatched blood.

Typing and cross-matching of donor and recipient red cells and plasma before a blood transfusion is essential except in dire emergencies. The object is to detect recipient antibodies that could agglutinate donor red cells. Agglutination of the recipient's red cells by donor plasma is rare but cross matching to exclude this possibility is also advisable. However, mistakes do occur for any one of many reasons, including human error and adverse transfusion reactions result.

Transfusion reactions due to ABO incompatibilities are immediate. Sudden back pain is a common first symptom followed by rigors, fever, chest and abdominal pains, dyspnea and hypotension. **The transfusion must be stopped immediately.** Retype and cross match the patient's blood with donor blood and with any residual blood in the bag. Check the blood and urine for free hemoglobin. Its presence indicates fairly significant intravascular hemolysis. Later complications include acute tubular necrosis of the kidneys with acute renal failure, and disseminated intravascular coagulation with an associated hemorrhagic diathesis.

Transfusion reactions involving white cells, platelets or plasma proteins are usually less severe and typically occur in individuals sensitized by previous transfusions or pregnancies. Rigors, fever and urticarial reactions are typical. Hemolytic reactions are not common. The safest course is to treat any adverse transfusion reaction as one would a suspected ABO incompatibility.

Transmission of infection.

It should be normal practice that all blood for transfusion is immunologically pre-examined for the hepatitis A, B and C antigens and for the human immunodeficiency virus. Microscopic examination to exclude bacteria and parasites, especially any one of the different forms of malaria, is also desirable. Unfortunately, occasional samples do escape detection and this is an ever-present danger.

An Internet statement by the IDRI in 2002 (www.idri.org etc.) suggested that screening for T.Cruzi should be included because of the many immigrants to North America from Central and South America. In that part of the world there is a high incidence of Chagas' disease caused by T.Cruzi infections. Accurate tests are available (see page 257 for references). The suggestion of the IRDI is reasonable as Chagas' disease is not a trivial myocardial infection. Perhaps testing of donated blood for T.Cruzi has now been implemented.

A not uncommon problem is transmission of infection by organisms that grow in the cold - gram-negative organisms such as pseudomonas and bacteria of the coli-aerogenes group. Typical consequences are shock, tachycardia, severe abdominal pain and occasionally, rapid death despite vigorous supportive measures. In the evaluation of any adverse transfusion reaction Gram-stains and cultures of the transfused blood are essentials.

The pros and cons of stored blood and fresh blood.

Fresh blood is blood used less than 8 hours after phlebotomy. Its principal advantages over stored blood are that it contains viable platelets (the counts are essentially similar to those of the donor), and that it also contains viable Factors V and VIII. These are important considerations when blood is given for thrombocytopenic syndromes, and for coagulopathies.

Another advantage is that there is little ammonia in fresh blood (approximately 50μg/dl as against some 700μg/dl in stored blood). The increased ammonia levels of stored blood can harm liver function when blood is given to individuals with advanced liver disease.

Miscellaneous transfusion reactions.

These include some that are obvious and some not so well known.

- Unidentifiable allergic reactions. In the days when rubber tubing was used for transfusion these were not uncommon. Plastic tubing has virtually eliminated this danger. A transfusion incompatibility reaction must be excluded before the transfusion is continued with antihistamine cover and careful monitoring.
- Overloading of the circulation.
- Air embolism.
- The temperature of the transfused blood is important. Blood must be stored at between 1-6°C (some state the upper figure is 10°C) and should be warmed to room temperature before transfusion. Rapid transfusion of cold blood can result in serious arrhythmias. Blood that has been stored at less than 0°C or warmed to more than 50°C will result in hemolysis when transfused.

Platelets.

The progenitor of the platelets are large marrow cells, the megakaryocytes. The mature platelet is a disk-shaped structure, approximately 2-3μ in diameter, and containing mitochondria, glycogen and granules. The granules contain factors that promote coagulation on contact with exposed collagen in the walls of damaged blood vessels. Adult blood contains 140-400 x 10^3 platelets per μL (SI units: 140-400 x 10^9/L). Each platelet survives for 8-10 days in the circulation after which it is ingested by liver and spleen phagocytes. About a third of the platelets are in the spleen at any one time. The probable reason is slow transit through the sinusoids. The figure can rise to 80% if there is any dysfunction resulting in congestive splenomegaly. Hence, a spleen that is enlarged from any cause can produce a spurious thrombocytopenia.

The functions of platelets.

The principal function of the platelets is to provide immediate and effective hemostasis when vascular injury occurs. They rapidly accumulate at the site of injury and their contents provide a temporary hemostatic plug when they come in contact with collagen. A more permanent seal results when Factor XII is activated by contact with collagen. Sequential reactions result in conversion of fibrinogen to a permanent fibrin plug (Chart

Chart 12-6: HEMOSTASIS AND THE BLOOD COAGULATION FACTORS

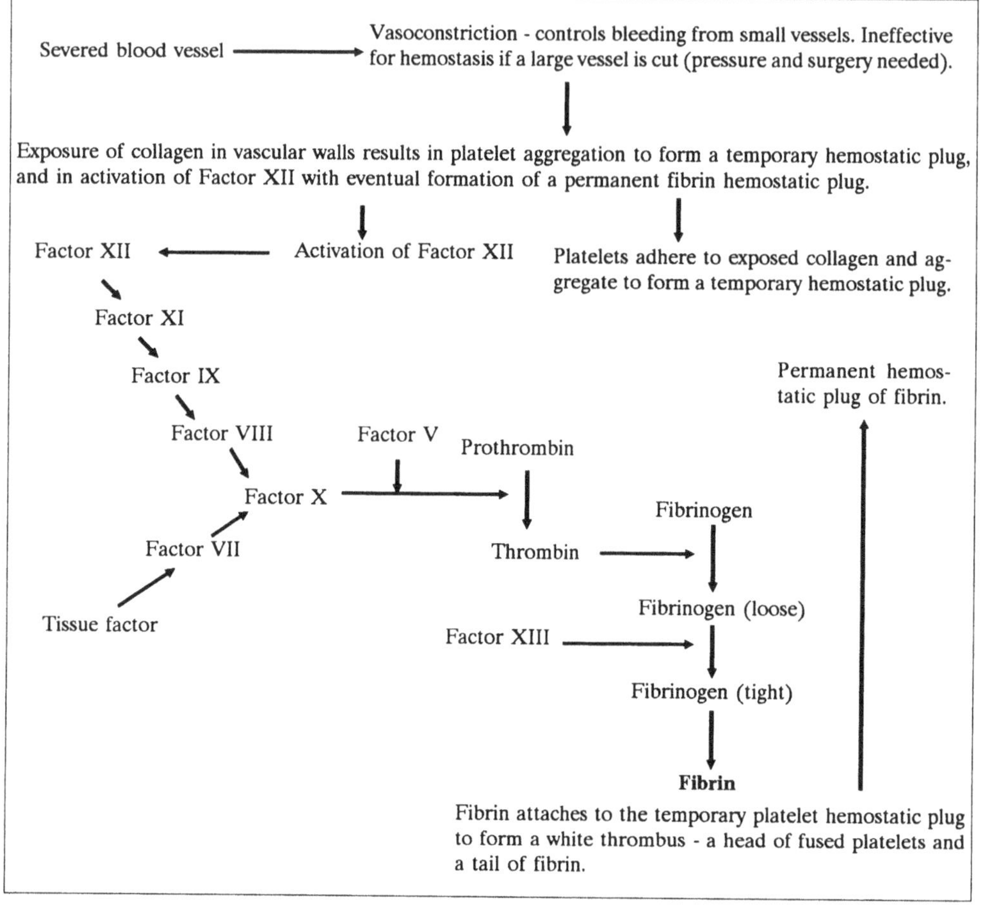

Severed blood vessel
Vasoconstriction - controls bleeding from small vessels. Ineffective for hemostasis if a large vessel is cut (pressure and surgery needed).
Exposure of collagen in vascular walls results in platelet aggregation to form a temporary hemostatic plug, and in activation of Factor XII with eventual formation of a permanent fibrin hemostatic plug.
Factor XII
Activation of Factor XII
Platelets adhere to exposed collagen and aggregate to form a temporary hemostatic plug.
Factor XI
Factor IX
Permanent hemostatic plug of fibrin.
Factor VIII
Factor V
Prothrombin
Factor X
Fibrinogen
Factor VII
Thrombin
Tissue factor
Fibrinogen (loose)
Factor XIII
Fibrinogen (tight)
Fibrin
Fibrin attaches to the temporary platelet hemostatic plug to form a white thrombus - a head of fused platelets and a tail of fibrin.

12-6). The smallest number of platelets required for normal hemostasis is about 50,000/μL but spontaneous hemorrhages are uncommon till the count decreases to about 20,000/μL.

When platelet counts are lower than about 50,000/μL individuals can develop petechiae from small changes in blood pressure or from insignificant trauma. It is suggested that this is because platelets are continually plugging vascular leaks resulting from vascular wall epithelial desquamations and that they cannot do so when their numbers are decreased.

The coagulation system.

Chart 12-6 graphically depicts the coagulation system. In actuality the process is somewhat more complex but the chart suffices to show the principal facts. Additional text is unnecessary. The eventual lysis of fibrin clots occurs as detailed in the section on disseminated intravascular coagulation (Chart 12-4). Alternatively the clot is eventually organized and replaced by the fibrosis of repair.

Inherited deficits of clotting factors.

Many inherited conditions of this type have been described. The commonest is **hemophilia.** It is an X-linked congenital disorder so that only males have the clinical disease but females can be carriers. The clinical features result from a Factor VIII deficiency or rather, from a functionally inactive Factor VIII analogue. Symptoms begin in childhood. Excessive bleeding is often first noted when the child is circumcised. Hemarthroses occur, eventually resulting in ankylosed joints. Other characteristic features are hemorrhages into soft tissues, hematuria, and occasional life-threatening intracranial bleeds. Symptom-free periods alternate with periods of serious bleeds. The disease is lifelong and requires regular infusions of active Factor VIII concentrates. Obviously, knowledgeable genetic counseling of the patient and the parents is imperative.

Another example of a coagulopathy due to inherited deficits is **Von Willebrand's disease** which shows decreased platelet adhesiveness and a reduction in Factor VIII. It is an autosomal dominant inherited bleeding disorder, is rare, and has features similar to classic hemophilia but in much milder form. When a hemophilia type syndrome affects females the probable diagnosis is von Willebrand's disease as this disease is transmitted as an autosomal dominant.

Numerous other diseases due to inherited deficits of clotting factors have been described. They are rare and their specific identification is the function of a specialist in hematology. It is enough for the average practitioner to realize that a bleeding diathesis exists and requires referral to a hematologist.

Abnormal and/or spontaneous bleeding.

There are many causes for abnormal and/or spontaneous bleeding due to thrombocytopenia or platelet dysfunctions. The following are some:

- **Probably the commonest cause of abnormal bleeding is aspirin.** It seems to be ingested by all who have heart disease, think they might have heart disease, or expect to have heart disease at some time in the near or distant future. The drug prolongs bleeding time by inhibiting platelet aggregation.
- **Purpura.**Most purpuras are benign. Examples are purpura without obvious cause (simple purpura), senile purpura which results from insufficient supporting tissue round the superficial blood vessels of the elderly, and purpura resulting from Vitamin C deficiencies.
- **More serious is allergic purpura (Schönlein-Henoch purpura)** which is a vasculitis of immunological origin directed against any one or more of many different antigenic stimuli. The ones often cited are the thiazide diuretics, antibiotics and tranquilizers. It is probably a Type III immunological reaction similar to acute glomerulonephritis. Fairly diagnostic is the biopsy of skin lesions when they coexist with purpura.

  Purpura is widespread and there is accompanying fever, arthropathies, abdominal pain, frequent gastrointestinal bleeding and occasional glomerulonephritis. In children it usually follows a respiratory tract infection and does not last long. In adults it is usually associated with exposure to various drugs. Most patients recover in 3-6 weeks but a few develop chronic renal failure. In a few others symptoms can last for a year or more.
- **Quantitative platelet abnormalities**: The normal platelet count is 140,000-400,000/μL (SI units: 140-400x10^9/L). Platelet counts have to be about 50,000/μL before significant bleeding is a risk. The risk is greater in the presence of infection, healing wounds, ulcerating neoplasms or pre-existing qualitative platelet abnormalitics.
- **Drugs.** Many have been implicated. I have personal experience of patients developing thrombocytopenia from thiazide diuretics and from gold injections for rheumatoid arthritis.
- **Infections.** Any bacterial or viral infection can result in thrombocytopenia.
- **The first indication of a gastrointestinal neoplasm (a benign polyp or malignant tumor) may be bleeding due to thrombocytopenia.** A more common cause is bleeding because of concomitant anticoagulant therapy.
- **Immunological causes.** This topic was discussed in Chapter 8. The usual cause is a Type 2 adverse immunological reaction (Chart 8-7 on page 184). Destruction of platelets by an immunological reaction con-

tinues to be called idiopathic thrombocytopenic purpura (ITP) despite its now presumed immunological etiology.

- **The hemolytic uremic syndrome and thrombotic thrombocytopenic purpura** (TTP) are probably the result of generalized immunological injury to vessel walls. The thrombocytopenias probably result from increased platelet deposition in cerebral and renal vessels. Associated widespread deposits of intravascular hyaline thrombi in small vessels are common. TTP is characterized by thrombocytopenia, hemolytic anemia, fever, neurological dysfunctions and frequent renal failure. Fortunately it is a rare condition.
- **Miscellaneous cause of abnormal bleeding include** alcohol and hypersplenism from any cause. Mechanical injury by prosthetic heart valves or severe aortic stenosis can also cause thrombocytopenia. The effect of hypersplenism is probably spurious as it possibly only causes thrombocytopenia by increasing the segregation of platelets in the spleen.
- **Another cause of spontaneous bleeding is therapeutic anticoagulation,** usually for previous deep vein thrombosis, for atrial fibrillation, or for individuals with prosthetic heart valves. Bleeding is always a possibility if the INR exceeds desired levels so that regular monitoring of blood INR (i.e., prothrombin) levels are essential. When and if the level of anticoagulation is too large a rapid return to normal levels is easy if Vitamin K_1 is injected or even taken orally.

Lymphoreticular neoplasms.

Concepts and treatments are continually changing. Therapy is best left to a specialist who treats hematological malignancies. It is enough for the generalist to recognize the possibility that a neoplastic condition exists. The following are grounds for suspicion:

- A lymph node that is palpably enlarged for no obvious reason. There is no adjacent infection, and no obvious primary malignancy in the afferent drainage area (always check the piriform fossa if a neck node is enlarged). The node may be smooth, discrete and mobile in Hodgkin's disease and most lymphomas or fixed and hard if it is a lymphosarcoma. The patient needs an ultrasound of the abdomen, a chest X-ray, and possibly a bone scan to exclude the presence of similar lesions in other sites. Certainly the persistence or increase in size of such a swelling after a period of about two weeks mandates biopsy or preferably, removal and histological examination if it is not a lesion infiltrating surrounding tissues.
- A patient who complains of tiredness and weakness and looks pale. A blood count may show abnormalities suggesting neoplasia in white cell, platelet, or red cell counts. Notable features are raised lymphocyte counts in the absence of any viral infection, a raised neutrophil count in the absence of any obvious bacterial infection and abnormal platelet counts. Suspicion is raised when a granulocyte count is raised because of an infection but fails to return to normal levels after the infection has resolved.
- Unexplained splenomegaly, hepatomegaly or multiple enlarge lymph nodes require investigations by blood counts, marrow aspirates and/or biopsies and determinations of leucocyte alkaline phosphatase levels to exclude leukemias.
- The presence of nucleated red cells in the circulation with a raised alkaline phosphatase is suggestive of widespread metastatic bone disease.
- If a chronic granulocytopenia exists chromosomal searches for the Philadelphia chromosome[1] are indicated. The Philadelphia chromosome is a marker for chronic granulocytic leukemia.

Therapeutic options for diseases and dysfunctions of the blood

The therapeutic options.

Most of the necessary decisions are implicit in the text of this chapter. Only a little textual amplification is needed.

Iron deficiency anemias. These are easy to treat with oral iron preparations - ferrous gluconate, fumarate or sulfate. The primary essential in an iron deficiency anemia is exclusion of bleeding from a gastrointestinal neoplasm that may be malignant or benign; benign polyps can bleed profusely. More common causes are gastroduodenal bleeding from ASA, the various non-steroidal anti-inflammatory drugs, ulcerations of hiatus hernias, and peptic ulcers. Another cause that requires exclusion is inflammatory bowel disease (Crohn's disease and ulcerative colitis). Patients can also bleed profusely from intestinal infections caused by any one or more causes, e.g., viral infections, bacterial infections (e.g., hamburger disease and Campylobacter infections) and parasitic infections. The cause of some iron deficiency anemias are never discovered. They are attributed to bleeding from angiodysplasias of the colon which are often not demonstrable unless there is an ongoing bleed.

When an anemia is associated with a low serum iron and ferritin the usual cause is an iron deficiency anemia. If the iron is low but the ferritin normal the problem is one of the so-called anemias of chronic disease or anemia due to renal failure. The latter responds to injections of erythropoietin. The former does not respond to any hematinic. It may disappear if the causative disease is cured but there is rarely an obvious cause. If a cause is not identified the anemia is usually ascribed to aging, assuming that the patient is elderly.

Macrocytic anemias They are readily treated with B_{12} or folate. Folate may restore the hemoglobin of B_{12} deficiency states to normal but not the neurological concomitants. A patient with a macrocytic anemia, a low B_{12} and a normal Schilling test usually has bacterial stagnation and B_{12} consumption in intestinal diverticula.

Stem cell transplants are in their infancy. It is possible that at some time in the future they will provide resolutions of aplastic anemias and many of the blood dysfunctions that result from inherited or fortuitous abnormal hemoglobins.

Supportive therapy. This includes relief of pain in sickle cell crises, preventions of infections in those with aplastic anemias and counseling for patients and relatives with inherited dysfunctions or infections such as AIDS or hepatitis C from tainted transfusions of blood or blood products.

The thalassemias. One has to include in this section a summarized version of the controversy regarding deferiprone which is an orally administered chelator of iron. A BMJ editorial[2] in 2004 summarizes the topic well. It was written by Julian Savulescu who holds the Chair in the Oxford Uehiro Centre for Practical Ethics at Oxford University. The following is a summary of his paper. Repeated transfusions of children with thalassemia major result in iron accumulations and subsequent hepatic cirrhosis, hemosiderosis and eventually fatal cardiomyopathies. Desferoxamine is an iron chelator but must be given by slow and often unpleasant daily injections. Deferiprone is oral medication that also chelates iron. Controversy about its uses began with a paper by Olivieri and associates[3]. It was not supportive of the drug. She and her associates claimed that it was less effective than desferoxamine and increased hepatic fibrosis. This is not the place to detail the subsequent antagonisms, controversies and charges of industry interference in clinical research. They were many and most were acrimonious.

Subsequent papers have detailed two large studies[4,5] that dispute the contentions of Olivieri and associates. They were not able to demonstrate the deleterious effects of deferiprone described by Olivieri and associates. The controversies continue and seem unending. At the time the BMJ editorial was published deferiprone was licensed for use in Europe (despite an unsuccessful intervention appeal by Dr. Olivieri in 2003 to the European Court of Justice), throughout Asia and recently in Australia but not in the United States or Canada. If the detractors of Olivieri's contentions are correct many children in the United States and Canada are being exposed to risk as compliance with desferoxamine injections wanes after a few years of daily injections. Eventually the truth must out, one way or another, regardless of nationalist, political and academic pressures.

Sickle cell anemia and other hemoglobinopathies. Sickle cell anemia is a distressing condition but the serious effects are only seen in homozygotes. As previously detailed the disease is genetically determined by a pattern which produces HbS. The trait is present in 40% of Africans but only in 10% of their American descendants. Fortunately less than 1% develop the homozygotic form with its unpleasant consequences which have been detailed in the text. Similar considerations apply to the hemoglobiopathies. Some result in structurally abnormal hemoglobins, others in hemoglobins which cannot be taken up by red cells in sufficient amounts and others in hemoglobins which do not release hemoglobin to cells in sufficient amounts. There are few therapies for these conditions apart from supportive measures to relieve pain and improve tissue oxygenation.

Anemias due to increased hemolysis of red cells, the coagulopathies and lymphoreticular neoplasms. The treatment of these conditions are best left to specialists dealing with hematological disease.

References for chapter 12

1. Nowell, P.C. and Hungerford, D.A. Science. 1960; 132:1497.

2. BMJ editorial by J.Savulescu. Thalassemia major: the murky story of deferiprone. BMJ 2004; 328:358.

3. Olivieri, N.F., Brittenham, G.M. et al. Long-term safety and effectiveness of iron-chelation therapy with deferiprone for thalassemia major. N. Engl. J. Med. 1998; 339:417.

4. Wanless, J.R., Sweeney, G. et al. Lack of progressive hepatic fibrosis during long-term therapy with deferiprone in subjects with transfusion-dependent beta-thalassemia. Blood 2002; 100:1566.

5. Cohen, A.R., Galanello, R. et al. Safety and effectiveness of long-term therapy with oral iron chelator deferiprone. Blood 2003; 102:1538.

13

Diagnosis: The Slave Systems
5. Systems for Maintenance of Homeostasis

Table of Contents

Notation

The notation ~P denotes phosphorous with a high energy bond. Depending on the context in which the term is used, ~P may also denote the energy liberated when a high energy phosphate bond detaches from ATP or ADP.

A comment on the methodology of clinical assessments.

The comments made **on page 119** about this topic are not repeated. They merit reading before proceeding with this chapter.

The objectives.

Intracellular homeostasis is the objective of the systems that regulate osmotic pressures, water and electrolyte contents of body fluids, and their temperatures and pH. The objectives are preservation or restoration of optimal physicochemical conditions for the actions of intracellular enzymes, especially those required for oxidative catabolism of environmental substrate (i.e., food and oxygen) to ~P. Some of the objectives are met by systems not dependent on enzymes. Examples are the free movements of water and gases across capillary and cell walls along concentration gradients.

The maintenance and preservation of homeostasis requires that the osmotic pressures, volumes, electrolyte contents, pH and temperature of fluids in the different body compartments remain within physiologically desirable and permissible limits. There are two groups of systems required. One is intracellular and the other is extracellular.

Intracellular systems remove unwanted and potentially toxic materials from the cell. Extracellular systems ensure that physicochemical conditions within the cell remain within physiologically desirable and permissible limits for osmotic pressures, intracellular volumes, electrolyte contents and electrical neutralities, pH levels and temperatures.

The resource systems for maintenance of homeostasis:

- **The intracellular Golgi apparatus, the lysosomes** and their catabolic enzymes.
- **Renal systems** for regulations of water balance, electrolyte contents and pH.
- **Hepatic systems** for detoxification of undesirable endogenous (e.g., heme) and exogenous materials (e.g., drugs and environmental toxins). Liver metabolism and detoxification are detailed in a later chapter on drug therapy (Chapter 16, pages 350-352).
- **The lungs** for elimination of volatile gases and carbon dioxide and for control of body fluid pH levels.
- **Systems which regulate body temperature.**

Each resource system has many minor system components which interact speedily, autonomously and automatically to attain the requirements of its resoure system.

Systems that assist the resource systems:

- **The rapid and easy diffusion of oxygen, carbon dioxide**, water and lipid soluble substances along pressure and concentration gradients created by the walls of blood vessels and the walls of surrounding cells.
- **The sodium pump systems of cell membranes.** They maintain intracellular negativity with respect to the extracellular environment. The sodium pump systems are numerous. A good review of sodium pumps and their mechanism is by Jorgensen and associates (Structure and mechanism of Na,K-ATPase: Functional sites and their interactions. Ann. Revu. Physiol. 2003; 65:817.) It seems that there are many such pumps on cell surfaces. The numbers differ according to the cell type. Estimates are that 20-25% of ~P produced in the cell is used to maintain the activity of the sodium pumps and up to 70% in nerve and muscle.
- **Voltage gated cell membrane ion channels** respond to neurotransmitters. These channels are distinct from the sodium pump channels. The Inhibitory Post Synaptic Potential, the IPSP (see page 121 for details) opens the potassium channel. K^+ moves out of the cell and intracelluar negativity increases. The Excitatory

Post Synaptic Potential, the EPSP opens the sodium channel. Na^+ ions move into the cell with a consequent decrease in intracellular negative charge. A change of +20 to +25mv at the axon hillock is required for initiation of the nerve impulse. The nerve impulse has a positive charge relative to the rest of the neuron and its axon extension. This lets it pass along the axon; unlike charges attract each other, like charges do not.

Without mechanisms for neural transfer, control of the integrated and coordinated activity of different systems by the CNS would not be possible. Physiological chaos and death would eventuate.

- **The porosities of the walls of the vascular system.** Most capillaries have walls with pore diameters which are smaller than the size of the smallest intravascular protein - albumin. Proteins exert an osmotic (oncotic) pressure and their presence in blood maintains intravascular volume because their contained proteins cannot egress from the vessels. Fluid is retained in the blood to maintain osmotic equivalence with the interstitial fluid. Osmotic equivalence is maintained by reduction of intravascular Cl^- to 105mEq/L from 115mEq/L in interstitial fluid and a change of protein from 15mEq/L in intravascular plasma to 5mEq/L in the interstitial fluid (Chart 13-4). Protein and cells which have leaked out in fenestrated and discontinuous capillaries are returned via lymphatics aided by tissue turgor.
- **The cell wall which is impermeable to most intracellular proteins.** Fluid is retained in cells and this water is essential for normal function. Intracellular proteins and organic acids have between 8-12MEq/L more protein than the interstitial fluid. Their electrolyte contents differ but Chart 13-4 shows how electrolyte differences preserve osmotic equivalence between the intracellular fluid (ICF) and the extracellular fluid (ECF). Note that there is electrical neutrality between cations and anions in each compartment.

Intracellular mechanisms for maintenance of homeostasis

The Golgi apparatus and its lysosomes and vesicles.

Lysosomes are irregularly round structures that derive from the Golgi apparatus. Each contains dozens of enzymes with different catalytic capabilities: proteases, lipases, nucleases and polysaccharidases.

Lysosomes take up and catalyze unwanted and degenerated intracellular materials. Examples are bacteria phagocytosed by neutrophils, foreign bodies, and degenerated organelles such as mitochondria and pump systems. The products of catabolism are extruded from cells by the lysosomes. The lysosomes also have a secretory capacity and produce the perforins used by cytotoxic T lymphocytes to destroy foreign cells.

Lysosomes are buds separated from the Golgi apparatus. The Golgi apparatus can also transport unwanted materials in vesicles which separate, bind to the cell membrane and then rupture and discharge their contents into the extracellular space. Thus, the Golgi apparatus is the basic resource for intracellular housekeeping.

Lysosomal storage diseases.

Numerous diseases that result from dysfunctions of lysosomal catabolism are described. They are rare and often difficult to diagnose. Any suspicion that a child's development is not normal is best referred to a specialist who deals with pediatric disease. Tay-Sachs disease is described below. It is an example of a lysosomal storage disease.

Tay-Sachs disease.

The disease results from the absence of a lysosomal enzyme (hexaminidase or Hex-A for short) which is needed for catabolizing a fatty waste substance in brain cells. When Hex-A is absent this material accumulates in the brain cells and results in their progressive damage. Death is the invariable end-result.

Symptoms first appear at about 4-6 months of age. There is no smiling, crawling, turning over, grasping or reaching out. Later the child becomes blind, paralyzed and unaware of its surroundings and eventually dies when 4-5 years old. At times the disease does not appear till the child is older. In these older children mental disease, vision and hearing are often not impaired but there are usually neurological deficits such as unsteady gait, slurred speech and muscle weakness and tremors.

It is said that one in thirty American Jews carries the Tay Sachs gene. The disease results from a recessive gene disorder. Carriers have one normal Hex-A gene and one Tay Sacks gene. Investigators claim that a comparable frequency extends to French-Canadians of the East St. Lawrence valley and to the Cajuns of Louisiana.

Carriers can be identified by blood tests and in the fetus the disease can be identified by examinations of amniocentesis fluids or by chorionic villus studies. The presence of Hex-A means that the baby will not have Tay Sachs disease.

Many other lysosomal storage disease are described. Examples are Gaucher's disease and Niemann Pick disease. This diversion to describe a clinical rarity is made to show the importance of the Golgi apparatus and its lysosomal buds in maintaining intracellular homeostasis. As of today there are no licensed and acceptable cures for these terrible afflictions.

The cell wall and intracellular DNA.

All cells have cell wall receptors for substances that enter by transport systems. Notable ones are those for the conjoint intracellular transport of sodium and glucose and the ones that bind LDL-cholesterol complexes. Intracellular mechanisms determine the numbers and avidities of these and many other receptors of the cell wall, always in concord with local microenvironmental conditions and intracellular needs. Perhaps most important of all is the intracellular synthesis by DNA of enzymes and of sodium and other pump systems to replace those that have degenerated.

Accurate DNA synthesis of materials needed by the cell is essential and errors of translation and transcription must be identified, repaired or deleted. All these activities require ~P for synthesis of enzymes and other proteins from DNA and for the repair or deletions of errors of transcription and translation. The objective of the systems that maintain intracellular homeostasis is provision of optimal intracellular physicochemical conditions for the enzymes which produce ~P by oxidative catabolism of substrate from the environment.

Extracellular mechanisms for maintenance of homeostasis

Chart 13-1: TYPICAL BALANCE SHEET FOR WATER INTAKE AND OUTPUT PER DAY[1]

Intake:		**Output:**	
Water and other liquids drunk	1,500ml	Insensible loss from skin	500ml
Water in food	800ml	Urine	1,500ml
Endogenous production during carbohydrate and fat metabolism.	300ml	Feces	100ml
		Total output	2,600ml
Total intake	2,600ml		

[1] Values are approximations for afebrile individuals living a sedentary life at a comfortable temperature and humidity.

Water and electrolyte balance.

Chart 13-1 summarizes the facts. Normally about 600mOsmo of solute are produced each day. With maximum antidiuresis, an afebrile individual living a sedentary life at a comfortable temperature and humidity, would need to pass about 500-800ml urine to excrete this solute load. The amount of water needed for normal water balance increases when renal concentrating capacity is decreased, if solute production increases because of increased catabolism, fever, trauma, or surgery, or if water loss increases because of hot weather, vigorous exercise or energetic manual labor.

Chart 13-1: INTERNAL TURNOVERS OF WATER [1]

Secreted:		Reabsorbed:	
Saliva	1,000ml	Jejunum	4,500 - 5,500ml
Bile	1,000ml	Ileum	3,000 - 3,500ml
Pancreas	1,500ml	Colon	100 - 1,000ml
Gastric juice	2,500ml	Total reabsorbed	8,000-10,000ml
Small intestine	2,000 - 3,500ml		
Total secreted	8,000 - 10,000ml		

[1] Values are averages of those given by three authors. Many of these values have been derived by extrapolations from animal experiments. For obvious ethical reasons accurate figures for humans are difficult to obtain. The potential magnitudes of losses from disease such as gastroenteritis or sequestrations of fluids in loops of obstructed or adynamic bowel are obvious.

Internal turnovers of water.

Large amounts of fluid are secreted into the gastrointestinal tract each day for digestion of ingested foods. Almost all is reabsorbed. Chart 13-2 summarizes these facts (it is a replica of Chart 9-2 on page 192, reproduced here for the reader's convenience). Normal water balance is lost when drinking water is in short supply or absent or when increased water losses result from pathology such as severe gastroenteritis, fistulae and ostomies or internal sequestrations of fluid in loops of adynamic, obstructed, or devascularized bowel.

Body water compartments.

Chart 13-3 summarizes the facts. Body water is about 60% of body weight. Approximately ⅔ is intracellular (ICF). The remaining ⅓ is extracellular (ECF). The intravascular fluid is part of the ECF and is approximately 5% of body weight, i.e., about 3.5L plasma in a 70Kg man. The remainder is interstitial fluid - about 15% of body weight or about 10.5L in a 70Kg man.

Osmotic pressure - the normal and the dysfunctions

What is osmotic pressure?

A semipermeable membrane is one which allows free back and forth movement of water and most electrolytes. A solution which contains solutes has less water per unit volume than one which has less solute. All biological solutions tend towards osmotic equilibrium. Hence, if the two solutions are separated by a semipermeable membrane water will flow from the compartment that has less solute to the one that has more, and consequently, less water. This is osmosis. The osmotic pressure is the force required to prevent this water movement.

Neither osmosis nor osmotic pressure depend on the nature of the solute particles separated by the semi-permeable membrane, only on their numbers after any ionic disassociations. Thus, the osmotic pressure of a solution containing 0.1M NaCl will be twice that of one containing 0.1M glucose because each molecule of NaCl dissociates to two ions (Na^+ and Cl^-) while glucose remains as a single undissociated molecule. For items which are not electrolytes, millimoles/L = milliosmoles/L. For electrolytes, milliosmoles/L = millimoles/L × the numbers of ions resulting from dissociation of a molecule of the electrolyte. All biological solutions

Chart 13-3: BODY FLUID COMPARTMENTS [1,2]

Total body water is about 60% of body weight in males and about 5-10% less in females (approximately 42 L in a 70 Kg. man). About ⅔ (28L) is intracellular and ⅓ (14L) extracellular.

The compartments of body water and the permeability characteristics of the membranes separating them (all values calculated for a 70 Kg. male).

Capillary wall → between intravascular and interstitial fluid; **Cell wall membrane** → between interstitial and intracellular fluid

Intravascular fluid	Interstitial fluid	Intracellular fluid
5% of body weight = 3.5 liters plasma in a 70 Kg. man.	**15% of body weight = 11.5 liters in a 70 Kg. man.**	**40% of body weight = 30 liters in a 70 Kg. man.**
Fluid is retained in this compartment because of the osmotic drag of its content of plasma proteins. The walls of most capillaries have tight junctions or fenestrations which are not large enough to allow egress of contained proteins. Water is retained to ensure an osmotic pressure similar to that in the interstitial fluid. There are exceptions where larger fenestrations allow large protein molecules and even cells to exit from vessels (detailed in the text).	Most interstitial fluid is in the form of a non-mobile gel consisting of a mesh of collagen fibers and an interstitium of water and hyaluronic acid. The suction of lymphatics, and the intracapillary reabsorption of leaked plasma proteins results in a negative interstitial fluid pressure of approximately -6.5mm Hg.	This is the largest fluid compartment of the body. Most intracellular anions are proteins and organic compounds. The cell membrane is impermeable to these substances. Water is retained in the cells to ensure osmotic equality with the extracellular fluids: an osmotic pressure of approximately 300mOsm/Liter.

[1] Other compartments exist (intralymphatic, intramitochondrial, etc.) but are small and only merit mention.

[2] Values of percentages and volumes in the chart are averagings of those given by five different authors.

have, or should have an osmotic pressure of about 280-300mOsm/L. The electrolyte compositions and osmotic pressures of fluids in the different body compartments are depicted in Chart 13-4. Note that the contents of each compartment have electrical neutrality because of equivalent contents of positive and negative ions.

The principle of osmotic equivalence.

The principal factor determining body water volume in the different body compartments are their electrolyte contents. They ensure that each has an osmotic pressure which is comparable to the osmotic pressures of the others - 280-300mOsm/Kg water. The principle of osmotic equivalence of different body fluids is a basic requirement of biology. Chart 13-5 summarizes the facts.

The walls of capillaries are semipermeable membranes.

Many items can traverse capillary walls but not the plasma proteins - in most tissues the spaces between the cells lining capillaries is less than the maximum size of an albumin molecule (MW 69,000 and radius of 7.5nm). Hence, in most parts of the vascular complex plasma protein oncotic pressure retains water in the circulation and thus preserves intravascular volume. The osmotic pressure of the intravascular compartment and the ECF are similar(Chart 13-4). Their protein and Cl^- contents differ to maintain osmotic equivalence; intravascular Cl^- = 105mEq/L and protein = 15mEq/L and interstial fluid Cl^- = 115 mEq/l and protein = 5mEq/L.

At any one time about 55% of the blood is in the venous and about 10% in the large arteries. The reminder is in the small arteries and the arterioles. These structures are essentially impermeable to proteins because of

Chart 13-4: ELECTROLYTE COMPOSITIONS OF BODY FLUIDS [1, 2]

Intracellular fluid [2]	
K^+	155 mEq./L.
Na^+	15 mEq./L.
Mg^{2+}	25 mEq./L.
Total cations	**~195 mEq/L**
PO_4^{3-}	115 mEq./L.
HCO_3^-	10 mEq./L.
Protein & organic acids :	70 mEq./L.
Total anions	**~195 mEq/L**

Interstitial fluid [2]	
K^+	4 mEq./L.
Na^+	138 mEq./L.
$Ca^{2+}+Mg^{2+}$	4mEq./L.
Total cations	**~146 mEq/L**
Cl^-	115 mEq./L.
HCO_3^-	26 mEq./L.
Protein & organic acids :	5 mEq./L.
Total anions	**~146 mEq/L**

Intravascular plasma [2]	
K^+	4.5 mEq./L.
Na^+	140 mEq./L.
$Ca^{2+}+Mg^{2+}$	~ 5 mEq./L.
Total cations	**~150 mEq/L**
Cl^-	105 mEq./L.
HCO_3^-	25 mEq./L.
Protein & organic acids :	15 mEq./L.
Total anions	**~150 mEq/L**

[1] Values given are the averages of those provided by different authors. They vary by ~ ± 5-10% from those given in this table.

[2] **The principle of electroneutrality:** in any given and finite volume of a normal body solution the total numbers of positive and negative charges must be equal.

their thick walls. Only about 5% of the circulating blood is in the capillaries at any one time. Most of the to-and-fro movements of water to maintain osmotic equivalence between the ECF and ICF takes place in capillaries with tight or fenestrated junctions between their lining cells. Water and gases traverse capillary and cell walls easily.

Chart 13-5: OSMOTIC EQUIVALENCE [1,2]

Intracellular water	Extracellular water (including plasma)
Volume of intracellular fluid in a 70Kg man = 30L	Volume of extracellular fluid in a 70Kg man = 15L
Total mOsm of dissociated and undissociated compounds in the intracellular fluid of a 70Kg man = 8700mOsm	Total mOsm of dissociated and undissociated compounds in the extracellular fluid (including plasma) of a 70Kg man = 4350mOsm
∴ osmolarity of intracellular fluid is $\frac{8700}{30}$ = 290 mOsm/L.	∴ osmolarity of extracellular fluid is $\frac{4350}{15}$ = 290 mOsm/L.

[1] Averages of values given by three different authors.

[2] Osmolarity values are higher than the totals of mEq/L in Chart 13-4 because both, intracellular and extracellular fluids contain compounds which do not dissociate but do contribute to osmolarity. They also contain electrolytes such as Ca^{2+}, Mg^{2+}, and PO_4^{3-}. These items dissociate to two or more ions each as do some of the protein contents of the body fluids. Osmotic pressures depend on the numbers of ionic and undissociated particles in a solution, not on their weights. The normal osmolarirty of the ECF, the ICF and its plasma components is 280-300mOsm/L.

The junctions between the cells lining capillaries do vary and continuity between adjacent cells may be lost in organs such as the liver and spleen. In areas where the fenestrations are greater than the size of albumin molecules protein and, at times, even cells escape into the tissues. Tissue turgidity returns some of these substances to the capillary blood and the remainder is removed by the lymph.

Some general comments on osmotic pressure dysfunctions.

Cell walls do not allow egress of intracellular protein unless there are special transport systems and biological structures such as lysosomes for removal of undesirable toxins and other degenerated materials. Water retained in the cells ensures osmotic equilibrium between intracellular and extracellular fluids.

A variety of dysfunctional syndromes associated with osmotic pressure changes are described: water depletion, water excess, electrolyte deficiencies and electrolyte excess syndromes. In reality there are few syndromes which are not combinations of water and electrolyte deficits or excesses. A pure syndrome of water deficiency exists when there is nothing to drink. Otherwise, a pure syndrome of water deficiency is uncommon without associated electrolyte disturbances. Sodium loss is usually the result of excess loss of body fluids from gastroenteritis, sequestration of fluids in obstructed loops of bowel, ileostomies, fistulae, and/or diuretics and is associated with loss of water. Sodium excess is a frequent concomitant of renal disease, congestive heart failure and cirrhosis of the liver, and in its purest form, the result of drinking hypertonic sea water by shipwrecked individuals.

Normal renal function is necessary for adequate compensations. It cannot compensate when extreme situations exist. Examples are the continued absence of drinking water and drinking of sea water by shipwrecked individuals. Often it cannot compensate for the water and salt retentions of congestive heart failure and hepatic cirrhosis; safety valves are accumulations of edema fluid in the interstitial spaces.

The initial response to water and electrolyte deficits.

The osmotic pressure in a body fluid compartment depends on its content of osmotically active solute. The main cation in the ECF is sodium. It comprises 90% of osmotically active cation in the ECF and is balanced by a mixture of osmotically equivalent anions. The ECF osmotic pressure must be equivalent to ICF osmotic pressure. In order to maintain this equivalence volumes and electrolyte contents in the ICF and ECF constantly change by small amounts as long as there are no major changes in body water and electrolytes. Because of the predominance of sodium as an osmotically active solute in the ECF the volume of the ECF mainly depends on its concentration in the ECF and, as a corollary, on the water content of the ECF.

This preamble helps to understand and predict the sequence which results from significant losses of water and electrolytes from the body. The early responses to fluid and solute losses because of vomiting, diarrhea, and sequestrations of fluids in loops of obstructed or adynamic bowel are to-and-fro movements of water and sodium between the ECF and ICF to maintain osmotic equivalences. The directions in which water and solutes move when there are deficits or excesses of one or both are only the initial responses for maintenance of osmotic equivalence between the ICF and ECF. They are of limited value as there are limits to the amounts of fluid which intracellular fluid can lose or gain without changes in intracellular osmotic pressures which are detrimental and dangerous, especially when they affect brain cells. Proteins cannot egress from cells except for specific purposes and they retain fluid in the cells to maintain ICF osmotic pressures and normal functions. When water in the ICF cells is reduced or increased beyond physiologically permissible and desirable limits there are neurological dysfunctions: confusions, and at times, convulsions, disorientations, coma and finally, death from brain failure.

Maxim.

Maintenance of ECF osmotic pressure takes priority over all other considerations in dysfunctions of water and electrolyte balances and pH and acid-base changes. The final osmotic pressures of the ECF and ICF must be equivalent. This requirement depends on renal function. It often results in a reductions of ECF volume and consequently in intravascular volume if there are uncorrected losses of water and/or electrolytes; isotonic hypovolemia. Renal control of water and electrolyte excretion is the final stabilizing mechanism for restoration or preservation of the isotonicity of the ECF and the plasma.

Renal control and regulation of water and sodium.

The kidneys control water and sodium retention and excretion and hence, the ECF osmotic pressure. It equates it with ICF osmotic pressure. Maintenance of isotonicity is effected by antidiuretic hormone-aldosterone cooperation in the distal nephron and collecting ducts (detailed later). If there are uncorrected water and salt deficits preservation or restoration of ECF isotonicity will often result in its contraction. This contraction will occur simultaneously in the intravascular volume which has the same osmotic pressure as the surrounding interstitial fluid. The results will be hypovolemia, hypotension and finally, if the deficits increase or are not corrected, cerebral hypoperfusion with confusional states progressing to hallucination, convulsions, coma and finally, death. Death in not merely a theoretical possibility for patients losing water and sodium because of uncontrolled and inadequately treated, or untreated gastroenteritis. **The WHO reports that each year 5-6 million deaths occur from diarrheal diseases.** Most of these deaths occur in young children (Internet: Diarrheal diseases. WHO fact sheet. http:/www.who.int/vaccine and the access “diarrheal diseases”).

A benefit for treating physicians is the knowledge that even if there is hypovolemia and hypotension the intravascular fluid will usually be isotonic. Replacement of volume does not require complex calculations because replacement with appropriate volumes of isotonic saline will usually suffice. Automatic internal adjustments of ECF and ICF electrolytes such as potassium are also usual but supplementation of intravenous fluids with potassium is needed when intravenous therapy is prolonged and in certain exceptional circumstances such as diabetic or starvation ketoacidosis where movements of potassium vary because of the disease and the consequences of therapy. Severe acidosis because of poisonings by methanol or ethylene glycol or excessive amounts of aspirin may also need additional corrective fluids.. Aging reduces renal function so that adequate compensations for water and salt loss may be deficient. There are two additional caveats The **first** is that prolonged intravenous therapy requires regular estimations of serum potassium and potassium supplements as needed. The **second** is that any decrease in urine output requires investigation to exclude renal failure. Intravenous saline is contraindicated if there is any suspicion of acute tubular necrosis and so is the administration of a potassium supplement.

If the ECF is hypertonic water is retained and solute (mainly sodium) is excreted. If it is hypotonic water is excreted and sodium retained. Water retention and excretion are coordinated by ADH and aldosterone (a detailed description follows later). ADH is responsible for body water homeostasis. It decreases water excretion and decreased ADH levels increases water excretion. Aldosterone promotes sodium retention and decreased aldosterone levels allows increased Na^+ excretion.

Preservation of ECF osmotic pressure by renal mechanisms often results in contraction of the ECF. This may spontaneously correct with time but frequently requires intravenous hydration with isotonic saline The preservation of ECF isotonicity results from interactions of ADH, aldosterone, and possibly ANP in the distal nephron and collecting ducts

The glomerular filtrate measures approximately 180L per day. Normally all but 1000-1500ml (the usual daily volume of urine) is reabsorbed. in the following ways:

1. **Passive water reabsorption with sodium.**

Sodium moves into tubular cells along its concentration gradient (Chart 13-6). Extracellular and hence, tubular fluid has a sodium concentration of about 149mEq/L and intracellular sodium is about 20mEq/L.

There is an accompanying passive intracellular movement of water from tubule to the lining cell to maintain osmotic equilibrium. The locus of this sodium and water reabsorption is the proximal tubule of the nephron. The luminal surfaces of the tubular cells are joined by tight junctions but lateral intercellular spaces exist. The sodium pumps of the tubular cell walls pump intracellular sodium into these spaces. The lateral intercellular space becomes hypertonic and water exits the tubular cells to restore normal tonicity. The water and sodium enter the interstitium and then the peritubular capillaries. This process of passive water reabsorption accounts for about **70-75% of the glomerular filtrate water which is returned to the interstitium and then to the blood.**

2. **Reabsorption of water by a countercurrent system in the rest of the tubule.**

The countercurrent system is complex and its detailed description is unnecessary, given the context of this monograph. It suffices to say that **approximately 15-20% of the glomerular filtrate water is absorbed by the countercurrent system.** This process and the one above leave about 5-10% of the glomerular filtrate water unabsorbed at the end of the distal tubule. The only clinically important fact about the counter current system for tubular reabsorption of water is that, in the ascending limb of Henle it involves the active transport of Cl^- out of the tubular lumen into the tubular cell and thence into the interstitium and peritubular capillaries. Sodium follows to maintain electrical neutrality.

Some loop diuretics act by decreasing this active transport of Cl^- out of the tubular fluid. The result is increased excretion of Na^+ and water.

3. **Hypothalamic antidiuretic hormone (ADH).**

The two previous processes of water reabsorption were essentially passive and automatic. It leaves about

5-10% of the glomerular filtrate water to reach the collecting ducts (i.e., 9-18L water/day).

Anti-diuretic hormone (ADH) controls renal water homeostasis by varying water reabsorption or excretion in

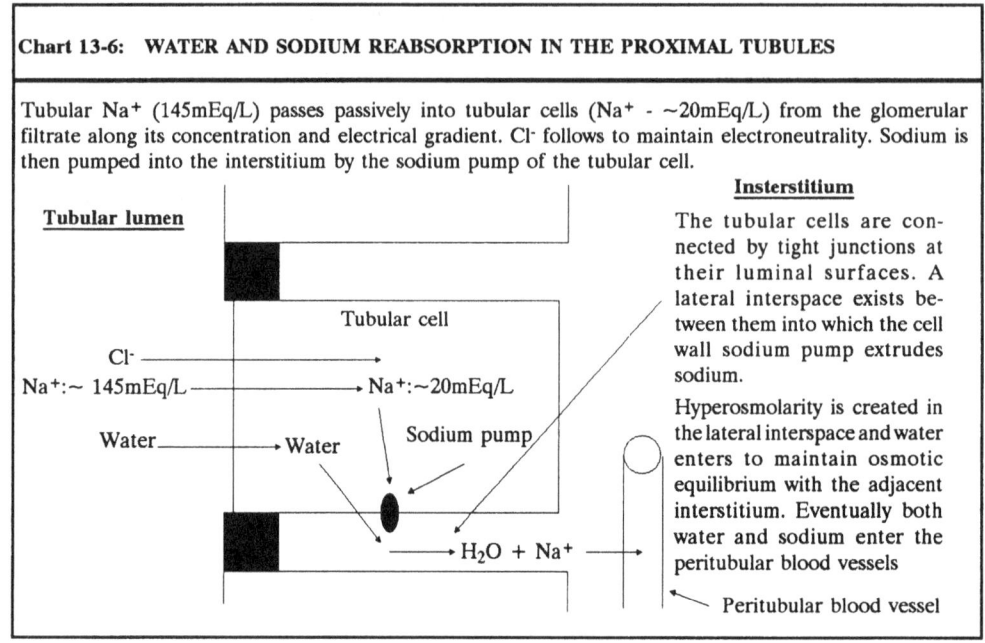

Chart 13-6: WATER AND SODIUM REABSORPTION IN THE PROXIMAL TUBULES

Tubular Na^+ (145mEq/L) passes passively into tubular cells (Na^+ - ~20mEq/L) from the glomerular filtrate along its concentration and electrical gradient. Cl^- follows to maintain electroneutrality. Sodium is then pumped into the interstitium by the sodium pump of the tubular cell.

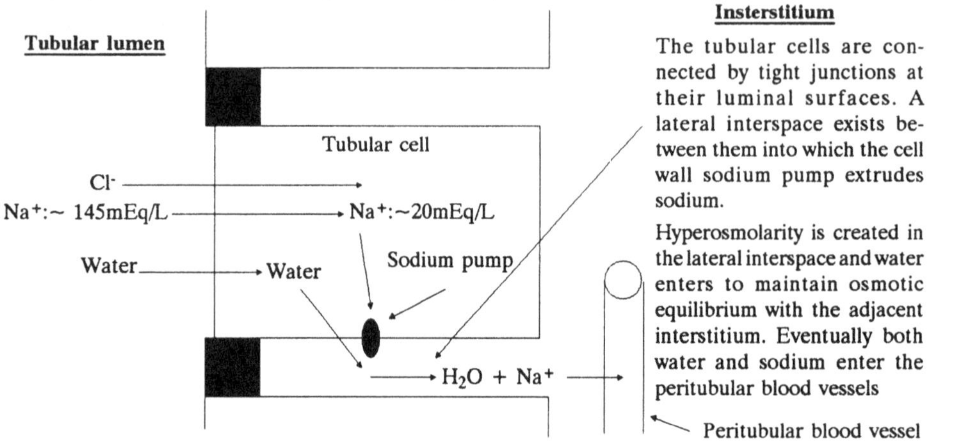
Insterstitium
Tubular lumen
Tubular cell
Cl-
Na+:~ 145mEq/L
Na+:~20mEq/L
Water
Water
Sodium pump
H2O + Na+
The tubular cells are connected by tight junctions at their luminal surfaces. A lateral interspace exists between them into which the cell wall sodium pump extrudes sodium.
Hyperosmolarity is created in the lateral interspace and water enters to maintain osmotic equilibrium with the adjacent interstitium. Eventually both water and sodium enter the peritubular blood vessels
Peritubular blood vessel

the collecting ducts. It is produced in hypothalamic neurons and stored as granules in the axon terminals of these neurons which are sited in the posterior pituitary. Control of production and delivery is by thirst mechanisms and feedback reflexes centered on hypothalamic osmoreceptors which sense osmotic pressure changes in perfusing blood.

When the osmotic pressure of the ECF is hypotonic it contains too much water. ADH activity decreases and water excretion increases till isotonicity is restored. The converse occurs when the ECF is hypertonic because there is an excess of solute. ADH activity increases, there is water retention and the ECF osmotic pressure returns to isotonicity.

ADH acts on water in the collecting ducts by varying the permeabilities to water of the epithelial linings of the distal nephron and the collecting ducts. It is a powerful hormone. In the absence of ADH (e.g., in primary diabetes insipidus) the daily urine output could exceed 18L per day. Maximum ADH antidiuresis can result in a urinary output as low as 600ml/day.

While ADH is controlling water homeostasis aldosterone is controlling sodium homeostasis. They act in concert, presumably by to and fro interactions till the osmotic pressure of the ECF is equal to that of the ICF.

4. Aldosterone and the renal mechanisms for sodium homeostasis.

Sodium loss in sweat and gastrointestinal secretions averages about 100mEq/day. Losses are greater if there are losses of sodium because of severe gastroenteritis, vigorous exercise, especially if losses of sodium in sweat are replaced with water alone, and in conditions such as Addison's disease. A basic intake of about 4 gm NaCl per day is appropriate. Renal sodium homeostasis is mainly a function of aldosterone control.

Adrenal aldosterone production is controlled by pituitary ACTH and by angiotensin produced by enzyme reactions based on renin production in the kidneys. Renin is produced by the juxtaglomerular (JG) cells which are epitheloid cells replacing the smooth muscle cells of the afferent arteriole just before it enters the glomerulus. They are stimulated to produce renin when blood pressure falls. The macula densa is a collection of specialized cells of the distal tubule located adjacent to the juxtaglomerular cells between afferent and efferent glomerular arterioles. They stimulate renin production by the JG cells when they sense decreases in tubular sodium.

Renin produced proceeds to activation of the potent vasoconstrictor, angiotensin II, (Chart 7-1, page 159) and angiotensin II in turn proceeds to production of Angiotensin III. Both angiotensins are vasoconstrictors and both stimulate aldosterone production by the adrenals. **Aldosterone increases Na^+ reabsorption in the distal tubule and is the regulator of renal sodium excretion.**

The glomerular filtrate contains approximately 26,000mEq of sodium each day. In the **proximal convoluted tubule 60-75% is isotonically absorbed** into the tubular cells. About 85% of the excreted $NaHCO_3$ is absorbed in the same segment. In the **ascending loop of Henle another 20-25% is passively reabsorbed** by following the active transport of Cl^- from tubular fluid to tubular cell. About 5-10% of the sodium in the glomerular filtrate is in the distal nephron. The amount excreted depends, in the main, on aldosterone which acts on the distal nephron and the collecting ducts. It can reduce sodium excretion to 1mEq/day. The amount of Na^+ excreted

Chart 13-7: ADH AND ALDOSTERONE INTERACTIONS FOR RESTORATION AND PRESERVATION OF THE ECF OSMOTIC PRESSURE

Control and preservation of ECF osmotic pressure is effected in the distal nephron and collecting ducts by the integrated actions of antidiuretic hormone (ADH) and aldosterone.

Water: The glomerular filtrate is about 180L/day. When it reaches the distal nephron and collecting ducts only 5-10% remains unabsorbed. ADH acts in this area by varying water excretion and reabsorption. An increase in ADH activity increases water reabsorption. A decrease allows water excretion. Absence of ADH, as in diabetes insipidus can result in a daily urine volume of 18L or more.

ADH production and delivery depend on reflexes centered on hypothalamic osmoreceptors and cerebral thirst mechanisms

Sodium: The glomerular filtrate contains about 126,000mEq/day. Of this only 5-10% remains when the filtrate reaches the distal nephron and collecting ducts. Aldosterone controls what is retained or excreted. The amount excreted can be as low as 1mEq/day or up to 400mEq/day if the diet contains lots of salt.

In summary, the mechanisms are as follows. When the macula densa senses low Na^+ in the tubular fluid it stimulates the JG cells to produce renin. Angiotensin and aldosterone production follow. Aldosterone acts on the sodium remnant in the distal nephron and collecting ducts by increasing sodium retention. A decrease or inhibition of aldosterone by a competitive antagonist such as spironolactone results in decreased reabsorption and increased excretion of Na^+.

Hypotonic ECF. Decreased ADH activity results in increased water excretion and increased aldosterone activity increases sodium retention.

↑

ADH and Aldosterone.

Integrated interactions for excretions and reabsorptions of water and sodium in the distal tubule and collecting ducts to preserve ECF osmotic isotonicity and equivalence with the ICF.

↓

Hypertonic ECF. Increased ADH activity decreases water excretion and decreased aldosterone production results in increased sodium excretion.

Isotonic ECF.

Same osmotic pressure as ICF (and incidentally of intravasular fluid). If there have been water and electrolyte losses the now isotonic ECF and intravascular fluid is often contracted.

If water and elctrolyte losses remain uncorrected the decreased intravascular volume can result in hypotension, a rapid pulse and deficits of cerebral perfusion with blood. Without corrections of water and salt deficits this hypoperfusion will progress to confusion, hallucinations, coma and finally, cerebral failure and death.

can be as high as 400mEq/day if the intake of salt is high, or there is disease of the adrenals such as Addison's disease which results in decreased or absent aldosterone production.

Renal interactions of ADH and aldosterone.

The distal nephron contains approximately 5-10% of unabsorbed water and unabsorbed sodium in the glomerular filtrate. Changes in this small portion of the glomerular filtrate determines the osmotic pressure of the ECF. The main mediators of control are ADH and aldosterone (Chart 13-7). Regardless of whether the losses are hypotonic, isotonic or hypertonic the end result of the ADH-aldosterone interactions should be restoration of the isotonicity of the ECF. If there have been losses of water and electrolytes from the body restoration of the isotonicity of the ECF will result in a reduction of volume and consequently the volumes of both interstitial and intravascular fluids will decrease. The reduction of intravascular volume will result in hypovolemia, hypotension, a rapid pulse and increased respiratory rate. The deficits of water and electrolytes must be replaced to avoid the consequences of cerebral hypoperfusion. The consequences of not replacing lost water and electrolytes are detailed in Chart 13-7; confusions, hallucinations, coma and eventual death. Cerebral failure is a too frequent end result of gastroenteritis in untreated children.

In the final analysis, renal function is the principal factor maintaining the osmotic pressure of the ECF. When the kidneys are diseased no amount of shuffling from one compartment of the body fluids to another will be able to maintain life. The alternatives are renal dialysis or a slow demise.

The role of atrial naturiuretic peptide (ANP)

ANP (de Bold, A.J., Borenstein, H.B. et al. A rapid and potent naturiuretic response to intravenous injection of atrial myocardial extract in rats. Life Sci. 1981; 5:28) is produced by atrial myocytes in response to atrial distension and also blood angiotensin II. It inhibits release or actions of aldosterone, angiotensin II and renin. It also increases salt and water excretion. In responses to water and elctrolyte losses important factors could be its release in response to angiotensin II and its ability to increase water and salt excretion. It would seem to interfere withe optimal functioning of the renin-angiotensin-aldosterone system. However, it is probably only a modulatory component of the main ADH-aldosterone interaction. In any case atrial distension is not a feature of water and electrolyte depletions though changes in renin and angiotensin levels are of consequence.

Assessment of body sodium deficiencies.

Renal mechanisms maintain the isotonicity of the ECF but often with contractions in volume. Hence, even if there are sodium deficits the serum sodium level may remain unchanged. A more appropriate estimation of a sodium deficit is the hematocrit which is the percentage of blood volume occupied by red cells.

Potassium balance

Potassium is widely distributed in foods. Hence, intake deficits are only seen in subnutrition and starvation, in some chronic gastrointestinal disturbances, in chronic alcoholics, and in patients on continuous intravenous fluids not supplemented with potassium.

The clinical consequences of potassium deficiency or excess are insidious and potentially life-threatening. Physiological levels of serum potassium are important for the normal functioning of smooth, skeletal and cardiac muscle. Most body potassium is in the ICF but the more physiologically important portion is in the ECF (3.5-5.5mEq/L).

The regulation of body potassium is mainly dependent on renal control; normal gastrointestinal and skin losses are negligible (approximately 10-15mEq per day). Renal excretion is about 80-100mEq per day. About 900mEq are filtered at the glomerulus each day. Most is reabsorbed in the proximal tubule (about 800-850mEq per day). **The distal nephron maintains potassium homeostasis by absorbing all but about 1% of what remains. It can also secrete potassium; normally about 100mEq daily but when necessary, up to 20% of the amount filtered at the glomerulus.**

K^+ excretion is increased in diabetic acidosis because the increase in circulating keto-acids is accompanied by increased K^+ excretion to maintain the electrical neutrality of the ECF.

Reasons for the dissimilar concentrations of K^+ in the ECF and ICF

The sodium pump. This cell membrane enzyme system pumps three Na^+ out of the cell for every two K^+ let in. One consequence is the intracellular electronegativity which is the basis for initiation and transmission of nerve impulses, and for reception of neurotransmitter-mediated commands.

The H^+ concentration. If there is acidosis H^+ enters the cell to be buffered and K^+ exits to maintain the electrical neutrality of the ECF.

Insulin. An increase in serum K^+ stimulates release of insulin which in turn promotes potassium uptake by muscle and liver cells. Decreased insulin secretion may result in increased serum potassium and the clinical features of hyperkalemia (described later). In the recovery phase of diabetic ketoacidosis injections of insulin force K^+ into cells and this often results in hypokalemia.

Aldosterone. An increase in serum potassium will increase aldosterone secretion. Aldosterone promotes the entry of potassium into cells and also increases renal excretion of the ion because of sodium retention.

Hypokalemia (i.e., a serum potassium less than 3.5mEq/L).

The following are some of the more common causes of hypokalemia.

Deficient intake. The causes include subnutrition and starvation, prolonged intravenous infusions with fluids not supplemented with potassium, and chronic alcoholism.

Diabetic acidosis. The increase in acetoacetate and hydroxybutyrate delivered to the kidney is not equaled, at least initially, by increased generation and excretion of ammonia. There is increased excretion of Na^+ and K^+ to preserve electrical neutrality.

Initial treatment consists of rehydration with isotonic saline and reduction of blood sugar with insulin. Insulin moves potassium into cells so that ECF hypokalemia, if not present initially, frequently develops after the first few hours of treatment. As a rule, if potassium cannot be taken orally, intravenous supplementation becomes necessary. Repeated ECG monitoring is essential for the control of blood potassium levels.

Vomiting, diarrhea and fistula formation. The amounts of K^+ in intestinal fluids is not large. However two factors contribute to K^+ deficiencies in these conditions. The first is increased aldosterone secretion. This increases renal potassium loss. The other is the loss of HCl and Na^+ in vomit resulting in an alkalemia. The plasma bicarbonate rises and the bicarbonate filtered at the glomerulus exceeds the capacity of the kidney for its reabsorption. There is increased secretion of K^+ at the distal nephron to preserve electrical neutrality and ECF hypokalemia results.

Uncommon renal and other conditions. Some examples are the Types 1 and 2 renal tubular acidoses, the late diuretic recovery phase of acute tubular necrosis, and familial periodic paralysis where potassium moves into cells after a carbohydrate meal

Clinical features of hypokalemia.

The clinical setting and findings should raise suspicion. Serum potassium levels are usually decreased but serum levels of potassium may not correlate with a clinically serious situation. At times clinical and ECG changes are better correlates. A low potassium due to diuretics or diabetic ketoacidosis is common.

The clinical features of hypokalemia include muscle weakness and flaccidity, intestinal ileus and distention of the colon, loss of reflexes and eventual paralysis. The ECG changes include decreased T wave amplitudes and the appearance of U waves (the U wave is an upward deflection from the isoelectric line after the T wave). The latter may become prominent with associated ST segment depression and inversion of the T wave. Ectopic activity involving atria and/or ventricles may appear later, especially if the patient is on digitalis. The final fatal conclusion could be an episode of ventricular fibrillation.

Hyperkalemia.

This is an insidious condition, often difficult to recognize, and potentially lethal. The following are some of the more common causes:

Over-treatment of hypokalemia. Oral replacement of potassium losses is always preferable to intravenous replacement. Whatever method of replacement is used repeated ECG and blood monitoring are essential to exclude hyperkalemia.

Chronic renal failure: A glomerular filtration rate as low as 5ml per minute is often sufficient to excrete the usual daily load of potassium. Any additional load as from increased intake or the increased catabolism associated with infections, fever, tissue damage or necrosis, hemorrhage or acidosis, may exceed the capacity of a diseased kidney to excrete enough potassium and result in hyperkalemia. Diuretics which inhibit potassium excretion (e.g., spironolactone and triamterene) can potentiate this effect.

Other renal causes.

Hyperkalemia is frequent in the early oliguric phase of renal failure due to acute tubular necrosis. It may complicate renal disease such as interstitial nephritis, or dysfunctions resulting from aldosterone deficits, muscle and/or tissue damage or necrosis, hemolysis of red cells in large hematomas, and acidosis from various causes.

Clinical features of hyperkalemia.

The clinical setting, the results of laboratory estimations and ECGs are the usual diagnostic criteria. The effects on skeletal and cardiac muscle are reductions of the resting potential of cells with consequent neuromuscular irritability which can proceed to depolarization block with paralysis affecting both skeletal and cardiac muscle. The cardiac manifestations include bradycardia, hypotension, and eventually, ventricular fibrillation and cardiac arrest. The ECG changes include tall, peaked, slender and symmetrical T waves. Later, the PR interval and the QRS duration are prolonged. The QRS complex is not symmetrical, often with one or more shoulders. Atrial and ventricular ectopic beats are common. Eventually, at about 10mEq/L the P waves disappear, the heart slows with wide QRS complexes and eventually there is asystole.

Treatment.

Rapid, vigorous and effective treatment is essential. Available therapy includes injections of calcium gluconate, intravenous sodium bicarbonate which causes potassium to move into cells, and intravenous glucose which raises insulin levels and in this way forces potassium into cells. However, deficits of insulin production may coexist with the hyperkalemia and many clinicians add a small amount of insulin (5-10 units of soluble insulin) to the glucose infusion. Finally, in acute situations where a high potassium does not respond to the above measures hemodialysis is required. After an acute phase has been controlled an oral cation resin such as Kayexalate can often control serum potassium levels. It is a polystyrene sulfonate resin which removes potassium from the body by a sodium-potassium exchange system.

Hydrogen ion controls - the normal and the dysfunctions

The sources of hydrogen ion are:

- **Volatile acid which is carbon dioxide,** a product of tissue metabolism. When hydrated it forms H_2CO_3 which dissociates to H^+ and HCO_3^-.
- **Fixed acid** which is derived from catabolism of sulfur-containing amino acids. The daily production is approximately 1mEq/Kg per day. Fixed acids cannot be removed by the lungs and must be excreted by the kidneys. Other sources of fixed acids are the ketoacids of uncontrolled diabetes, and lactic acid produced during vigorous and prolonged exercise. Removal of fixed acids from the body results in loss of bicarbonate in the glomerular filtrate. This bicarbonate must be recovered and complex renal mechanisms exist for this purpose (described later in this chapter).

Carbon dioxide removal.

Ambient air is virtually free of CO_2 (Chart 10-2, page 225). The pCO_2 of alveolar air is 40 mm Hg because it mixes with residual air in the lungs. Arterial blood has about the same tension. Intracellular pCO_2 is higher so that CO_2 diffuses into venous blood which acquires a pCO_2 of about 46 mm Hg. The venous return to the heart enters the pulmonary arteries via the right atrium and the tricuspid valve. Blood perfusing the lungs has a pCO_2 of 46mm Hg. The difference of about 6mm Hg between the pulmonary arterial blood pCO_2 of 46mmHg and alveolar pCO_2 of 40mmHg. results in pulmonary elimination of about 210 ml CO_2/min by diffusion along the concentration gradient.

The buffers.

Between production of H^+ ion and its removal from the body there must be mechanisms for preventing unacceptable changes in the pH of body fluids. This is done by binding H^+ to buffers. The principal intracellular buffers are proteins and phosphates. There is some extracellular buffering by the plasma proteins but the carbonic acid-bicarbonate buffer system and hemoglobin are the most important buffers of the extracellular fluids.

About 5-8 % of the CO_2 which enters venous blood remains in solution in the plasma. About 5-10% combines with hemoglobin to form carbamino-hemoglobin ($HbCO_2$). This reaction is reversible and its direction depends on the pCO_2. An increase drives the reaction to right with production of more $HbCO_2$. A reduction decreases the amount of $HbCO_2$. The rest of the CO_2 enters the red cells (approximately 80% of total CO_2 in the blood) and combines with water to form H_2CO_3. .The reaction is catalyzed by carbonic anhydrase, an enzyme which is plentiful in red cells. Dissociation of H_2CO_3 follows with formation of $H^+$and HCO_3^-. The H^+ combines with hemoglobin to form HHb. The HCO_3^- moves into the plasma along a concentration gradient and Cl^- moves into the erythrocyte to maintain electrical neutrality (the chloride shift).

Like oxygen, the amount of carbon dioxide carried by blood is related to its partial pressure. The relationship is expressed by a CO_2 dissociation curve. The relationship is curvilinear but within the physiological ranges of tensions may be regarded as linear. In addition, the relationship is affected by oxygen tension (called the Haldane effect); the unloading of oxygen in the tissues facilitates the loading of CO_2 there and the opposite occurs in the lungs.

The removal of fixed acids and bicarbonate recovery.

Fixed acid production of H^+ is about 1mEq/Kg per day; about 70mEq/day for a 70Kg man. Additional H^+ derives from any respiratory insufficiency which might exist.

Fixed acids are first buffered by blood bicarbonate. The daily glomerular filtrate contains about 4,500mEq of bicarbonate. Bicarbonate recovery in the kidneys is essential or all bicarbonate would be consumed in a few days.

When serum bicarbonate is less than 26mEq/L almost all is reabsorbed. The process of bicarbonate reabsorption is complex. About 85-90% of bicarbonate is recovered in the proximal tubule by a series of reactions which results in recovery of $NaHCO_3$. In the process Na^+ is extracted from the tubular fluid and H^+ is actively secreted into it. The rest of the bicarbonate is recovered in the distal nephron by many complex reactions.

Phosphate and ammonia control of renal acid excretion.

The kidneys help to maintain body fluid pH at about 7.35-7.45 by reabsorbing bicarbonate and excreting H^+ ions. The maximum amount of free H^+ that can be excreted is limited by the fact that urine pH cannot be reduced below 4.5 by excretion of H^+ alone. This is equal to a urine concentration of less than 1mEq/L of H^+.

H^+ ions which would require a urine pH lower than 4.5 combine with phosphate buffer or secreted ammonia; about ⅓ with the former and ⅔ with the latter. Buffering with phosphate removes H^+ in the distal tubule and also returns bicarbonate to the blood. This replaces bicarbonate used for buffering of fixed acids and not recovered in the proximal tubule.

The phosphate buffering system. Most buffering by phosphate occurs in the distal tubule. H^+ ion is secreted into the urine and Na^+ enters the cell to maintain electrical neutrality. H^+ ion combines with Na_2HPO_4 in the tubule to form NaH_2PO_4 which is excreted as an addition to urine acidity.

The ammonia excretion system is more effective. Ammonia is produced in cells of the renal tubule by removal of amide from glutamine, and also from asparagine and other amino acids. The ammonia is produced in the form of a gas. The gaseous form, NH_3^-, diffuses easily across membranes. The NH_4 form does not. NH_3^- enters the tubule and combines with H^+ ion excreted by the tubular cell. NH_4 is trapped in the lumen and then excreted. When there is chronic acidosis the amount of ammonia produced rises so that it plays a more important role in H^+ ion excretion.

Some clinical dysfunctions of acid-base balance.

A variety of dysfunctions of acid-base balance are described. Chart 13-8 summarizes the causes, clinical features and biochemical changes of the principal ones.

Respiratory acidosis.

Chart 13-8: **A SUMMARY OF THE CLINICAL AND LABORATORY FEATURES OF DIFFERENT ACID-BASE DYSFUNCTIONS [1,2]**

The acid-base dysfunctions	Common causes	Biochemical changes
Respiratory acidosis	Respiratory insufficiency	pCO_2 ↑ ↓ HCO_3^- ↑ ↓ pH normal or ↑
Metabolic acidosis	**Increased H^+:** Diabetic ketoacidosis, lactic acidosis, advanced renal failure, aspirin overdose, accidental or deliberate drinking of methanol or ethylene glycol. Anion gap increased. **Loss of HCO_3^-** : Diarrhea, biliary or pancreatic fistulae, ostomies, renal tubular acidosis, etc. Anion gap normal or decreased.	HCO_3^- ↓ ↓ hyperventilation ↓ pCO_2 ↓ ↓ Eventual fall in pH
Respiratory alkalosis	Usually psychogenic hyperventilation or over-ventilation by a respirator. Other causes are aspirin overdose and advanced CNS and liver disease.	pCO_2 ↓ ↓ HCO_3^- ↓ ↓ Normal or raised pH
Metabolic alkalosis	Vomiting of gastric fluid, excess diuretics such as the thiazides and furosemide (both result in almost equal losses of Na^+ and Cl^-) and rare causes such as hyperaldosteronism and hypercorticism	HCO_3^- ↑ ↓ pCO_2 ↑ ↓ Normal or raised pH

1 pH does not change if buffering is adequate.

2 The anion gap is serum ($Na^+ + K^+$) - ($Cl^- + HCO_3^-$). A raised AG suggests metabolic acidosis due to organic acids; diabetic ketoacidosis, lactic acidosis, uremia and salicylate poisoning are examples. The normal anion gap is about 8-12mmol/L.

Chronic elevations of pCO_2 are often present in patients with lung pathology such as chronic obstructive lung disease. The kidneys respond by increasing excretion of acid with a corresponding increase in bicarbonate reabsorption. The serum bicarbonate is raised and pH increases because of reduced H^+ concentration.

Metabolic acidosis.

The causes are either increased serum H^+ or loss of HCO_3^-. Causes of increased serum H^+ are diabetic keto-acidosis, excessive ingestion of aspirin, advanced renal failure, and lactic acidosis. Common causes for increased HCO_3^- losses are diarrhea, biliary or pancreatic fistulae, various ostomies and uncommon renal diseases such as renal tubular acidosis.

The clinical picture may be one of trivial changes or of extreme dysfunctions. A typical example of severe metabolic acidosis is diabetic ketoacidosis; deep and rapid respirations (Kussmaul breathing), dry mucus membranes, a characteristic fruity odor, and drowsiness leading to coma and death if untreated. Metabolic acidosis is occasionally seen in chronic alcoholics who have deliberately or mistakenly drunk methanol or ethylene glycol. Typically, the pulse is rapid and the blood pressure low, as are the bicarbonate, the pCO_2 and pH.

The anion gap (AG) helps to determine the nature of a metabolic acidosis. It is the sum of measured cations less the algebraic sum of measured ions: $(Na^+ + K^+) - (Cl^- + HCO_3^-)$. The normal value is 8-12mmol/L. It increases when there is a metabolic acidosis due increased H+ production. Chart 13-8 lists the common causes

Therapy of metabolic acidosis always requires that one remembers that correction of acidosis without correction of an associated potassium deficit can result in serious and occasionally fatal consequences from hypokalemia.

Respiratory alkalosis.

The causes include hyperventilation from hysteria or a panic attack, excessive ventilation by respirators, gram negative shock, and occasionally hypermetabolic states such as fever and thyrotoxicosis. The pCO_2 is decreased and the pH increased. The symptoms of hysterical overbreathing are readily relieved by repeated rebreathing into a paper bag.

Metabolic alkalosis.

The two commonest causes are vomiting of gastric contents, or water and salt depletion due to excessive intake of diuretics. Uncommon causes include primary hyperaldosteronism or hyperadrenocorticism.

When associated with contraction of the ECF the pulse is fast, the blood pressure is low, and there is latent tetany. The hematocrit may exceed 50%, serum sodium and potassium are often low, and the blood bicarbonate and pH are increased. Treatment is simple; NaCl solutions and potassium supplements as needed to correct hypokalemia.

Regulation of body temperature.

Most in vitro chemical reactions can be accelerated by heat. In the body this is not possible. Too much heat could denature and inactivate enzymes and too much cold will retard their activities.

Normal body temperature. In humans normal body temperature is 37°C ± 0.2°. Rectal temperature measures core temperature and is usually about 0.5^0C higher than oral temperature. Measurement of temperature by a thermometer placed in the axilla has dubious accuracy.

Control of temperature. Temperature control is determined by a central thermostat in the hypothalamus. Most of the afferent input is determined by temperature sensitive surface and internal receptors. The efferent hypothalamic output is via somatic and autonomic nerves.

The sources of body heat. Heat is a product of the many metabolic activities of normal biology. It is also produced by muscle contraction during exercise and by the calorigenic effects of dysfunctions such as hyperthyroidism.

Mechanisms for responding to temperature change.

Excess heat. Loss of excessive heat is by radiation, direct conduction by contact with cooler surfaces, convection, cutaneous vasodilation and sweating. Sweat cools by vaporization from the body surface - the vaporization of 1g water results in a heat loss of about 0.6KCal heat. Sweating comes in two forms, often, both are active simultaneously. The first is insensible sweating. Normal human insensible sweating measures approximately 500ml per day. Sweating in response to excess heat, as after vigorous exercise in hot environments can amount to more than 1L/hour. Panting also increases heat loss.

Cold. Warming can be achieved in a variety of ways. The following are some examples: cutaneous vasoconstriction, warm clothing, shivering, and reflex increases in catecholamine secretions.

Renal failure.

There are two types of renal failure: acute renal failure which is usually synonymous with acute tubular necrosis or bilateral cortical necrosis, and chronic renal failure which is a frequent end-stage syndrome of diabetic nephropathy, angiosclerotic nephropathy, some cases of polycystic kidneys and miscellaneous primary and secondary glomerulonephritic diseases.

The renal dysfunctions that can result from immunological reactions were detailed in a previous chapter. For now it suffices to state that **acute glomerulonephritis and the renal failure of Goodpasture's disease (Types 3 and 2 adverse immunological reactions: pages 183-185)** can infrequently result in a rapidly progressive form of acute renal failure.

Acute tubular necrosis.

Any one of two pathologies can result in acute tubular necrosis: nephrotoxins or decreased vascular perfusion. The first includes items such as heavy metals and chance reactions to various drugs; e.g., sulfonamides and the aminoglycosides. The second includes shock and prolonged hypovolemia due to any one of many causes; major trauma with muscle damage, blood loss, loss of plasma from extensive burns, intestinal obstructions with fluid segregated in loops of distended bowel and acute gastrointestinal fluid losses from viral or bacterial infections. The essential pathological lesion is tubular cell necrosis. In nephrotoxic acute tubular necrosis death of tubular cells and subsequent regeneration are more easily demonstrable than in the disease which results from hypoperfusion.

Clinical features.

Typically, there are three phases: the oliguric phase followed by the diuretic phase and then a recovery to normal or near normal function. In the **oliguric phase** the urine output falls to less than 20ml/hour. There is uremia with progressively rising serum creatinine and urea, hyperkalemia and acidosis. The patient is easily overhydrated. The possibility of fatal infections are always present and the patient looks and feels ill, vomits and has frequent nausea. Another hazard is gastrointestinal bleeding. Renal dialysis is often needed in the oliguric phase to control hazardous biochemical changes such as hyperkalemia.

The oliguric phase usually lasts 7-10 days. If the duration exceeds 3 weeks a biopsy is advisable to exclude bilateral cortical necrosis as the cause of oliguria or anuria. Its causes are similar to those of acute tubular necrosis but recovery does not follow. The patient will require long-term dialysis and when possible, available and acceptable, an eventual renal transplant.

The **diuretic phase** begins as the tubular epithelium regenerates. At first there is diuresis because the ability to concentrate urine is absent or decreased. Large amounts of sodium and potassium may be lost and careful monitoring and fluid replacements are necessary at this stage. This phase may last up to two weeks or so.

Eventually there is **recovery of renal function**. It might not be complete but will usually provide adequate renal function. The treatment of acute tubular necrosis requires careful monitoring of water intake, diet and calories, electrolyte intake, and supplementary dialysis as and when needed. The expectation is that appropriate supplementary treatment will prevent death till the kidneys recover.

Chronic renal failure.

Causes. The common causes are end-stage diabetic nephropathy, arteriosclerotic nephrosclerosis, any one of the glomerular nephropathies, nephrotic syndromes and end-stage polycystic kidney disease. Acute and progressive failure can be precipitated in a previously stable dysfunction by any one or more of the following: fever, infections of any sort, anemia, endocrine dysfunctions such as thyrotoxicosis, excessive intake of water and/or salt, and binge eating and binge drinking of alcohol. Nephrotoxins and hypotension and/or hypovolemia can also precipitate failure in a previously stable situation.

Clinical features.

Common symptoms include nausea and vomiting, a loss of appetite and neurological deficits ranging from lethargy and somnolence, twitchings and cramps, to psychotic behavior, with eventual coma and death.

Many abnormalities are seen in the blood and urine; a raised creatinine and urea, sodium depletion, hypokalemia or hyperkalemia, anemia (usually due to a erythropoietin deficit), and an inability to concentrate the urine so that urine osmolarity is fixed near the level in plasma (~300mOsm/L). Urinary casts of different types are frequent.

An abnormal bleeding tendency is frequent as is congestive heart failure due to water and sodium retention by the kidney. An increased intake of calories is often needed but with protein restriction. Endogenous protein catabolism is reduced if the diet has little protein but enough fat and carbohydrate to meet energy requirements.

Chronic renal failure often ends with chronic dialysis and a subsequent renal transplant if an organ is available and suitable. Alternatively, there is progression to death if the patient does not meet the requirements to qualify for a transplant or does not wish to continue dialysis or succumbs to some cardiac catastrophe.

The generated responses to acute hypovolemia.

This chapter would not be complete without a summary of the physiological responses to acute hypovolemia. Sudden hypovolemia can result from loss of blood, loss of plasma as in severe burns, or loss of body water and electrolytes in severe gastroenteritis or from sequestrations of fluids in dilated adynamic, obstructed, or devascularized loops of bowel.

The response to an acute hemorrhage typifies the response to sudden hypovolemia. Initially, the responses are primarily directed to maintaining cerebral perfusion with oxygen and glucose. The sequential responses are as follows:

The immediate response is rapid and starts in about fifteen seconds of an acute fall in blood pressure. It is mediated by the neuromediators of autonomic nerve impulses and results in peripheral vasoconstriction and tachycardia and an increase in the respiratory rate. The reflexes are optimal in specific blood pressure ranges. Those mediated by baroreceptors and chemoreceptors in the 80+mm Hg range, by chemoreceptors alone in the 40-80mm Hg range and by the central nervous system response to brain stem ischemia in the <50mm Hg range.

The next stage begins within a minute or so of the hemorrhage and continues till blood pressure is restored. There are two mechanisms:

First, the renin-angiotensin vasoconstriction. A fall in blood pressure results in renin release from the kidneys and the subsequent conversion of plasma substrate to active angiotensin: a potent vasoconstrictor.

Second, the passive transvascular fluid movements. When blood pressure falls below normal fluid passively moves from extracellular fluid to the intravascular compartment as transvascular Starling forces change. This mainly takes place in the peripheral capillaries.

The next stage is one of stabilization and return to normal. The previously produced **angiotensin** stimulates aldosterone secretion. The result is retention of water and salt and an increase in extracellular fluid.

The final stage is stimulation of erythropoietin production because of renal hypoxia. There is increased red cell maturation and production till eventually, normal blood values return.

Therapeutic options for corrections of water and electrolyte dysfunctions

Most of the therapeutic options have been mentioned in the text, The diuretics and the solutions available for intravenous therapy are the main therapeutic options for maintenance of homeostasis when abnormal conditions prevail.

Diuretics.

The loop diuretics such as thiazide and furosemide. The loop diuretics inhibit the Cl^- egress from the tubule in the ascending loop of Henle.. Na^+ remains in the tubule and this results in diuresis. Different diuretics inhibit in different areas; metolazone and the thiazide diuretics in areas which are not the same as those where furosemide acts. Hence, useful additive effects can be obtained in difficult situations by using diuretic combinations which act in different ways and in different parts of the loop of Henle.

Spironolactone and **Triamterene** are competitive antagonists of aldosterone at the distal tubule and in this way promotes sodium excretion. They may result in hyperkalemia.

Solutions for intravenous therapy.

A 70Kg resting individual needs about 2L fluid daily to compensate for water losses from skin and lungs and to provide enough water to excrete the daily load of solute. Obviously the amounts needed increase if there is fever, trauma, severe infections or if the individual is in a postoperative phase.

The amounts of water and salt lost in water and salt deficiency syndromes are not constant or predictable. At times more water is lost and at other times the opposite occurs. If renal compensation is normal the result will be an isotonic but contracted ECF and intravascular fluid compartment.

Isotonic sodium chloride (0.9%NaCl) provides the principal extracellular ion in physiological concentration. It is the parenteral solution of choice when adequate oral rehydration is not possible because of vomiting, an inability to drink the large amounts needed or semicomatose or comatose states (e.g., in diabetic ketoacidosis). The solution is readily absorbed when given subcutaneously if a vein cannot be found or the child or adult resists the intravenous infusion. No untoward effects occur if given subcutaneously as long as there are no additives which can cause inflammatory effects. Glucose and potassium must never be added to saline solutions which are to be given subcutaneously. The subcutaneous route has a certain safety as the bump produced by the injection is readily absorbed if dehydration is severe. Apart from the needle prick it is painless and can be given two to three times in 24 hours; about 50ml each time depending on the size of the child. The rate at which the bump decreases slows as hydration improves.

Mixed sodium chloride and glucose solutions are often used when dehydration is stabilized but oral hydration is not possible for any one of many reasons, especially in the postoperative period after abdominal surgery. At this stage the favorite of many physicians is 5% dextrose in 0.45% saline. The solution is slightly hypertonic (406mOsm/L). It pulls fluid and electrolytes from the interstitial fluid into the intravascular compartment. The effects are stabilization of blood pressure, an increased urinary output and reduced edema if any exists. It should not be given if there is any evidence of intracellular dehydration. It has the advantage over isotonic saline of providing some calories, but only 170KCal/L.

Dextrose solution (5%) is given when there has not been any significant electrolyte loss and only water needs replacement. They replace water and provide some calories.

Intravenous alimentation. If intravenous therapy extends over 4-5 days intravenous alimentation must be considered to provide the necessary daily caloric requirements of the patient.

Potassium supplements. As far as possible oral replacement therapy is best. Potassium is available in tablet or liquid form. Potassium for intravenous use usually comes as a 10% solution of potassium chloride. If the intravenous route is used 10-20mEq per hour should not be exceeded. Regular monitoring of serum potassium levels and ECGs is desirable. Intravenous potassium is not routinely needed except in conditions such as diabetic ketoacidosis where the keto acids require increased excretion of K^+ and insulin injections promote entry of K^+ into cells.

This ends the chapter on the slave systems that maintain homeostasis.

14

Diagnosis: The Slave Systems

6. The Musculoskeletal System

Table of Contents

Notation.

The notation ~P denotes phosphorous with a high energy bond. Depending on the context in which the term is used, ~P may also denote the energy liberated when a high energy phosphate bond detaches from ATP or ADP.

General comments.

The comments made on page 119 about the methodologies of clinical assessments are not repeated. They merit reading before proceeding with this chapter.

The musculoskeletal system is a slave system controlled by the brain and spinal cord, hormones and microenvironmental control systems. Bone and joint dysfunctions are too numerous to detail, except in summary. Any of the causes of disease detailed on pages 75 and 76 can affect bones and joints. The more common dysfunctions are detailed here but the text concentrates on the basic physiology of bone. Comparisons of clinical findings with these facts will provide the bases for diagnostic suspicions, diagnoses, assessment of the qualitatives of dysfunction and the responses to therapy.

Bones are levers which articulate with each other at joints. Muscles attach to bones and their contractions move bones at their articulations with joints. Most striated muscle contractions are responses to commands from the CNS, or to reflexes with center points in the brain or spinal cord. The end result of all these activities is the smooth, precise, purposeful and coordinated movements of animates, and the maintenance of static postures and of balance and postures during movements.

Bone must have tensile strength to bend and spring back, and lightness and resistance to stress. It cannot be so brittle that slight stress would normally result in a fracture. The histologies of bone satisfy these requirements.

Bone is also important for eating as this requires movements to obtain food and then transfer it to the mouth by hands or utensils. It requires precise and complex movements of the hands and joints of the upper body. Bone and related joints are also needed for ingestion and mastication of food.

Bones provide the rigid but mobile frame which is essential for the respiratory oxygenation of blood and exhalation of carbon dioxide. In addition bones provide the anatomical arrangements for orderly transport of ingested material from one metabolic area to another. The aorta is attached to a bony framework of vertebrae and the viscera hang from vessels emerging from this large vessel. Bone also protects viscera, vascular structures and of special importance is its provision of a rigid covering which protects the brain.

Bone structure.

Normal bone has six components: the matrix, the minerals, osteoblasts, osteoclasts, the Sharpey's fibers and blood vessels.

The matrix. Approximately 95% of the matrix is Type 1 collagen fibers. The rest is mineral, mainly a complex crystalline hydroxyapatite which is a complex of calcium and phosphorous obtained from the blood. It constitutes about half the weight of normal adult bone (Chart 14-1). The crystals are deposited along the collagen fibrils. Control of mineral synthesis is by the effects of vitamin D, by parathyroid hormone and to a lesser degree, by estrogens and growth factors.

The osteoblasts produce the collagen fibers and ground substance of the matrix and are also responsible for calcification along the collagen fibers and in the matrix. They can secrete and also absorb the matrix. Osteoblasts are located in the matrix or on the surfaces of osteoid. They form collagen I which comprises some 90-95% of the organic component of bone. It is deposited in a multilayer weave pattern when bone formation is rapid as it is in the fetus. Woven bone is also characteristic of pathologies such as hyperparathyroidism and fibrous dysplasia. Mature bone has collagen deposited in concentric or parallel layers.

Osteoblast activity is controlled by parathyroid hormone, estrogen and growth factors. They have receptors for these substances. Physical activity is another stimulator of osteoblast activity.

The osteoclasts are large multinucleated cells, probably derived from monocytes. They break down the matrix by secreting osteolytic agents such as lysozymes, hydrolytic enzymes and other chemicals.

They can absorb bone, and are usually multinucleated cells located in Howship lacunae which are small spaces where bone absorption is occurring. Osteoclasts do not have receptors for parathyroid hormone and osteoclast mediated bone absorption probably does not proceed when osteoblasts are absent. Canaliculi allow the processes of osteocytes to interact with each other and with the central Haversian canal.

The Sharpey's fibers anchor ligaments to bones. They are fibers of collagen which extend into bone and become continuous with the collagen fibers of the matrix.

Blood vessels are plentiful in bone. They enter at one or more points on their surfaces and ramify widely in bone via the Haversian and Volkmann's canals.

Compact bone and cancellous bone.

Compact bone is formed of structures called osteons. Each osteon has concentric collagen fibers with a central Haversian canal which contains blood vessels and nerves. To increase strength the long axes of the collagen lamellae of an osteon orient at different angles to each other though the osteon itself is usually oriented parallel to the long axis of the bone. The Haversian canals are linked to form a network of blood vessels by canals which connect them to adjacent canals (the Volkmann's canals).

Cancellous bone is a network of trabeculae with interstices filled with marrow. Its cellular and matrix composition is similar to that of compact bone but the collagen lamellae are not arranged concentrically around a central Haversian canal but usually lie parallel to each other or in other patterns.

In long bones most of the diaphysis is compact bone. A little cancellous bone lines the marrow cavities. The epiphyses are mostly cancellous bone covered by a thin layer of compact bone. The flat bones of the skull are complexes of compact and cancellous bone. A layer of compact bone covers the upper and under surfaces with a layer of cancellous bone between.

Turnover and remodeling of bone.

Bone turnover and remodeling occurs throughout life with areas of focal bone removal by osteoclasts and formation of new bone by osteoblasts. Total bone mass increases as the individual matures. It remains constant for the next two to three decades and then, after the age of 40 or 50 begins to decline. Over the next three or

Chart 14-1: FACTORS AFFECTING BONE FORMATION AND LOSS

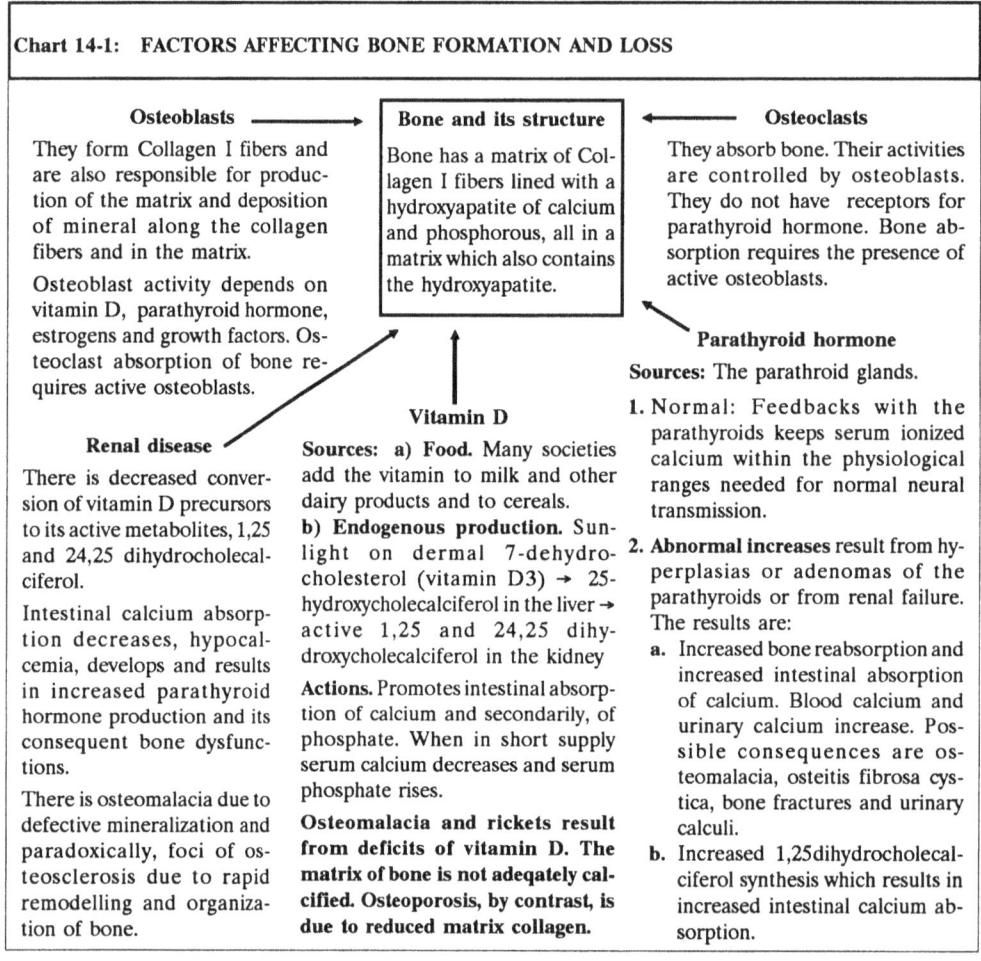

Osteoblasts →

They form Collagen I fibers and are also responsible for production of the matrix and deposition of mineral along the collagen fibers and in the matrix.

Osteoblast activity depends on vitamin D, parathyroid hormone, estrogens and growth factors. Osteoclast absorption of bone requires active osteoblasts.

Bone and its structure

Bone has a matrix of Collagen I fibers lined with a hydroxyapatite of calcium and phosphorous, all in a matrix which also contains the hydroxyapatite.

← **Osteoclasts**

They absorb bone. Their activities are controlled by osteoblasts. They do not have receptors for parathyroid hormone. Bone absorption requires the presence of active osteoblasts.

Renal disease

There is decreased conversion of vitamin D precursors to its active metabolites, 1,25 and 24,25 dihydrocholecalciferol.

Intestinal calcium absorption decreases, hypocalcemia, develops and results in increased parathyroid hormone production and its consequent bone dysfunctions.

There is osteomalacia due to defective mineralization and paradoxically, foci of osteosclerosis due to rapid remodelling and organization of bone.

Vitamin D

Sources: a) Food. Many societies add the vitamin to milk and other dairy products and to cereals.
b) Endogenous production. Sunlight on dermal 7-dehydrocholesterol (vitamin D3) → 25-hydroxycholecalciferol in the liver → active 1,25 and 24,25 dihydroxycholecalciferol in the kidney

Actions. Promotes intestinal absorption of calcium and secondarily, of phosphate. When in short supply serum calcium decreases and serum phosphate rises.

Osteomalacia and rickets result from deficits of vitamin D. The matrix of bone is not adeqately calcified. Osteoporosis, by contrast, is due to reduced matrix collagen.

Parathyroid hormone

Sources: The parathroid glands.

1. Normal: Feedbacks with the parathyroids keeps serum ionized calcium within the physiological ranges needed for normal neural transmission.
2. **Abnormal increases** result from hyperplasias or adenomas of the parathyroids or from renal failure. The results are:
   a. Increased bone reabsorption and increased intestinal absorption of calcium. Blood calcium and urinary calcium increase. Possible consequences are osteomalacia, osteitis fibrosa cystica, bone fractures and urinary calculi.
   b. Increased 1,25dihydrocholecalciferol synthesis which results in increased intestinal calcium absorption.

four decades the decline in bone mass could amount to 30-50% of skeletal mass. The decline seems to be faster in women than in men. Studies with radioactive calcium and quantitative x-rays suggest that the bone mass decrease results from increased osteoclastic activity while the rate of new bone formation by osteoblasts is at the levels found in normal adults.

The synovium.

Bones articulate at joints. The articular surfaces are covered with cartilage which does not have a perichondrium and are joined to each other by a capsule. The outer layers of the capsule are fibrous tissue which usually extend some distance along the diaphysis of the bones. The innermost layer is the synovial membrane. It lines the inner surface of the capsule and is reflected onto bones up to their articular cartilages. The synovial membrane is a sheet of connective tissue, abundantly supplied with blood vessels and nerves. It has cells that secrete the hyaluronic acid which lubricates joint surfaces. It also has cells which phagocytose unwanted materials and debris.

Parathyroid hormone.

This hormone is produced by the parathyroid glands. It increases blood calcium by its actions on bone, kidney and intestine. The hormone increases urinary phosphate excretion and increases Ca^{++} absorption in the distal tubule. It also increases 1,25-dihydroxycholecalciferol synthesis. The active metabolites of 1,25-dihydroxycholecalciferol increase the intestinal absorption of Ca^{++}. Normal blood levels of serum ionized calcium are essential for orderly conduction of nerve impulses.

Control of parathyroid hormone production and of blood calcium levels is by a simple feedback mechanism between the two. The blood component of this feedback system is the level of serum ionized calcium and the parathyroid component is a cell membrane Ca^{++} receptor.

Vitamin D.

Sources: Food is a poor source of Vitamin D (fish liver oils are not a favored food). Hence, many societies add the vitamin to milk, dairy products and cereals to compensate for environments which lack adequate sunlight or exclude sunlight because of social customs (e.g., those wearing the head to toe purdah). Sunlight is an important requirement for an adequacy of Vitamin D; rickets has been described as a common disease of "smokey cities and cloudy skies".

Vitamin D_3 (cholecalciferol) is produced in the skin by the effects of sunlight on 7-dehydrocholesterol. Vitamin D_3 is converted to 25-hydroxycholecalciferol in the liver. Next the kidney converts 25-hydroxycholecalciferol to the biologically active metabolites of Vitamin D: 1,25 and 24,25 dihydroxycholecalciferol.

The active metabolites of vitamin D promote intestinal and renal absorption of calcium. When they are in short supply intestinal absorption of calcium decreases and serum calcium decreases. The serum phosphate rises but the serum calcium decreases to levels which do not permit adequate mineralization of osteoid. The decreased serum calcium increases parathyroid hormone secretion and the result could be the superimposed changes of osteitis fibrosa. The vitamin increases osteoblast activity and is needed for matrix calcification

Calcium homeostasis.

The calcium content of a young adult is 1000-1500g. The skeleton contains 99% of this calcium while about 1% is in the blood. Some of the blood calcium binds with protein. The remainder is in an ionized unbound form (2.2-2.5mmol/L). This ionized unbound calcium is a requirement for normal nerve transmission, muscle contraction and blood clotting.

About 100mmol of bone calcium is exchangeable with calcium in blood. There is a to-and-fro movement of about 500mmol between bone and blood calcium each day. The remaining 27,000-28,000mmol of bone calcium is not exchangeable with calcium in the blood. It is used for the repeated internal reabsorptions and depositions of bone.

Calcium enters the blood from absorbed food content and from the bone. It is lost in urine and feces, by deposition in bone, and a little is lost in sweat. Estimates are that about 500mg calcium enter and leave the skeleton each day.

Almost all (98-99%) of the calcium in the glomerular filtrate is reabsorbed; about 60% in the proximal tubule and the remainder in the loop of Henle and distal tubule. The latter portion is subject to parathyroid hormone regulation.

About 50% of the calcium in blood is not bound to plasma proteins. This is the biologically important component. A decrease increases neuromuscular irritability and may induce tetany. The principal danger from tetany is development of bronchospasm and laryngeal spasm. The Chvostek and Trousseau signs are positive and the ECG Q-T interval increases.

In sum, two items are needed for calcium homeostasis and regulation: parathyroid hormone and vitamin D.

Some bone and joint dysfunctions.

Fractures.

The most common bone dysfunction is a fracture due to trauma. Pathological fractures are fractures due to pre-existing disease. The commonest cause is a metastatic malignancy. Other cause include the fractures of osteoporosis and osteomalacia, fractures due to benign tumors and cysts and primary malignant bone tumors. Another cause is an excess production of parathyroid hormone which results in osteomalacia or osteitis fibrosa cystica. Finally, some rare bone dysfunctions that cause pathological fractures are genetically determined. Examples are the dysfunctions of osteogenesis imperfecta which are the result of mutations affecting production of Collagen I. An example is fragilitas ossium.

A fracture is a break in bone. Various terms are used to describe the anatomical features of a fracture: fractures without displacement; with or without impaction; comminuted fractures (a fracture with multiple fragments); stress fractures (fractures resulting from repeated stresses on a normal bone such as a metatarsal); compound fractures (fractures where the overlying skin is open because of the nature of the trauma and/or because of penetration of overlying skin by one or more fragments of the fracture); and pathological fractures which are fractures resulting from existing bone pathology.

The process of repair begins with invasion of the blood clot by granulation tissue which is arcades of new capillaries with interspersed fibroblasts. Adjacent periosteal osteoblasts proliferate and deposit osteoid in the granulation tissue. Next, the osteoid is mineralized and forms a bridge of woven bone immobilizing the fractured bone surfaces. Finally, the woven bone is replaced by lamellar bone. Firm union is established and remodeling by osteoclasts and osteoblasts restores a contour which resembles, but usually not exactly, the original contours.

The complications of fracture healing.

Many factors affect the speed and effectiveness of repair: the type of fracture; its severity; the correct choice and application of therapy; the presence of infection; the age of the patient; the vascularization of the area; subnutrition and malnutrition; concomitant unrelated disease (some examples are diabetes, infections, anemia, and chronic cardiac, neurological, pulmonary, renal or hepatic disease); and pathology affecting the bone and causing the fracture, especially metastatic or primary malignant bone tumors.

Each type of fracture has specific therapeutic requirements. The basic one is immobilization till there is union unless dealing with a fracture which needs no treatment, e.g., the stress fracture of a metatarsal. Methods of immobilization range from strapping, immobilization in a plaster cast and, when appropriate, surgical stabilization with metallic plates and pins.

Malunion, delayed union or non-union are usually the result of inappropriate alignment, inadequate or insufficiently long immobilization, or unsuspected interposition of soft tissues between the fractured surfaces. Other contributing factors are infections of the fracture site, bone necrosis, and underlying bone disease such as tumor.

Metabolic bone disease.

There are many causes of metabolic bone disease. The principal ones are osteoporosis and osteomalacia.

Osteopenia and osteoporosis.

Osteopenia describes radiologically demonstrable loss of bone density. The causes include:

- Disuse atrophy.
- Osteoporosis.
- Osteomalacia and rickets.

- Endocrine disease and other chronic diseases (e.g., hypercortisolism and hypogonadism, hyperthroid disease and hyperparathyroidism, chronic renal failure and malabsorption syndromes).
- Subnutrition and malnutrition, especially scurvy from vitamin C deficits.
- Diffuse metastatic malignant disease, leukemia and multiple myeloma.
- Corticosteroids.
- Rare hereditary diseases (e.g., the osteogenisis imperfecta variants).

Osteoporosis.

Osteoporosis is a common disease, often with disabling consequences because it is the cause of many of the fractures of elderly people.

Osteoporosis is a decrease in bone density due to a decrease of collagenous bone matrix. The bone itself is mineralized normally. As mentioned previously, the disease results from decreased osteoblast activity but enough remains for continued osteoclastic bone absorption. The end result is gradual reduction in the collagenous framework of bone. The condition is more common in elderly females than in males. It is postulated that the reason is reduction of estrogen in postmenopausal women with concurrent reduction in osteoblast activity; osteoblasts have receptors for estrogen. The symptoms and complications include the following:

- Fractures, especially collapse fractures of vertebral bodies and fractures of the wrist (Colle's fracture) and hip.
- Back pain, often of recent onset, gradual decreases in height, and a progressive thoracic kyphosis.

Routine laboratory investigations are usually normal but radionuclear scans show the characteristic features of osteoporosis. They also provide some information about the immediate risk for femoral neck and wrist fractures.

Therapy for osteoporosis is often disappointing. The numbers of claims for therapeutic benefits of different agents is legion. Equally numerous are claims which refute. **Estrogen** does help to prevent progression and to stimulate osteoblastic activity but the results of recent studies on hormone replacement for postmenopausal symptoms preclude its use. Contrary claims have been made about the value of **calcium and vitamin D** administration in individuals with osteoporosis; Chapuy and associates have claimed a beneficial effect[1] but Lips and associates dispute this claim[2].

Similar conflicting claims have been made for the **biphosphonates** such as etidronate, alendronate and many others. These drugs have an affinity for bone apatite and are potent inhibitors of bone reabsorption. They do seem to slow progression but restoration to normality does not occur.

Raloxifene (Evista; Lilly) inhibits the action of estrogen on the breast and endometrium. It acts as an estrogen agonist on osteoblasts. The MORE study (Multiple Outcomes of Raloxifene Evaluation)[3] involved 7705 women with osteoporosis. There was a significant reduction in vertebral fractures but no effect on non-vertebral fractures.

It is difficult to know whether or not to give therapy to osteoporotic individuals. Good and harmless advice (unless the patient has lactase deficiency) is to drink milk, get some exposure to sunlight, but not enough to induce tumors, and to exercise. Trials of the different therapies mentioned above will depend on the physician's interpretation of results in the literature. Estrogens certainly did retard progress of the disease but its current use would be inappropriate. The one advantage of raloxifene is its putative ability to reduce the incidence of breast cancer[4].

Osteomalacia and rickets.

Both diseases are due to vitamin D deficiencies. In countries where foods are not supplemented with vitamin D the effects of deficits are seen in premature infants, the elderly, the poor, and those with dietary fads. Other causes of vitamin D deficits are hepatic disease, especially biliary obstruction and biliary cirrhosis which reduce bile acid excretion from the liver. These acids are needed for the intestinal absorption of vitamin D. Decreased absorption is also a frequent concomitant of chronic pancreatitis and small intestine malabsorption syndromes (eg., celiac disease, Crohn's disease, sprue and extensive small bowel resection). Phenytoin sometimes interferes with intrahepatic vitamin D metabolism and results in deficits of the vitamin.

Vitamin D.

This is a topic detailed on page 312 and summarized in Chart 14-1. Additional text is not needed.

The role of phosphate in causing osteomalacia and rickets.

Occasionally osteomalacia and rickets result from decreases in blood phosphate. The precipitating causes are uncommon and often of congenital origin (e.g., the Fanconi syndrome, renal tubular acidosis, x-linked hypophosphatemia and the autosomal recessive vitamin D-dependent rickets).

The pathology and clinical features of osteomalacia and rickets.

The principal lesion in osteomalacia is decreased mineralization of osteoid, at times, with production of excess osteoid. Osteoporosis results from decreased collagen in the matrix.

Osteoid is pre-osseous tissue. It is composed of collagenous tissue in an amorphous matrix of protein and polysaccharide. In vitamin D deficiencies there is a failure to adequately mineralize and the osteoid often becomes excessive.

Muscle weakness and diffuse joint pains are common presenting features. Clinical features due to defective mineralization of osteoid appear later. In children the osteoid excess is responsible for the frontal bossing, the rachitic rosary which is due to beading at the costochondral junctions, and the fractures and deformities of softened bones caused by defective mineralization at the epiphyses. In adults fractures and bone deformities are the principal features. As mentioned previously, pelvic deformities are common in pregnant women excluded from sunlight. Often it is necessary to perform Cesarian sections on women with perfectly normal pregnancies but with anatomical deformities of the pelvis which preclude normal vaginal deliveries. Eventually, and unfortunately, customs dictate that any female progeny are similarly affected by lack of vitamin D.

The diagnosis. There is a decreased serum calcium, an increased serum alkaline phosphate, a decreased serum vitamin D and decreased urine calcium excretion in a 24 hour specimen of urine. X-ray characteristic of osteomalacia are bands of radiolucency (termed pseudofractures or Looser's zones). A bone biopsy may be needed if no dietary or sunlight deficits are identifiable because rare cause are due to congenital metabolic dysfunctions.

Paget's disease of bone.

It is said that Paget's disease is the second most common bone disease in the USA. Osteoporosis is the first. In poor countries osteomalacia usually places first. Fractures are probably evenly distributed throughout the world but probably not their final outcomes. Affluence always has advantages.

Paget's disease is a common skeletal disease characterized by random bone breakdowns and over-formations. The new bone is dense but fragile. Contrary to popular medical belief Paget's disease affects both women and men. The usual age of onset is in the early 50s or later.

Any bone can be affected but the common sites are the pelvis, the spine and the bones of the legs. Symptoms may be absent. Alternatively, there is bone pain, arthritis, fractures, a characteristic bowing of the limbs and hearing loss when the disease affects the skull.

The cause is unknown. Some suggest that it results from a slow virus infection of bone but no evidence supports this hypothesis. There is also a hereditary factor as more than one member of a family can be affected.

The only treatment of any use seems to be exercise to preserve mobility and muscle strength. Analgesics are often needed to alleviate pain.

Hyperparathyroidism.

Causes. The diseases results from an excess of circulating parathyroid hormone. The cause could be a tumor (usually a benign adenoma) of one gland or hyperplasias of all four. Secondary excess of parathyroid hormone may result from renal failure which causes hypocalcemia and hyperphosphatemia. Finally, unrelated neoplasms can produce parathyroid hormone-like substances which mimic the features of the primary disease - conditions termed pseudohyperparathyroidism or ectopic hyperparathyroidism.

Pathology: An excess of parathyroid hormone results in increased bone reabsorption and raised serum and urinary excretion of calcium. The characteristic pathological lesions are diffuse or focal areas of increased osteoclastic activity and a reactive fibrous tissue reaction, hence the name of the disease - "osteitis fibrosa cystica". "Cystica" because in some cases cyst-like lesions (the"brown tumors") are present in bones and may be a cause of fractures. The cystic lesions usually appear in diaphyses of long bones and the jaw and skull. Histologically, they closely resemble giant cell tumors of bones and a differentiation can be difficult. Giant cell tumors usually occur in epiphyses and do not have changes in serum calcium and parathyroid hormone levels. In hyperparathyroidism any new bone is usually of the immature woven type. There is hypercalcemia and raised serum parathyroid hormone blood levels.

Clinical features: Symptoms are vague complaints of weakness, fatigue and gastrointestinal symptoms. Often the condition is first recognized when a routine examination shows a high serum calcium or the patient presents with a fracture or with bilateral renal stones.

Renal osteodystrophy.

Chronic renal failure usually results in a decrease in functioning renal parenchyma. There is a decreased conversion of vitamin D to its active metabolites, a consequent decrease in intestinal absorption of calcium, hypocalcemia, renal retention of phosphate and increased parathyroid hormone secretion. The metabolic acidosis of chronic renal failure also decreases the conversion of vitamin D to its active metabolite.

A variety of abnormalities can result. They include osteomalacia due to defective mineralization of osteoid, the bone changes of hyperparathyroidism and paradoxically, osteosclerosis due to the rapid remodeling and organization of bone. The blood changes include decreased serum calcium and increased serum phosphorous, alkaline phosphatase and parathyroid hormone.

Treatment includes vitamin D and a reduction of serum phosphate by intestinal binders such as aluminum hydroxide.

Some common joint dysfunctions.

Joint dysfunctions are many and the scope of this book only permits detailing of a few. Any of the items listed in the section on etiology (Chapter 3) can affect joints. They include trauma, infections by any one of many agents, tumors, arthropathies due to neurological diseases which cause sensory deficits (an example is the Charcot arthropathy of tabes dorsalis or syringomyelia) and arthropathies due to metabolic dysfunctions (gout is an example).

The autoimmune arthropathies.

Another group is the autoimmune arthropathies; or at least, arthropathies presumed to result from autoimmunity. They were itemized and summarized on pages 185-186. Rheumatoid arthritis is well described in standard texts as are other joint dysfunctions presumed to be the result of autoimmune reactions. In contrast to osteoarthritis which is described in the next section, autoimmune disease of joints are diseases which primarily affect synovial membranes.

Rheumatoid arthritis.

Rheumatoid arthritis is the most common of these arthropathies. The typical lesion is an infiltration of lymphocytes and plasma cells with focal vascular changes which include a proliferation of endothelial cells with narrowing of vessels, vasculitis, fibrinoid change and necrosis of vessel walls. Decreased vascularities can result in ischemic symptoms and microinfarcts.

The disease begins in the synovium which is thickened. Next the pathology spreads over the articular cartilage as a "pannus". There is adherence between opposing cartilaginous surfaces with restriction of movement. Progression results in destruction of the underlying cartilage. Eventually as the pannus ages fibrosis and contraction leads to a type of slightly flexible false ankylosis.

The disease can be difficult to diagnose if the blood rheumatoid factor is negative as it is in about 10-15% of patients (sero-negative rheumatoid arthritis). The disease is usually multiarticular though in the early stages it might seem to affect a single joint. There is swelling and often a doughy feel to the joint. Effusions are common. Pain and limitation of movement predominate and in the late stages there is a false ankylosis. There may be splenomegaly and leucopenia - described as Felty's syndrome.

Initial therapies are ASA or a NSAID. Subsequent modalities include corticosteroids, gold injections and immunosuppressive such as methotrexate. Often the ESR is a good guide for assessing severity and responses to therapy.

The arthritis of rheumatic fever.

This is an acute and transient non-specific synovitis affecting many joints but most commonly the knees, ankles and wrists. It begins about 2-3 weeks after a throat infection with Group A streptococci and is thought to be an autoimmune reaction to a bacterial antigen. The arthritis usually subsides after a few weeks without residual change. Subcutaneous nodules are common and chorea may also develop. The main danger is a carditis with characteristic Aschoff bodies in the infiltrates. The carditis often involves the valves with residual scarring of one or more valves, and subsequent stenoses and/or incompetences.

Osteoarthritis.

This common joint disease has been given a variety of names: osteoarthritis, osteoarthrosis, osteoarthropathy and degenerative joint disease. The usual picture is that of a polyarticular arthropathy. Secondary osteoarthritis is the result of previous trauma, infection, surgery or congenital and acquired focal deformities.

The most common form is primary osteoarthritis. It is a degenerative joint disease insofar as its incidence increases with age. Almost all over the age of 60 are afflicted in one form or the other.

At times one joint's disease predominates and the disease appears to be monoarticular. In fact many other joints are affected at the same time though seemingly symptomless. The joints of the fingers are often affected, especially in individuals such as seamstresses who do fine but repetitive manual work with their fingers. The metacarpo-phalangeal and interphalangeal joints are affected. Joint deformities and nodules are characteristic.

The pathology begins with degeneration and disintegration of articular cartilage. The underlying bone becomes sclerotic and proliferates with subchondral lipping by bony outgrowths which further distort the joint anatomy.

Pain and limitation of movements are the principal clinical features. Radiological studies show subchondral sclerosis and spur formation at the margins. Palpation may reveal nodularities, crepitus on movement and limitations of mobility. The pain and limitations are often severe enough to require surgical replacement of joints such as the hips and knees with prostheses.

There is no therapy for this disabling degeneration of aging apart from pain relievers and surgery when appropriate. It is necessary to exclude other causes of polyarthropathy before concluding that the clinical picture is that of osteoarthritis. In order to exclude autoimmune arthropathies basic studies should include estimations of erythrocyte sedimentation rates, rheumatoid factor, anti-nuclear antibodies and, if appropriate, anti-DNA estimations.

This ends a brief summary on bone and joint physiology and pathology.

Chapter 14 references.

1. Chapuy, M.C., Arlot, M.E., et al. Effect of calcium and calciferol treatment for three years on hip fractures in elderly women. Brit. Med. J. 1994; 308:1081.
2. Lips, P., Graafmans, W.C., et al. Vitamin D supplementation and fracture incidence in elderly persons: a randomized, placebo-controlled trial. Ann. Intern. Med. 1996; 124:400.
3. Ettinger, B., Black, D.M., et al. Reduction of vertebral fracture risk in postmenopausal women with osteoporosis treated with raloxifene: results from a three year randomized clinical trial. JAMA 1999; 282:637.
4, Cummings, S.R., Eckert, S., et al. The effect of raloxifene on risk of breast cancer in postmenopausal women: results from the MORE randomized trial. JAMA 1999; 281:2189.

15

Therapy

1. The Prevention of Disease

Table of Contents

Socioeconomic measures

Socioeconomic conditions are commensurate with the affluence of the country where the patient lives. In wealthy nations most people have enough material needs for comfortable and healthy living. Distribution of affluence is seldom equable but most have comfortable housing, clean and safe water, personal safety, protection from inclement weather, and enough food. In poor countries they do not. Poor socioeconomic conditions are uncomfortable and unpleasant. Additionally, they predispose to the development of infections that might not occur in the inhabitants of more affluent countries.

The figures for deaths from preventable diseases in poor countries are horrifying. Unicef reports (www.unicef.org/immunization/index_measles.html) that measles infects 30-40 million children each year and kills more than 500,000. Many who survive have lifelong neurological dysfunctions. This is a disease which is preventable by an inexpensive vaccine. Malaria kills even more people. There are 300 million cases worldwide each year with more than a million deaths annually (www.globalhealthreporting.org/malaria.asp). The topic of childhood diarrhea was extensively discussed on pages 199-201. It kills 5-6 million children each year (WHO fact sheet: http//www.who.int/vaccines and then access "diarrheal diseases"). Many of these deaths are preventable by good hygiene, rehydration and education of how disease spreads and the need to boil drinking water. One estimate is that about 12 million people die each year from treatable and preventable diseases. These are the common illnesses of poverty and a significant number, if not the majority of those who die are children. UNICEF reports that in 2004 4,000 died every day because of dirty water or poor sanitation and the UN's Food and Agriculture Organization estimates that in that same year some 850 million people were chronically hungry. Neither I nor the readers of this book belong to these groups of disadvantaged people but it is not enough to commiserate from a distance. All of us who are fortunate are obligated to do all that is within our capabilities to remedy or, at least ameliorate these horrifying statistics.

Digging wells for clean water is not difficult. Unfortunately the initial responses of optimism and gratitude are occasionally marred by later unpleasant assertions of hierarchical superiorities in the village, by local politics, by corruption and by myths, superstitions and suspicions. In practice, the main problem is lack of local technical expertise to create wells and unintended contaminations of new wells.

Disease perpetuation because of poor socioeconomic conditions.

Tuberculosis exemplifies the role of adverse socioeconomic conditions in perpetuating disease. It is a disease caused by bacteria but additional and important causes are poverty, poor nutrition, overcrowded living conditions, and the other many causes of ill health in the populace of impoverished countries. In affluent societies treatment can cure. Not so in countries that are not affluent. In those countries active disease can usually be cured and controlled by drugs. Many countries do provide free anti-tuberculosis medications to the indigent as a way of maintaining public health. However, dormant but potentially active bacteria usually persist. Disagreeable socioeconomic living conditions and diseases such as AIDS almost guarantee eventual recurrence, additional treatments, additional recurrences, and often, eventual death. The WHO[1] estimates that 1.64 million individuals die each year from this disease.

Acquired human immunodeficiency disease. This disease is a scourge of modern times comparable to the lethal pandemics of previous centuries. HIV/AIDS is a disease that favors infections by dormant bacteria such as M.Tuberculosis. It also favors opportunistic infections by usually non-pathogenic organisms that may or may not be normal body commensals. These organisms do not cause disease when normal defense mechanisms are unimpaired. Impoverished individuals with AIDS are more likely to contract and die from such infections than the rich because of adverse socio-economic conditions and the lack of monies to buy needed medications. These are the principal reasons why AIDS is decimating the population of Africa. AIDS is currently incurable but life can be prolonged with appropriate therapy. The socioeconomically disadvantaged are likely to die earlier than the affluent. They do not have money for drugs and their resistance to opportunistic infections is often negligible.

Currently, political pressures, charitable donations and relatively inexpensive generic drugs are beginning to ensure that the people in poor countries receive enough anti-AIDS drugs. Will this effectively prolong life? Perhaps, but one doubts if the end result will compare favorably with the fates of those in affluent societies. As mentioned above, many, if not most AIDS-related deaths are the result of opportunistic and often untreatable infections. Bad socioeconomic conditions predispose to development of such infections. Without better nutrition, less overcrowding, better hygiene, improved shelters and the many other factors that make life bearable, if not pleasant, the impoverished will remain at greater risk of dying from opportunistic infections than the affluent. Perhaps anti-AIDS drugs when available and affordable will reduce the numbers but poor socioeconomic conditions will always favor development of opportunistic infections. They remain the principal determinants of eventual fatalities.

The role of the physician.

There is usually little the individual physician, acting alone, can do to control infections except by providing therapy and attempting to control the reservoirs and vectors of infection. But the physician, as a member of a pressure group can press for improvement or change. The individual physician also has a role as advisor, at times an agitator, and always an educator. It is not difficult to advise people about basic hygiene; the need to boil drinking water if there is any possibility of its contamination by pathogens; the ways that contamination of clean water by humans or animals can be avoided; the need to wash foods before cooking; the ways to prevent bacterial contamination of food; and other related matters. When presented with tact and sensitivity advice is usually received with thanks, even when dealing with the poorest of villages in an underdeveloped country. Believe it or not, even in this age many living in small villages (the majority of the inhabitants of poor or developing countries) do not know that pathogens exist, that infections are caused by pathogens, nor that illnesses due to pathogens can be spread by the secretions and excretions of humans and animals.

The prevention and control of infections

Infections are a frequent cause of morbidity, disability and often, death. Prevention and control requires assessments of the following:

Where is the reservoir of infection?

What are the vector or vectors that transmit the infection?

Who is the host? In clinical medicine it is usually a human.

What are the numbers and virulence of the infecting organisms?

Are there any factors that reduce the ability of the host to resist infection by innate protective mechanisms and/or generated immune responses? Some examples of such factors are:

- Advanced age.
- Inherited or acquired immunological deficits such as those due to HIV/AIDs infections, long-term corticosteroid administration, anti-cancer chemotherapy and radiation. M.Tuberculosis is a frequent dormant pathogen in many individuals. It is readily activated to produce disease by unfavorable socioeconomic conditions such as insufficient food, a lack of potable water, poor housing, overcrowding and a number of other factors which result in disagreeable living conditions.

  Opportunistic pathogens are dormant bacteria that are usually not pathogenic or are part of the normal flora of humans. Normally they do not cause disease. When immune responses and/or natural defense mechanisms are compromised they can cause infections, termed opportunistic infections.
- Chronic disease or failure affecting any organ system (e.g., congestive heart failure, respiratory failure and renal or hepatic failure).
- Malignant disease. Especially extensive metastatic disease and lymphoreticular neoplasms.
- Anemia.
- Jaundice.
- Foreign bodies from injuries, indwelling intravenous and intravesical catheters, and endotracheal intubation for assisted ventilation.

The reservoirs of infection.

Common reservoirs of infection are humans, arthropods (they are more likely to be vectors, other animals, food, contaminated drinking water, contaminated water used for washing and bathing, pools of stagnant water, cows giving milk containing M.Bovis or the organisms that cause brucellosis, and the environments of hospitals. The reservoirs contain the pathogens and the vectors transmit them.

The vectors of infection.

Humans are common vectors of infection.

- **Transmission by coughing.** Tuberculosis, influenza, smallpox, other viral infections, and bacterial pneumonia are examples of diseases spread by coughing. Droplets 1-5 microns in diameter remain suspended in the air when coughed up by an infected person. They are inhaled by uninfected individuals, phagocytosed by macrophages and deposited in the lung parenchyma where infections result if local conditions are conducive.
- **Person to person transmission.** An example is smallpox which spreads by person to person transmission by coughing or contact in any one of many ways. There is no intermediate vector and this fact has helped the eradication of smallpox by vaccination.
- **Transmission by food and water.** Examples are meat contaminated with E. Coli resulting in so-called "hamburger disease". Tuberculosis and brucellosis transmitted in milk. Fecal-oral contamination, either directly by unwashed hands or via contaminated food and/or water. Viral dysenteries, poliomyelitis, amebiasis, tape worm infestations and trichinosis are examples of disease spread by fecal-oral contamination.
- **Infections due to penetration of epithelial surfaces by pathogens.** Examples are wound infections and infections resulting from penetration of intact skin by pathogens such as schistosomes and hookworms.
- **Infections by transfused blood.** Transmission of AIDS, hepatitis B and C and other infections by transfused blood are ever-present dangers. The risks can be minimized but not eliminated by screening before transfusion.
- **Sexually transmitted infections.** The most dangerous of these is AIDS, a disease not exclusive to homosexuals but increasingly common in heterosexuals. A condom provides some protection but the statement that it is "safe sex" misleads. The safety is certainly nowhere near 100%; inadvertent events can never be avoided, nor the possibility that virus can escape from the appliance in amounts sufficient to produce disease. An increasingly common cause of AIDS is self-injection of contaminated "recreational" drugs and the use of previously contaminated needles and syringes. Gonorrhea, syphilis and chlamydia infections can be cured by appropriate antibiotics. Herpes and papilloma infections remain major problems.
- **Infections can be transmitted in utero or at the time of parturition.** The consequences of syphilis, rubella and toxoplasma infections of the mother during pregnancy are often seen in the offspring. Infection by Group B streptococci during vaginal delivery can results in fatal consequences for the fetus.
- **Nosocomial infections.** A nosocomial infection is defined as one that was not present when an individual was admitted to a health-care facility[2]. Infection occurring some 72 hours after admission will exclude most infections incubating prior to admission. Nosocomial infections are particularly common in intensive care units where patients are usually debilitated, elderly and often immunocompromised. Other factors are the use of ventilators and indwelling catheters.

  The organisms responsible for nosocomial infections are varied. Mixtures of gram positive and negative organisms, yeasts and viruses are usual. Predisposing conditions include diabetes mellitus, alcoholism and/or other drug addictions, subnutrition and malnutrition, chronic lung disease and, as previously mentioned, aging and immunocompromised states. Major surgery and extensive burns are two other important negatives.

  Mortality and morbidity figures are difficult to evaluate as hospitals and health-care facilities vary according to the types of patients treated, the size, if any, of their intensive-care units, and the seriousness of the diseases treated. Figures for nosocomial infections in intensive care units vary from 10%-35% of patients treated. The three most common sites of infection are the lungs, the urinary tract and the blood stream.

The topic of nosocomial infections is extensively reviewed in a paper by the National Nosocomial Infection Surveillance[3]. A total of 498,998 patients were studied and the paper presents much informative analyses of nosocomial infections.

— **Disease transmission by arthropods.** Transmission by arthropods could be from one human to another (e.g., malaria and yellow fever) or from animals to man (e.g., plague, and most rickettsial infections).

— **Anaerobic wound infections.** The usual cause of anaerobic wound infections are C.Tetani, C.Welchii and the other organisms of the gas gangrene group. Promotion of infection results from an impaired blood supply, deep penetrating wounds providing anaerobic conditions, dead tissue, foreign bodies, local edema and concomitant infection by aerobic organisms which create anaerobic environments.

Anaerobic infections are usually the result of wound contamination by soil or occasionally, feces. They contain spores and, at times, bacteria. In anaerobic conditions the spores germinate to pathogens. C.Tetani results in little local tissue destruction but produces a toxin that causes the clinical features of tetanus. The gas gangrene organisms can cause extensive destruction of tissue, often with the characteristic crepitus of confined gas. The organisms also produce toxins. These can result in profound toxemias and even death.

The prevention of tetanus and gas gangrene is immediate removal of dead tissue, exposure of infected tissues to aerobic conditions and establishment of an adequate blood supply. The average incubation period of tetanus is about 8 days so that if there has not been prior immunization antitoxin as well as toxoid should be given as soon as possible after infection if the possibility of tetanus infection is significant. Penicillin is effective against Clostridial infections. However it does not reduce toxin production by C.Tetani or the gas gangrene organisms.

The prevention of infections.

The following are some requirements for prevention of infections:

— **Hygiene.** The most effective and easy way to protect against infections is good hygiene. Hand hygiene is the most important as the hands are the vectors of many infections. Numerous studies have shown that hands of health care personnel are often contaminated with pathogens[4]. The licking of fingers to facilitate the flipping over of sheets of papers is dangerous and should be avoided.

Hand washing is especially important after urination, defecation or changing of menstrual protections. It is also essential after handling sick patients, changing their bed linens and their dressings. Washing of hands before examining patients protects the sick. Washing hands after the examination only protects the examiner. It is said that rubbing hands with antiseptic alcohol-based solutions is equally, and perhaps more effective than a soap-and-water rinse[5]. Maybe so but the latter is the traditional way of cleaning hands. Perusal of CDC suggestions for hand hygiene is strongly recommended[6].

Equally important are general cleanliness of the body and the abode, proper disposal of human and animal wastes, clean clothing, trimmed finger nails and a host of other factors that reduce the chances of infection transmissions by humans.

— **Protection against insect vectors.**

The following are the more important measures for controlling vectors which transmit infections:

- Eliminate or control pathogens in their **reservoirs.**
- Eliminate or control the **vectors** of infection
- **Immunize** to provide prevention against the establishment of pathogens.
- **Improve socioeconomic conditions:** Clean water, improved nutrition, adequate shelters and miscellaneous other measures that can improve general resistance to infection.
- **Treat established disease with appropriate drugs.** This topic is detailed in the next chapter. It discusses antibiotics and other methods of treating infections.

Malaria - an illustration of how to prevent and protect against infections.

Malaria and its prevention illustrate many of the factors mentioned above. Protective vaccines are still not available so that prevention by immunization is not possible. Prevention of other diseases by immunization is detailed later in this chapter.

The natural history of malaria is chosen to illustrate the frequent complexities of reservoirs, vectors and pathology. In any case it is sufficiently common and potentially lethal to earn consideration on its own merits - one to two million deaths from the disease each year. Malaria illustrates the importance and frequent difficulties encountered when trying to control reservoirs and vectors of infection.

The natural history of malaria.

In a 2002 publication the WHO (http://www.who.int/vaccine) stated that malaria was the most important tropical parasitic disease and that it killed more than 1.1 million people each year. Children were especially affected with one child dying of malaria every 30 seconds. The Economist of August 22, 2002[7] went even further, stating that malaria infects more than 500 million people each year, killing about 2.7 million individuals. Three quarters of the fatalities were children under 5. The enormity of these numbers is outrageous. It is the children who are most in need of protection. Anders has suggested the following rationale for this statement:

> ".... most human deaths from malaria are in children under the age of four. After that symptoms become less severe and people develop significant immunity and suffer less severe, briefer episodes of parasitaemia than non-exposed individuals. Those who have acquired immunity may be making antibodies against secreted toxins ... rather than against structural antigens." (Nova: Science in the News. http-//ww.science.org.au/nova)"

He could be right. If correct, this concept could contribute to the development of effective anti-malaria vaccines.

Malaria is caused by one or more of four species of plasmodia: P.Falciparum, P.Vivax, P.Malariae and P.Ovale. The natural **reservoirs of the organism are humans and pools of stagnant water.** Occasionally organisms are present in birds, monkeys and reptiles. The **vector is the Anopheles mosquito.**

The organism has **two life cycles, an asexual and a sexual phase.**

The asexual phase occurs in humans. Mosquito bites introduce sporozoites that are parasitized by red cells. Development proceeds with formation of trophozoites and then merozoites. Erythrocyte destruction releases merozoites and the products of cell destruction into the circulation and these are the causes of the fever and toxemia of malaria. Some of the trophozoites in the red cells develop into male and female gametocytes that enter the mosquito when it bites humans and this starts the sexual phase.

The sexual phase begins with mosquitoes sucking up gametocytes while feeding on human blood. Male and female gametocytes unite to form zygotes, and finally, sporozoites. Some sporozoites are stored in the mosquito's salivary glands and enter humans when the mosquito bites, and so the cycle starts again.

Clinical features identify two different types of malaria. **One is** infection with P.Vivax, P.Malariae and P.Ovale. These infections are rarely fatal. There are rigors, fever and generalized weakness. The disease usually resolves in 10-14 days. Infections with P.Vivax and P.Malariae tend to recur if not adequately treated when they first occur.

The other is infection with P.Falciparum. It results in a more severe infection and kills about 2% of those infected. A characteristic feature is accumulations of parasitized red cells in capillaries. Possible consequences are ischemic infarcts. The spleen, bone marrow, brain and lungs are the tissues usually affected by such infarcts. The most serious complication is cerebral clumping, with encephalopathies resulting in neurological deficits, confusions, hallucinations and disorientations which often end in coma or death.

Occasionally the clumps hemolyse. Hemoglobin enters the blood and when free hemoglobin exceeds the conjugating capacity of the blood it is excreted in the urine. The result is the characteristic dark urine of "blackwater fever". P.Falciparum infection is the commonest form of malaria in subSaharan Africa. Unfortunately it is also becoming more common in places such as India. Previously, P.Vivax infection was the usual form of malaria in India.

The prevention of malaria. Uninfected individuals can be protected when traveling to countries with endemic malaria by any one of a number of different therapeutic regimens. Recommendations frequently change so no specific regimen is recommended here. Information about the latest recommendation is easily obtained from a local public health authority. **Prevention in areas where malaria is endemic is controversial.**

DDT usage.

The mainstay of protection from malaria in countries where the disease is endemic, and often epidemic, is destruction of mosquitoes by pesticides. But which pesticide? **DDT (Dicloro-diphenyl-trichloroethane)** remains a commonly used but controversial pesticide.

The advantages and disadvantages of DDT.

The pros and cons of DDT usage are presented in some detail for three reasons. **First** to itemize its advantages and disadvantages for prevention of a widespread disease with high annual mortality. **Second,** to show how resistance to protective pesticides invariably develops after prolonged use. **Third,** and equally important, to show the counter-productive, but perhaps well meant coercions that International agencies can exert. They have tried to exert political and financial pressures to coerce the recipients of aid in small and politically weak countries, to comply with the opinions of environmentalists in affluent donor countries. Currently, DDT is banned in many industrialized countries and the United Nations Environmental Program is currently promoting a global ban. The Stockholm Convention of 2001 was signed by 91 countries and the European Community and was designed to eliminate persistent organic pollutants (POPs). Fortunately it included an opt-out provision that allowed for continued use of DDT. More than 20 countries applied for and were granted exemptions, including China, India and the Russian Federation.

Many effective agents are available for treatment of clinical malaria. Prevention remains the ideal for no anti-malaria vaccines are available. Protection is limited to destruction of mosquito reservoirs, protections of homes by pesticides and of humans by barriers such as mosquito nets.

There are many advocates for effective control by mosquito nets, well tucked in under the mattress at all places. One recommendation is to impregnate them with an insecticide such as Permethrin or one of the newer agents such as Deltamethrin that is said to persist on the net even after twenty washings. Unfortunately individuals in affluent societies often do not realize that those who are most in need cannot afford the purchase and cleaning of mosquito nets; in fact, often they cannot even afford the luxury of a mattress. Additionally, in hot countries mosquito nets are frequently discarded during the night because they make people hotter and more uncomfortable.

Despite controversies about its safety DDT remains a commonly used pesticide. Malaria control by DDT is more than fifty years old. Its early effectiveness was recorded in many ways. Peer approval was award of the Nobel prize to Muller in 1948 for his work on DDT and in 1970 the National Academy of Sciences[8] issued the following statement:

> "To only a few chemicals does man owe as great a debt as to DDT ...... In little more than two decades, DDT has prevented 500 million human deaths, due to malaria, that would otherwise have been inevitable."

This statement was made when widespread malaria in Europe and the United States had been controlled. In May 1955 the Eight World Health Assembly adopted a Global Malaria Eradication Campaign that included widespread use of DDT for prevention. By 1967 malaria had been eradicated in all developed countries.

The controversy about the use of DDT began with Rachel Carson's 1962 book, "Silent Spring". In that book she claimed that DDT was affecting egg shell thickness, and the reproduction and survival of birds. It was also supposed to have caused a decline in the bald eagle population and to have increased the incidence of cancer in humans. Rachel Carson's book was published in 1962. By 1970 DDT was not a requisite for malaria control in developed countries. Shortly thereafter (1972) pressure by environmentalists succeeded in having DDT banned in the United States.

At that time, and up to the present, no studies suggest that DDT is a carcinogen in humans. DDT does act as a hepatic carcinogen in mice when given in large doses but there is no evidence that it does so in humans[9]. With respect to breast cancer, no increase was found in North Vietnamese women who had raised serum DDT levels after exposure to anti-malarial sprays[10]. Why Vietnam? Probably because the pesticide is banned or inaccessible in most western nations. In any case the current incidence of malaria in western nations is too small for any conclusive studies. A paper written in 2000 by Curtis and Lines[12] states that after critical examination of relevant data the toxicity of DDT for humans and its purported adverse effects on the environment remain unproven. In the same paper they showed that there is a rapid increase in the incidence of malaria in a country that stops using DDT as a wall spray - this is the vector-control procedure - (current WHO guidance is that houses should be sprayed with 2gm DDT per m^2 every six months). Unfortunately, there is no perfect solution to the control of malaria for pesticide-resistant species do develop with prolonged use of any pesticide, including DDT. The reference cited above as well as other publications (e.g., Smith[11] - Lancet Editorial) conclude that the carcinogenicity of DDT is minimal or non-existent. Smith writes as follows:

> "In summary, DDT can cause many toxicological effects but the effects on human beings at likely exposure levels seems to be very slight."

A caustic comment is recorded by Desowitz in his book:"Malaria Capers"[13]. He claimed that advocates of population control blamed DDT for increasing the populations of the Third World. He also claimed that the International agencies believed that the solution to the population problem was the death from malaria of 40% of the children in impoverished countries. An official of the Agency for International Development was quoted as saying: "Rather dead than alive and riotously reproducing" Unfortunately, this expectation is being realized. The WHO and UNICEF report (Africa Malaria Report of 2003) states that malaria is the biggest killer of young children in Africa and the most significant health threat to pregnant women and newborns in those countries (quoted from Internet: Africa Fighting Malaria, 2004). With AIDS killing millions of able-bodied people on that continent one wonders with great trepidation and sympathy about the future for these unfortunate people who share this planet with us, especially the many with immune systems compromised by HIV/AIDS.

At present the manufacture and widespread use of DDT continues in two countries where a third of humanity lives - China and India. The latter produces more than 9,000 metric tonnes of DDT each year and its export markets include the United States. Figures for Chinese production are not available.

The disadvantages of DDT.

The preceding discussion is probably irrelevant except to show how political and other considerations can intrude on the abilities of poor and weak nations to make their own decisions. Irrelevant because resistance to any pesticide is inevitable after prolonged use. In India many vector species have become resistant to DDT and malathion, either sprayed separately or in combination (Sharma, V.P. Current scenario of malaria in India. Parassotologia 1999; 41:349). DDT is no longer used for malaria control in Indian urban centers; malathion and other synthetic pyrethroids are favored and resistance to malathion has developed in certain areas. Even mosquitoes in rural areas are becoming resistant to DDT and about 65% of Indian malaria is located in these areas. The problem is not trivial as the country spends a large part of its health budget on malaria control.

Alternative methods are being tried. Examples are the introduction into ponds of biological larvicides, polystyrene beads coated with larvicides designed to kill larvae and pupae, and fish that eat larvae.. Such methods were in use for centuries before being overshadowed by DDT. In two papers published in the 1980s there were reports that bioenvironmental control had decreased by 70% the incidence of malaria in the two states of Karnataka and Maharashtra in India[15]. More recently, at the Indian Science Congress of 2003 Dr. V.P. Sharma also reported on the use of guppies to eat mosquito larvae. In some areas the fish had almost eliminated all Anopheles mosquitoes carrying malaria but in other areas the results were disappointing. Obvious additional measures are the elimination of stagnant pools of water and the vigorous destruction of mosquitoes and larvae.

There is a great need for development of vaccines against malaria. Most adults in areas where malaria is pandemic seem to be relatively immune. Most of the deaths occur in children and Anders has suggested this is because adults have immunity to the secretions of anopheles mosquito products (see page 324). Could the preventive we look for be in the blood or serum of adults in these areas?

Recently, South Korean scientists have reported that a fish, the muddy loach, can completely remove mosquito larvae from rice fields within a day (details accessible on the Internet in an article by Liu Li Cheng at http://www.i-sis.org.uk). They could probably do the same in lakes and ponds but the fish are too large for use where the Anopheles commonly breed, i.e., in small pools of stagnant water.

Finally, there is continual need for development of new pesticides that are safe and effective. Some do exist at the present but high costs preclude many countries from switching to the more expensive organophosphates, the carbamates, and the various commercially available pyrethroid insecticides. Until vaccines are available the sequence of pesticide-resistance followed by the development of new pesticides will probably continue.

As previously mentioned, recent WHO guidance suggests that houses should be sprayed with 2gm DDT per m^2 every six month. Some mosquitoes may be resistant to DDT but others will die and the incidence of the disease reduced. In those countries where malaria is an ever-present danger and DDT is used as a pesticide, few worry about Rachel Carson's predictions of decreased egg shell thicknesses or decreased avian reproduction. Human survival is more important.

Immunizations

With the exception of vaccines directed against Hepatitis B (more about that later), all vaccines are produced by one of two methods. One is the inactivation of viruses or bacterial toxins with formalin or propriolactone by methods that retain the immunogenicity of their pathogenic antigens. The other is production of attenuated viruses that are unable to produce the disease of the parent virus but retain its content of antigens that are immunogenic but not pathogenic. When orally or parenterally introduced into the body a protective immune response results.

Most vaccines are packaged with small amounts of antibacterials (usually detailed on the accompanying instruction sheet) and many of the attenuated viruses are grown on egg media. Before giving a vaccine ask about hypersensitivities and allergies to eggs. In addition vaccines should not be given if there is any concurrent infection as infections are said to decrease immune responses.

Thimerosal in vaccines and refusals of immunizations.

Vaccines are required to have small amounts of antibacterials that prevent microbial and fungal contaminations of repeatedly punctured multi-dose vials. Till recently thimerosal which is about 50% mercury by weight was used for this purpose. In recent years there have been concerns about development of neurodevelopmental disorders such as autism and attention deficit hyperactivity disorder in children given vaccines containing thimerosal. The topic has been investigated by many groups. The consensus is that these fears are without substance. However, there is current real and persistent concerns about almost all vaccines. Some are concerns about the neurological dysfunctions which occasionally follow most immunizations. An encephalitis (subacute sclerosing panencephalitis or SSPE) is a rare sequel to immunization against measles. The risk is about one per million doses of vaccine. Additional comment on SSPE is made later in this section.

Parental concerns about the mercury in thimerosal are now addressed. Vaccines recommended for infants and children are now available in formulations that do not contain thimerosal. The concerned parent can find a list of these formulations on the Internet (US Food and Drug Administration. Thimerosal in vaccines. www.fda.gov/cber/vaccine/thimfag.ht.)

There are two caveats regarding refusal of immunization. Many mothers are currently refusing immunizations for their children because they fear neurodevelopmental disorders in their offspring. This they have a right to do in many jurisdictions. If measles-mumps-rubella immunization is refused and the child gets mumps or measles it is the parent's responsibility to get appropriate care and to prevent the spread of the infection to other children. Before accepting the refusal it is a good idea to tell them that measles infections can result in long-term neurological and pulmonary dysfunctions and that it is a disease that can kill and does kill 500,00 children annually. The disease and its pulmonary and neurological complications can occur in any location and affect any individual; rich and poor equally.

The second is that if an unimmunized child gets rubella and comes in contact with a pregnant woman congenital deformities in the newborn are real dangers. Mothers who refuse immunization for their children should be advised about this. Costly litigation can follow if the child of the pregnant woman has any of the deformities associated with in utero infection with rubella. The diagnosis can be missed as the usual symptoms and signs of a rubella infection are those of trivial viral infection with an unremarkable rash, both only lasting a few days. It is often accompanied by various lymph node enlargements.

Pregnant women should have laboratory estimations of anti-rubella titers. If they are absent they should be warned of the dangers of coming into contact with children who are unwell. As mentioned above, rubella is often difficult to diagnose and is usually a trivial illness lasting only a few days. Often there are few diagnostic clinical features detectable by the untrained. Anti-rubella immunization before contemplating another pregnancy is essential for all women who are negative for anti-rubella antibodies. Needless to say, all teachers should ensure they are adequately immunized against rubella.

Immunization with attenuated viruses.

The first attenuated virus used for immunization was the natural cowpox virus used by Jenner to protect against smallpox. The virus was an attenuated small pox virus. It had the same immunogenic antigens as the small pox virus but did not cause the same disease. Jenner's discovery was extensively detailed on page 8. The use of this non-toxic variant for immunization established an important principle. Attenuated viruses could be used, or developed for use as immunogens against disease produced by the parent virus.

The following are some examples of vaccines that are attenuated viruses:

The measles-mumps-rubella (MMR) vaccine.

Ideally immunization should begin at the end of the first year of life; each country seems to have its own subsequent immunization schedule guidelines. If begun earlier the measles immunity could be reduced because of persistent maternal anti-measles antibody in the child.

Vaccines of attenuated live organisms should not be given to individuals with immune responses impaired by radiotherapy, chemotherapy, corticosteroids or AIDS. Neither should they be given to individuals with tumors of the reticulo-endothelial system (e.g., lymphomas) or leukemia.

MMR should not be given to pregnant females and if de novo immunization of young women is needed a beta-HCG estimation is advisable a day before the immunization. Avoid pregnancy for the subsequent three months.

Post-immunization encephalitis. An encephalitis (subacute sclerosing panencephalitis or SSPE) has been reported as a sequel to immunization against measles in children with no current or previous history of measles. The risk is about one per million doses of injected vaccine. The CDC has postulated that measles vaccine reduces rather than increases the incidence of the encephalopathy. The incidence of SSPE in previously unimmunized children with measles is about 6-22 per million cases. Nevertheless, even in those jurisdictions where immunization is mandatory physicians would be wise to caution and, when necessary, obtain specific consent from parents before injecting the vaccine.

Anti-Yellow fever vaccine.

This is another example of a vaccine derived from attenuated viruses and it is also a vaccine that, on rare occasions, results in an encephalitis. It is an effective vaccine with immunity lasting several years. International Health Regulations only require revaccination after 10 years.

Poliomyelitis vaccine.

Two dissimilar vaccines are available; an inactivated polio virus vaccine developed by Salk in 1955 and a live attenuated oral polio vaccine developed by Sabin in 1961.

Each has advantages and disadvantages and every country seems to have dissimilar recommended, and often mandatory, immunization schedules.

The Sabin vaccine (OPV) is given orally and is relatively inexpensive. It protects by producing antibodies in the blood as well as a local immune response in the intestinal mucus membranes. The latter response is ideal for stopping person-to-person fecal-oral transmission in an epidemic. Virus that is not adequately attenuated could cause clinical poliomyelitis. The incidence of infection by inadequately attenuated virus shed in the stools is low; about 1 for every 2.5 million immunized individuals given OPV.

Immunizations with vaccines that do not contain live organisms.

The Salk inactivated polio vaccine (IPV) is derived from inactivated virus. It is given by injection. IPV confers immunity by producing protective antibodies. When injected it prevents paralytic polio but only induces low levels of intestinal immunity. Virus can multiply in the intestine and be shed in feces. Hence, when sanitation is poor or there is a local epidemic OPV is the preferred choice. Even in countries that rely on IPV alone for immunization additional OPV was often given in epidemics. This was the procedure used in an outbreak in the Netherlands in 1992.

Currently there are global programs for the total eradication of poliomyelitis by 2005. There is no reason why this should not be possible. It has been done for smallpox where the reservoir was in humans and the vector direct or aerial transmission between humans. Poliomyelitis is not too different. The reservoir is man, transmission is by contaminated water, food, or both. Immunization (especially with OPV) is simple and cheap.

The anti-diphtheria, anti-tetanus and anti-pertussis triad.

The anti-diphtheria and anti-tetanus components are derived from the toxins of these bacteria. Acellular pertussis vaccines have been used to effectively control pertussis in Japan since 1981. Acellular anti-pertussis vaccine is now widely accessible (Infanrix: SmithKline Beecham) and could eliminate the rare neurological complications that were the occasional sequelae to pertussis immunizations. In any case neurological complications resulting from clinical pertussis are far more common than those resulting from immunization against the disease.

The Hib vaccine.

Hemophilus Influenza B infection occurs primarily in children under 5. A significant number of the infected develop meningitis. The total mortality is around 5% but about 35% of the survivors of meningitis have neurological sequelae ranging from convulsions and deafness to mental retardation. The vaccine is made from the polysaccharide capsule (PRP) of the organism and anti-PRP activity correlates well with the protective effect of the vaccine.

Vaccines produced by genetic engineering.

The introduction of genetically engineered anti-Hepatitis B vaccine probably ushers in a new era in vaccine development and production. The HBsAg gene from the Hepatitis B virus has been cloned into Saccharomyces cerevisiae. The HBs antigen produced is extracted by complex processes and used for immunization after inactivation. It is marketed as Engerix-B (SmithKline Beecham) and seems to provide the same protective effects as plasma-derived vaccines.

Other vaccines not mentioned.

Vaccines directed against other entities include anti-chicken pox vaccine, anti-influenza vaccines, anti-pneumococcal vaccines, and anti-anthrax vaccines. It is uncommon for vaccines direct against influenza viruses, Anthrax and Pneumococci to provide complete protection. Their principal value is reduction of the severity of any infection contracted.

The challenges.

So far the text has detailed the available vaccines. Immunizations have reduced mortalities and residual disabilities throughout our world. Three important challenges remain. Effective vaccines against three of the major killers of people remain undiscovered: vaccines against tuberculosis, human immunodeficiency virus and malaria. Vigorous research to develop such vaccines are sponsored and financially supported by many International organizations and private charities. Individuals infected with M.Tuberculosis are more fortunate than the others. If they survive the primary infection fairly effective generated immunity can protect against reactivations or new infections. Those infected with HIV or malaria are not so fortunate. Infection does not confer immunity and no vaccines of proved effectiveness are available.

Immunization - precautions and contraindications.

The following summarizes the WHO recommendations for immunization (some have been previously mentioned but for completeness all WHO recommendations are presented):

- An anaphylactic reaction is always possible after immunization. Ask the recipient to remain in the office for 20-30 minutes after the injection (my recommendation) and always have epinephrine available for injection. I have personal experience of two patients who developed severe anaphylactic reactions 10-25 minutes after immunization against tetanus. Both required immediate epinephrine and oxygen.
- If the sequel to injection of a vaccine is an adverse reaction such as anaphylaxis, collapse, shock, non-febrile convulsions, or any neurological dysfunctions, subsequent injections of the same vaccine should never be given. Give the patient written information about the reaction. It can be provided to any other physician who feels immunization is necessary but is unaware of previous reaction to the vaccine.
- Immunization should be postponed if there is evidence of an acute illness, especially one accompanied by fever and/or toxemia.
- The disinfecting agent (usually alcohol) used to clean the site of immunization must dry prior to injection.
- Do not use the intramuscular route if the patient has a bleeding disorder such as hemophilia or thrombocytopenia or is on anticoagulants.
- In order to avoid harming the fetus, live attenuated virus vaccines should not be given to pregnant women unless circumstances are exceptional.
- Live attenuated virus vaccines should not be given to individuals with lymphoid or reticuloendothelial malignancies or to individuals with immune responses impaired by disease (e.g., AIDS), radiotherapy, anticancer chemotherapy or prolonged administration of corticosteroids.
- The WHO recommends that both, asymptomatic and symptomatic HIV-positive children and women of child-bearing age receive anti-diphtheria, tetanus, pertussis, hepatitis B and oral polio vaccines.

  The risk of disease from live attenuated viruses do exist, but the incidence and mortality of measles is significant in these children. An American publication[17] provides appropriate recommendations and so does the Internet (http://www.aidsmap.com/en/docs). The general opinion is to withhold vaccine from adults with CD4 counts less than 200/mm^3 and for children, withhold vaccine when those aged 1-5 have CD4 counts less than 500/mm^3 and children less than one year old have CD4 counts less than 750/mm^3.

  BCG is of no value in preventing reactivation tuberculosis in patients with AIDS, and yellow fever vaccine is best avoided unless the HIV-positive patient is asymptomatic or the risk of yellow fever is high.

Immunization against tuberculosis.

There is no conclusive proof of the efficacy of any vaccine directed against tuberculosis - certainly not of BCG. BCG is a live vaccine derived from an attenuated strain of M.Bovis. It is often given to children at birth in poor countries to protect against the severe forms of tuberculosis such as miliary and meningeal infections. It cannot protect against reactivation infections in adults. Individuals with AIDS often die from reactivation tuberculous infections. BCG inoculation is not safe in individuals with AIDS because their compromised immunological systems may be unable to protect against disseminated BCG disease. However, both the WHO and UNICEF advise giving BCG at birth to asymptomatic HIV-infected children living in areas where tuberculosis is endemic. It should not be given if there is symptomatic HIV infection. The pros and cons of BCG immunization are complex and, if possible, a physician who is thinking of giving BCG to a patient would be well advised to consult a physician especially cognizant of tuberculosis and its treatment before giving the inoculum.

The role of BCG in the prevention of tuberculosis is controversial. Many trials have been conducted over the last 50+ years with results showing protection that varied from 0% to 80%. Almost all have been the subjects of controversy. A fairly recent study by Colditz and associates[18] does suggest that the vaccine is about 50%

effective but currently there is decreasing interest in BCG vaccination to protect against tuberculosis.

Meanwhile the toll continues. In a 1995 Lancet conference on "The challenge of tuberculosis:" Mwinga claimed that there will be 15 million new cases of tuberculosis in sub-Saharan Africa in the next five years[19]. The prediction has been met. The WHO estimates that of the infected about 8 million will develop clinical disease but only about 1.6 million individuals will die of tuberculosis[20] because of the immunity conferred by the initial infection.

Nutrition and diet

Satisfactory nutrition is an important requisite for the prevention of disease. It is a constant consideration for patients receiving drugs, or continuous intravenous infusion of electrolyte solutions and glucose without supplements. Infusions without adequate calories have deleterious effects when prolonged for more than 4-5 days. When calories are insufficient protein wasting because of gluconeogenesis begins after this period.

The conversions of environmental energy substrate to energy usable for biological activities were detailed in Chapter 4. It is stored as high energy phosphate bonds in ATP and/or ADP till needed.

Calculation of the calories needed for adequate nutrition.

The numbers of calories required for adequate nutrition depend on the individual's basal metabolic needs, additional caloric needs for different levels of activity, plus additional caloric needs for any existing disease or trauma, and for the specific dynamic action of food.

The basal metabolic rate (BMR) is the caloric requirements of a fasting individual at physical and mental rest, living at a comfortable temperature of about 20^0C. The BMR (in KCal/m^2/hour) is estimated from the formula:

BMR = 37 - ((Age - 20) ÷ 10) KCal/m^2/hour.

Chart 15-1: NOMOGRAM FOR DETERMINING BODY SURFACE AREA[1]

HEIGHT	BODY SURFACE	WEIGHT
140 cm. (56 in.)–		–40 Kg. (88 lbs.)
145 cm. (58 in.)–	1.4 m^2	–45 Kg. (99 lbs.)
150 cm. (60 in.)–		–50 Kg. (110 lbs.)
155 cm. (62 in.)–	1.5 m^2	–55 Kg. (121 lbs.)
160 cm. (64 in.)–		–60 Kg. (132 lbs.)
165 cm. (66 in.)–	1.7 m^2	–65 Kg. (143 lbs.)
170 cm. (68 in.)–		–70 Kg. (154 lbs.)
175 cm. (70 in.)–	1.9 m^2	–75 Kg. (165 lbs.)
180 cm. (72 in.)–	2.0 m^2	–80 Kg. (176 lbs.)
185 cm. (74 in.)–		–85 Kg. (187lbs.)
190 cm. (76 in.)–	2.2 m^2	–90 Kg. (198 lbs.)
195 cm. (78 in.)–		–95 Kg. (209 lbs.)
200 cm. (80 in.)–	2.3 m^2	–100 Kg. (220 lbs)
205 cm. (82 in.)–		–105 Kg (231 lbs.)

[1] Surface area in square meters = $W^{0.425} \times H^{0.725} \times 71.84 \times 10^{-4}$ where W = Weight in kilograms and H = Height in centimeters (modified equation from Du Bois and Du Bois, Arch. Int. Med.: 17:863, 1916 as abstracted from Documenta Geigy, Sixth Edition, 1962).

Body surface area is determined from a nomogram (Chart 15-1) or the formula in the footnote of the nomogram.

The formula looks difficult but is easily programmed into a hand held calculator.

Daily basal metabolic needs are:

BMR in KCal/m^2/hour x Body surface area in m^2 x 24.

To the daily basal metabolic needs add:

For fever: 10% of the basic BMR per degree centigrade.

For bad infections, major trauma and surgery and postoperative recovery: 30-50% of basic BMR

For burns exceeding 50% of body surface: 100% basic BMR

For cardiac failure: 20% of the basic BMR.

For pregnancy and lactation: 500KCal to 24 hour BMR.

To the corrected daily basal metabolic needs add:

For sedentary living: 500KCal/day.

For light work: 1,000KCal/day.

For moderately heavy work: 1,500-2,000KCal/day.

For heavy work: 2,500-8,000KCal/day depending on the work.

For energy lost because of specific dynamic action of food.

Add 10% of total metabolic needs.

Chart 15-2: ENERGY NEEDS: METHOD OF ESTIMATION IN A SAMPLE SITUATION [1, 2]

Example:

Calculate the 24 hour energy needs of a 60 year old man hospitalized with multiple trauma. The patient is 180 cm. (72") tall and weighs 85 Kg. (187 lbs.).

BMR = 37 - ((Age - 20) ÷ 10) = 37 - ((60 - 20) ÷ 10) = 37 - 4 = 33KCal/m^2/hour.

Surface area from nomogram is approximately 2.1m^2 and from formula in Chart 15-1 = $85^{0.425}$ x $180^{0.725}$ x 71.84 x 10^{-4} = 2.05m^2.

Total daily basal metabolic requirements: 24 x 33 x 2.05 = 1623.6KCal/day.

Additional basal energy needs required because of multiple trauma (50% of basal energy requirements) = 1623.6 + (0.5 x 1623.6) = 2435.4KCal.

Increase the basal level by the energy needed for activity: 500KCal (needs for sedentary person as patient is confined to bed) = 2435.4 + 500 = 2935.4KCal..

Additional energy needs related to specific dynamic action of food: 10% of total energy needs = 0.1 x 2935.4 = 293.54KCal.

Total daily energy needs of this hospitalized man with multiple trauma = 2935.4 + 293.54 = 3228.94 KCal/day.

1 Adapted and modified from: Wilmore, D.W. The Metabolic Management of the Critically Ill. New York. Plenum, 1977.

2 Surface area in m^2 = $W^{0.425}$ x $H^{0.725}$ x 71.84 X 10^{-4} where W is the weight in kilograms and H the height in centimeters (modified equation from Du Bois and Du Bois, Arch. Int. Med.: 17:863, 1916 - abstracted from Documenta Geigy, Sixth Edition, 1962). A hand held calculator is easily programmed to make this calculation from the formula.

for fat and about 6KCal/100KCal for carbohydrates. About 10% of total energy needs is an estimate used to calculate the SDA needs. It must be added to the caloric requirements when calculating total energy needs.

Final estimation of 24 hour metabolic needs:

Chart 15-2 is an example that shows how one determines the energy needs of an individual with arbitrarily chosen age, height, weight and disease.

There are significant differences in the water contents of different foods. Milk (whole pasteurized milk) has a water content of about 85% and a caloric content of about 65KCal/100g. Eggs and cooked rice each contain approximately 75% water, bread and meats about 30-50%, and at the other extreme, cooking oils have practically no water. Caloric values per unit weight are based on calculations which include the weights of these water contents.

For example, potatoes contain about 75% water and have a caloric content of about 85KCal/100g. I specifically mention potatoes and milk because a friend (a physician) once told me that potatoes and milk constituted a perfect combination diet, one used in Ireland for many years, presumably with occasional supplements of eggs and meat. My friend claimed that starvation and mass migration from Ireland occurred because of starvation resulting from failure of a potato harvest! This may or may not be true. Certainly, cow's milk does contain all the essential amino acids and one could devise an adequate, albeit a dreadfully monotonous and unpleasant diet, based on cow's milk and potatoes.

The essential components of a diet.

The following summarizes the essentials of a satisfactory diet.

Proteins and the essential amino acids.

Ten amino acids are essential for an appropriate diet: arginine, histidine, leucine and isoleucine, lysine, methionine, phenylalanine, threonine, tryptophan and valine. Two of the ten, histidine and arginine, are only required for normal growth. The essential amino acids are constituents of body proteins and are called essential because ionine, phenylalanine, threonine, tryptophan and valine. Two of the ten, histidine and arginine, are only required for normal growth. The essential amino acids are constituents of body proteins and are called essential because the body cannot synthesize them, or can only do so in insufficient amounts.

Proteins are often classified as Grade 1 and Grade 2 proteins. The former are the proteins of meat, dairy products, fish and eggs. They contain all essential amino acids in appropriate proportions. Most Grade 2 proteins are plant proteins that lack one or more essential amino acids or contain them in wrong proportions. Nevertheless, if their intake is sufficiently varied and large, amino acid needs can usually be met. Proteins should constitute some 20-25% of the calories in a normal diet. When calculating dietary needs it is common to calculate protein needs first. The remainder can be split (ideally in a ratio of about 3:2) between carbohydrates (45%) and fat (30%) according to taste and available monies; most carbohydrates (for example bread, pasta, potatoes, and rice) are much cheaper than other types of food. Carbohydrate consumption creates hunger, probably because of the hypoglycemic dips within a few hours of eating. This is probably why the poor are often fatter than the affluent; carbohydrate is cheap but it creates hunger.

Essential fats.

Two fatty acids are considered essential dietary components: linoleic acid and arachidonic acid. The latter can be synthesized in vivo from the former. Most of the dietary needs are readily met from vegetable seed oils (sunflower, safflower, soybean, peanut, etc.).

Saturated and unsaturated fats.

Fats contain saturated as well as unsaturated compounds. Fatty acids are chemicals with long side chains of hydrocarbons: $-CH_3-CH_2-CH_2$....(15-24 carbons long)..CH_2 The last carbon atom attaches by separate bonds to O or to OH. The bonds between carbon atoms are covalent bonds.

Saturated fatty acids have no double bonds between carbon atoms. **Unsaturated fatty acids** have at least one double bond in the hydrocarbon side chain this bond lets them bend. They tend to be liquids at room temperature.

Saturated fats are thought to raise blood cholesterol more than the unsaturated variety. Saturated fats are the fats from meat, milk and dairy products; abstinence can be difficult and probably nutritionally undesirable for both, vegetarians and meat-eaters. Dietary moderation of meat, milk and dairy product consumption is the best solution. Vegetarians should consume adequate amounts of dairy products to compensate for avoiding meat products.

Partially hydrogenated vegetable oils are often used in the manufacture of margarine and shortening. They contain a variety of **unsaturated fat known as trans-fatty acids.** Trans fatty acids are also supposed to raise blood cholesterol though not as much as saturated fats.

Monosaturated and polyunsaturated fats are present in most vegetable oils. Olive and canola oils have the highest levels. But most other vegetable oils, nuts and fatty fish have high levels of polyunsaturated fats. Both monosaturated and polyunsaturated fats are said to reduce blood cholesterol when they replace saturated fats in the diet.

Omega-3 is a polyunsaturated fatty acid present in fish fat. It is said to decrease the risk of coronary artery disease but the postulate remains unproven.

Carbohydrate.

There are no essential dietary carbohydrates. Stored and dietary fat can supply energy for all biological activities except those performed by the CNS. Glucose is the almost exclusive source of energy for the brain (after 4-5 days of fasting the brain can use ketones for some of its energy needs). Glucose can be synthesized from protein (the alanine-glucose cycle), from the metabolism of glycerol and from odd-chain fatty acids. Enzymes for conversion of even-chain fatty acids do not exist in the body and only 5% of body fatty acids are odd-chain compounds so that fat contributes little to gluconeogenesis. Protein wasting is a consequence of supplying the brain with glucose when the diet contains insufficient carbohydrate. Muscular weakness results and the failure of respiratory muscle function is the usual cause of death after prolonged fasting or starvation.

Vitamins.

The vitamins are essential for maintenance of health. Some such as Vitamin D can be synthesized in the body as long as there is sufficient exposure to sunlight. Intestinal bacteria can synthesize others such as Vitamin K. Hence, the need to reduce anticoagulant dosage when patients receive oral antibiotics that may kill these bacteria. In general, vitamins are essential components of diet.

There are two main groups of vitamins. A water-soluble group that is easily absorbed (Vitamin B complex and Vitamin C) and the fat-soluble vitamins (Vitamins A, D and K - also Vitamin E, a vitamin of uncertain activity). Deficits of fat-soluble vitamins contained in eaten fat can develop if obstruction at the ampulla of Vater or marked cholestasis blocks intestinal entry of biliary or pancreatic lipase or bile salts. The bile salts are responsible for emulsification of water-insoluble fat so that the area available to lipase is increased. They are also required for the formation of the micelles that keep the water-insoluble products of fat digestion in solution till they are absorbed into the intestinal mucosa.

Minerals.

Various minerals must be ingested for maintenance of health. They include the following: chromium, cobalt (for vitamin B_{12} production), copper, fluorine, iodine (deficiencies result in thyroid dysfunctions), sodium, manganese, molybdenum, nickel, potassium (it is almost impossible to have a diet that does not contain sodium and potassium), selenium, silicon, tin, vanadium and zinc[21]. Deficiency syndromes are rare as few diets do not supply an abundance of these trace elements. They may occur if there are deficiencies in solutions used for long-term intravenous alimentation.

Water and oxygen.

Water and oxygen needs have been detailed in previous sections. Both are essential requirements for production of energy that can be used for biological needs, i.e., ~P.

Syndromes of nutritional dysfunction.

The most common dysfunctional syndromes responsible for disease are obesity, malnutrition, subnutrition, and abnormalities of lipid metabolism. The overfed are prone to diseases with multifactorial causes: heart disease, diabetes, respiratory disease, and arthritis are some.

Subnutrition and malnutrition result in weak, apathetic and stunted individuals. They tire easily, the smooth contours of the body are absent and the bony protuberances are prominent. When children are affected there is good evidence that there is retarded mental development in addition to subnormal growth.

Nutritional marasmus is the eventual pathetic result of prolonged subnutrition. Typical is the wasted body, devoid of muscle and fat, generalized weakness, growth retardation, and eventual death.

Many syndromes characterize deficiencies of specific dietary components and some are detailed below. Notable examples are the different protein, iron and vitamin-deficiency syndromes.

Iron,Vitamin B_{12} and folate deficiencies.

These topics were detailed on pages 274-277. Additional text would be repetitive.

Protein-energy malnutrition and Kwashiorkor.

Causes: A diet rich in carbohydrate but deficient in protein. Factors which adversely affect the condition are often present. They include infections, parasite infestation, gastroenteritis, and childhood exanthems.

Clinical features: Typical features are edema (usually due to low serum albumin), apathy, wasted and weak muscles, various skin lesions, deficits in growth and motor development, and hepatomegaly.

The WHO[22] calls protein-energy malnutrition a "silent emergency" that is an accomplice in at least half of the 10.9 million child deaths each year. Protein-energy malnutrition affects every 4th. child in the world. Of them 150 million (26.7%) are underweight while 182 million (32.5%) are stunted. More than 70% of these children live in Asia, 26% in Africa and 4% in Latin America. The WHO seems to distinguish between protein-energy malnutrition and kwashiorkor. It ascribes the latter to natural or man-made emergencies

The clinical features of kwashiorkor are more severe than those seen in protein-energy malnutrition. Typical features are edema (usually due to low serum albumin) of the legs, torso, and face, apathy and weakness, muscle wasting, skin that is cracked, peeling and prone to infections, deficits in growth and motor development, hepatomegaly, and sparse blonde hair.

Pellagra - a niacin deficiency syndrome

Nicotinic acid (niacin) is present in grains, dairy products, meat and vegetables. It can also be synthesized endogenously from tryptophan and then converted to nicotinamide, an essential component of normal metabolism. It is a requirement for many anabolic and catabolic processes - glycolysis, and fatty acid, protein and amino acid metabolism.

A deficiency occurs when a specific type of diet is eaten. Typical was the diet of the slave plantations where the main staple food was corn. The diet was deficient in tryptophan and existing niacin was endogenously bound and biologically unavailable. The clinical features were summarized as the four ds: diarrhea, dementia, dermatitis and eventually, death.

Vitamin A deficiency:

Sources: Vitamin A and its provitamin, β-carotene are present in vegetables and in fruit and dairy products but not in meat or grains.

Causes: Vitamin A is a fat soluble vitamin and deficiencies can result from failures of absorption due to any one or more of the following: pancreatic or biliary tract obstructions, chronic diarrhea, malabsorption syndromes and cystic fibrosis. Other causes are the dietary deficiencies that are seen in some parts of Asia where rice devoid of carotene is the staple food and the diet is deficient in protein with consequent protein-energy malnutrition.

Deficiency syndrome: Vitamin A deficiency is the main cause of blindness in our world. The unfortunate victims are often young children. Surprisingly, it is commonest in countries where plant carotenoids are plentiful: e.g., India, Indonesia, and Central America. Maternal education on diet is essential. Vitamin A deficiency results from of lack of food and potable water, and a diet which does not include essential nutrients such as Vitamin A. Undoubtedly, malabsorptions due to chronic gastrointestinal infections and lactase deficits are additional important factors. The effects of Vitamin A deficits are probably preventable by eating lots of uncooked vegetables or fruits and supplementing food with Vitamin A. The supplements are not without danger and have caused fatalities in at least one WHO trial in India (S. Desai in http://www.indiasocial.org/ogi/news.asp).

In 1992 an online WHO bulletin by Humphreys and associates (http://whqlibdoc.who.int/bulletin/1992) claimed that Vitamin A deficiency resulted in millions of cases of xerophthalmia and a half million cases of irreversible blindness each year. Things have improved because of education and supplements. An early symptom of Vitamin A deficiency is the appearance of Bitot spots which are gray foamy spots in the whites of the eyes. Night blindness is an early symptom. The characteristic corneal lesions develop later: dryness, ulceration, corneal destruction (keratomalacia), scarring and eventual loss of vision.

Vitamin B-complex deficiencies.

Sources: These vitamins are present in most foods: meat, grains, dairy products and vegetables.

Thiamine (Vitamin B_1) deficiency.

Thiamine is an essential requirement for Kreb's cycle metabolism. It is mostly present in the outer layers of seeds. Consumption of polished rice used to be a common cause of thiamine deficiency in rice-eating countries. In alcoholics deficiency syndromes result from a combination of an inadequate intake of thiamine and increased excretion of this water-soluble vitamin. The clinical syndromes vary. Dry beri-beri is characterized by peripheral neuropathies, muscle wasting and weaknesses, and uncommonly, eventual paraplegia.

In wet beri-beri the target tissue of the deficit is the heart and the condition is characterized by tachycardia, edema and other signs of cardiac failure. The response to therapy can be surprisingly prompt. An example case history was detailed on page 259.

Wernicke's encephalopathy is almost exclusive to thiamine deficiency in alcoholics of European descent. Typical is the triad of confusion, ataxia and ophthalmoplegia. Psychosis, confabulation, and poor memory and cognition are other common features.

Riboflavin (Vitamin B_2) deficiency.

Riboflavin is present in dairy products, meat and grains. Deficits occur as part of generalized subnutrition or malnutrition states and in alcoholics. The clinical features are not characteristic: angular stomatitis, glossitis and sore throats.

Vitamin C deficiency.

The vitamin is plentiful in citrus and other fruits, leafy vegetables and tomatoes. The principal defects result from deficient collagen synthesis. The result is generalized small hemorrhages. The following are some of the clinical features; swollen and bleeding gums, petechiae. follicular hyperkeratoses with perifollicular hemorrhages, fatigue and aching muscles. In extreme cases there are hemorrhages into pleural and pericardial cavities subperiosteal hemorrhages and separations of epiphyses or costochondral junctions. The X-ray appearances are characteristic.

Children develop scurvy when bottle fed with boiled milk or milk substitutes lacking Vitamin C. Typically symptoms are seen at about eight months of age. The legs are slightly flexed, painful and tender as are the costochondral junctions. Petechiae and hemorrhages may be present but the gums show little change till teeth erupt. They then become swollen and hemorrhagic.

Treatment of adults and children is simple and effective. Orange juice and/or ascorbic acid tablets are the remedies.

Vitamin D deficiency.

A deficiency of Vitamin D is the cause of osteomalacia and rickets. The topic was discussed in a previous chapter that detailed the normal and abnormal biologies of bone (pages 311-312). Additional text is not needed.

Iodine deficiency.

Iodine deficiency was and perhaps still is the world's commonest cause of mental retardation. It is especially common in mountainous areas such as the Himalayas, the Alps and the Andes where glaciation has washed away iodine and there is no iodine supplementation of salt.

Iodine deficiency during pregnancy may result in stillbirths, abortions and cretinism. Cretinism is a serious and irreversible form of mental retardation affecting children born in iodine-deficient areas of Africa and Asia. With growth other features often become demonstrable - dwarfism, puffy features, dry skin and hair, squints, deaf mutism and a characteristic motor spasticity.

The goiter of individuals living in areas of iodine deficiency is a hyperplastic response to iodine deficiency. Characteristically, it is a smooth and diffuse goiter. Later nodules may develop and, at times, nodules with autonomous production of thyroid hormones. Therapy of non-toxic goiters due to iodine deficiency is supplemental iodine. At times individuals receive L-thyroxine to decrease goiter size. It suppresses TSH stimulation of the thyroid. TSH stimulation of the thyroid is a major cause of iodine deficiency goiters in areas where iodine is deficient. Thyroxine is best not given to elderly patients unless there is evidence of myxedema or hypothyroidism caused by some other dysfunction such as Hashimoto's disease. I_{131} has been used to decrease thyroid size but has its own dangers. Pressure effects from large goiters may need surgical reductions.

Prevention is simple - iodination of salt. Universal salt iodination (USI) (70mcg/g) was started in 1993. Now more than 70% of individuals living in iodine deficient areas have access to iodized salt and global rates of mental retardation and cretinism are falling fast as is the incidence of iodine-deficiency goiter. Dropping iodine into well water is a practical solution in many developing countries.

Disordered uric acid metabolism.

Uric acid is formed from ingested purines as well as those formed by endogenous metabolism. By far the commonest manifestation of disordered uric acid metabolism is gout. The specific cause is undetermined and the condition is a consequence of over-production and/or decreased excretion of uric acid.

Gout occurs in two forms: acute and chronic. Primary acute gout, occurring for no obvious reason, is the common form. It results from deposition of urate crystals in cartilage, articular bone, and periarticular structures with a surrounding inflammatory reaction. Its manifestation is a monoarticular acute arthritis with pain, swelling, redness, heat, and fever. The first metatarso-phalangeal joint is affected in about half those affected but no one joint is immune. The condition is readily treated with colchicine or a non-steroidal anti-inflammatory, e.g., indomethacin, and if untreated, is self-limiting. Colchicine is preferable if there are any cardiac dysfunctions. Indomethacin and other non-steroidal anti-inflammatories can result in water retention with development of congestive heart failure in previously well controlled and stable cardiac dysfunctions.

A chronic form of gout is common if high blood levels of uric acid are not adequately controlled. Features include gouty tophi, chronic gouty arthritis with characteristic radiological features, a high incidence of renal calculi, and chronic renal disease.

Secondary gout results when hyperuricemia results from causes which are known to produce the metabolic dysfunction. Examples are myeloproliferative disorders, extreme obesity, chronic renal disease, and situations where therapeutic drugs raise blood uric acid levels (e.g., chemotherapy for treatment of leukemias). The last results in urate release from destroyed white cells.

All patients with a history of gout and persistently high levels of blood uric acid should receive allopurinol. This drug blocks production of xanthine oxidase. Xanthine oxidase is the enzyme which converts hypoxanthine to xanthine and then to uric acid.

Allopurinol should also be given to all patients receiving chemotherapy for white cell neoplasms. Destruction of white cells raises blood uric acid levels and can result in gout as well as renal uric acid stones.

Disordered amino acid metabolism.

Most of these conditions are uncommon genetically transmitted diseases. They are rare and for more information on the subject specialized texts should be consulted.

Exercise

The value of exercise is recognized by most cardiac rehabilitation centers. It reduces the incidence and severity of myocardial infarctions and there is some evidence that exercise enhances opening up collaterals.

Isotonic and isometric exercise.

Isotonic exercise.

Isotonic exercise consists of voluntary muscle movements characterized by alternate contractions and relaxations of muscle groups. Examples are walking, jogging and swimming.

Isometric exercise.

Isometric exercise is static exercise in which muscles are kept in a state of continued contraction. A typical example is weight-lifting. It is inferior to isotonic exercise because energy expenditure is less than in isotonic exercise and undesirable hemodynamic changes can occur.

Training.

Trained athletes have a larger stroke volume, a lower heart rate and a larger heart than the untrained. An important effect of exercise is an increase in maximal oxygen consumption (VO_{2max}). It reflects cardiac output and O_2 usage by muscles and other tissues. The normal VO_{2max} is about 32ml/Kg/min. This works out to about

2.2L/min of oxygen for a 70Kg man. Ideally, training sessions should aim for VO_{2max} levels of at least 60%. Unfortunately facilities for measurement are usually not available.

The following are some of the benefits of a training program:

- Reduction of body weight and body fat percentage and an increase in lean body mass.
- Increased mobility of joints - this is especially valuable in the elderly.
- An increase in work capacity that results when VO_{2max} increases by 10-30%. This increase results mainly from increased cardiac output and increased pulmonary ventilation. An additional cause is an increased extraction of oxygen from arterial blood. Commensurate with the increase in heart rate, cardiac output and ventilation, the venous oxygen saturation decreases as more oxygen is extracted and used in the cells,
- At similar work loads trained individuals will have lower heart rates and a more rapid post-exercise recovery of heart rate.
- With training higher oxygen debts can be incurred and for the same amount of work there is less accumulation of lactate.
- The systolic pressure and diastolic pressures of trained individuals are lower and there is evidence that training can reduce hypertension.
- The improved psychology and social adjustments of exercise training are important.

Exercise for patients with cardiac disease.

Physical inactivity is an independent risk factor for coronary artery disease. The usual recommendation is isotonic exercise and some limited isometric exercise.

A warm-up and cool-down phase are said to be especially important in patients with cardiac disease as they seem to reduce the incidence of ischemia and ventricular arrhythmias[24]. There are few absolute contraindications to exercise for patients with coronary artery disease though obvious ones are a recent myocardial infarct, especially if accompanied by serious arrhythmias. Another qualified contraindication is a low ejection fraction; nothing more vigorous than light exercise is acceptable for these patients.

Adaptations that result from exercise are predominantly peripheral and located in exercising muscle. However, the beneficial effects of exercise for patients taking beta blockers could in part result from increased cardiac contractility. The heart rate cannot increase much in these patients so that there must be some increase in cardiac contractility and output during exercise to supply the increased demands of the peripheral vasculature.

Reducing the intensity and increasing the duration of exercise, and breaking up the sessions are valuable options for the elderly and for patients in poor condition. The total work done is unchanged.

Lifestyle changes

Many diseases result from inappropriate habits and lifestyles, especially, many cardiac, respiratory, and neurological diseases and malignancies. Examples are smoking, taking so-called "recreational" drugs, drinking excessive amounts of alcohol, and risky sexual relations. The function of the physician is to advise. The patient must be told what possible consequences could result from any one or more forms of the intemperate behaviors practiced. Gentle and repeated persuasions are generally more effective than demands for change. Unfortunately any change in habit is unusual.

This ends a short summary of therapeutic measures that help to prevent or, at least, ameliorate diseases.

References to Chapter 15.

1. WHO Global tuberculosis control: surveillance, planning, financing. WHO report 2003; Geneva. WHO
2. Garner, J.S., Jarvis, W.R., et al. CDC definitions for nosocomial infections. Am. J. Infect. Control 1988; 16:128.
3. Richards, M.J., Edwards, J.R., et al. Nosocomial infections in combined medical-surgical intensive care units in the United States. Infect. Control Hosp. Epidemiol. 2000; 21:510.

4. Pittet, D., Dharan, S., et al. Bacterial contamination of hands of hospital staff during routine patient care, Arch. Int. Med. 1999; 159:821.

5. Maury, E., Alzieu, M., et al. Availability of an alcohol solution can improve hand disinfection compliance in an intensive care unit. Am. J. Respir. Crit. Care Med. 2000; 162:324.

6. Boyce, J.M., Pittet, D. Guidelines for hand hygiene in health care settings. MMWR Recomm. Rep. 2002; 51:1.

7. Preventing malaria. Another jab. The Economist 2002; August 22. (http://www.economist.com/research/backgrounders).

8. National Academy of Sciences, Committee on Research in the Life Sciences of the Committee on Science and public policy. 1970.

9. Smith, A.G. Chlorinated hydrocarbon insecticides. In Hayes, E.J., Laws, E.R. (Eds.): Handbook of pesticide toxicology. San Diego. Academic Press, 1991.

10. Schechter, A., Toniolo, P., et al. Blood levels of DDT and breast cancer risk among women living the North of Vietnam. Arch. Enviro. Contamin. Toxicol. 1997; 33:453.

11. Smith, A.G. How toxic is DDT. Lancet 2000; 356:267.

12. Lines, J.D. Should DDT be banned by International treaty? Parasitol. Today 2000; 16:119.

13. Desowitz, R.S. Malaria Capers. W.W. Norton & Company, 1992 (quote obtained from "100 things you should know about DDT." by Edwards, J.G., Milloy, S.: http://www.junkscience.com).

14. Sharma, V.P. & Sharma, R.S. Cost Effectiveness of Bioenvironmental Control of Malaria in Kheda District of Gujarat. Ind. J. Malariology 1986; 23:141.

15. Sharma, V.P. Laboratory experiments on the effectiveness of Expanded polystyrene beads in mosquito control. Ind. J. Malariology 1984; 21:115.

16. Polio vaccines: http://www.polioeradication.org/vaccines/polioeradication/all/background/vaccines.asp.

17. Halsey, N.A., et al. Measles immunization in HIV-infected children. Pediatric 103: 1057; 1999

18. Colditz, G.A., Brewer, T.E., et al. Efficacy of BCG vaccine in the prevention of tuberculosis: meta-analysis of the published literature. JAMA 1994; 271:698.

19. Mwinga, A. Treatment in developing countries. In: Enarson, D.A., Grosset, J., et al. (Eds.).The challenge of tuberculosis: statements on global control and prevention. Lancet 1995; 346:812.

20. WHO web page for vaccines. http://www.who.int/vaccine_research/diseases/tb/en/.

21. Ulmer, D.D. Trace elements. N. Engl. J. Med. 1977; 297:318.

22. WHO Web site for nutrition. "Alleviating protein-energy malnutrition".

23. WHO Web site for "Micronutrient deficiencies."

24. Foster, C., Anholm, J.D. et al. Left ventricular function during sudden strenuous exercise. Circulation 1981; 63:592.

16

Therapy
2. Drugs and Surgery

Table of Contents

Notation.

The notation ~P denotes phosphorous with a high energy bond. Depending on the context in which the term is used, ~P may also denote the energy liberated when a high energy phosphate bond detaches from ATP or ADP.

Chart 16-1:	A SUMMARY OF THE POSSIBLE REASONS FOR NOT OBTAINING A DESIRED AND EXPECTED THERAPEUTIC RESPONSE
A.	**THE CHOICE OF THERAPY WAS WRONG:**
1.	Incorrect interpretation of the history.
2.	Mistakes in the clinical examination.
3.	Erroneous interpretations of ancillary findings and/or failure to do other necessary and appropriate investigations.
4.	Insufficient or mistaken knowledge.
5.	Not knowing that additional information related to the problem exists and/or where to find it.
6.	Insufficient objectivity.
7.	Failure to consult books, journals, colleagues and specialists as and when necessary.
8.	Failure could be the result of abnormal drug metabolism, or clinical responses which are less than those expected because of any one or more different causes. Many possibilities are detailed in the text. Try increasing the dose but with close clinical and, if possible and available, monitoring of blood levels. Alternatively, try another drug which is expected to have the same clinical effects as the one which has failed.
B.	**THE CHOICE OF THERAPY WAS CORRECT BUT THE PATIENT'S RESPONSE WAS POOR:**
1.	Check for patient's compliance with therapy.
2.	Cause of disease cannot be treated, controlled or eliminated. Disease can take any one of three forms: curable and controllable; incurable but controllable; or incurable and uncontrollable. When disease is both incurable and uncontrollable a fatal termination is inevitable if biologically essential systems are affected. Thus, osteoarthritis is usually incurable and often uncontrollable but is not, per se, an eventually fatal condition. Progressive and incurable neurological, respiratory, cardiac, renal or hepatic failure are.
3.	Biological and pharmacogenetic variations in physiology, pharmacology, and response to therapy.
4.	Intercurrent dysfunctions which might have precipitated failure is a previously stable situation:, e.g., fever, anemia, infections, compromised immunological competencies (e.g., in patients with AIDS), thyrotoxicosis, binge eating and/or drinking of food, water, and/or alcohol, and the taking of drugs which adversely affect the ability of the CNS to compute, control and command (therapeutic drugs and also the so-called "recreational" drugs).
5.	Unsuspected and undiagnosed additional disease such as diabetes, infections such as tuberculosis or AIDS, or occult primary or metastatic malignancy.
6.	Age related failures in response to therapy and in compensatory and protective mechanisms. The functional reserves of most organ systems decrease with the individual's aging. The physiological deficits which accompany aging were documented on pages 74-75.
7.	Adverse reactions to drugs: toxic, idiosyncratic or allergic, expected or unexpected, in any one or more combinations. Adverse drug reactions are comprehensively detailed and described later in this chapter.
8.	Disease too advanced to respond to treatment.
9.	Insufficient functional reserve in diseased tissues.
10.	The functional responses of compensatory mechanisms are not providing adequate compensation or control. They may be adversely affected by the disease being treated or by the therapy being given, or by some other different etiology. Alternatively they may be already performing to their limits.

The objectives.

This chapter details the two principal modalities for the treatment of disease: drug therapy and surgery. Often, both are required in combination. The objectives are two:

- **First, the elimination of the cause of the disease or dysfunction, and/or retardation of its progression. If neither is possible the only therapeutic objectives are relief of pain and suffering,** **(Contd. on page 343)**

Chart 16-2: THE ITERATIVE LOOP FOR EVALUATION OF THERAPEUTIC RESPONSES

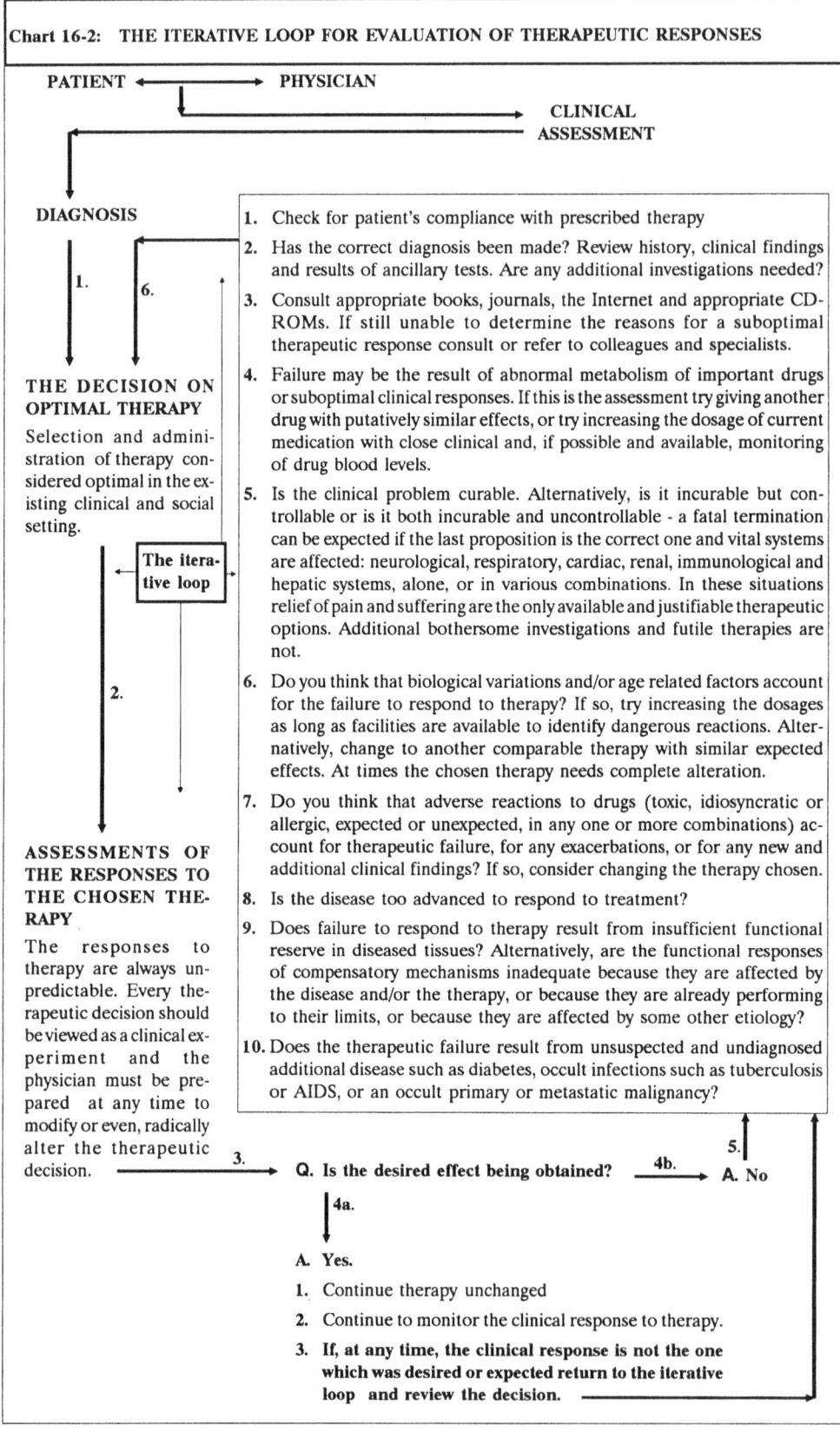

PATIENT ↔ **PHYSICIAN** → **CLINICAL ASSESSMENT** → **DIAGNOSIS**

DIAGNOSIS

1. ↓ 6. ↓

THE DECISION ON OPTIMAL THERAPY

Selection and administration of therapy considered optimal in the existing clinical and social setting.

The iterative loop

2. ↓

ASSESSMENTS OF THE RESPONSES TO THE CHOSEN THERAPY

The responses to therapy are always unpredictable. Every therapeutic decision should be viewed as a clinical experiment and the physician must be prepared at any time to modify or even, radically alter the therapeutic decision. — 3. → **Q. Is the desired effect being obtained?** — 4b. → **A. No** — 5. ↑ (to the iterative loop)

1. Check for patient's compliance with prescribed therapy
2. Has the correct diagnosis been made? Review history, clinical findings and results of ancillary tests. Are any additional investigations needed?
3. Consult appropriate books, journals, the Internet and appropriate CD-ROMs. If still unable to determine the reasons for a suboptimal therapeutic response consult or refer to colleagues and specialists.
4. Failure may be the result of abnormal metabolism of important drugs or suboptimal clinical responses. If this is the assessment try giving another drug with putatively similar effects, or try increasing the dosage of current medication with close clinical and, if possible and available, monitoring of drug blood levels.
5. Is the clinical problem curable. Alternatively, is it incurable but controllable or is it both incurable and uncontrollable - a fatal termination can be expected if the last proposition is the correct one and vital systems are affected: neurological, respiratory, cardiac, renal, immunological and hepatic systems, alone, or in various combinations. In these situations relief of pain and suffering are the only available and justifiable therapeutic options. Additional bothersome investigations and futile therapies are not.
6. Do you think that biological variations and/or age related factors account for the failure to respond to therapy? If so, try increasing the dosages as long as facilities are available to identify dangerous reactions. Alternatively, change to another comparable therapy with similar expected effects. At times the chosen therapy needs complete alteration.
7. Do you think that adverse reactions to drugs (toxic, idiosyncratic or allergic, expected or unexpected, in any one or more combinations) account for therapeutic failure, for any exacerbations, or for any new and additional clinical findings? If so, consider changing the therapy chosen.
8. Is the disease too advanced to respond to treatment?
9. Does failure to respond to therapy result from insufficient functional reserve in diseased tissues? Alternatively, are the functional responses of compensatory mechanisms inadequate because they are affected by the disease and/or the therapy, or because they are already performing to their limits, or because they are affected by some other etiology?
10. Does the therapeutic failure result from unsuspected and undiagnosed additional disease such as diabetes, occult infections such as tuberculosis or AIDS, or an occult primary or metastatic malignancy?

4a. ↓

A. Yes.

1. Continue therapy unchanged
2. Continue to monitor the clinical response to therapy.
3. **If, at any time, the clinical response is not the one which was desired or expected return to the iterative loop and review the decision.** →

(Contd. from page 341)

not additional unnecessary investigations and unpleasant therapies and medications. The response to therapy is determined by comparing physiologically permissible and desirable limits of function with those that exist in the sick person. If they are returning to normal therapy is succeeding. If not, it is failing for any one or more of the reasons cited in Chart 16-1.

The object is to restore clinical disease and dysfunctions to functions that are within normal limits. Chart 16-1 provides a check-list for identifying possible causes for therapeutic success or failure. When there seems to be therapeutic failure it is a good idea to go through the chart to try and identify a possible reason or reasons.

Evaluations of responses to therapy need iterations of previously designed loops. Chart 16-2 on page 341 showed how iterative loops can be used for evaluating the response to therapy.

- **The second objective is therapy which which does not result in adverse effects and residual disabilities in:**
  - **Tissues affected by the disease.**
  - **Systems that are compensating** for the physiological dysfunctions resulting from the disease and
  - **Systems not affected by the presenting disease and unrelated to the one primarily affected.** Any damage to the function of such systems could easily decrease inter-system coordination and in this way jeopardize the normal coordinated integrations of sensory, intellectual and motor functions.

The start of therapy

The most important decision in the therapeutic decision is the first one.

The Economist of March 9, 2002 published an article citing the views of Mr. Welch, then Chief Executive Officer of General Electric. He quoted from a letter written by a senior manager to Fortune magazine. The quote was based on a book written in 1832 by an eminent Prussian military strategist, Carl von Clausewitz and titled, “On War”. The quote stated:

> “Von Clausewitz summed up what it had all been about in his classic “On War”. Men could not reduce strategy to a formula. Detailed planning necessarily failed, due to the inevitable frictions encountered: chance events, imperfections in execution, and the independent will of the opposition. Instead, the human elements were paramount: leadership, morale, and the instinctive savvy of the best generals.”

The Prussian general staff, under the elder von Moltke, perfected these concepts in practice. They did not expect a plan of operations to survive beyond the first contact with the enemy. They set only the broadest of objectives and emphasized seizing unforeseen opportunities as they arose. Strategy was not a lengthy action plan. It was the remembering of basic and essential objectives despite continually changing circumstances.

The uncertainties and unpredictabilities of medicine require that the physician proceed in the same way when initiating therapy and evaluating the results. When the clinical situation is complex and especially when the patient is elderly, it is most unlikely that all will go according to plan for any one or more of the reasons detailed in Chart 16-2. Always be ready to change, to look for desirable and undesirable changes, to combat changes that are undesirable, and to seize on unexpected advantages. Optimal therapy often requires modifications and changes as therapy progresses. These are the only effective weapons in a war against disease and premature death, for it is a war.

Unfortunately, for every human a final defeat is inevitable for all humans are mortals. When faced with defeat, accept its inevitability, cease unnecessary, uncomfortable and useless investigations and therapies and concentrate therapeutic endeavors on relieving pain and suffering till the inevitable end.

Three maxims of good therapy follow. The first derives from the above, the others from what follows in this chapter.

— **Maxim 1: In treating disease the choice of initial therapy is the most important consideration. If it is**

incorrect failure is almost certain. Sometimes resolution and recovery do occur even when the choice of therapy is wrong. This type of recovery usually results from innate and spontaneous resistances and resolutions. Useless therapy has failed but the internal resources of the patient have succeeded.

- **Maxim 2: Any drug can do anything, at any time, at any dose, to any patient, regardless of the disease being treated. Unpredictables and uncertainties are inherent to any form of therapy. Always evaluate clinical responses and decisions in the frame of this caveat.**
- **Maxim 3: Every therapeutic decision is a clinical experiment with unpredictable outcomes. It may cure, have no effect or worsen the clinical picture. Repeated monitoring is essential using iterative loops of the type depicted in Chart 16-2. When necessary be prepared to modify or radically alter the therapy. The reasons for the unpredictabilities and uncertainties of clinical therapeutics were listed in Chart 16-1.**

The scope of drug and surgical therapy.

Some therapeutic regimens **cure,** admittedly, at times, without assurance of permanent cure. For example, when surgery is performed for conditions such as malignant disease or coronary artery disease the initial perception of cure is often followed by subsequent recurrences of disease and symptoms.

Other therapies only **control.** Their failure to cure does not detract from their value in clinical therapeutics. When I was a resident many of the individuals in hospital wards had preterminal congestive heart failure with dyspnea at rest and gigantic swollen, edematous legs. All we had to offer were digoxin and injections of a painful, and not too effective mercurial diuretic (mersalyl), two or three times a week.

The advent of diuretics has completely altered the picture. I have treated patients with congestive heart failure who have survived more than fifteen years with judicious control of symptomatology using diuretics, digoxin or beta blockers, and more recently, the ACE inhibitors. For those who experienced the situation fifty years ago the changes verge on the miraculous.

Fifty years ago hypertension was essentially untreatable. It often progressed to a malignant phase with papilledema, cardiac and renal failure, and eventual death. All that could be offered in acute situations were potent hypotensives used by the anesthetists. In less acute phases bizarre diets were prescribed. I well recall one that was called the rice diet and consisted, if I remember correctly, of a diet of rice and orange juice, exclusive of anything else. All has changed. Now most essential hypertension is easily controlled by any one or more drugs and death from uncontrolled hypertension has become a rarity unless unrecognized, or when the subject does not wish to take the requisite medications, or does not have the means to purchase them. Unrecognized or uncontrolled hypertension is a significant risk factor for hemorrhagic cerebrovascular strokes.

Currently, control of cardiovascular disease is of major importance. The WHO MONICA (MONItoring C-Ardiovascular disease) project claims that ⅓ of global deaths result from cardiovascular disease. Their estimate includes all patients with congenital heart disease, coronary artery disease, cerebrovascular disease, hypertension, cardiomyopathy, rheumatic heart disease and disease of the peripheral vessels. Cardiovascular disease kills 16.5 million individuals each year. It is not exclusive to affluent developed countries. The WHO estimates that by 2010 cardiovascular disease will be the leading cause of death in developing countries. Many of these deaths are unnecessary but lack of physicians, lack of drugs, and lack of monies to purchase drugs for long-term use are important negatives. Not only do 16.5 million people die each year but about 20 million survive and require costly future care. Drugs that control cardiovascular disease are valuable therapeutic agents even if they do not cure, but many are expensive.

Encouraging therapies are dialysis which is life-saving but has inherent disadvantages. The same applies to renal and liver transplantation. Control of endocrine hypofunction by replacement therapy is a bright spot as is therapy of endocrine hyperfunction. With respect to cancer, comments must be guarded. Chemotherapy seems to work well in the cancers of young people. An example is the remarkable recovery of many children with leukemia given chemotherapy. A well recognized triumph of chemotherapy is the cyclist, Lance Armstrong. Treatment with chemotherapy resulted in resolution of metastatic malignancy (I think the primary was a seminoma) and he has subsequently won the Tour de France on many occasions. With adult cancers the outlook is not as bright. Some control of recurrent breast cancer by chemotherapy does seem to be an actuality. I find it difficult to identify the exact percentage of patients who derived benefit from chemotherapy because of the many different therapeutic and clinical permutations and combinations in reported trials on breast cancer treatments and survivals. Certainly the outlook for patients with lung and stomach cancers[1] getting chemotherapy is bleak

The modes of action of drugs

The following describes the different ways in which drugs act. It includes some suggestions and caveats on the use of drugs and ways to deal with the uncertainties and unpredictables of drug use.

Approximately 50% of drugs act on cell membrane receptors, about 30% on enzyme systems and about 5% alter cell membrane ion channel permeabilities[2]. The remainder have diverse modes of action; examples are the cytotoxic agents used in cancer chemotherapy. New innovative drugs and also, drugs imitating the actions of those currently available, regularly appear on the market. In this text it is often impossible to avoid mentioning specific drugs by name without inadequately illustrating and documenting important principles. At all times the emphasis is on general principles for one knows that the future development and uses of new drugs and therapies is an inevitable ongoing process. Many of those in current use have limited shelf lives. A recent example is hormone replacement for post-menopausal symptoms, so actively promoted a few years ago

1. **Drugs that act on cell membrane receptors.**

The following are examples of drugs that act on cell membrane receptors:

a) **The agonists.**

Agonists are drugs that activate cells by binding to receptors on cell membranes. When an agonist (a stimulator) binds to a receptor the conformation of the latter changes and this stimulates specific cell activity. The receptor is specific for its agonist, presumably because of its shape. Many agonists have desirable as well as undesirable effects. Much pharmacological research is directed to altering the structure of agonists so that unwanted effects are decreased while the desired effects are retained or enhanced.

— **The artificial agonists.** One of the aims of pharmacology has been the development of drugs that resist quick removal of agonist from receptor because the synthetic drug resists the usual metabolic degradation of the natural agonist at the receptor. Perhaps the most commonly used drug of this type is salbutamol, an agent that stimulates respiration by stimulating β_2 adrenergic receptors and thus relaxing bronchial smooth muscle. The therapeutic effect results from its longer binding to the receptors than the natural agonist. Its bronchodilator effect can be potentiated by an anti-cholinergic drug having bronchodilator properties. An example is ipratropium bromide (Atrovent; Boehringer Ingelheim).

Occasionally tissue selective agonists are developed. An example is Raloxifene (Evista; Eli Lilly), a drug widely prescribed for treatment of osteoporosis. It inhibits the action of estrogen on the breast and endometrium but acts as an estrogen agonist on osteoblasts. The MORE study (Multiple Outcomes of Raloxifene Evaluation)[3] evaluated the effects of raloxifene on 7705 women with osteoporosis. A significant reduction in vertebral fractures was noted.

— **The natural agonists. A number of natural agonists exist in the body.** Notable examples are the hormones: insulin, thyroxine, the steroid hormones, the subtypes of histamine, and the many physiological peptides and neurotransmitters. Many natural agonists are of clinical use when there are deficiencies. Examples are insulin, thyroxine, the corticosteroids, norepinephrine and epinephrine. The last two are inhibitors of the histamine released in anaphylaxis; they also inhibit the release of mast cell histamine and kinins in anaphylactice reactions The bindings of natural agonists and their receptors are characterized by rapid separation of receptor from agonist once the latter has had its effect. This is a necessity for precise control of biological activity.

b) **The competitive antagonists.**

The competitive antagonists usually have a structural similarity to the agonist and can therefore bind to the specific receptor of the agonist. However, they do not stimulate the receptor. This inability to stimulate the receptor is usually only relative; a natural agonist can stimulate the receptor if the amount of competitive antagonist is not sufficiently large.

When the action of a natural agonist is prevented the body increases its production. Hence, if blockage of a receptor by a competitive antagonist is suddenly stopped excessive agonist effects. An example is the development of severe angina, and even congestive heart failure because of the effects of increased levels of norepinephrine when a beta blocker given as therapy is suddenly stopped. Cessation of treatment with competitive antagonists should be gradual so that sufficient time is available for the natural agonist to return to physiological levels. Competitive antagonists are probably the commonest of all drugs and those currently available act on most of the receptors identified to date. The following are some of those most commonly used:

- **Competitive antagonists that inhibit at the adrenergic alpha and beta receptors.**An example is the beta-blockers. Dichloroisoproterenol was the first beta-receptor antagonist used in humans but its use was discontinued because it had too much agonist activity which often resulted in tachycardia. Modifications of its catechol groups produced propanolol, a drug with increased anti-agonist activity but with almost no agonist activity. Propanolol is a non-specific beta-adrenergic receptor blocking drug. Subsequent research has introduced drugs such as atenolol that are said to only block the cardio-specific β_1 adrenergic receptor. There is often some spill-over to blockage of β_2 receptors so that the use of these so-called cardio-selective drugs is contraindicated if there is any clinical respiratory dysfunction.
- Ipratropium bromide (Atrovent; Boehringer Ingelheim) attaches to respiratory alpha adrenergic receptors and blocks the attachment of acetylcholine to these receptors. Thus, it is a drug which negates the constrictor effects of acetylcholine at the muscarinic receptors on bronchial muscle. Other competitive antagonists that inhibit at cholinergic receptors are atropine that inhibit at muscarinic receptors and curare that inhibits at nicotinic receptors.
- **Competitive antagonists that inhibit at histamine receptors.** Examples are anti-H_1 and anti-H_2 drugs. The H_1 competitive antagonist are anti-allergic drugs that block H_1 receptors. The H_2 competitive antagonists reduce gastric acidity by blocking gastric H_2 receptors. Examples of the latter are cimetidine and ranitidine.
- **Competitive antagonists that inhibit at opiate receptors.** In clinical practice naloxone that inhibits at the Mu receptor is of importance for diagnosis and treatment of opiate overdoses.
- **Competitive antagonists that inhibit hormones.** This is an important group of drugs and merits more detailed discussion than the previous competitive antagonists.

  Perhaps the commonest example of hormone inhibition therapeutics is the **birth control pill.** Typically, the pill is a combination of an agent with estrogenic activity (e.g., ethinyl estradiol) and one with progestational activity (e.g., levonorgestrel). Administration results in gonadotropin suppression and consequent suppression of ovulation.

  Tamoxifen is a hormone-antagonist that is anti-estrogenic because it competes with estrogen for binding sites in the breast and uterus. It is widely and effectively used in various phases of breast cancer. Unfortunately, the drug itself has estrogen-like effects on some tissues, notably, the endometrium, bone, and the blood lipids. The effect on the endometrium has the potential for inducing malignancy and regular monitoring of individuals taking tamoxifen as adjuvant therapy for breast cancer is essential.

  Aromatase inhibitors such as anastrazole (Arimidex; Zeneca) are alternatives that prevent de novo estrogen synthesis thus eliminating the estrogenic side effects occasionally seen with tamoxifen.

  Flutamide inhibits androgen uptake by target tissues and also inhibits intracellular binding of androgen to nuclear contents. When used in combination with an inhibitor of gonadotropin production (see below) inhibition of the progression of prostate cancer is enhanced.

  Inhibitors of gonadotropin production.[4] These drugs are analogs of gonadotropin releasing hormone

(GnRH or LHRH). Examples are leuprolide acetate (Lupron; Abbott) and goserelin acetate (Zoladex; AstraZeneca). They are potent inhibitors of gonadotropin production. A consequence is suppression of gonadal steroid production: ovarian as well as testicular. In women these agents are often used for treatment of endometriosis which is a frequent cause of infertility and in men, for treatment of prostatic malignancy, often in combination with an anti-androgen such as flutamide.

How do they act? The postulate is that the continual presence of these analogs at their pituitary receptors prevents the receptors from identifying the normal fluctuations in hypothalamic gonadotropin releasing factor levels. The receptors eventually become insensitive to the native hormones though there may be an initial flare reaction with increased LH and testosterone production. Eventually testosterone secretion stops in the face of continuous stimulation by the gonadotropin analog. The analog is often used with flutamide which blocks testosterone receptors. Remarkable remissions of metastatic prostatic cancer can be obtained. The following is an example of a patient with metastatic prostate cancer which regressed with Zoladex injections.

Case history

Male aged 77 seen because of dysarthria and dysphagia and deviation of the tongue. History of total prostatectomy for prostatic cancer 3 years previously. Clinically the findings were consistent with a jugular foramen syndrome: paralysis of 9th. to 12th. cranial nerves. An X-ray showed slightly increased density at the jugular foramen but the CT scan of the skull was normal. However, an MRI and a radionuclear scan showed extensive destruction of the base of the skull (in such situations never be fooled by near normal X-rays or normal CT scans). Always rely on the clinical assessment and follow through with a nuclear scan and a MRI if one is available. Treatment was one injection of goserelin acetate (Zoladex; Zeneca) every two weeks for the first two months and then once a month. Dysarthria and dysphagia began to decrease in two months. After a year a nuclear scan showed some reossification of the base of the skull. Complete reossification was demonstrable after three years. Dysarthria and dysphagia improved but never returned to normal. After a year he was articulate and understandable and could eat soft foods. He remained alive and well for seven years after starting Zoladex. Eventually control of cancer was lost but fortunately there was no painful ending as he died in his sleep at the age of 85, eight years after initiation of the gonadotropin-releasing hormone analog.

This case history is presented in some detail to show what surprising results are achievable by administration of a gonadotropin analog. Obviously, regression similar to that described above is not usual but some prolongation of life is, especially when the patient is elderly.

2. **Drugs that act on enzymes.**

Drugs that inhibit enzymes are widely used in clinical practice. The following are some of the more common ones:

-- **The angiotensin-converting enzyme (ACE) inhibitors.** ACE inhibitors such as captopril, lisinopril, and enalapril are widely and effectively used for treatment of hypertension and congestive heart failure. They act by suppressing the conversion of Angiotensin I to Angiotensin II by angiotensin converting enzyme (ACE). Angiotensin II is a potent vasoconstrictor. The ACE inhibitors reduce arteriolar resistance. Systolic and diastolic pressures decrease. Afterload and preload decrease and cardiac output and stroke volume increase. Decreased aldosterone production results in increased renal sodium output with water following passively. The uses of ACE inhibitors were extensively detailed in previous Chapters 7 and11. Their use in cardiovascular diseases is now well established and many publications attest to this. Recently a new class of drugs has been introduced. They are blockers of the angiotensin receptors. An example is Losartan potassium (Cozaar-Merck). It remains to be shown that they are superior to conventional ACE inhibitors for the treatment of cardiac dysfunctions and hypertension.

-- **Allopurinol** is another example of a commonly used enzyme-inhibiting drug. It inhibits xanthine oxidase and thus reduces in vivo synthesis of uric acid. The drug is widely used as prophylaxis in situations where high levels of uric acid exist (e.g., in gout) or when it is anticipated (e.g., in the treatment of hematological malignancies).

- **The monoamine oxidase (MAO) inhibitors.** Monoamine oxidases are enzymes that break down catecholamines in the circulation and the tissues. Most are found in neural tissues and the liver. In the liver they inactivate circulating catecholamines as well as circulating monoamines and monoamines absorbed from the intestine, notably tyramine.

  Inhibitors of these enzymes are occasionally used for treatment of depressions resistant or intolerant to other drugs or unsuitable for ECT. An important toxic reaction to these enzyme inhibitors is the **hypertensive crisis**. Monoamines, and especially tyramine absorbed from the gut escape deamination in the liver because of MAO inhibition. Tyramine that has not been deaminated by monoamine oxidase stimulates catecholamine release from nerve tissues where they have accumulated because of monoamine oxidase inhibition. Normally, monoamine oxidases break down catecholamines. The release of catecholamines into the circulation because of the failure of tyramine deamination can result in a hypertensive crisis. There is an acute elevation of blood pressure with severe headaches, fever, arrhythmias, pulmonary edema and occasionally, cerebrovascular hemorrhages, at times resulting in death.

  An average meal of cheese contains enough tyramine to precipitate a hypertensive crisis. Other substances implicated are many - beer, wine, chocolate, pickled herrings, coffee, cream and citrus fruits are some examples. Any patient given a MAO inhibitor must be given a list of foods to avoid, and close relatives should be advised on the symptoms suggestive of a hypertensive crisis and of appropriate dietary restrictions.

3. Drugs that act on cell membrane pumps and ion pores.

This class of drugs acts by its effects on macromolecules (the ionophores) that transport ionic material across cell membranes. Examples of drugs that exert their effects by acting on membrane ionophores include common anti-epileptics, and some drugs that are cardiac anti-arrhythmics.

Others function by an effect on membrane pumps. An important example is digitalis. This drug is widely used in patients with cardiac problems and therefore merits a little additional comment.

- **Digitalis.** The drug probably acts by inhibition of the cell membrane pump and ion channel for sodium transport. It does this by inhibiting cell membrane Na^+/K^+-ATPase which provides the energy (~P) for maintenance of the cell membrane pumps and ion channels. The intracellular entry of Na^+ increases because of a concentration gradient. The result is an increased uptake of calcium by the sarcolemma to maintain the osmotic balance between intracellular and extracellular environments. The amount of calcium released to the myofilaments during excitation is increased and the result is a positive cardiac inotropic effect. One consequence of this positive effect is an increase in the oxygen needs of the myocardium. Other effects of digitalis include slowing of the heart rate. The margin separating toxicity from therapeutic effectiveness is small as compared with most other drugs. Hence, the need for regular monitoring of the clinical status, the serum digoxin levels and the ECGs of patients receiving digitalis. This is important if there is any evidence of renal dysfunction as digoxin is removed from the body in the urine. Aging is one cause of reduced renal function.

  The use of this drug for cardiac disease seems to be out of fashion at present. However, many clinical trials in the 1980s[5] confirmed the value of digoxin in cardiac disease. The publication cited is only one of many which also confirm the clinical value of digoxin in cardiac disease. They have shown that digitalis can reduce the dyspnea, the fatigue, the cardiomegaly, and the pulmonary and peripheral edema of congestive heart failure in both, patients with normal sinus rhythm or atrial fibrillation.

- **The proton-pump inhibitors.**These are drugs recently introduced for the treatment of peptic ulcer without evidence of H. Pylori infection (or failure to respond to therapy for H.Pylori infection), or severe gastroesophageal reflux (e.g., the reflux in patients with esophageal progressive systemic sclerosis). The proton pump inhibitors include the drugs omperazole (Losec; Astra), lansoprazole (Prevacid; Abbott) and pantoprazole (Pantaloc; Solvay Pharma). New imitating drugs continue to appear for this is a lucrative market. All act by inhibiting the parietal cell H^+/K^+-ATPase enzyme that provides the energy (~P) from local ATP for proton pump basal and post-prandial gastric acid secretion by the parietal cells.

4. Drugs that act within the cell.

Most other drugs that act within the cell are able to do so because of their lipid solubility and their ease of transfer across cell membranes. Examples are the general anesthetics, and the tricyclic antidepressants. The latter, because of their lipid solubility, can inhibit the amine pump in the nerve endings of adrenergic nerves. Lipid solubility is probably the only factor responsible for transport of general anesthetics across cell membranes. Some drugs that cross the cell membrane also have nonspecific toxic intracellular effects of therapeutic value. Many are used for cancer chemotherapy.

The antibiotics, antifungals, anti-parasite and anti-helminth drugs.

The modes of action of these drugs is diverse; some inhibit bacterial growth, others kill bacteria, some inhibit fungi, helminths and parasites while others kill them. It is beyond the scope of this monograph to specify the ranges of activity and the indications for use of each of these agents.

Three subjectively chosen exceptions are made; comments on the beta-lactamase sensitive antibiotics, on antibiotics effective against Mycoplasma Pneumonia and H.Influenza and the developments of antibiotic resistance.

- **The beta-lactamase sensitive antibiotics.** They include penicillin with predominant activity against Gram positive organisms, its later derivatives (ampicillin and amoxicillin) with activity against Gram positive and Gram negative organisms and the cefalosporins. The penicillins are bactericidal and act by inhibiting a transpeptidase needed for linkage of the monomeric units required for bacterial cell wall synthesis. The cephalosporins act in a similar way.

  Many beta-lactamase sensitive antibiotics are inactive if the infecting bacteria produce penicillinase or other beta lactamases. **Beta-lactamase inhibitors such as clavullinic acid** will provide the necessary inhibition of any beta-lactamases. Commercial combinations of clavullinic acid and either ampicillin or amoxicillin are marketed). **Cloxacillin** is a penicillin that is resistant to staphylococcal penicillinase.

- **Antibiotics effective against Mycoplasma Pneumoniae.** The three principal antibiotics in this group are erythromycin, clairithromycin and tetracycline. Undoubtedly additional ones will appear as time passes. These antibiotics are active against Gram positive organisms and some that are Gram negative. Their principal value is their ability to inhibit Mycoplasma P., Legionella P., and H. Influenza. Various studies have shown that Mycoplasma pneumonia causes 15-50% of all pneumonias in adults and an even higher percentage in school children[6]. Treatment is erythromycin, clairithromycin, or tetracycline. The last should not be given till all teeth have erupted and grown for earlier administration can result in their yellow discoloration.

- **Bacterial resistance to antibiotics - MRSA and others.** According to the CDC (Centers for Disease Control and prevention. http://www.cdc.gov/drugresistance/community/) some 2 million patients in the United States gets a hospital infection each year. About 90,000 of these patients die each year because of their infection. They correctly suggest that some 70% of the bacteria that cause hospital-acquired infections are resistant to at least one, if not more, of the drugs used to treat the infection.

  There are many publications which detail development of bacterial resistance to antibiotics. So many that it would be invidious to select any single one for reference. Resistance is especially dangerous when it develops against drugs used to treat tuberculosis and the so-called methicillin resistant staphylocococcus aureus (MRSA). I use the term so-called because methicillin was the antibiotic used many years ago to treat S. Aureus infections. It is no longer used and MRSA now denotes antibiotic-resistant S.Aureus. Many of these organisms are now even resistant to vancomycin which is often an antibiotic of last resort. Increased use of vancomycin for treating such infections have resulted in the appearance of vancomycin resistant strains of S.Aureus and enterococci which can cause cardiac infections and bacteremia.

  The literature on the subject of antibiotic-resistance is large and those interested can find hundreds of publications on the Internet. Drug resistance to anti-tuberculosis therapy can be a major problem.

How do bacteria develop resistance? They are unicellular organisms which multiply frequently. Antibiotic treatment can fail to destroy a resistant mutant. The other sensitive organisms are inactivated but the mutant keeps multiplying till the whole colony is resistant to the antibiotic.

The message is **do not give patients antibiotics when they are not clinically necessary**. Antibiotics for young healthy patients with viral infections are contraindicated. They may be necessary as prophylactic therapy in the aged and those with dysfunctions of the heart. Their use in COPD is controversial and the pros and cons were detailed on page 237 in Chapter 10.

Is the development of new and potent antibiotics likely?

The following is a verbatim quote from the Economist of November 5, 2005:

> "Antibiotics are not big earners for the pharmaceutical companies. Drugs for chronic conditions are far more profitable because they keep working and remain saleable - unlike antibiotics. .... An American study last year found that out of 506 drugs in development, only five were new antibiotics."

The future looks bleak with little more than the currently available antibiotics to combat infections and drug resistance. Pathogenns resistant to available antibiotics are a major problem in hospitals because they have many patients with serious antibiotic.-resistant problems. It is gradually becoming an increasingly difficult problem in community-based practices where most pneumonias and acute exacerbations of COPD are treated

Intrahepatic metabolism of drugs

Polar and non-polar compounds.

Chemical bonding is the union of atoms by shared electrons to form molecules.

Non-polar bonds.

The oxygen molecule is a simple example. Each atom consists of eight negatively charged electrons of negligible mass circling a nucleus containing eight positively charged protons, each with an atomic mass of 1, and eight electrically neutral neutrons, each with an atomic mass of 1. The result is an atom that is electrically neutral with an atomic mass of 16. When two oxygen atoms unite to form a molecule of O_2, bonding is between two electrons of one atom with two adjacent and similar electrons of the other. **This is a non-polar bond.** The shared electrons are equidistant from each nucleus and the molecule is therefore, electrically neutral. If bonding is between many different atoms and the end result is an electrically non-polar neutral compound.

Non-polar compounds are soluble in lipids but not in water. They cannot be excreted in the urine unless and until converted to polar metabolic products. Lipid solubility lets them traverse lipid membranes and enter cells but their removal from the body requires initial metabolic conversion to water soluble compounds (mainly in the liver) to products that can be excreted in the urine or bile. The intermediates of metabolism can have toxic effects.

Polar bonds.

The simplest example is the union of two dissimilar atoms. The electrons of the bond are shared but one member of the bond will contain more protons, and consequently, more positive charge than the other. Electrons are negatively charged. They are pulled towards the side that has greater electrical charge and they take with them their nucleus. A polar structure results with one pole relatively positive to the other.

Polar compounds are soluble in water and body fluids and can be excreted intact in the urine. They are insoluble in lipid membranes and, for this reason rarely enter cells except when special mechanisms exist for transfer (e.g., receptors and active transport mechanisms). Those that act by affecting membrane enzyme systems (e.g., inhibition of Na^+/K^+-ATPase by digitalis) do not need to enter the cells.

In sum, **polar compounds** are soluble in blood and urine but insoluble in the lipid of membranes. They are usually excreted intact in the urine though occasionally broken down first by enzymes. **Non-polar compounds** are insoluble in blood and urine but can traverse lipid membranes. Before removal from the body they are first broken down, mainly in the liver, to water soluble substances that can be excreted. In the process biological activity is generally lost. At times metabolism converts the non-polar compound to toxic intermediate metabolites before their final degradation to polar compounds that can be excreted in the urine.

The initial hepatic metabolism of drugs.

As mentioned previously, whatever the mode of administration, a portion of drug in the circulation binds to serum albumin. The fraction may be as high as 80-90%. The unbound fraction is the pharmacologically active fraction. At each circuit of the blood a fraction of non-polar drug that is not bound to albumin crosses the liver cell membrane because of its solubility in lipid. It is then bound in the liver cell to proteins called Y and Z proteins and catabolized. In this way the diffusion gradient between extracellular and intracellular drug is maintained so that there is continuous intracellular ingress and degradation of the drug with the extracellular unbound fraction gradually decreasing as it is used.

Intrahepatic catabolism is the principal mechanism for degradation and elimination of foreign water-insoluble non-polar compounds. It also removes endogenous waste products such as the heme of dead red cells that is excreted in the bile after initial degradation. Hepatic intracellular reactions catabolize non-polar drugs to blood and water soluble polar metabolites that can be excreted in the urine. In the process the biological activity of the drug is also destroyed. As previously mentioned, some of the intermediates of metabolism can exert toxic effects before removal from the body.

Phases 1 and 2 intrahepatic metabolism of drugs.

The principal intrahepatic drug metabolism reactions are designated Phase 1 or Phase 2 reactions. Most Phase 1 reactions use the Cytochrome P450 system. Some do not. Most Phase 2 reactions are conjugation reactions.

Phase 1 reactions that use the Cytochrome P450 system.

Only a summarized outline of the chemistry of reactions using Cytochrome P450 is relevant, given the context of this book. The cytochrome P450 system[8] is a large gene with 14-20 known mammalian gene families that can encode for more than 500 distinct enzymes. They function as the terminal microsomal oxidases in drug metabolism. Drug metabolism is mainly effected by members of the CYP1, CYP2, and CYP3 groups. The biochemical events are complex. Two enzymes are involved; NADPH Cytochrome P450-reductase and the Cytochrome P450 enzyme complex (a complex of some 10-20 related enzymes). Both are located in the intracellular endoplasmic reticulum of liver cells and are associated with a microsomal electron transport system. The reduction of NADPH by the enzyme NADPH Cytochrome P450-reductase results in production of Cytochrome $P450^{++}$ which then binds to drug substrate and oxygen. One atom of oxygen attaches to two of hydrogen to produce a molecule of water. The other atom of oxygen attaches to substrate. This oxidized drug complex is then usually hydroxylated or dealkylated to water soluble compounds that can be excreted in the urine. Cytochrome P450 returns to its original form and another cycle of drug degradation starts.

Phase 1 reactions that do not use the Cytochrome P450 system.

Some examples are the oxidation of purines to uric acid by xanthine oxidase; oxidation of secondary and tertiary amines by amine oxidases of the endoplasmic reticulum; deamination by mitochondrial enzymes of catecholamines, serotonin, and drugs with comparable structures; and ethanol breakdown by aldehyde dehydrogenase.

Phase 2 reactions.

They detoxify by conjugations. The product is a drug that is inactivated and also made water soluble and excretable in the urine. Production of toxic intermediates is uncommon. A variety of conjugations are possible. The commonest are conjugation with glucuronic acid (probably the principal conjugating agent in man), with sulfate, with glutathione, or by acetylation. A single drug can be conjugated in different ways.

Another important function of these conjugation reactions is detoxification of metabolic intermediates produced in Phase 1 reactions. Important examples vis-a-vis clinical medicine are conjugation by glutathione of toxic epoxides formed during catabolism of unsaturated ring structures by the Cytochrome P450 complex.

A clinically important example is the hepatic metabolism of acetaminophen. The drug itself can conjugate with glucuronic acid or sulfate. Toxic intermediates formed during its metabolism by the Cytochrome P450 complex can be detoxified by conjugation with glutathione. At first, about 4% of the the drug conjugates with glutathione. As the dose of acetaminophen increases the capacity for conjugations with glutathione, glucuronic acid and sulfate are sated. The Cytochrome P450 system takes over. Any toxicity of the oxidation products are neutralized by conjugation with glutathione. Serious consequences result if large amounts of acetaminophen are taken. Exhaustion of the amount of available glutathione can result in persistent toxic intermediates. In general the dose of acetaminophen taken by an adult should not exceed about 4gm per day.

The uncertainties and unpredictables of clinical therapeutics

Almost all therapies have innate uncertainties and unpredictables[7]. Indeed, it is the uncertainties and unpredictables of clinical medicine that justify the existence of trained physicians. In the absence of these two factors any person, given the symptoms, the physical signs, the results of ancillary investigations and a computer could be a competent physician, secure in the knowledge that the prescribed therapy would ensure recovery from sickness. This is clearly not correct. Appropriate clinical decisions require in-depth knowledge of the causes of clinical uncertainty, and the ways to deal with their consequences, tempered with the knowledge that one day therapy will certainly fail and death ensue. The physician cannot provide immortality but can often delay the end. When the day inevitably comes when this is not possible, the function of the physician is to alleviate pain and suffering; not to engage in additional unnecessary investigations and useless additional therapies.

Most of the causes of therapeutic failure were listed in Chart 16-1. There are three main groups of causes:

- **Therapeutic failure because of drug-related problems.**
- **Therapeutic failure because of adverse drug reactions.**
- **Therapeutic failure because the disease is too advanced, or incurable because no therapy is available for it, or simply because no therapy is available for the inevitable preterminal state which one day afflicts all animates.** No additional comment is made or needed on the last of these three possible causes for therapeutic failure.

Therapeutic failure because of drug-related problems

The following are some possible causes:

1. **The choice of therapy was wrong.**

   If therapy does not start to restore the qualitatives of dysfunctions to physiologically permissible and desirable levels an unemotional and objective reassessment of the clinical picture and therapeutic decision is needed. Chart 16-1 and 16-2 provide some helpful suggestions.

2. **Correct therapy but the patient did not respond.**

   The following text expands on the possibilities:

   a) Non-compliance.

   Patients often do not comply with therapy they have agreed to take. Forgetting to take the medication is a common cause. Other common causes are lack of sufficient money to buy and the inability to accept expected side effects. Most should have been detailed to the patient at the start of therapy. Examples are the blurring of vision that sometimes accompanies taking of anti-depressants and the impotence and cold extremities that often accompany taking of beta blockers. When non-compliance results from any of the above try a different drug with comparable effectiveness. Inexplicable and bizarre intolerances occur.

   Often compliance can be increased by decreasing the frequency of dosing. An example is the preferential use of the once a day atenolol rather than the original inderal as a beta blocker in the treatment of cardiac disease. Another is the use of one a day ACE inhibitors in preference to the original captopril.

b) Variations in intestinal and hepatic first pass metabolism of drugs.

A portion of an orally administered drug may be inactivated in the gut, the gut wall or the liver before it enters the circulation. This process is called **first pass metabolism.**

Degradation of proteins and peptides by digestive enzymes is another important factor limiting oral administration of drugs such as insulin and catecholamines. The residuum of gases used in anesthetic practice are readily inactivated and exhaled by the lungs so that continuous administration is needed.

Apart from normal biological variations first-pass metabolism is affected by liver pathology. In acute and chronic liver disease liver function is adversely affected and a frequent consequence is a decrease in the capacity to metabolize drugs. Alcohol related liver disease also reduces the ability of the liver to metabolize drugs.

For any drug first pass metabolism shows significant variations from one individual to another and this is of clinical importance as some drugs have a high first pass metabolism and cannot be given orally. An example is lidocaine. Because of high first pass clearance it cannot be orally administered for the treatment of arrhythmias. Other commonly prescribed oral drugs that have high first pass clearance are acetaminophen, propanolol and imipramine. The degree of degradation is not enough to vitiate oral administration but the high first pass clearances and the fact that this can vary significantly between individuals means that the response to therapy needs monitoring and adjustment of dose.

c) Variations in absorption of drugs given orally.

Two principal factors are responsible.

First, variations in water and lipid solubility of orally administered drugs. In order to be absorbed across the gut wall drugs must first dissolve in water and have lipid solubility in order to traverse cell walls. Many drugs are not readily soluble in water. Important examples are digitalis and the corticosteroids. Manufacturers respond in various ways: compacting particles of small size, adding fillers that function as lubricants, and agents that disaggregate. A coating may be added to improve storage, and dyes and flavoring to facilitate identification and increase palatability. It is not unusual to find more than ten inactive ingredients in a pill. Many are potentially toxic or allergenic ingredients.

Problems arise when the product of another manufacturer is substituted. The absorption characteristics may differ resulting in a decreased response or, more seriously, an increased response; an increased response could have disastrous effects when a drug such as digitalis is taken. The moral is, use substitution only when essential and with subsequent initial clinical monitoring of the patient's response.

Many gastrointestinal disturbances can affect the absorption of orally administered drugs: difficulty in swallowing, nausea, vomiting, diarrhea, intestinal immobility (postoperative ileus is a common example), malabsorption syndromes, and short bowel syndromes resulting from surgery are some examples. There are many more.

Second, variations in the avidity of the absorbed drug for plasma proteins; the unbound fraction is the biologically active portion. A portion of most drugs in the circulation bind to serum albumin. Usually the individual variations in albumin binding are small. It is the free fraction of the drug that is its functionally active part. This fraction may be increased if the albumin binding sites are occupied by an excess of endogenous substances as is possible in advanced hepatic and renal disease. An example where this can lead to major clinical problems is phenytoin that is normally 90% bound to albumin. In advanced renal disease decreased binding to 80% is possible with an increase in the active unbound material. Binding to serum albumin can also be saturated by injection of intravenous bolus doses. Another factor that requires consideration is an increase in unbound drug when albumin synthesis is decreased because of impaired liver function.

d) Variations in drug-target interactions.

There are many causes for abnormal drug-target interactions. The following are some.

- **Variations in levels of intrahepatic microsomal drug-inactivating enzymes.** This is an important consideration in clinical medicine, especially in individuals receiving warfarin anticoagulants. Intracellular hepatic microsomal enzymes inactivate drugs by oxidation and are integral and essential components of the Cytochrome P450 system. The activity of these enzymes can be increased (a process termed induction) by a number of agents. Over 100 such agents have been implicated to date. They include alcohol and barbecued foods, and tobacco smoke! More serious is induction by certain drugs; of practical importance are the drugs, phenytoin, progesterone and rifampicin. One consequence of induction of hepatic microsomal oxidation enzymes can be increased breakdown of drugs such as warfarin anticoagulants and the estrogen in oral contraceptives. In the former case the therapeutic agent would lose its effect. More serious, if the dose was increased to maintain prothrombin times (the INR) at therapeutic levels a dangerous situation could arise because of increased anticoagulation if the inducing agent were withdrawn. Another example is the occurrence of pregnancy in individuals on rifampicin for tuberculosis who are simultaneously taking oral contraceptives. I have heard of one such case from another physician.
- **Variations in the excretory removal of drugs from the body.** Polar compounds are soluble in blood and urine but insoluble in the lipid of membranes. Non-polar compounds are insoluble in blood and urine. Non-polar compounds must be broken down in the liver to water soluble and biologically inactive substances before excretion in urine (occasionally toxic intermediate compounds form but are usually rapidly inactivated). Renal disease is not a hazard if hepatic drug metabolism has resulted in a product that is harmless, inactive and not toxic. It is a hazard if the drug to be excreted is a polar water-soluble compound with potential for biological activity. A notable example is digoxin. Other drugs that are excreted unchanged by the kidney are aminoglycoside antibiotics such as gentamicin, neomycin and streptomycin, diuretics (e.g., triamterene and amiloride), lithium, potassium, and benzyl penicillin.
- **Variations in blood flow.** The rapidity of action, and the effectiveness of a drug will depend to a significant degree on the blood flow through the target organ. For example, the treatment of infections affecting a limb with vascular insufficiency is often difficult, protracted, and usually, ineffective. Healing of wounds is likewise delayed and, often unsuccessful. Examples are surgical amputations that do not heal because they are too low and the surgical treatment of infected ingrowing toe nails in a limb with inadequate blood supply; the effects of surgery often do not heal and may progress to gangrene.
- **The blood-brain barrier.** Brain capillaries are lined by cells connected by tight junctions. To gain access to brain tissue drugs must pass through endothelial cells. Lipid soluble substances can easily pass across and so can substances like glucose that has its own transport system. Difficulties arise with antibiotics and catecholamines such as dopamine. **Catecholamines,** would be of value in the treatment of Parkinson's disease if they could cross the blood-brain barrier. Dopamine deficiency is though to be a principal etiological factor in Parkinson's disease. Dopamine cannot cross the blood-brain barrier. Fortunately, a precursor, levo-dihydroxyphenylalanine (L-dopa) can. In the brain it is decarboxylated to dopamine. To avoid peripheral dopamine side effects (cardiac arrhythmias, anorexia, constipation, etc.) it is usually given with carbidopa as a levodopa-carbidopa combination (Sinemet; Bristol-Meyers Squibb). Carbidopa is an inhibitor of peripheral L-Dopa decarboxylase.
- **Variations in effects due to interactions between drugs.** The subject is considered in detail in the section on adverse drug reactions. The consequences of any such interactions may be synergistic, additive, or subtractive. The following are two examples.

  Indomethacin given to a patient with acute gout has the side effect of water retention. In a patient with well-controlled congestive heart failure this can result in destabilization unless there is close monitoring and a possible increase in the dose of diuretic given.

  Antibiotics given to a patient with well-controlled coumadin anticoagulation can result in increased anticoagulation if the antibiotics are able to destroy intestinal vitamin K-producing bacteria.
- **Variations in cell wall and intracellular interactions between drugs and their targets.**

  If the Y axis represents the response to a drug and the X axis its concentration a hyperbola forms. At low concentrations no effect is seen. As the concentration increase there is a rapid increase in response till a maximum is reached. After that increasing drug concentration has little effect. The response at any drug concentration will depend on whether the curve moves to the right or left.

Many factors could cause such shifts: the number of available receptors; the sensitivity of the receptor for the drug; the avidity of the receptors for the drug; the number of receptors that need to bind the agonist, the antagonist, or any other item required to produce an effect; changes in the avidity of the receptor (the continued presence of an agonist can decrease sensitivity and its absence can increase sensitivity); the activity of cell membrane pump systems; the intracellular concentration and/or activity of systems responsible for the pharmacological effects of drug-target interaction; and many other possible factors. Few are readily identifiable or quantitatively or qualitatively measurable. It is because such variations are possible that the effect of any drug is always unpredictable. Continual monitoring is need ed. Therapy given to a patient initiates a clinical trial with an outcome that is never certain.

Failure of therapy because of adverse drug reactions

The WHO has defined adverse drug reactions as follows[11]:

> "a response to a drug that is noxious and unintended and occurs at doses normally used in man for the prophylaxis, diagnosis or therapy of disease, or for the modification of physiological function."

There have been criticisms of some of the terminology used in this definition but, in general it is good and accurate. The WHO continues to provide valuable monitoring of adverse drug reactions through a program in Uppsala[12].

Adverse drug reactions are a serious problem in clinical practice, especially in hospitalized patients; probably because they are more sick and receive more potentially toxic drugs than out-patient ambulating patients. The incidence of adverse drug reactions was studied by Lazarou and associates in 1998[13]. A meta-analysis of 39 prospective studies from USA hospitals indicated that about 6.7% of hospitalized patients had adverse drug reactions and that in 0.32% the reactions were fatal; a very small percentage but one which resulted in about 100,000 deaths per year of hospitalized patients. The figures are startling but probably less horrific than they appear at first glance. Many hospitalized patients are terminally sick and heavily dosed with narcotics and other medications to relieve pain and suffering. In such circumstances death from therapy is common - the alternative is to withhold palliative drugs and allow the patient to die in a natural but often extremely unpleasant manner.

Classifications of adverse drug reactions.

The literature on adverse drug reactions is voluminous. Each author seems to provide a personal point of view and a related classification. Many feel that the Rawlins-Thompson[11] classification is superior to the standard classification of adverse drug reactions. The standard classification describes them as being toxic, idiosyncratic, or allergic. The Rawlins-Thompson classification is less rigorous as to etiology. The following summarizes its principal features:

Type A reactions (Rawlins-Thompson classification).

Types A and B reactions. Type A reactions are predictable, related to the pharmacological actions of the drug, and not uncommon. About 80% of adverse drug reactions are Type A reactions. **Examples are:**

- **Organ or systems toxicity** from an overdose of therapeutic agents. An example is digitalis toxicity. The dose does not have to be excessive to produce cardiac dysfunctions in susceptible individuals. Those especially at risk are patients who are elderly and/or those who have impaired renal function.
- **Expected and common side-effects.** Examples are the visual blurring experienced by many taking tricyclic anti-depressants, the systemic side effects of beta blockers and the sedative effects of antihistamines.
- **Drug interactions.** There are two sorts of drug interactions. The less common are direct adverse interactions such as theophylline toxicity when a patient is given erythromycin.

  Other examples are rises in prothrombin times in patients receiving oral antibiotics and warfarin at the same time. The antibiotic destroys vitamin K-producing bacteria in the intestine with consequent reduction of hepatic vitamin K stores. The result is an increase in previously controlled prothrombin times without any change in warfarin dosage.

Another example is precipitation of congestive heart failure in a previously well controlled patient who develops gout. Indomethacin is given, water retention results and the dose of diuretic that previously sufficed to control cardiac dysfunction no longer suffices. There is water retention and edema as well as exertional and nocturnal dyspnea. Colchicine is a better drug for these patients.

-- **The inappropriate administration of drugs** can have disastrous consequences in certain clinical situations. An example is administration of a beta-blocker to an individual with asthma or some other form of chronic obstructive pulmonary disease. Beta-blockers slow the heart rate. When combined with a drug such as verapamil that slows conduction through the A-V node dangerous bradycardia can result.

Giving sedatives to individuals with central nervous system disease that is not preterminal needs caution. So also is giving a sedative to individuals with a known previous history of some form of intolerance to that same drug or to a patient in status asthmaticus. A relative of mine with distressing status asthmaticus got off an airplane in a major European airport and was immediately seen by the local airport physician. He mistook the status asthmaticus for a panic attack and gave a dose of vallium intravenously. About five minutes later the patient stopped breathing and died. No mechanical life support equipment was available at this major airport to sustain life till the effects of the vallium had dissipated.

-- **Secondary effects.** They are common. A typical example is the the epigastric discomfort and at times, the diarrhea that is a frequent accompaniment of oral antibiotics. The former because of gastric irritation and the latter because of the alterations in intestinal bacterial flora.

Type B reactions (Rawlins-Thompson classification).

Type B reactions are not predictable, not related to the pharmacological actions of the drug, relatively uncommon and usually unrelated to the dose given. Many authors group all Type B reactions into a single category: **idiosyncratic reactions:. There are six principal causes for these "so-called" idiosyncratic reactions:**

-- **Reactive metabolites.**

-- **Genetic abnormalities** (i.e., pharmacogenetics).

-- **Abnormal immunological responses.**

-- **Resistance to antibiotics and other drugs.**

-- **Teratogenic effects.**

-- **Carcinogenic effects.**

1. Reactive metabolites.

During the breakdown of drugs toxic intermediates may form. Examples are the formation of free radicals that disrupt the structures and function of intracellular and pericellular membranes by peroxidizing unsaturated fatty acids in a self-sustaining chain reaction. This is the way carbon tetrachloride damages liver and it is probably one way that halothane exerted its toxic effect. With isoniazid the situation is more complicated. The drug is first acetylated and then hydrolyzed to acetyl hydrazine which is next broken down by the cytochrome P450 system to one or more toxic intermediates. Another factor affecting isoniazid catabolism is genetic; 80% of Orientals are fast acetylators and isoniazid induced liver injury is more common in this group.

There is much evidence to support the view that many idiosyncratic drug reactions result from the effects of metabolites produced during drug catabolism. One hypothesis is that the reactive metabolite acts as a hapten that binds to a body protein and that this protein is recognized as a foreign substance by the immune system. Why do some metabolites result in idiosyncratic reactions in some individuals and not in others? The danger hypothesis[14] is an attractive concept. The theory hypothesizes that the immune system only responds to a seemingly foreign protein if the protein is associated with a danger signal derived from dead and necrotic cells.

2. Pharmacogenetics.

Differences in drug metabolism due to inherited chromosomal abnormalities are legion. Many of the adverse reactions that, in the past, have been ascribed to biological variations probably result from inherited chromosomal abnormalities and polymorphisms. Only ones that have frequent clinical consequences are mentioned here.

- **Inherited deficiencies.** The example usually quoted is an inherited deficiency of cholinesterase. Prolonged muscle relaxation follows suxamethonium administration.
- **Abnormal acetylation.** The rate of acetylation of a drug is under genetic control. As mentioned above, 80% of Orientals are fast acetylators and isoniazid induced liver injury is more common in this group. In circumstances where there is a decrease in the activity of the liver enzyme, N-acetyltransferase, slow acetylators will tend to develop a peripheral neuropathy when given isoniazid .
- **Polymorphisms of the liver drug-metabolizing enzyme cytochrome P450.**
  - **Polymorphism at the CYP2D6 locus** is an example. Its results include variations in the metabolic breakdown of antidepressants. Antidepressant toxicity occurs in poor metabolizers and ineffectiveness in rapid metabolizers.

    Another example is variations in the breakdown of codeine. About 10% of codeine is O-demethylated to morphine. This path is deficient in poor metabolizers so that there will be no pain relief from codeine in the 5-10% of the population who are poor metabolizers. More than 70 variant alleles of the CYP2D6 locus have been described. Those interested in the many consequences are referred to standard publications such as the one by Meyer[9].
  - **Polymorphism at the CYP2C9 locus.** Variants at this locus are especially important for individuals receiving the anticoagulant, warfarin[10]. The CYP2C9 alleles with decreased enzyme activity are associated with lower warfarin requirements to reach therapeutic prothrombin levels.

I have had patients who showed marked variations in their needs for warfarin anticoagulation. One 82 year old patient with COPD and deep vein thrombosis following surgery for a fractured hip required only 1 mg warfarin daily to maintain an INR between 2-3. Another of the same age and proportions required 8 mg daily while a third, a woman with respiratory failure and paroxysmal fibrillation, showed no change in INR with a dose of 10 mg daily. At that point it was suggested she merely continue with a daily dose of ASA.

3. Adverse drug reactions due to immunological processes.

Many Type B adverse drug reactions are due to abnormal immunological reactions. They include the Types 1-4 adverse immunological reaction described by Coombs and Gell and detailed on pages 182-186. Some examples are anaphylaxis, the various autoimmune hemolytic anemias and, the various putative autoimmune lupus-type diseases.

The Type 3 reaction is the most frequent. It results from complexes of antigen, IgG or IgM and complement. Presumably the antigen is the drug or some part of it. The results can be an immune complex nephritis with proteinuria and/or maculopapular skin rashes from deposition of soluble immune complexes of IgM and antigen in the skin.

Serum sickness syndrome.

This is a Type 3 immune reaction. Immune complexes of IgG and antigen can cause **serum sickness** after exposure to drugs such as aspirin, penicillin and sulfonamides. Symptoms begin 7-12 days after treatment has begun and consists of fever, arthralgia, urticaria and lymphadenopathy. Additional features are cervical lymphadenitis and skin rashes that may be as innocuous-looking as an exanthem or as life-threatening as a Stevens-Johnson syndrome. Organ involvement is common; any combination of liver, kidney, central nervous system, intestinal or lung dysfunctions are frequent. Treatment consists of immediate cessation of therapy, supportive measures and oral corticosteroids (there is some dispute as to whether or not corticosteroids help). Any subsequent administration of the causative agent will result in the syndrome appearing within a day.

Other presumed immunological reactions.

The Type 1 reaction is responsible for many of the allergic responses to drugs. I have seen it as an acute manifestation of penicillin sensitivity. The immunological Types 1-4 reactions were described in detail on pages 183-186. Additional text would be repetitive.

Presumed autoimmune reactions. The drug induced lupus-like syndromes have positive antinuclear factor, LE cells, arthralgia and fever. However, unlike spontaneous lupus, anti-DNA antibodies are uncommon and CNS manifestations are rare. Drug induced lupus has been reported with isoniazid, and with drugs rarely used such as procainamide and hydralazine.

Cell-mediated immunity (type 4 reactions). Most rashes that appear where drugs have been applied locally are probably mediated by immune T cells interacting with antigen in the local environment.

Pseudoallergic reactions. Typical examples are reactions to dyes used for radiological or nuclear medicine studies. The reactions mimic allergic reactions but are considered to be of non-allergic etiology.

4. Resistance to antibiotics.

This topic was discussed on page 348. It is an increasingly common cause for adverse drug reactions and failed therapy

5. Teratogenic effects and other Phase 4 reactions.

An example of a Phase 4 reaction was the epidemic of phocomelia caused by administration of thalidomide in the early weeks of pregnancy. Dilantin taken during a pregnancy increases the incidence of hare lip and cleft palate. Many antitumor chemotherapeutic agents are also teratogenic. A deficiency of folic acid during pregnancy is said to increase the incidence of neural tube defects in the newborn. Many other examples exist.

Watch the literature for reports of Phase 4 adverse effects. When a new drug enters the market it is assumed that regulatory agencies are satisfied that the Phases 1-3 trials have shown that the drug is effective and safe within the perimeters of advertised cautions. The Phase 4 reaction is an infrequent adverse effect, often recognized some time after the drug is approved for clinical use and prescribed. Many examples come to mind: the thalidomide tragedies first, suggested in a 1960 paper[19] and in 1961 essentially confirmed by McBride[20]; the cervical and vaginal tumors in the daughters of women given stilboestrol for repeated miscarriages some twenty years previously[21,22]; and more recently, the uncommon deaths from myonecrosis in a few patients receiving statins to control blood cholesterol. Many other examples of Phase 4 adverse reactions exist. It is difficult to predict a Phase 4 reaction. Unless essential, physicians are well advised to use a new drug only after its general acceptance and usage and especially some time after its introduction.

6. Carcinogenic effects.

Variations of the Ames test are used to determine the in vitro carcinogenic potential of drugs. The most frequently used variation uses salmonella strains that are deficient at the His operon and cannot synthesize L-histidine which is an essential amino acid. The bacteria only grow if this compound is present in the medium. If organisms grow in the presence of the drug being tested for mutagenicity the assumption is that the drug has induced mutations that have the His operon needed for L-histidine production. The addition of rat liver microsomal preparations increases the sensitivity of the test. Because of the difficulty, time, ethics and expenses of carrying out tests in animals this test has replaced animal testing for mutagens and, by implication, carcinogens.

Testing is really for in vitro mutagenic potential, not necessarily for carcinogenicity. An in vitro test does not necessarily equate with in vivo consequences and, in any case absence of mutagenicity does not necessarily mean that the drug might not be carcinogenic.

Carcinogenicity of a drug is difficult to prove or disprove because of the time lapse before any tumors appear. An extreme and strange example is the appearance of uncommon cervical neoplasms in the daughters of women given stilboestrol twenty years or so previously for repeated miscarriages[15]. Estrogens by themselves can be carcinogenic and there is an increased incidence of breast[16] and endometrial cancers in postmenopausal women receiving hormone replacement therapy. Not surprising as one of the first experimental tumors was produced in 1932 by Lacassagne who gave estrogens to mice of both sexes. Breast malignancies developed in a certain proportion of animals in both groups. Interestingly the incidence varied from breed to breed, a finding similar to the racial and genetic differences noted in humans. It is one's opinion that the carcinogenicity, or lack of it, of any drug will be extremely difficult to decide on except over long periods of administration and epidemiological observation. The Ames test and its variations must suffice for the moment.

How does one identify the agent or agents that caused the adverse drug reaction?

It is often difficult to be certain that the clinical picture is the result of an adverse drug reaction. Suggestive features are clinical findings that are unlikely to be the result of the disease being treated or other concurrent disease. The manifestations of adverse drug reactions are diverse and may mimic the symptoms of disease affecting any one of the many biological organ systems. At times the diagnosis is obvious but often, the culprit is not, especially when many different drugs are being taken. Reactions typical of adverse drug reactions include anaphylactic reactions, urticaria and other types of skin rashes, abnormalities in the blood counts and hemoglobin levels, gastrointestinal symptoms such as epigastric discomfort or diarrhea, any features of the drug hypersensitivity syndrome, and any symptoms or signs that are not normally associated with therapeutic administration of the suspected drug. The temporal relationship between drug administration and onset of the clinical picture provides an important clue, as does amelioration of the reaction when the drug is stopped.

It is not only the drug but also the non-therapeutic excipients added at the time of manufacture to facilitate absorption and increase bulk that may be responsible for adverse drug reactions. For example, two patients, a wife and husband, with hypertension were given atenolol for control. The husband had had a previous myocardial infarct and angioplasty and was already taking the generic form of the drug. When the couple tried to share medication the wife found she could not tolerate the generic brand but had no problems with the brand name drug subsequently prescribed by me.

A caveat. Always ask the patient to name or show you all medications being taken. Especially include all medications viewed as harmless by the patient, especially herbal preparations, multivitamin pills, and any of the various items recommended for healthy life styles.

How does one treat adverse drug reactions?

Emergency measures (adrenalin and oxygen) are occasionally needed as for example when there is anaphylaxis. If the cause of the adverse drug reaction is known a risk-benefit assessment is needed before stopping the drug. If many drugs are being taken some detective work is needed to identify the culprit. If the adverse reaction started soon after a particular drug was taken the best option is to give another drug with similar therapeutic effects. If no specific agent is identifiable start with stopping drugs that are not essential. I know that the term "unnecessary drug" sounds like an oxymoron but it is frequent except when a placebo is given deliberately.

A dose-related reaction is readily remedied by reducing the dose; this is commonly required when the difference between therapeutic and toxic doses are small. Common examples are digitalis and warfarin. If possible, especially in the elderly, start with the lowest dose that could have a therapeutic effect. For example an elderly individual who does not require rapid digitalization should start with a daily dose of .0625 mg digoxin and gradually work up till the desired therapeutic response is obtained.

Finally, there are situations when adverse side effects must be accepted. A typical example is the use of chemotherapy in the treatment of malignant disease. The side effects and toxic effects are often horrendous but usually require acceptance by the patient. Of course, informed consent must be obtained prior to starting therapy. A requirement for informed consent is that the patient knows all possible and probable consequences of the proposed therapy, and the risk-benefit ratio. Patients often agree to chemotherapy because they are given hope even if there is none, and often there is none.

Some important final caveats about drug therapy.

Continuous vigilance, evaluations and assessments are always necessary when treating a patient with drugs, however benign they might appear to be. How does one minimize the chances of unpredictable and/or uncertain outcomes of drug therapy?

The following are some suggestions:

1. **Lack of knowledge.** It is impossible for any one individual to know all the possible interactions and adverse effects of a multitude of drugs. In clinical practice a rapid decision on therapy is often needed A solution is to restrict ones regular use to a limited number of drugs. I only use about 30 drugs on a regular basis. An additional requirement is as much knowledge as possible about their modes of action, contraindications and potential adverse effects.

2. **A new drug** should only be added to ones personal pharmacopoeia if it satisfies an obvious need. An example was the initial introduction of the calcium channel blockers (diltiazem, nifedipine and verapamil). At first they were widely used for all sorts of cardiac dysfunctions, especially for patients with cardiac disease who needed beta blockers but could not be given them because of respiratory insufficiency. Only later did we learn of their undesirable effects when given to a patient with a damaged myocardium or congestive heart failure[17]; in these situations the effects on symptoms and survival were both adverse. One should still prescribe them when indicated but judiciously and with full knowledge about their possible adverse effects. Fortunately the ACE inhibitors have reduced most of the needs for calcium channel blockers.

3. **The recommended use of beta blockers for congestive heart failure** needs continual clinical re-evaluations of the subjects. The MERIT study[18] studied the effects of a beta blocker on patients with congestive heart failure. It records that:

   "Study group drug was permanently stopped early in 13.9% of the metoprolol CR/XL group ..... ."

   No reasons are given for stopping the drug but one presumes that it was because of adverse responses to the therapy.

4. **A harmless placebo** is always an option when there is no clear need for any drug therapy though the patient feels there is. A common example is a patient with a viral respiratory tract infection who insists that a potent antibiotic be prescribed. The use of placebos in such situations often generates controversy. Many feel that this is a form of chicanery while others are proponents of placebos in clinical medicine. However, in a clinical study Beecher found that placebos were effective in some 30-40% of subjects. According to White et al.[23] it appears to be especially effective after therapy. The placebo effect probably results from a combination of anticipated symptomatic and clinical improvement combined with the ability of natural defense mechanisms and systems to correct pathophysiological dysfunctions.

   I was once asked by an 80 year old patient with severe COPD for something strong to make him sleep as all the pills previously given were useless - because of his advanced COPD they were intentionally weak hypnotics and low in dosage. I told him I would prescribe the best available hypnotic and wrote a prescription for one. When the patient left I phoned the pharmacist and asked him to disregard the prescription and instead give the patient lactose powder in a colorful capsule. The patient was not aware of this as he was a senior citizen who did not have to pay for medications and this particular pharmacist always waived the dispensing fee for this family. A month later the patient came to the office and asked for a repeat as he had never slept so well for years till he took his new medicine!

   A pithy and hopefully, tongue-in-cheek (though perhaps not) summary was the comment of Montaigne in his Essays. It may appropriately describe the benefits of occasional placebo administration. It was contained in a 1958 reprint of his Essays[24]:

   "Why do doctors begin by practicing on the credulity of their patients with so many false promises of a cure, if not to call the powers of the imagination to the aid of their fraudulent concoctions? .... there are men on whom the mere sight of medicine is operative."

5. **At all times be ready to give epinephrine and oxygen** to any one you have given a drug, especially if it has been given intravenously; anaphylaxis is an ever-present danger, regardless of the drug. The patient of a colleague died in his office from anaphylactic shock following intramuscular injection of vitamin B_{12}.

6. **Identify and remember potentially lethal complications of the drugs you use.** Examples of such potentially

lethal combinations are tranquilizers such as diazepam given to individuals with severe asthma. Beta blockers given to individuals with lung disease. Narcotics given to patients with head injuries or advanced disease of the nervous system. Anticoagulants or steroids given to individuals with a history of duodenal ulcer. At times there are no alternatives. As an example I once had a patient of 24 who had had a mitral valve replacement and subsequently developed a duodenal ulcer. Anticoagulants had to be continued to prevent embolic stroke but when combined with a proton pump acid inhibitor to decrease the chance of hemorrhage all went well. She was a fit happy mother when I last saw her some 5 years ago before she left for another town, five years after treatment with proton pump inhibitors started.

7. **Give drugs with potentially lethal complications only when an alternative is not available.** A prime example was phenylbutazone. It is rarely used or available now but could cause death from marrow failure; acetylsalicylic acid (aspirin) and other nonsteroidal anti-inflammatories are equally effective and relatively nontoxic. Another is chloramphenicol. It is best reserved for severe hemophilus influenza infections that are insensitive to other antibiotics.

8. **Remember the drug combinations that can cause serious consequences,** either from additive effects (e.g., hypnotics, barbiturates, tranquilizers and opiates), or negative effects (e.g., inhibition of warfarin anticoagulation because of the induction of liver microsomal enzymes). A previous section detailed some of the many agents that can induce these enzymes.

9. **Remember the drugs that can cause serious adverse reactions** in the presence of disease; for example, anticoagulants in individuals with ulcerated lesions that cannot be protected by another drug such as a proton pump inhibitor of gastric acid secretion. Common examples are ulcerated malignant lesions. I well remember a patient on anticoagulants for previous deep vein thrombosis (possibly, in retrospect, due to a paraneoplastic process) who presented with life-threatening melena as the first symptom of a colonic neoplasm. In general, corticosteroids should not be given to individuals with tuberculosis unless this is imperative as in post-transplant therapy. Give digitalis with care and continuous monitoring if the patient has any degree of renal failure.

10. **Assume that any unexpected reaction in a patient receiving a drug is due to an adverse reaction to that drug.** Stop the drug and if necessary replace it with an equivalent. Examples are frequently seen with antibiotics and with tricyclic antidepressants that have an anticholinergic effect. The response to the latter may vary. For example, many patients who cannot take amitriptyline have no problem with imipramine and vice versa.

11. **If there is no alternative to a drug that has a side effect which is undesirable, unnecessary and cannot be tolerated, the side effect in question should be negated by another drug if this is possible.** An example is carbidopa negating the peripheral effects of dopa. Another is the use of drugs such as cogentin to negate the peripheral effects of phenothiazines given to schizophrenics.

12. **Remember that serious withdrawal effects may occur if habituating drugs are suddenly stopped,** especially benzodiazepines, barbiturates and many of the drugs prescribed by psychiatrists. To avoid complications and to ensure patient compliance do this slowly. Similar caveats apply to beta blockers given for angina. There have been many reports showing that sudden discontinuation of beta blockers given for treatment of angina may result in severe exacerbations of angina, and/or myocardial infarction or a ventricular arrhythmia - the latter two may occur with or without preceding exacerbation of angina. Discontinuation of the drug must be by gradual reduction of dosage over a period of about a week. Patients often stop taking drugs because of side effects. If they are taking drugs that could have undesirable consequences when suddenly stopped they should be warned of the possible consequences of sudden discontinuation.

13. If a desired result is not being obtained **verify that the agent is being taken correctly and at the appropriate times.** An example is insulin. If the blood sugar and hemoglobin A_{1c} are still too high despite insulin dosage that is seemingly correct, before altering the dose or type of insulin ensure that the patient is correctly drawing up and injecting the insulin, and also that the patient is correctly measuring the response. In addition satisfy yourself by personally supervising a repeat of the methods the patient uses to take insulin.

14. **Remember the half lives of commonly used drugs.** Drugs with long half-lives steadily accumulate with daily dosing and take a long while to reach a steady state concentration. Examples are diazepam (half life of 48 hours), warfarin (half life of 42 hours), digoxin (half life of 36 hours) and at the extreme chloroquine with a half life of 120 hours. If a rapid action is needed the agent has to be given intravenously (e.g., digoxin) till a steady state concentration has been reached with orally administered drugs. Another example is giving heparin for the first 48 hours after commencement of oral warfarin; one expects that a steady state warfarin effect would have begun within 48 hours. Of course this is not necessary if the need for anticoagulation is not urgent, e.g., after an episode of paroxysmal atrial fibrillation.

There are many other injunctions and caveats that could be added to the above list. The principal ones have been detailed. Others were deliberately omitted because of limitations of space, and others inadvertently or from ignorance.

Drug therapy in special situations

Drug therapy during pregnancy.

Special precautions are necessary when pregnant women and individuals with renal and/or hepatic failure need drugs. **Details of drugs that are to be avoided and those that can be given in specific situations are fully detailed in the WHO Model Formulary[25].** It is too long to detail here.

Major congenital malformations occur in 2-4% of live births and some 15% of pregnancies end in miscarriages. Most are not related to drug therapy but, when given, drugs pose the greatest risk to the fetus in the first trimester. During the last two trimesters they may affect fetal growth and functional development. In general all medications should be avoided in pregnancies unless therapy is absolutely essential.

Severe infections during a pregnancy may require antibiotics. Penicillin and its derivatives (e.g., amoxicillin ± clavullinic acid) as well as erythromycin are not known to be teratogens and are the drugs of choice. Absence of teratogenic activity has not been clearly established for the others. The WHO states that the broad spectrum antibiotics, ceftazidime and ceftriaxone are not known to be harmful but manufacturers of both caution that safety in pregnancy has not been established. They are effective agsinast gram negative organisms and if necessary may have to be prescribed but always with the informed consent of the mother.

Diabetic pregnant women always present a problem. The WHO recommends that all oral medication be stopped and insulin substituted for all pregnant diabetics. Often this is not a problem as the affected mother usually has a juvenile-onset type diabetes already controlled with insulin alone.

Pregnant women receiving on-going treatment for epilepsy pose a problem. Valproic acid should be avoided if possible because of an increased incidence of neural tube defects. There is evidence for teratogenic abnormalities if more than one anti-epileptic is given at the same time. Phenytoin is a potential teratogen and so is phenobarbital. All patients on either one of these anti-epileptics should receive folic acid supplements. Discussion with the mother is essential. A seizure during pregnancy could easily harm the fetus because of direct trauma or anoxia during the seizure. On the other hand most anti-epileptic medications are potential teratogens. Any final decision must eventuate from a joint discussion with the mother and a neurologist about the pros and cons of continuing or discontinuing medication.

Pregnant women with pre-existing or de novo cancer may require chemotherapy. These drugs are known teratogens and fetal death is always a danger when they are given. However, at times all goes well. A 35 year old patient developed de novo breast cancer in the third month of the pregnancy. She refused abortion but accepted surgery for the cancer and postpartum chemotherapy with a fatalism born of deeply held religious beliefs. A healthy baby was born and she remained disease free when last seen five years ago before she moved to another country.

The fetal alcohol syndrome.

Fetal alcohol syndrome (FAS) and associated neurological abnormalities (ARND - Alcohol Related Neurodevelopmental Disorder) affect some 40-50,000 infants each year - more than the combined totals of newborns with Down's syndrome, cystic fibrosis, spina bifida and sudden infant death syndrome.

Alcohol is a teratogen. When the mother drinks alcohol it enters the fetal blood and causes abnormalities. The final picture is evident at birth or only at a later date. The facial abnormalities may be present at birth and include small eye openings, short and upturned nose, flat nasal bridge, a characteristic skin web between the eyes and the base of the nose and eyes which do not move in similar directions. Often these facial abnormalities are not present at birth.

More commonly FAS and ARND are only recognized when functional and mental retardation are demonstrable as the infant grows. Often, in addition to the cognitive retardation there are behavioral and learning problems and difficulties with memory, attention and judgment. Neurological deficits are often associated with these mental abnormalities. Examples are poor motor skills and coordinations.

The obvious solution is abstention from alcohol during pregnancy to avoid fetal brain damage. There are those who maintain that moderation is all that is needed. It is best to advise the mother of the pros and cons and usually she is compliant.

Drug therapy for patients with renal and/or hepatic disease or failure.

The liver and kidneys are the principal detoxifiers and excretors of drugs, their metabolites, and endogenous toxic materials such as the products of hemoglobin breakdown. In both renal and hepatic failure there may be decreased capacities to detoxify drugs and to excrete any non-polar compounds or water soluble toxic metabolites of hepatic detoxification.

In addition, renal function declines with age so that drug therapy in the elderly must be carefully monitored at all times by blood levels (especially digoxin and any drugs given for psychiatric disorders) and repeated assessments of clinical responses. For example, the margin separating the toxic and therapeutic levels of digoxin is small. As mentioned previously, when giving digoxin to the elderly start with a small dose, e.g., 0.0625mg daily and gradually increase dosage till the desired effect is obtained or toxicity (best measured by an ECG and serum digoxin levels) develops. It is a water-soluble drug excreted by the kidneys. The same caveat applies to an anti-depressant given to an elderly patient unless the dose is minimal, e.g., 10mg of amitriptylline

All drugs that are actually or potentially nephrotoxic or hepatotoxic should be avoided. Few hard and fast rules can be laid down for drug therapy given to patients with renal and/or hepatic failure. Most of these patients have other consequential or associated diseases and dysfunctions. Repeated risk-benefit assessments and, when possible, monitoring of blood levels of drugs and the clinical responses to therapy are all that can be done to minimize adverse reactions due to overdosage.

A WHO web page[26] extensively details drugs that are permissible in renal and/or hepatic failure, those that are not, and those that require close and frequent monitoring if given. The material is too large to present here. When faced with unknowns this web page is a good one to reference for information. Try to familiarize oneself with the possible complications associated with the use of a few of the drugs you commonly use, if and when these are given to patients with hepatic and/or renal disease or failure. Notable examples are digoxin, diuretics, ACE inhibitors, beta-blockers, medications for psychiatric disease and pain (especially NSAIDs and opiate derivatives), antibiotics and corticosteroids. When giving drugs to individuals with renal and/or hepatic disease or failure try to only use those familiar to you. If other drugs are needed the physician is well advised to access the WHO web page referenced to obtain information about possible adverse effects in renal or hepatic dysfunctions.

Surgery.

Most of the basic decisions have been made once the patient is referred to a surgeon Only the surgeon can decide whether the decision is acceptable and this is done on the basis of knowledge, individual judgment. experience and recognition of personal competence and limitations.

However, it is necessary that the patient's regular physician recognize situations where surgical consultation is required. The patient's primary care physician also needs to know the common postoperative complications.

Patients with minor complications such as wound infections, hematomas and postoperative lung and urinary infections can be treated by the individual's regular physician or, if the physician prefers, sent back to the treating surgeon. It would be polite to inform the surgeon of the complication you intend to deal with before proceeding.

Major complications need rapid hospitalization. Examples are wound rupture, leakage from anastomoses, intracranial, intrapleural or intraabdominal hemorrhages and infections, ruptured bronchial stumps, severe sepsis, hypovolemic shock, myocardial dysfunctions and a variety of other dysfunctions. All should be recognizable by the primary care physician.

References for chapter 16.

1. Preusser, RP., Achterrath, W., et al. Chemotherapy for gastric cancer. Cancer Treatment Reviews 1988; 15:257.
2. Drews, J., Ryser, S. The role of innovation in drug development. Nat. Biotechnol. 1997; 15:1318.
3. Ettinger, B., Black, D.M., et al. Reduction of vertebral fracture risk in postmenopausal women with osteoporosis treated with raloxifene: results from a three year randomized clinical trial. JAMA 1999; 282:637.
4. Huirne, J.A.F., Lambalk, C.B. Gonadotropin-releasing-hormone-receptor antagonists. Lancet 2001; 358:1793. (Review article).
5. Guyatt, GH, Sullivan, M.J.J., et al. A controlled trial of digoxin in congestive heart failure. Am. J. Cardiol. 1988; 61:371.
6. Mycolasma pneumonia. http://health.allref.com/mycoplasma-pneumonia-info.html.
7. Logan, R.L., Scott, P.J. Uncertainty in clinical practice: implications for quality and costs of health care. Lancet 1996; 347:595.
8. Guengrich, F.P. Reactions and significance of P450 enzymes. J. Biol. Chem. 266; 10019, 1991.
9. Meyer, U. Drugs in special patient groups: clinical importance of genomics in drug effects. In: Carruthers, G., Hoffmann, B., et al. (Eds.), New York. McGraw-Hill, 2000.
10. Aithal, G., Day, C., et al. Association of polymorphism in the cytochrome P450CYP2C9 with warfarin dose requirement and risk of bleeding complications. Lancet 1999; 353:717.
11. WHO. International drug monitoring: the role of national centers. Tech. Rep. Ser. WHO, 1972, no. 498.
12. Edwards, I. What are we doing in medicines safety? A perspective from the Uppsala Monitoring Center. In:Dukes, M. and Aronson, J. (Eds.): Meyer's side effects of drugs. An encyclopedia of adverse reactions and interactions, 14th. Edition. Amsterdam. Elsevier, 2000.
13. Lazarou, J., Pomeranz, B., et al. Incidence of adverse drug reactions in hospitalized patients: a meta-analysis of prospective studies. JAMA 1998; 279:1200.
14, Uetrecht, J. New concepts in immunology relevant to idiosyncratic drug reactions: the danger hypothesis and innate immune system. Chem. Res. Toxicol. 1999; 12:387.
15. Scully, R.E., Robboy, S.J., et al. Vaginal and cervical abnormalities including clear-cell adenocarcinoma related to prenatal exposure to stilboestrol. Am. Clin. Lab. Sci. 1974; 4:223.
16. Hulka, B.S., Stark, A.T. Breast cancer: cause and prevention. Lancet 1995; 346:883. (Review paper.)
17. Goldstein, R.E., Boccuzzi, S.J., et al. Diltiazem increases late-onset congestive heart failure in postinfarction patients with early reduction in ejection fraction. The Adverse Experience Committee; and the Multicenter Diltiazem Postinfarction Research Group. Circulation 1991; 83:52.
18. MERIT-HF Study Group. Effect of metroprolol CR/XL in chronic heart failure: Metoprolol CR/XL Randomized Intervention Trial in Congestive Heart Failure. Lancet 1999; 353:2001.
19. Leslie., F.A. Is thalidomide to blame? BMJ 1960; ii:1954.
20. McBride, W.G. Thalidomide and congenital abnormalities. Lancet 1961; ii:1358.
21. Herbst, A.L., Ulfelder, H., et al. Adenocarcinoma of the vagina: association of maternal stilboestrol therapy with tumor appearance in young women. N. Engl. J. Med. 1971; 284:878.
22. Herbst, A.L., Scully, R.E. Adenocarcinoma of the vagina in adolescence. A report of seven cases including six clear cell carcinomas (so-called mesonephromas). Cancer 1970; 25:745.
23. White, L., Tursky, B. Schwartz,G.E. (Eds.): Placebo theory, research, and mechanisms. New York. The Guildford Press,1985.
24. de Montaigne, M. On the power of the imagination. In: Essays. Harndsworth, U.K. Penguin, 1958.
25. Fetal alcohol syndrome. http://www.nofas.org/main/what_is_FAS.htm
26. Internet WHO http://mednet3.who.int/mf/modelFormulary.

17

Therapy

3. Clinical Trials and Comments on the Pharmaceutical Industry and Medical Journals

Table of Contents

New knowledge.

When can one use new knowledge? New knowledge and new information derive from any one or more of the following:

— Empirical observations.

— Findings derived from laboratory studies.

— Controlled clinical trials based on hypotheses generated from the above.

Assessment of new knowledge.

The following are the criteria for assessments of the validity or otherwise of new knowledge:

— Are the observations statistically significant but biologically unimportant.

— Do they demonstrate some hitherto unobserved principle?

— If they do is the same principle demonstrable if a different methodology is used?

— Are the observations repeatable?

- If they are the results of animal experiments can similar results be obtained using different animal species?
- Does knowledge of clinical medicine, physiology and pathology suggest that the postulated facts are Are they likely to be of clinical value? The results of clinical trials often need peppering with variable amounts of cynicism, common sense and critical assessment.
- Are the consequences of error too hazardous to permit of a clinical trial?
- Has a well designed clinical trial shown that the results are repeatable when applied to human subjects?

Only if all the answers to the above questions are affirmatives can the new knowledge be incorporated into the body of medical knowledge.

The objectives and requirements for clinical trials

The clinical trial.

The clinical trial is experimentation on humans but it is, or certainly should be, experimentation performed ethically, with the informed consent of the participants, with the approval of a review committee of peers and with the objective of improving therapy.

The objectives.

1. To test a hypothesis that appears reasonable.

A clinical trial is only justifiable when it alone can tell whether a hypothesis is correct or not. Needless to say the hypothesis should be one that could have significant and desirable clinical consequences. All participants in the trial must be fully informed of the objectives, the methodologies, and the possible dangers of the trial. Needless to say, all participants must provide signed informed consent for inclusion in the trial.

Perhaps the most important function of an ethics committee is to be sure that all participants in a clinical trial have enough information to provide informed consent. The information needed by participants in a clinical trial is usually more than that needed by individuals being treated with therapy that has the sanction of general usage and acceptance. In the latter instance, after due deliberation, a course of action, frequently based on previous clinical trials, is recommended to the patient because the physician feels that it is optimal therapy. In a clinical trial the human is a guinea pig. The results of the trial are unpredictable, otherwise no trial would be needed. The participant must be informed of all possible beneficial, as well as adverse consequences that could eventuate. Also, that the clinical trial might not show any benefit as compared with current therapy or that it might show an effect that is unfavorable.

There are those who feel that ethical standards may be unnecessarily rigid at times. Thus, in 1963 Bradford Hill[1] in a lecture decried the labeling of observational studies as experimental even if no experimentation was involved - this seems to be a valid objection.

Others decry the composition of many ethics committee, made up as they are, not only of physicians but also of ethicists (usually self-proclaimed), lawyers, bureaucrats and politicians. Ingelfinger[2] has commented on this; he wrote that just as there were unethical physicians who persuaded their patients to have inappropriate treatments for personal financial gain or career advancement, so also were there unethical ethicists who defamed medicine and physicians for similar reasons. This is an extreme view, though possibly, partially correct. Certainly, it is difficult to describe findings based on observations as unethical. William Withering's studies on digitalis (described in detail in page 9) were harmless observational studies of great benefit to humanity (William Withering: An account of the foxglove and some of its medical uses: with practical remarks on dropsy and other diseases. London. G.G.J. & J. Robinson, 1785.). His findings were made in a remote corner of England and were based on observations. He noted that local villagers drank an infusion of the foxglove (a plant) to reduce the edema of cardiac failure and identified digitalis as the ameliorating agent.

However regardless of any inconveniences or seemingly ridiculous constraints, all participants in clinical trials must have maximum protection. This is only possible if all pros and cons have been detailed and consented to. Observational studies should probably be exempt from such rigid constraints.

The Nuremberg Code has summarized well the requirements for a clinical trial in articles 2-10; article 1 relates to the subject of informed consent and was detailed on page 4 (Chapter1) of this book. Articles 2-10 summarize the other requirements for an ethical clinical trial:

Article 2: The experiment should be such as to yield fruitful results for the good of society, unprocureable by other methods or means of study, and not random and unnecessary in nature.

Article 3: The experiment should be so designed and based on the results of animal experimentation and a knowledge of the natural history of the disease or other problem under study that the anticipated results will justify the performance of the experiment.

Article 4: The experiment should be so conducted as to avoid all unnecessary physical and mental suffering or injury.

Article 5: No experiment should be conducted when there is **an priori** reason to believe that death or suffering will occur; except, perhaps, in those experiments where the experimental physicians also serve as subjects (I think it would have been better to omit the word "also").

A physician doing the initial experiment on himself is an ideal that has been realized in the past. An example was Werner Forssman, a German urologist, who did the first catheterization of the heart on a human, and this on himself. Apparently he just inserted the catheter into the antecubital vein for some 35cm and then walked with the catheter to the X-ray department to see where it was located. Soon after this he returned to the practice of urology. In 1966 he shared the Nobel prize with transatlantic colleagues Andre Cournand and D.W. Richards for their work. A retrospective of the importance of their original work was a paper by Cournand in 1975 (Cournand, A. Cardiac catheterization; development of the technique and its contributions to experimental medicine and its initial application in man. Acta Med. Scand. Suppl. 1975; 579:3).

Article 6: The degree of risk to be taken should never exceed that determined by the humanitarian importance to be solved by the experiment.

Article 7: Proper preparations should be made and adequate facilities provided to protect experimental subjects against even remote possibilities of injury, disability or death.

Article 8: The experiment should be conducted only by scientifically qualified persons. The highest degree of skill and care should be required through all stages of the experiment of those who conduct or engage in the experiment.

Article 9: During the course of the experiment the human subject should be at liberty to bring the experiment to an end if he has reached the physical or mental state where continuation of the experiment seems to him to be impossible.

Article 10: During the course of the experiment the scientist in charge must be prepared to terminate the experiment at any stage, if he has probable cause to believe, in the exercise of good faith, superior skill and careful judgment required of him, that a continuation of the experiment is likely to result in injury, disability, or death to the experimental subject.

To the many female physicians I apologize that the Nuremberg Code is not gender sensitive but this was how it was written - male is the only gender referred to.

2. To compare a therapeutic regime with another or with a placebo.

The object is to determine whether the drug or therapeutic regimen improves the response to therapy of a specific disease or clinical dysfunction.

- **To see whether the results of laboratory experiments done on animals are applicable to humans.**
- **The testing should not be done to satisfy curiosity but to provide an answer to a significant clinical problem;** for example, amelioration or eradication of malignant disease or occlusive vascular disease.

3. To confirm the validity or otherwise of a fortuitous observation.

Without clinical trials improvement of therapy for disease would be difficult. For example, thirty years ago the most common major operations were surgeries for peptic ulcer. The observations of Lykoudis[3] published in 1966 showed that a frequent cause of peptic ulceration was bacterial infection that was successfully treatable with antibacterials. His "Elgaco" medication contained unabsorbable quinolones. Confirmation by "science"[4] in 1984 was required before the principles postulated got general acceptance and usage. Peptic ulcers are now treated and heal with antibiotic therapy or are controlled by potent antacids - surgery for peptic ulcer is now uncommon and usually reserved for complications resulting from long-standing disease.

The clinical trial of today has **rigorous requirements.** This we owe to those who succumbed and suffered in the many state-approved and sponsored atrocities of recent times; it is with regret and shame that one records that physicians were often initiators, participants and perpetrators in these atrocities.

The following are some of the basic requirements of the modern clinical trial:

— **A reasonable and important basic proposition** that requires testing. There should always be a possibility of clinical benefit. No clinical trial, apart from one that is merely observational, is justifiable if the only object is satisfaction of academic curiosity.

— Assurance that **unqualified informed consent** will be obtained from all participants in the trial.

— **A protocol considered by a panel of disinterested individuals (an ethics committee) and found acceptable.** The following are some requirements:

- A **low risk-benefit ratio.**
- **Acceptable methods of randomization** for purposes of comparison.
- **Statistical methods and sample sizes appropriate for the clinical trial.** Ideally, statisticians unconnected with the study should predetermine if the proposed statistical methods are appropriate. Ideally, the study should also ask them to verify the validity of the conclusions.
- **Baseline characteristics of participants.** All relevant details of the baseline characteristics of participants in each trial group must be detailed and get approval from the Ethics Committee before the trial starts. The baseline characteristics of patients in trial and control groups should be comparable. This is particularly important when variables can be numerous. An example is a clinical trial on patients with breast cancer.
- **The placebo.** If the control group gets a placebo the nature and manner of its administration must be detailed. The literature has too many publications where these facts are not detailed. Statistics always require consideration of a null hypothesis or a conclusion opposite to what was hoped for. There can never be certainty that any improvement in the trial group was not due to worsening of the condition by the placebo. Alternatively, some negation of the beneficial effects of the therapy being received in addition to the trial material.

  The ALLHAT trial on the use of statins (The ALLHAT Officers and Coordinators for the ALLHAT Collaborative Research Group. Major outcomes in moderately hypercholesterolemic, hypertensive patients randomized to pravastatin vs usual care. JAMA 2002; 288:2998.) is especially persuasive about this point. The study had 10,335 participants divided into two comparable groups. One group was given a statin and "usual care" and the other got "usual care" only, i.e., no placebo. It was the only major study of the statins that did not give a placebo to control groups. There was no difference between the two groups with respect to coronary artery disease. All other meta-analyses of this topic that I have studied gave a placebo (usually not described in any detail in the text) to participants and all found statistically significant differences between experimental and control groups. They all claimed superiority for the statin studied. These topics were extensively reviewed on pages 18-22.
- **Publication and dissemination of all information obtained in the trial.** This includes information that does not support the hypothesis being tested, as well as information detailing all undesirable consequences and effects.

  A widely read medical journal is the best vehicle for dissemination of important material. In most cases all material that is not merely anecdotal should be peer reviewed before publication. Anecdotal findings rarely have the numbers and other criteria required for rigorous peer review and this is unfortunate as it results in the loss of many important observations which result from ad hoc therapies by qualified physicians. An example was the dismissal of findings made by Lykoudis[3] on the treatments and presumed etiology of peptic ulcerations of the stomach and duodenum.

- **Criteria for terminating the trial.** Before the clinical trial starts decisions must be made as to the criteria for terminating the trial if, during the course of the clinical trial, an obvious beneficial or harmful effect is found in one of the test groups.
- **A statement of the conclusions reached.** This conclusion could differ from that of the physician studying the reported results. The physician can only judge well if the publication includes all information obtained in the clinical trial.

The use of placebos in clinical trials.

The World Medical Association First Declaration of Helsinki was revised in 2000. **Article 29** reads as follows:

> "The risks, burdens and effectiveness of a new method should be tested against those of the best current prophylactic, diagnostic and therapeutic methods. This does not exclude the use of placebo or no treatment, where no proven prophylactic, diagnostic or therapeutic method exists."

In other words, placebos should not be used in clinical trials if there is an effective option to the procedure or therapy being tested. One completely concurs with this recommendation but with certain caveats.

They are two.

The first is that if placebos are given to control groups publications must state the precise nature of the placebos. Often they are only described in general terms.

The second is that some evidence must be provided to show that any apparent beneficial effect from the therapy in the study group did not reflect a deleterious effect from the placebo in the other group. The placebo could have reduced the effects of therapy and thus shown a spurious improvement in the study group.

The ALL-HAT study previously mentioned is persuasive. It compared groups given "normal care" with groups given "normal care and a statin". No difference was noted while differences were demonstrated (always in favor of the statins) in meta-analyses in which control groups got some placebo.

Unethical clinical trials - an example

Many such trials are conducted. Even in countries where constitutional mandates require unfettered recognition of the rights of humans.

One such example was a US-sponsored clinical trial in Africa, the Dominican Republic and Thailand. The trials were initiated by the US National Institutes of Health and the Centers for Disease Control. The studies were done on pregnant HIV positive women in Africa, the Dominican Republic and Thailand. The object was to compare prevention of maternal-fetal HIV transmission by a less costly alternative to the treatment then current. A placebo-controlled group was included. Even if informed consent was obtained it is difficult to believe that any woman would knowingly consent to be part of a study where effective therapy was already available, though costly. Women in the placebo-treated groups did not receive any treatment to prevent HIV transmission to their children. Criticism of this study is the subject of a paper by Lurie and Wolfe[5] and the ethics of clinical research in the third world are the subjects of a paper by Angell[6]. These studies were US Government sponsored, presumably vetted by ethics committees, and yet allowed to proceed. I guess that the value judgments on the worth of human lives were geographically determined by these ethics committees; or perhaps they were not able to find enough American women who were misguided enough to participate in such a trial.

The pharmaceutical industry and clinical trials.

The Nuremberg Code was written at a time when pharmaceutical companies were not major initiators or financial supporters of clinical research. They are today and because of possible conflicts of interest, restrictions on their roles in clinical research are necessary.

When judging on the merits or otherwise of a clinical trial it is advisable to see if, at the end of the publication, any mention is made of sponsorship or assistance of any sort by a pharmaceutical company. If this exists it does not make the study invalid but does make it worthy of a little more scrutiny.

Maxim.

Always give a little more attention when assessing the published data of clinical trials that have had assistance or sponsorship from a pharmaceutical company, even if the assistance only consists of donated drugs or other materials. This is not intended to be an unfair accusation directed against the pharmaceutical industry. Reputable and ethical pharmaceutical companies would welcome close scrutiny of any sponsored clinical trials.

The pharmaceutical industry is not a charitable organization. Its mandate from shareholders is to maximize profits ethically and within the framework of the law of the land where it functions. The expenses of marketing a drug are large. Advertising and the salaries of pharmaceutical company representatives are part of the cost. Not insignificant is the largesse they provide to physicians, usually by informal methods, in order to persuade recipients to prescribe their products: monies paid for "attendance at spurious conventions", for giving lectures, and for company-sponsored symposia where food, drink and occasionally, paid honoraria are disbursed. This has been going on for many years and continues despite the revelations made by Senator Kennedy[7] as far back as 1990. On December 11 and 12, 1990, he told a United States Congressional committee, that, by his calculations, in 1988 16 major pharmaceutical companies had spent approximately $165 million on physician gratification. The gratifications took the form of "holiday seminars", gifts, honoraria and various other assorted benefits. These practices continue and have been detailed by many publications since then. In 2003 the American Medical Association issued guideline E-8.061 on the subject of gifts to physicians from industry.

The report states that it was developed by the AMA and industry representatives; at least nine companies were named, all prominent members of the pharmaceutical industry. The recommendations were good but not too specific. In January 2005 the AMA issued a helpful and detailed Internet statement described as "Opinion E-8.601: Clarifying addendum." (http://www.ama-assn,org/ama/publcategory/4001.html). Unfortunately guidelines are not law and a determined physician or member of the industry can ignore the recommendations without fear of consequences or, at best, a lawsuit of interminable duration, usually financed by the physician's Insuring agency. Similar guidelines have been issued by many other national and provincial licensing bodies[8].

The solution to this problem is difficult and has to rely on the individual physician's ethics. Once a patient consults a physician the interests of the former must override any conflict of interest. The potential for such conflict exists when there is any interaction between the physician and the industry representative that could result in recommendation of treatment that is acceptable but not optimal.

The following are suggested guidelines for clinical research sponsored by pharmaceutical companies.

- **The results of every clinical trial (whether or not financed by a pharmaceutical company) must be published in toto,** in a well-regarded medical journal, and without statistical manipulations of results. Before the trial is started there should be unanimous and written agreement by all parties that there will be full publication of the findings, even if there is a null or adverse effect.
- **If the research is initiated or financed by a pharmaceutical company the organization must be named as well as its contributions to the study;** this includes the supply of drugs at no cost and the names of the individuals who received financial assistance. The exact amounts do not require detailing. Any financial assistance must be viewed as a potential conflict of interest and the published results, and especially, the published conclusions, merit more than the usual scrutiny given to published material.
- **Obviously, the sponsoring company may and should indicate the objectives of the proposed research; never the desired conclusions.** They should not be involved in designing the protocol nor in viewing the results as they appear. However, they should have the option of viewing the proposed protocol before the trial begins. At this stage they should also have the option of withdrawing and terminating their intent to participate in the trial.
- **The sponsoring company should not be able to prevent publication of results,** be they advantageous to

their financial interests or not. Always get the parent Institution to sign any contract with a pharmaceutical company. They have access to good legal advice and are responsible for paying any damages if any are awarded. In years gone by the pharmaceutical industry did not participate in clinical research as much as they do now. Scientists knew that the basis for scientific advancement was the sequence of research, publication, and then confirmation or refutation by others. It still is but interference in the sequence in order to increase shareholder and corporate incomes must be resisted by all physicians. An example detailed in Chapter 12, page 289, described the disputations between Apotex and Dr. N. Olivieri about deferiprone. How much better if her findings were published with the approval of the sponsor with subsequent papers confirming or refuting her findings. The case of Dr. Betty Dong is detailed below as another inappropriate exercise of industrial privilege.

The case of Dr. Betty Dong.

This research worker at the University of California Medical Center in San Francisco agreed with Boots Pharmaceutical to compare the therapeutic values of synthroid and generic levothyroxine. At the time synthroid was one of Boots' most lucrative products. She found no difference between the therapeutic effects of the two products. Boots found ways of stopping publication of the results and so did Knoll Pharmaceutical after acquiring Boots. The results were not published for seven years. Eventually she presented her paper to the JAMA where, after peer review, it was accepted for publication. Two weeks before publication she withdrew the paper because of impending legal action. It was only after publicity in the Wall Street Journal that Knoll Pharmaceutical gave permission for publication in the JAMA (JAMA 1999; 277:1205).

Why all this trouble. This was an unnecessary study. Surely the companies must have known that there would be no difference between generic thyroxine and their product. Unfortunately, in the contract she signed there was a clause which stated: "Data obtained by the investigator while carrying out this study is also considered confidential and is not to be published or otherwise released without written consent." How unwise, especially as the chances of showing that synthroid was better than thyroxine were almost non-existent.

Clinical trials in developing countries.

A disturbing trend is clinical trials initiated and controlled by Pharmaceutical Multinationals and conducted in developing countries which are poor. India is a favored site for these trials. It is a practice which I decry for two main reasons. First, the lack of an effective infrastructure and second, because of the potentials for patient abuse and coercion.

At various times the industry has claimed that it takes $500 million to bring a drug to market. About a third of this cost is the expense of conducting Phase 3 trials, i.e., trials on individuals with the disease being investigated. Clinical trials in India cost 50-60% less. The potential increase in shareholder value is obvious. Against this is the utilization of the numerous sick, indigent and often homeless individuals in poor countries to improve the profits of the affluent nations. It sounds a bit like 21st. century colonial exploitation by affluent nations, conducted by the affluents of the countries being exploited, as was the case in previous centuries.

The following are comments about the design of the clinical trials and the available infrastructures. Common baseline characteristics of trial and control groups are difficult to establish because of the heterogeneity of the population. In addition, there has been little training and experience in the meticulous keeping of records which is crucial for assessing the results of clinical trials.

Dr. Arun Bal, head of the Association for Consumers Action on Safety and Health in Mumbai claims that many participants in these clinical trials must sign consent forms written in English, even though they may not know the language. He also claimed that women are pressured into signing by their families. Add to all this the inability of those with minimal education to know what the trial is about except that they might receive free medicine for their ailment if they are in the trial group. In addition, socio-economic conditions show significant differences from one part of the country to another and many hospitals do not have ethics committees which actively monitor the welfare of participants in the trial. Finally, many participants often just return to their native villages in the middle of the trial and thus cease being participants in the trial. Indian promoters of these trials claim that they only include patients who have access to the best hospitals. This again introduces an undesirable variable because it selects for the socially acceptable and excludes a large rural population. The Government of India does not help. It can take up to two years for regulatory permission.

Finally, do the pharmaceutical companies think that the regulating bodies in North America or Europe are going to accept the results of flawed and marginally unethical clinical trials as a basis for licensing a drug for general use? I doubt that they will. A message to Pharmaceutical Multinationals - in general, do your clinical research at home on your own population, on diseases common to them and in the ways that you are required to do them. Let the Pharmaceuticals of poor nations do their own clinical trials on diseases in their own countries, diseases which the major pharmaceuticals of the world have neglected till it has now become politically correct to show interest in these diseases. Suggestions for clinical trials will always be welcome whether the country is affluent or poor with unsatisfactory socio- economic conditions

Interpretation and misinterpretation of the results of clinical trials.

Any one of many factors can result in misinterpretation of the results of a clinical trial. At times the clinical trial refutes widely accepted dogma. The following are some examples of both:

1. **Most incorrect conclusions are the result of clinical trials that are deficient in design and protocol.**

Any one or more of the following could be responsible: the analysis contains too many variables; unsuitable methods for randomization of control and study groups; inappropriate choice of participant baseline characteristics; insufficient reporting of the baseline characteristics of control and study groups; inappropriate choice of statistics; incorrect selection of sample sizes for the statistics used; insufficient and inaccurate reporting of the results - as far as possible all results should be reported in toto, albeit with a summary that reflects the assessments of the observers. The in toto reporting includes results that do not support the hypothesis or therapeutic regimen being tested. Another requirement is that there must be no minimization and insufficient reporting of undesirable and other serious, as well as harmless, consequences and adverse effects of the therapy being tested. Clinical trials can be effective tools for challenging and altering dogma. An example follows.

The Heart and Estrogen/Progestin Replacement Study (HERS).

This is an example of a recent well designed clinical trial that refuted previous widely held, and acted upon, clinical assumptions. In 1992 the American College of Physicians published guidelines that recommended Hormone Replacement Therapy (HRT) for all postmenopausal women, and especially for those with any history or risk of coronary artery disease[9]. Many later publications concurred. The HERS[10] was designed to determine if HRT altered the chances of myocardial infarction or death from coronary artery disease. There were 2763 women in the study, divided into two groups, one given an estrogen/progestin combination and the other a placebo. After 4 years the incidence of cardiac incidents was almost identical in the two groups, one given HRT and the other a placebo. In fact there were more coronary events in the treated group. The American Heart Association[11] has attempted to provide various explanations for the adverse effects of HRT in the HERS study - none convincing, in my opinion.

Support for the HERS study comes from another publication[12]. The findings of the HERS study plus the increased incidence of breast[13] and endometrial cancers in postmenopausal women receiving hormones must be cogent considerations, for patient and physician, when prescribing HRT for relief of menopausal symptoms.

2. **Unintentional misrepresentation and outright fraud.**

   The causes are numerous:

   - **Publish or perish.**

     After the second world war Governments all over the world provided large sums of money to researchers in the belief that this would find cures for all sorts of ills. Numerous experiments were performed, much new knowledge accumulated, was published and now remains moldering on the bookshelves and in the basements of libraries throughout the world (my own publications included). In academia publish or perish became the order of the day. It still is. As an example, as far back as 1987 Stewart and Feder[14] recorded word-for-word a memorandum from the Director of one of the world's leading research institutions to a junior colleague. This is an old reference but the language is choice and unfortunately, could easily be written in similar terms today. The memorandum went as follows:

> "There is no demand that these be literary masterpieces in first line journals; journeymen works for publication in second, third or fourth line archival publications will be quite satisfactory. Upon proper completion and submission of (two) manuscripts, (a technician's) appointment will be extended to April 1, 1984. During that time it is expected that an additional manuscript on (subject) will be completed and submitted. If so the period of employment will be extended an additional three months and again an additional manuscript on (subject) is an anticipated result of the extended employment."

This is a philosophy that places great pressure on individual scientists to repeatedly rechurn data, often of meager content and equally meager import, into one paper after another. It is only necessary to change the format of the text on each occasion. I believe that there are some 1000 or more medical publications current so that it is not too difficult to get a forum for publication; publications are entrepreneurial enterprises and those of lower grade must lower the criteria for acceptance if they are to survive.

- **Fraud.**

A more serious consequence of the "publish or perish" philosophy is fraud. The paper authored by Stewart and Feder also documents in detail an investigation of a case of fraud by one, Dr. John Darsee (www.unmc.edu/ethics/data/darsee.htm). Investigating committees found that fabricated data had formed the basis of more than 100 of his publications over a period of three years. Fabrication fraud continues to be a problem in biomedicine. Another case of fraud has been studied by Engler and associates[15]. This paper also philosophizes on different aspects of misrepresentation. They define "fraud" as intentional misrepresentation. The paper includes much philosophizing about the reasons for scientific fraud. One suspects that these reasons are not complex. There are, and always will be individuals who cut corners to achieve advancement and/or increase capital. Not all. A few do so to benefit the interests of their patients and are subsequently vilified for this altruism by a hierarchy dedicated to exact maintenance of the conditions of a clinical trial[16,17]. The vilification often continues despite indisputable analyses which show that the purported fraud did not affect the conclusions reached when the cases inappropriately included in the trial were excluded. Engler and associates propose the following as additional causes of misrepresentation:

- **Understandable and justifiable mistakes.**

Understandable and justifiable mistakes occur when the scientist had no reason for believing that the statements made were incorrect.

- **Carelessness.**

There was no intention to deceive. Results and information were available but not published because it was felt they were superfluous or valueless. This is specially important if the omitted negative information might have invalidated the postulated conclusions of the clinical trial.

- **Wrong conclusions.**

The incorrect assessment and reporting of conclusions reached in clinical trials are subjects detailed and discussed in many publications; representative early examples are listed in the references at the end of this chapter[18,19,20,21,22] - additional examples continue to be published each year. They include papers published in prestigious and scrupulous journals - glaring examples are published conclusions that are not supported by the methodology or results of the clinical trial[20,21]. For example, the paper by Tyson and colleagues reports that of a total of 86 controlled trials in four journals dealing with pediatrics and obstetrics the conclusions reached were justified in only 10% of the reported trials. In 71% information provided was not enough to make any judgment. Other representative publications on this subject routinely appear year after year. Many of the journals cited are prestigious publications which claim rigorous peer review of all published material.

The paper of Altman and Doré[22] merits additional comment. The authors selected and analyzed the first 20 randomized clinical trials published after January 1, 1987 in each of four medical journals of quality: the Annals of Internal Medicine, The New England Journal of Medicine, The Lancet and the British Medical journal. The authors noted significant deficiencies in design, reporting, or both in a noteworthy percentage of cases; deficiencies in randomization, in selection of sample size, and in not reporting, or not making adjustments for variations in baseline characteristics. Publications of a similar nature appear each year.

- **Incorrect and inadequate peer review.**

  What is the message of the preceding paragraph? The peer review process is flawed. Journals which claim prestige because of rigorous peer review are fooling themselves, printing erroneous material and generally creating confusion in the medical community. Who and what do we believe and when? The following is a sobering incident:

  The radioimmunoassay of peptide hormones - five rejections followed by a Nobel prize.

  A paper published by Russo[30] quotes S.Z.Hirschman as recounting that the paper describing radioimmunoassay for peptide hormones such as insulin, growth hormone and parathormone, developed by Solomon Berson and Rosalyn Yalow in the **1950s, was rejected five times by different journals before getting published. For this work the 1977 Nobel Prize in Physiology and Medicine was awarded to Rosalyn Yalow. Berson had died a few years earlier or he would undoubtedly have been a corecipient**

  This was peer review at a performance nadir.

  From a practical point of view this and the preceding section mean that treatment of patients should not change unless one knows enough about statistics to judge on the design of the trial, and enough about the subject to evaluate the conclusions with care. For those who have neither, a good plan is to wait until the conclusions have received general acceptance and usage. Incorporation in standard textbooks of quality is usually a good test of validity but one which could delay use of useful findings by many years!

The value of pharmaceutical research.

Pharmaceutical companies must receive their due. They cannot be rapacious marketers of substandard or harmful medications or devices; the financial consequences could be devastating. New medicines cost a lot to develop, manufacture and market. The Association of Pharmaceutical Research and Manufacturers of America accessed on the Internet[23] claims that it takes $500-600 million, and 12 to 15 years to market a new drug, and that only one of 5,000 to 10,000 compounds screened will become a prescription drug. An article in the Economist of July 16, 2002 provides some corroboration for these figures. The following summarizes relevant material in the article:

> "According to an oft-quoted figure from the Tufts Center for the Study of Drug Development, in Medford, Massachusetts. The entire process of getting a drug to market is $900m dollars and takes 15 years....... Only one in 1,000 compounds tested make human trials and only one in five of these emerges as a drug."

It is difficult to verify these claims without access to the books. The following are some relevant questions. Did listed expenses include the contributions of basic research done in universities and hospitals supported by taxpayers? Were various tax reliefs, subsidies and other taxpayer-funded goodies included in the calculations?

Nevertheless, regardless of the above comments, the amounts required to bring an effective agent to market are large. A major part of this expenditure is on clinical trials and marketing but without clinical trials which showed amelioration of diseases Regulatory approval for marketing and use would not be possible, and without marketing recovery of costs and profit-making would also be impossible. Even after successful marketing dangers continue. Infrequent but dangerous adverse reactions of a drug or appliance such as an IUD (i.e., Phase 4 reactions) could be missed in clinical trials that did not involve large numbers of subjects over long periods. Subsequent litigation could be financially devastating for the manufacturer.

The pharmaceutical industry walks a tight rope. Their mandate is to provide shareholders with an appropriate return on investment. A single error can result in bankruptcy and they certainly have provided the world with valuable therapeutic agents, albeit, many of their recent products are not innovations but copy-cat drugs for diseases of the affluent. Examples are the nonsteroidal anti-inflammatories, the statins and the gastric proton pump inhibitors. Drug prices do not necessarily reflect costs but rather whatever the market can bear; drugs produced in America are often more costly in America than in countries that receive exports of the same drugs. Manufacturers claim that the cost of drugs is high because of the costs of research. However the WHO/WTO secretariat[24,25] has estimated that the costs of advertising and promotion usually exceed expenditure on research - research usually based on taxpayer funded basic research done in universities and hospitals.

A major part of the cost of producing a new drug is the long period needed for its development and clinical testing. I present one example of the delay in, and the cost of development of the first ACE inhibitor - captopril. Subsequently numerous other ACE inhibitors have appeared.

The development of the ACE inhibitors.

The story begins in the 1890s when Tigerstedt and Bergman (Inagami, T. In memorial to Robert Tigersted: the centennial of renin discovery. Hypertension 1998; 32:223.) showed that injecting kidney extracts into rabbits resulted in an increase in blood pressure. They called the active substance renin.

In 1932 Goldblatt showed that progressive constriction of both renal arteries of a dog resulted in hypertension. Constriction of other major vessels did not. The results were published in the Journal of Experimental Medicine (1934; 59:347). Goldblatt's postulate that the kidney produces a secretion that causes vasoconstriction was not received with enthusiastic acceptance. Nevertheless, many attempts were made to isolate renin. Increased purity of renin extracted from kidneys resulted in decreased ability to produce hypertension.

Eventually in 1939 Eduardo Braun-Menendez in Brazil and Irvine Page in the USA deduced that the decreased hypertensive effect of purified renin was due to the loss of substrate. The conclusion was reached that renin was an enzyme which converted a plasma substrate to a hypertensive which they called angiotensin. Actually, not quite that simple for there were other steps to get to the real hypertensive as shown in Chart 7-1 on page 159. Subsequent investigations showed that the effect of renin was to convert circulating renin substrate (angiotensinogen) to angiotensin I which was physiologically inactive. The next step in the cascade was conversion of angiotensin I to angiotensin II by angiotensin converting enzyme (ACE). Angiotensin II was a potent vasoconstrictor and stimulator of aldosterone secretion. The final step was development of the first ACE inhibitor - captopril - by a group at Squibb laboratories which included Charles Smith and John Vane. Captopril only got FDA approval in the early 1980s.

Almost a hundred years from Tiegerstadt and Bergman to captopril. Now the market is flooded with ACE inhibitors. The cost to synthesize the original drug was about a million dollars a kilo and Smith and Vane record (The FASEB Journal 2003; 17:788) that Smith was often asked how R&D could justify spending so much money on a drug in which only Vane and Laragh (a clinician) had confidence. Vane (seemingly a trans-atlantic consultant for Squibb at the time) was already a Nobel Laureate and this probably helped to sway the R&D spenders. The gamble certainly paid off.

The selection of drugs for development.

These days gambles like those made by Squibb are not numerous. Pharmaceutical companies choose to develop drugs for disorders with high prevalence in rich countries. Examples are the many statins developed to reduce blood cholesterol. They all pretty well have comparable effects and none are affordable by the poor. Another similar example is the many expensive nonsteroidal anti-inflammatory drugs developed to allay the musculoskeletal aches and pains of the affluent. ASA is probably comparable in effectiveness and in toxic effects such as gastrointestinal bleeds.

The "10/90 gap".

The phrase "10/90 gap" is used to exemplify a major problem[26,27]. It reflects the fact that 90% of the health problems of this world (mainly the health problems of impoverished or developing countries) are not funded or researched because the pharmaceutical companies cannot profit from their development and marketing. A report by Medecins Sans Frontieres in 2001[28] reports similar conclusions.

There are two basic problems. First, the neglect of research and development of therapy for diseases of the poor, and second, the high price of drugs developed for diseases that affect the affluent and the impoverished alike; a contemporary example is AIDS. Can drug prices be lowered? The answer is a qualified yes, but it requires modification of the patent laws of the jurisdiction.

Henry and Lexchin report[29] that there was a 97% reduction in the price of combination anti-retroviral drugs after production and marketing by Indian pharmaceutical companies. Why? A change in the patent laws was responsible. The Indian patent law of 1970 allowed pharmaceutical companies to market any patented drug so long as the method of manufacture was quite different. In 2001 one corporation, Cipla, offered an anti-AIDS combination cocktail of lamivudine, stavudine and nevirapine to Medecin Sans Frontieres at a cost of US$350 per patient per year for distribution anywhere in Asia or Africa, and US$1200 per year for individuals who were not impoverished. The average cost of this cocktail in western countries at that time was US$10,000-15,000 per year.

Incidentally, the Indian pharmaceuticals were not entirely copy-cat drugs. The methods of production differed from those used by established pharmaceutical countries but the initial research on AIDS and its therapeutic requirements had been done in Universities and other Institutions funded by foreign tax-payer money. The Indian pharmaceutical industry benefited from not having to pay for the R&D which identified and developed the drugs used, the necessary clinical trials, the rigors of getting regulatory approvals from Governments and the promotion of these drugs. To this extent it must be admitted that it was unfair competition.

It remains to be seen what happens now that India has joined the WTO and agreed to abide by its rules on patent infringement. The Indian system of pharmaceutical patenting was supposed to end in January 2005. By that date the TRIPS agreement of the WTO required patents to extend to the chemical entities and processes involved in production. There have been many protests about this but if the manufacturing processes were really dissimilar it should not be a problem to patent each item and the way it is used in production. An option of extending the deadline to 2016 was given to "least developed countries" but excluding India. The transfer of production to "least developed countries" or other methods of bypassing the decrees of the European/US coalition should not be difficult. In any case the patents on most of the lucrative drugs are likely to end within a few years.

A new Indian copyright law was passed in December 2004 to meet the January 2005 deadline. The law does not completely satisfy the wishes of multinational pharmaceuticals nor the objections of the local Communist Party of India which is a coalition partner of the current government. In any case delay is inevitable for there are more than 12,000 patent applications to be processed and this will take at least eight months, if not more. The law has provisions for compulsory licensing in cases of national emergencies or exporting medicines to countries which have public health emergencies.

Regardless, the production of inexpensive medications will continue for every successful entrepreneur industrialist is an inventive person. One suspects that the "least developed countries" will get new factories to produce inexpensiive generics. Inexpensive drugs will remain available and the status quo will not change. The entrepreneur's profit will remain and perhaps increase. The "least developed countries" get employment and other benefits. All will be happy except those who sit in the paneled boardrooms of affluent Multinational Pharmaceuticals.

Unintentional perpetuation of the 10/90 gap by medical journals.

Few medical journals are non-profit publications. The objectives of the owners of for-profit journals are dissemination of peer reviewed medical information and maximization of shareholder value. Few physicians in developing countries can afford the more reliable, and hence, prestigious journals. Consequently the contents of these journals are directed to the needs of physicians in affluent societies and the diseases they are likely to encounter. The diseases of poor countries are neglected. Millions die each year of malnutrition, subnutrition, and infections such as malaria, tuberculosis and viral, bacterial and parasitic infections of the gastrointestinal tract. Papers on these topics are uncommon in prestigious general journals such as the New England Journal of Medicine and the Lancet. Likewise, advances in the management of Chagas' disease are negligible and unreported in the major medical journals. It is a disease that inflicts chronic cardiac and intestinal disease on some 16-18 million people and results in some 50,000 deaths each year; needless to say this disabling and often lethal infection by Trypanosoma Cruzi is a disease of the impoverished countries of Central and South America.

Is this all? No. Physicians in affluent countries regularly affirm their convictions that clinical practice must be based on "evidence-based medicine". The difficulties of conducting meaningful studies of this type in poor but emerging nations have been detailed in previous paragraphs. In any case few publications from poor countries could survive the standardized, and often inappropriate rigors of peer review mandated by prestigious journals, and usually conducted by individuals who vigorously and regularly defend the status quo of medical convictions.

It is not enough to throw up one's hands in despair and accept the status quo. Physicians in under-developed countries are not incompetent or uneducated (most are not, some are). They just do not have access to information because they cannot afford to buy medical journals and few have access to the meager materials provided by their local medical school libraries. For example, my annual payment for the Lancet is $155.00 (US). The institutional rate is $711.00 per year. Subscriptions to the New England Journal of Medicine are comparable, though a bit higher. Few medical school libraries in the poorer countries of the world can afford more than a handful of such journals (I gather that some reductions of the costs are possible, based on needs). In addition, funds for large clinical comparative studies are rarely available in poor countries. The students who will become future doctors must rely on teachers and textbooks which are expensive and usually not affordable when new. The textbooks are handed down at progressively decreasing prices from one graduating class to the next. Eventually students are learning from editions which are 10-15 years old. The clinical features of diseases are well described in most of these books but not the ancillary investigations and therapies currently available. The consequences are obvious. The physician learns to be a diagnostician but does not have the means to treat. Even if the physician knows what treatment to prescribe the patient is often unable to afford the investigation or the product.

Some of the major advances in medicine have resulted from anecdotal findings; examples are digoxin, quinine and vaccination against smallpox. If anecdotal information is repeatedly rejected by journals it is inevitable that eventually such information will be posted on the Internet in blogs and this is already happening. Given the botherations of peer review and delays in publication, increasing amounts of otherwise publishable material will eventually gravitate to blogs. The exceptions will be publications which depend on obtaining grants from funding agencies on the bases of the numbers of their publications in prestigious journals. At present anyone can find a reference to support a view which requires support, however unorthodox or incorrect the postulate.

Medical chaos is beginning. Physicians are starting to distrust publications, even those in prestigious journals, for reasons already detailed. The additional confusion created by many unreviewed blogs will compel those who practice clinical medicine to only use material published in standard texts. Unfettered scientific advances in medicine will end. The amount of material presented as Internet blogs is astounding. **I recently asked Google to search for Internet blogs on statins. They found 55,400 blogs on the topic!**

Chart 17-1: THE INFORMATION EXPLOSION

	Google search	PubMed
Childhood diarrhea	356,743 ref.	1,730 ref.
EPSPs[1]	19,584 ref.	6,444 ref.
Breast cancer	27,727,445 ref.	141,775 ref.
Atrial fibrillation	354.146 ref.	22,432 ref.
Use of memory for reasoning	6,620,000 ref.	827 ref.

[1] EPSPs are Excitatory Post Synaptic Potentials

The information explosion in medicine.

The information currently available is mind-boggling (Chart 17-1). The references in PubMed are probably fewer than those identified by the Google search engine because they reflect publications in scientific journals only. The search engine does not discriminate but includes all; advice to lay persons, personal stories and opinions from those who are informed and also from those who are not.

At present there are some cogent problems regarding new information. Numerous publications have correctly described deficiencies in the review and verifications of published material, including information published in prestigious journals.

The problem is not that there is insufficient information available. It is that there is too much to use and digest.

This is inevitable. Scientific research is extremely wasteful of endeavor and labor but this is an essential element of the process of discovery. Thousands of papers may only produce a single fact of importance. The process is a sequence of research followed by publication or presentation followed by refutations and arguments. As a rule some sort of consensus is eventually reached. Later, usually many years later, if the consensus holds it appears in one or more standard textbooks. By that time new information has accrued and the textbook is out of date and so the cycle is repeated again and again over the years; this even when research is targeted as it is in most pharmaceutical firms. A previous section detailed some facts about the industry. Only one of 5,000 to 10,000 compounds screened will become a prescription drug.

The search for an exotic item such as EPSPs (i.e., excitatory post synaptic potentials) on the Internet. It showed 6,444 items available. Being a curious person I looked up the first hundred of these. There was really nothing new compared with the original Hodgkin-Huxley model of nerve transmission. The papers were all variations on the basic theme using different biological materials, varying conditions and testing hypotheses, often hypotheses which were ridiculous. Interestingly, the further back I went the more obvious it became that much current research is variations on facts published in the 1940s and even earlier. Information about how memory is used for mentation and decision-making is one of the most important questions of human biology. Little new information is available on this topic. In a similar vein any physician wanting to identify optimal treatment for a specific breast malignancy would only find confusion if opting for a resolution on the Internet. I suspect that oncolologists are similarly confused and rely on treatment protocols issued by hierarchies.

Case history.

Schizophrenic patient age 46 (perimenopausal symptoms present but normal FSH) with impalpable breast cancer diagnosed by mammogram. With great difficulty she was persuaded to have a local excision. About two weeks later I got a phone call from the radiation oncologist. Apparently the patient had refused postoperative radiotherapy because she felt the machines would brain wash her and deliver bizarre commands. I told the radiotherapist that before trying to persuade the patient to have radiotherapy I would like to know what effect it would have on her long-term survival. She said it would not prolong life but only reduce the chances of a local recurrence. I searched the Internet for confirmation of this statement. She was correct though many of the publications had many "if" and "but" qualifications.

On the basis of these facts and the statement of the radiation oncologist I did not pursue the topic with this already difficult patient. There is total confusion on the topic of postoperative radiation for breast cancer and the facts remain unresolved. A local recurrence can always be readily excised and whatever the subsequent course of the disease, survival will not be prolonged by postoperative radiation. The cynic might conclude that, as usual, the advice given to patients by physicians is often related to considerations other than advising on optimal therapy. The patient is alive and well twelve years later. She was given an anti-estrogen fom the day before surgery. She could not tolerate tamoxifen and is taking an aromatase inhibitor (Arimidex) instead.

Peer review.

Most physicians believe that peer review is an essential requirement for medical publications that can be trusted. There are pros and cons regarding this belief and each individual's belief will differ in degree or in totality. Peer review is not infallible but it usually provides a fairly good judgment on the merits of a paper.

Unless reviewers deliberately check for specific items much can be missed. The previously cited papers by Tyson and associates[20] and by Altman and Doré[19] show how deficient peer reviews can be. Even as experienced and knowledgeable a person as Dr. Braunwald was fooled for a time by the publications attributed to John Darsee. The repeated rejections of the paper by Berson and Yalow and the subsequent Nobel prize for the contents of the rejected paper were detailed on page 373. It also casts doubt on the process of peer review.

These facts do not mean that peer review is valueless and often faulty. It does mean that the reader must retain a certain amount of skepticism when reading a much acclaimed publication. It also means that Editors must ensure that the reviewers conscientiously review and question every omission, doubtful contention or controversial finding in the paper. This can be a daunting task as those who do research and publish findings seem to relish words and paper and are allowed to publish material which could be reduced by half without omission any significant findings.

What is to come?

Very few people in the health sciences and few people in the publishing industry realize what changes will eventuate from the advent of the Internet, the electronic dissemination of information and increasing largesse from Governments for biomedical research.

Changes will certainly occur, not excluding the possibility that medical journals as we know them today will become extinct. Attempts are being made to provide open access. The Public Library of Science publishes papers in PLoS Medicine. The contents are peer reviewed articles. The public has free access but the author must pay $1000-1500 for each article printed. One presumes these charges are for handling, processing and publishing. They do seem excessive but I presume the assumption is that costs are not too important as the monies will come from taxpayer funded research grants to the authors. The fee does not seem to be a "take it or leave it" ultimatum as PLoS states: "the ability of authors or their institutions to pay publication charges will never be a consideration in the decision whether to publish.". Another comparable service is BioMed Central where the charge is $500 per article though "waivers will be considered on a case by case basis and may be granted in cases of lack of funds". Another means test. Tests of this sort make authors uncomfortable. They certainly make me feel uncomfortable.

The Public Access to Science Act.

This Act was introduced in the US House of Representatives on June 26, 2003. I do not know if it has been passed but if it has, established journals will need to modify their current modus operandi. The proposals in the bill are worth itemizing:

1. The United States Government funds basic research with the intention and belief that the new ideas and discoveries that result from research will improve the lives and welfare of the people of the United States and around the world.
2. Works of the United States are beyond the reach of copyright protection so that they will be freely available for the benefit of the people of the United States (unfortunately the bill does not include copyright protection for the rest of the world - my comment).
3. The United States Government spends $45,000,000,000 a year to support scientific and medical research whose product is new knowledge for the public benefit;
4. The Internet makes it possible for this information to be promptly available not only to every scientist and physician who could use it to further the public good, but to every person with access to the Internet at home, in school, or in a library; and
5. United States Government funded research belongs to, and should be freely available to, every person in the United States (and by extension, the whole world as the reach of the Internet is global - my comment).

People are just tired of paying taxes and not receiving value but I doubt that this law will ever be passed without considerable modification because of financial considerations related to copyright protections. Even a modified version will require many changes in the functioning of medical journals, including the ones that are the most popular and prestigious.

At present there are many reasons for pessimism. Much of the information in first second or third level journals or in Internet blogs is not believed or believable. The amounts of information progressively increase but most are variations on themes published in the last century, some in the early years of that century. Either because of inadequate peer review or for monetary reasons entrepreneurial journals continue printing this regurgitated material.

Some new information printed in journals is not harmless. Physicians are being advised to practice therapies which are found to be dangerous a few years later. An example is hormone replacement therapy for the symptoms of the menopause. What are we to make about the deferiprone controversies? What considerations justify that this drug is licensed for use in Asia, Europe and Australia but not in the USA or Canada? And the list goes on and on.

I end this book on a pessimistic note. I do not know how we can deal with the vast amount of information currently available. Currently, many physicians and scientist descibe their findings in Internet blogs, often because they have controversial views or because they do not have the patience for a long period of peer review followed by a longer period for alterations and publication. This book is a self-published monograph for all the above reasons. Many of the views expressed are controversial and certain to conflict with the views of reviewers. I wish to express them and am not inclined to argue with the dissenters. Hence, the solution of desk-top writing, repeated home computer editing of language and punctuation and subsequent self publication.

References to Chapter 17.

1. Hill, A.B. Medical ethics and controlled trials. Brit. Med. J. 1963; i:1043.
2. Ingelfinger, F.J. The unethical in medical ethics Ann. Intern. Med. 1975; 83:264.
3. Lykoudis, J. The truth about gastric and duodenal ulcer. Athens, Greece. 1966.
4. Marshall, B.J., & Warren, J.R. Unidentified curved bacilli in the stomach of patients with gastritis and peptic ulceration. Lancet 1984; i:13115.
5. Lurie., R.P. & Wolfe, S.M. Unethical trials of interventions to reduce perinatal transmission of the human immunodeficiency virus in developing countries. N. Engl. J. Med. 1997; 337:853.
6. Angell, M. The ethics of clinical research in the third world. N. Engl. J, Med. 1997; 337:853.
7. Gifts to physicians from industry. Accessed on-line at hhtp://www.ama-assn.org/ama/pub/category.
8. MD relations with drug companies. hhtp://www.cpso.on.ca/policies/drug_relation.htm.
9. American College of Physicians. Guidelines for counseling postmenopausal women about preventive hormone therapy. Ann. Intern. Med. 1992; 117:1038.
10. Hulley, S., Grady, D., et al. Randomized trial of estrogen plus progestin for secondary prevention of coronary heart disease in postmenopausal women. JAMA 1998; 280:605.
11. Mosca, L., Collins, P. et al. Hormone replacement therapy and cardiovascular disease. A statement for health care professionals from the American Heart Association. Circulation 2001; 104:499.
12. Herrington, D.M., Reboussin, D.M., et al. Effects of estrogen replacement on the progression of coronary artery atherosclerosis. N. Engl. J. Med. 2000; 343:522.
13. Hulka, B.S., Stark, A.T. Breast cancer: cause and prevention. Lancet 1995; 346:883. (Good review paper.)
14. Stewart, W.S. & Feder, N. Nature 1987; 325:2077.
15. Engler, R.L., Covell, J.W., et al. Misrepresentation and responsibility in medical research. N. Engl. J. Med. 1987; 317:1383.
16. Angell, M., Kassirer, J.P. Setting the record straight in breast cancer trials. N. Engl, J. Med. 1994; 330:1448.
17. Fisher, B., Redmond, C.K. Fraud in breast cancer trials. N. Engl. J. Med. 1994; 330,1458.
18. Engler, R.L., Covell, J.W. et al. Misrepresentation and responsibility in medical research. N. Engl. J. Med. 1987; 317:1383.
19. Altman, D.G. Statistics in medical journals. Stat. Med. 1982; 1:59.
20. Tyson, J.E., Furzan, J.A., et al. An evaluation of the quality of therapeutic studies in perinatal medicine. J. Pediatr. 1983; 102:10.
21. Pocock, S.J., Hughes, M.D.et al. Statistical problems in the reporting of clinical trials. N. Engl. J. Med. 1987; 317:426.
22. Altman, D.G. & Doré, C.J. Randomization and baseline comparisons in clinical trials. Lancet 1990; 335:149.
23. www.phrma.org/publications/publications/10.08.2001.528.cfm.
24. Summary report of the WHO/WTO Secretariat Workshop Differential Pricing and Financing of Essential Drugs. Norway. Geneva, WHO 2001 (accessed on the Internet).
25. Laing, R.D. Health and pharmacy systems in developing countries. In: WTO/WHO Workshop Differential Pricing and Financing of Essential Drugs, Norway. Geneva WHO 2001 (accessed on the Internet)
26. Global Forum for Health Research. The 10/90 report on health research 2000. Global Forum for Health Research. Geneva, 2001. (accessed on the Internet).
27. Ramsay, S. No closure in sight for the 10/90 health-research gap. Lancet, 358:1348, 2001.
28. Drugs for Neglected Diseases Working Group, Medecins Sans Frontieres. Fatal imbalance: the crisis in research and development for drugs for neglected diseases. MSF, Geneva. 2001 (accessed on the Internet).
29. The pharmaceutical industry as a medicines provider. Lancet, 2002; 360:1590.
30. Russo, E. Bypassing Peer Review. The Scientist 2000; 14:1.3

INDEX

www.ingramcontent.com/pod-product-compliance
Lightning Source LLC
Chambersburg PA
CBHW081103170526
45165CB00008B/2313